Pearson Nursing Reviews & Rationales

Pathophysiology

Third Edition

SERIES EDITOR

MaryAnn Hogan, MSN, RN

Clinical Assistant Professor
School of Nursing
University of Massachusetts–Amherst
Amherst, Massachusetts

CONSULTING EDITORS

Margaret M. Gingrich, RN, MSN

Professor
Harrisburg Area Community College
Harrisburg, Pennsylvania

Karen Hill, RN, BS, MSN, PhD

Associate Professor
Southeastern Louisiana University
Hammond, Louisiana

Toni Scialdo, RN, PhD, MSEd, MSN, CNE

Nursing Instructor
San Antonio College
San Antonio, Texas

Lisa A. Wolf, PhD, RN, CEN, FAEN

Director, Institute for Emergency Nursing Research, Emergency Nurses' Association
Clinical Assistant Professor
University of Massachusetts–Amherst
Amherst, Massachusetts

PEARSON

Boston   Columbus   Indianapolis   New York   San Francisco   Upper Saddle River
Amsterdam   Cape Town   Dubai   London   Madrid   Milan   Munich   Paris   Montréal   Toronto
Delhi   Mexico City   São Paulo   Sydney   Hong Kong   Seoul   Singapore   Taipei   Tokyo

Director of Readypoint™: Maura Connor
Executive Editor: Jennifer Farthing
Developmental Editor: Elisa Rogers
Editorial Assistant: Deirdre MacKnight
Director, Digital Product Development: Alex Marciante
Media Product Manager: Travis Moses-Westphal
Vice President, Director Sales & Marketing: David Gesell
Senior Marketing Manager: Phoenix Harvey
Marketing Coordinator: Michael Sirinides
Director of Media Production: Allyson Graesser
Media Project Manager: Rachel Collett

Managing Editor, Production: Patrick Walsh
Production Liaison: Maria Reyes
Production Editor: GEX Publishing Services
Manufacturing Manager: Lisa McDowell
Art Director/Cover Designer: Christopher Weigand
Cover Image: Monkey Business Images / Shutterstock.com
Cover Designer: Dina Curro
Composition: GEX Publishing Services
Printer/Binder: Edwards Brothers Malloy
Cover Printer: Lehigh/Phoenix Color Hagerstown

Notice: Care has been taken to confirm the accuracy of the information presented in this book. The authors, editors, and the publisher, however, cannot accept any responsibility for errors or omissions or for the consequences for application of the information in this book and make no warranty, express or implied, with respect to its contents.

The authors and the publisher have exerted every effort to ensure that drug selections and dosages set forth in this text are in accord with current recommendations and practice at time of publication. However, in view of ongoing research, changes in government regulations, and the constant flow of information relating to drug therapy and drug reactions, the reader is urged to check the package inserts of all drugs for any change in indications of dosage and for added warnings and precautions. This is particularly important when the recommended agent is a new and/or infrequently employed drug.

The authors and publisher disclaim all responsibility for any liability, loss, injury, or damage incurred as a consequence, directly or indirectly, of the use and application of any of the contents of this volume.

Library of Congress Cataloging-in-Publication Data

Hogan, Mary Ann, MSN.
 Pathophysiology / MaryAnn Hogan ; consulting editors, Margaret M. Gingrich ... [et al.]. -- 3rd ed.
  p. ; cm. -- (Pearson nursing reviews & rationales)
 Includes bibliographical references and index.
 ISBN-13: 978-0-13-324977-4 (pbk.)
 ISBN-10: 0-13-324977-8 (pbk.)
 I. Gingrich, Margaret M. II. Title. III. Series: Pearson nursing reviews & rationales series.
 [DNLM: 1. Nursing Assessment--methods--Examination Questions. 2. Nursing Assessment--methods--Outlines. 3. Pathology--Examination Questions. 4. Pathology--Outlines. WY 18.2]

 616.075--dc23
                    2012041768

10 9 8 7 6 5 4 3 2 1

PEARSON

ISBN-13: 978-0-13-324977-4
ISBN-10: 0-13-324977-8

Contents

Welcome to the Pearson Nursing Reviews & Rationales Series!

This series has been specifically designed to provide a clear and concentrated review of important nursing knowledge in the following content areas:

- Anatomy & Physiology
- Nursing Fundamentals
- Nutrition & Diet Therapy
- Fluids, Electrolytes, & Acid–Base Balance
- Medical-Surgical Nursing
- Pathophysiology
- Pharmacology
- Maternal-Newborn Nursing
- Child Health Nursing
- Mental Health Nursing
- Health & Physical Assessment
- Leadership & Management

The books in this series are designed for use either by current nursing students as a study aid for nursing course work, for NCLEX-RN® licensing exam preparation, or by practicing nurses seeking a comprehensive yet concise review of a nursing specialty or subject area.

This series is truly unique. One of its most special features is that it has been developed and reviewed by a large team of nurse educators from across the United States and Canada to ensure that each chapter is edited by a nurse expert in the content area under study. The series editor, MaryAnn Hogan, designed the overall series in collaboration with a core Pearson team to take full advantage of Pearson's cutting-edge technology. The consulting editors for each book, also experts in that specialty area, then reviewed all chapters and test questions submitted for comprehensiveness and accuracy. Finally, MaryAnn Hogan reviewed the chapters in each book for consistency, accuracy, and applicability to the NCLEX-RN® Test Plan.

All books in the series are identical in their overall design for your convenience. As an added value, each book comes with a comprehensive support package, including access to additional questions online, complete eText, and a tear-out *NursingNotes* card for clinical reference and quick review.

What's New in this Edition

- Completely updated review material reflecting the 2013 NCLEX-RN® Test Plan
- Online access to NursingReviews and Rationales.com where students can complete quizzes on the computer to practice for the NCLEX® experience
- Includes a fully searchable eText version of the book as well as valuable note-taking and highlighting tools
- 850 updated or brand-new NCLEX®-style practice test questions
- Features new alternate-item format questions
- The latest test prep advice from MaryAnn Hogan, trusted expert in what nursing students need to know

Study Tips

Use of this book should help simplify your review. To make the most of your valuable study time, also follow these simple but important suggestions:

1. Use a weekly calendar to schedule study sessions.
   - Outline the timeframes for all of your activities (home, school, appointments, etc.) on a weekly calendar.
   - Find the "holes" in your calendar, which are the times in which you can plan to study. Add study sessions to the calendar at times when you can expect to be mentally alert and follow your plan!
2. Create the optimal study environment.
   - Eliminate external sources of distraction, such as television, telephone, etc.
   - Eliminate internal sources of distraction, such as hunger, thirst, or dwelling on items or problems that cannot be worked on at the moment.
   - Take a break for 10 minutes or so after each hour of concentrated study both as a reward and an incentive to keep studying.
3. Use pre-reading strategies to increase comprehension of chapter material.
   - Skim read the headings in the chapter (because they identify chapter content).

- Read the definitions of key terms, which will help you learn new words to comprehend chapter information.
- Review all graphic aids (figures, tables, boxes) because they are often used to explain important points in the chapter.

4. Read the chapter thoroughly but at a reasonable speed.
   - Comprehension and retention are actually enhanced by not reading too slowly.
   - Do take the time to reread any section that is unclear to you.
5. Summarize what you have learned.
   - Use the accompanying online resource, NursingReviewsandRationales.com, to test yourself with hundreds of NCLEX-RN®-style practice questions.
   - Review again any sections that correspond to questions you answered incorrectly or incompletely.

Test-Taking Strategies

Test-taking strategies accompany the rationales for every question in the series. These strategies will assist you to select the correct answer by breaking down the question, even if you don't know the correct response. Use the following strategies to increase your success on nursing tests or examinations:

- Get sufficient sleep and have something to eat before taking a test. Avoid eating concentrated sweets, though, to prevent rapid upward and then downward surges in your blood glucose. Avoid also high-fat foods that will make you sleepy.
- Take deep breaths during the test as needed. Remember, the brain requires oxygen and glucose as fuel. Avoid concentrated sweets before a test, however, to avoid rapid upward and then downward surges in blood glucose levels.
- Read the question carefully, identifying the stem, all the options, and any critical words or phrases in either the stem or options.
  - Critical words in the stem such as "most important" indicate the need to set priorities, since more than one option is likely to contain a statement that is technically correct.
  - Remember that the presence of absolute words such as "never" or "only" in an answer option is more likely to make that option incorrect.
- Determine who is the client in the question; often this is the person with the health problem,

but it may also be a significant other, relative, friend, or another nurse.
- Decide whether the stem is a true response stem or a false response stem. With a true response stem, the correct answer will be a true statement, and vice-versa.
- Determine what the question is really asking, sometimes referred to as the issue of the question. Evaluate all answer options in relation to this issue, and not strictly to the "correctness" of the statement in each individual option.
- Eliminate options that are obviously incorrect, then go back and reread the stem. Evaluate the remaining options against the stem once more to make a final selection.
- If two answers seem similar and correct, try to decide whether one of them is more global or comprehensive. If the global option includes the alternative option within it, it is likely that the more global response is the correct answer.

The NCLEX-RN® Licensing Examination

Upon graduation from a nursing program, successful completion of the NCLEX-RN® licensing examination is required to begin professional nursing practice. The NCLEX-RN® licensing examination is a Computer Adaptive Test (CAT) that ranges in length from 75 to 265 individual (stand-alone) test items, depending on individual performance during the examination. The blueprint for the exam is reviewed and revised every three years by the National Council of State Boards of Nursing according to the results of a job analysis study of new graduate nurses practicing within the first six months after graduation. Each question on the exam is coded to a *Client Need Category* and an *Integrated Process*.

Client Need Categories. There are four categories of client needs, and each exam will contain a minimum and maximum percent of questions from each category. Two major categories have subcategories within them. The *Client Needs* categories according to the NCLEX-RN® Test Plan effective April 2013 are as follows:

- Safe, Effective Care Environment
  - Management of Care (17–23%)
  - Safety and Infection Control (9–15%)
- Health Promotion and Maintenance (6–12%)
- Psychosocial Integrity (6–12%)
- Physiological Integrity
  - Basic Care and Comfort (6–12%)
  - Pharmacological and Parenteral Therapies (12–18%)

- Reduction of Risk Potential (9–15%)
- Physiological Adaptation (11–17%)

Integrated Processes.   The integrated processes identified on the NCLEX-RN® Test Plan effective April 2013, with condensed definitions, are as follows:

- Nursing Process: a scientific problem-solving approach used in nursing practice; consisting of assessment, analysis, planning, implementation, and evaluation.
- Caring: client–nurse interaction(s) characterized by mutual respect and trust and that are directed toward achieving desired client outcomes.

- Communication and Documentation: verbal and/or nonverbal interactions between nurse and others (client, family, health care team); a written or electronic recording of activities or events that occur during client care.
- Teaching and Learning: facilitating client's acquisition of knowledge, skills, and attitudes that lead to behavior change.

More detailed information about this examination may be obtained by visiting the National Council of State Boards of Nursing website at http://www.ncsbn.org and viewing the *2013 NCLEX-RN® Test Plan*.[1]

[1]Reference: National Council of State Boards of Nursing, Inc. *2013 NCLEX-RN© Test Plan*. Effective April, 2013. Retrieved from https://www.ncsbn.org/2013_NCLEX_RN_Test_Plan.pdf.

HOW TO GET THE MOST OUT OF THIS BOOK

Each chapter has the following elements to guide you during review and study:

Chapter Objectives describe what you will be able to know or do after learning the material covered in the chapter.

Objectives

➤ Define key terms associated with hepatobiliary health problems.
➤ Identify risk factors associated with the development of hepatobiliary health problems.
➤ Explain the common etiologies of hepatobiliary health problems.
➤ Describe the pathophysiologic processes associated with specific hepatobiliary health problems.
➤ Distinguish between normal and abnormal hepatobiliary findings obtained from nursing assessment.

NCLEX-RN® Test Prep

Use the accompanying online resource, NursingReviewsandRationales, to test yourself with hundreds of NCLEX®-style practice questions.

Review at a Glance contains a glossary of key terms used in the chapter, with definitions provided up-front and available at your fingertips, to help you stay focused and make the best use of your study time.

Review at a Glance

ascites increased amount of fluid in abdominal cavity

bile a thick, yellow-green fluid secreted from biliary tract and duodenum; responsible for digestion of food, absorption of fats and fat-soluble vitamins, and stimulation of peristalsis

fulminant hepatitis necrosis and shrinking of liver, possibly resulting in liver failure; a complication of viral hepatitis

hemochromatosis a genetically transmitted disease where iron is excessively absorbed and accumulated

pancreatitis inflammation of pancreas

portal hypertension increase in pressure in portal vein caused by obstruction or congestion; a complication of cirrhosis of liver

splenomegaly an enlarged spleen

Pretest provides a 10-question quiz as a sample overview of the material covered in the chapter and helps you decide in what areas you need the most—or the least—review.

PRETEST

1 The nurse is reviewing a client's liver biopsy report, which confirmed a fatty liver and the diagnosis of nonalcoholic fatty liver disease (NAFLD). The nurse checks laboratory data expecting to find elevation of which value?

1. Bilirubin
2. Triglycerides
3. Amylase
4. White blood cell count (WBC)

Practice to Pass questions are open-ended, stimulate critical thinking, and reinforce mastery of the chapter information.

Practice to Pass

A client asks, "How can I keep from developing hepatitis B?" What should the nurse tell him?

!

NCLEX® Alert identifies concepts that are likely to be tested on the NCLEX-RN® examination. Be sure to learn the information highlighted wherever you see this icon.

Case Study, found at the end of the chapter, provides an opportunity for you to use your critical thinking and clinical reasoning skills to "put it all together." It describes a true-to-life client case situation and asks you open-ended questions about how you would provide care for that client and/or family.

Case Study

M. S. is a 55-year-old female presenting as a hospital admission for surgery in the morning. She is a divorced mother of 3 adult children and has smoked 1 pack of cigarettes daily for 30 years. In the past month, she has lost 20 pounds, cannot sleep lying on her back, and is unable to tolerate solid foods. The client became jaundiced in the past 48 hours and computed tomography (CT) scan confirmed a mass in the pancreas.

1. What are the primary risk factors present for pancreatic cancer?

2. Where is the likely location of the tumor based upon the client's symptoms?

3. What are the primary preoperative nursing interventions?

4. What are the primary postoperative nursing interventions?

5. What is the likely prognosis for this client?

For suggested responses, see page 464.

Posttest provides an additional 10-question quiz at the end of the chapter. It provides you with feedback about mastery of the chapter material following review and study. All pretest and posttest questions contain comprehensive rationales for the correct and incorrect answers, and are coded according to cognitive level of difficulty, NCLEX-RN® Test Plan category of client need, and integrated process.

POSTTEST

1 When considering risk factors for pancreatitis, the nurse determines that which assigned client is most likely to develop chronic pancreatitis?

1. 59-year-old male with a history of excessive alcohol use
2. Client with renal problems and hypocalcemia
3. Client recovering from a myocardial infarction with hypercholesterolemia
4. Client with a stone lodged in the pancreatic duct

NCLEX-RN® Test Prep: NursingReviewsandRationales.com

For those who want to prepare for the NCLEX-RN®, practicing online will help you become more familiar with the computer-based testing experience, especially for new alternate item formats such as audio, media-enhanced, hot spot, and exhibit questions. With this new edition, use the code printed inside the front cover of the book to access Nursing Reviews & Rationales, which offers 850 practice questions using all NCLEX®-style formats. This includes the practice questions found in all chapters of the book as well as 30 additional questions per chapter. Nursing Reviews & Rationales allows you to choose two ways to prepare for the NCLEX-RN®. Both approaches personalize your practice experience according to what stage you are at in your NCLEX® preparation.

Nursing Reviews & Rationales includes the eText version of *Pearson Nursing Pathophysiology: Reviews and Rationales*, third edition. This eText is fully searchable and includes features like notetaking, highlighting, and more. The eText allows you to take your review with you anywhere you have an internet connection to NursingReviewsandRationales.com.

NursingNotes Card

This tear-out card provides a reference for frequently used facts and information related to the subject matter of the book. This is designed to be useful in the clinical setting, when quick and easy access to information is so important!

About the Pathophysiology Book

Chapters in this book cover "need-to-know" information about pathophysiology of a wide variety of health problems. They include health problems that relate to the respiratory, cardiovascular, neurological, musculoskeletal, gastrointestinal, endocrine, renal, reproductive, and integumentary systems. Other chapters address immunological, hematological, oncological, and infectious health problems. Finally, the last two chapters review two unique areas, genetically transmitted health problems and multisystem health problems. Mastery of the information in this book and effective use of the test-taking strategies described will help you be confident and successful in testing situations, including the NCLEX-RN®, and in actual clinical practice.

Acknowledgements

This book is a monumental effort of collaboration. Without the contributions of many individuals, this edition of *Pathophysiology: Reviews and Rationales* would not have been possible. Thank you to all the contributors and reviewers who devoted their time and talents to the third edition. The contributors for this edition are Margaret M. Gingrich, RN, MSN, Professor, Harrisburg Area Community College, Harrisburg, Pennsylvania; Karen Hill, RN, MSN, PhD, Associate Professor, Southern Louisiana University, Hammond, Louisiana; Toni Scialdo, RN, PhD, MSEd, MSN, CNE, Nursing Instructor, San Antonio College, San Antonio, Texas; Lisa A. Wolf, PhD, RN, CEN, FAEN, Director, Institute for Emergency Nursing Research, Emergency Nurses' Association and Clinical Assistant Professor,

University of Massachusetts, Amherst, MA. The reviewers for this edition are Sonia Rudolph, RN, MSN, ARNP, FNP-BC, Jefferson Community and Technical College, Louisville, Kentucky; Daryle Wayne, PhD, ARNP, FNP-BC, Coordinator Generic RN Nursing Program, Professor of Nursing, Pasco-Hernando Community College, New Port Richey, Florida.

Thanks also to the contributors and reviewers who assisted with the previous editions of this book: Karen Hill, RN, MSN, PhD, Associate Professor, Southern Louisiana University, Hammond, Louisiana; Julie A. Adkins, RN, MSN, FNP, Family Nurse Practitioner, West Frankfort, Illinois; Jana G. Brannan, MN, RN, CNAA, Assistant Professor, Louisiana State University Health Science Center, New Orleans, Louisiana; Carol D. Clark, MS, RN, ANP, GNPC, Associate Professor, Indiana Wesleyan University, Marion, Indiana; Cathy Cormier, MN, RN, C, Instructor, Southeastern Louisiana University, Hammond, Louisiana; Mical DeBrow, PhD, RN, Vice President/ Healthcare Services, Gulf South Health Plans, Baton Rouge, Louisiana; Joseann Helmes DeWitt, MSN, RN, C, CLNC, Assistant Professor, Alcorn State University School of Nursing, Natchez, Mississippi; Lynn H. Doyle, RN, MS, CPNP, Assistant Professor Pediatrics, Marian College, Fond du Lac, Wisconsin; Pam Hamre, RN, MS, CNM, Assistant Professor, College of St. Catherine, St. Paul, Minnesota; Ann Harley, EdD, RN, Professor, Carson Newman College, Jefferson City, Tennessee; Sherry Hendrickson, RN, PhD, CS, Assistant Professor of Clinical Nursing, The University of Texas at Austin, Austin, Texas; Barbara Moffett, PhD, RN, Professor, Southeastern Louisiana University, Hammond, Louisiana; Patsy Rider, RN, MSN, CS, Instructor, The University of Texas at Austin, Austin, Texas; Diane E. Smith, MSN, RN, Assistant Professor, Baton Rouge, Louisiana; Susan K. Steele, MN, RN, AOCN, Oncology Clinical Nurse Specialist/ Assistant Professor, Louisiana State University Health Science Center, New Orleans, Louisiana; Betty Jane Sylvest, BSN, RN, MSN, University of Southern Mississippi, Hattiesburg, Mississippi; Eugenia H. Tickle, RN, MSN, EdD, Associate Professor, Midwestern State University, Wichita Falls, Texas; Janie Butts, DSN, RN, Assistant Professor, University of Southern Mississippi, Hattiesburg, Mississippi; Christine A. Cannon, RN, PhD, Associate Professor, University of Delaware, Newark, Delaware; Linda Covington, PhD, Associate Professor, Middle Tennessee State University, Murfreesboro, Tennessee; Barbara Daniel, MEd, MS, CRNP, Professor, Cecil Community College, North East, Maryland; Ann M. Findley, PhD, Associate Professor, Department of Biology, University of Louisiana at Monroe, Monroe, Louisiana; Diane Ford, RN, MS, FNP, CS, Assistant Professor, Andrews University, Berrien Springs, Michigan; Wanda Gifford, RN, MSN, CS, FNP, Family Nurse Practitioner/Instructor, St. Josephs College, Rensselaer, Indiana; Sandra Smith Huddleston, RN, PhD, Associate Professor, Berea College, Berea, Kentucky; Robin Kirschner, RN, MA, CPAN, Professor, Scottsdale Community College, Scottsdale, Arizona; Jane Koeckeritz, RN, PhD, Professor, University of Northern Colorado, Greeley, Colorado; James A. Metcalf, PhD, Professor, George Mason University, Fairfax, Virginia; Mercy Mammah Popoola, RN, CNS, PhD, Professor, Georgia Southern University, Statesboro, Georgia; Elizabeth Ann Rettew, MSN, RN, FNP-BC, Associate Professor, Malone College, Canton, Ohio. Their work will surely assist both students and practicing nurses alike to extend their knowledge in the area of pathophysiology.

I owe a special debt of gratitude to the wonderful team at Pearson Nursing for their enthusiasm for this project, as well as their good humor, expertise, and encouragement as the series developed. Maura Connor, Director of Readypoint™, was unending in her creativity, support, encouragement, and belief in the need for this series. Jennifer Farthing, Executive Editor, Readypoint™ coordinated this revision with insight, talent, and zeal, and fostered a culture of true collaboration and team work. Elisa Rogers, Developmental Editor, devoted many long hours to coordinating different facets of this project, and tirelessly and cheerfully encouraged our efforts as well. Her high standards and attention to detail contributed greatly to the final "look" of this book. Editorial Assistant, Deirdre MacKnight, helped to keep the project moving forward on a day-to-day basis, and I am grateful for her efforts as well. A very special thank you goes to the designers of the book and the production team, led by Patrick Walsh, Managing Editor, and Maria Reyes, Project Manager, who brought the ideas and manuscript into final form.

Thank you to the team at GEX Publishing Services, led by Project Coordinator Michelle Durgerian, for the detail-oriented work of creating this book. I greatly appreciate their hard work, attention to detail, and spirit of collaboration.

Finally, I would like to acknowledge and gratefully thank my children, Michael Jr., Kathryn, Kristen, and William, who donated time that would have been spent with them, so this book could be revised. I would also like to thank my students, past and present, for continuing to inspire me with their quest for knowledge and passion for nursing. You are the future!

–MaryAnn Hogan

Respiratory Health Problems

Chapter Outline

Risk Factors Associated with
   Respiratory Health
   Problems
Obstructive Pulmonary
   Disorders

Restrictive Pulmonary
   Disorders
Pneumonia
Pulmonary Tuberculosis (TB)
Pleural Effusion
Pleuritis (Pleurisy)

Pneumothorax/Hemothorax
Pulmonary Embolism (PE)
Pulmonary Hypertension
Lung Cancer
Respiratory Failure

Objectives

➤ Define key terms associated with respiratory health problems.
➤ Identify risk factors associated with the development of respiratory
   health problems.
➤ Explain the common etiologies of respiratory health problems.
➤ Describe the pathophysiologic processes associated with specific
   respiratory health problems.
➤ Distinguish between normal and abnormal respiratory findings
   obtained from nursing assessment.
➤ Prioritize nursing interventions associated with specific respiratory
   health problems.

NCLEX-RN® Test Prep

Use the accompanying online resource,
NursingReviewsandRationales, to test
yourself with hundreds of NCLEX®-style
practice questions.

Review at a Glance

asthma an obstructive airflow disorder where narrowing and inflammation of airways cause respiratory distress

atelectasis collapse of a portion of lung with limited gas exchange

bronchiectasis an irreversible state of bronchial dilation and destruction of bronchial walls

bronchitis inflammation of mucous membranes of bronchial airways; another term for chronic bronchitis is "blue bloater" because of hypoxemia that leads to cyanosis

chronic obstructive pulmonary disease (COPD) a group of pulmonary diseases involving obstruction of airflow that is chronic and recurrent, usually associated with emphysema and chronic bronchitis

cor pulmonale a disorder manifested by hypertrophy of right ventricle caused by pulmonary hypertension; manifests as right heart failure

cystic fibrosis (CF) autosomal recessive disease of exocrine glands that manifests itself in multiple organs, characterized by excess production of mucus and COPD in early childhood

emphysema a chronic disorder of lungs resulting in overinflation of air spaces, loss of elasticity, and decreased gas exchange; another term for chronic emphysema is "pink puffer" because client does not become cyanotic until end stages of disease

flail chest instability of chest wall usually caused by trauma or fractured ribs with a reverse in chest wall movement

from normal; chest wall contracts on inspiration and expands outward on expiration

hemothorax collection of blood or fluid in pleural space

obstructive pulmonary disorders any respiratory disorder where airflow is hindered to lungs, may be chronic or acute

pleural effusion increased accumulation of fluid between visceral and parietal pleura of lung

pleuritis inflammation of parietal space of lungs, also known as pleurisy

pneumonia inflammation of lungs caused by bacteria, viruses, fungi, or other pathogens

pneumothorax collapse of a portion or all of lung due to trapping of air in pleural space

pulmonary embolism (PE) blockage of a pulmonary artery by an embolus of blood, fat, amniotic fluid, air, or foreign substance

pulmonary hypertension a sustained elevation of pulmonary artery pressure, greater than 20 mmHg

restrictive pulmonary disorders any disease that limits expansion of lungs or chest wall movement

sleep apnea having periods of delay or lack of breathing (usually longer than 10 seconds) during sleep

status asthmaticus an acute emergency of a prolonged or repetitive asthma attack

tuberculosis (TB) infection of lung with an acid-fast bacillus, Mycobacterium tuberculosis

PRETEST

1 A 67-year-old male client with chronic respiratory acidosis from end-stage chronic obstructive pulmonary disease (COPD) is receiving oxygen at 1 L/min per nasal cannula. Which statement by the nurse best explains to the client's daughter how this therapy prevents respiratory depression?

1. "Your father's breathing effort is driven by lower oxygen levels."
2. "Your father's breathing effort is driven by a low carbon dioxide level."
3. "Your father will retain metabolic acids if the oxygen level is too high."
4. "Your father will breathe best when he has a moderately high oxygen level."

2 A client presents to the emergency department with acute respiratory distress and the following arterial blood gases (ABGs): pH 7.35, PCO_2 40 mmHg, PO_2 63 mmHg, HCO_3 23 mEq/L, and oxygen saturation (SaO_2) 93%. The nurse concludes that which of the following represents the best analysis of the etiology of these ABGs?

1. Tuberculosis (TB)
2. Pneumonia
3. Pleural effusion
4. Hypoxia

3 When assessing a client with impaired oxygen perfusion from pulmonary emboli, the nurse would expect to note which symptoms? Select all that apply.

1. Warm, dry skin
2. Anxiety
3. Tachycardia
4. Dyspnea
5. Bradycardia

4 A client who is 1 day postoperative reports shortness of breath. The respiratory rate (RR) is 35 and slightly labored, and there are no breath sounds present in the right lung base. The nurse would suspect which of the following conditions?

1. Cor pulmonale
2. Atelectasis
3. Pulmonary embolus
4. Cardiac tamponade

5 A client with an acute case of pneumonia has a dry, hacking cough, temperature of 100.6° F, white blood cell (WBC) count of 12,000/mm³, decreased breath sounds, and pain upon deep inhalation or coughing. Which of the following would indicate positive results after a respiratory treatment of normal saline, acetylcysteine (Mucomyst), and albuterol (Proventil)? Select all that apply.

1. Reduced crackles and moderate amount of productive sputum
2. Absent breath sounds in bases and normal breath sounds in upper lobes
3. Wheezing, nonproductive cough
4. Increased coughing but with thinner and easier to expectorate sputum
5. Reduced anxiety and verbalization of improved ability to breathe

6 The nurse prioritizes that which client is in need of *immediate* medical attention and emergency intervention?

1. Client reporting sharp pain upon taking a deep breath and excessive coughing
2. Client exhibiting yellow, productive sputum, low-grade fever, and crackles
3. Client with a shift of the trachea to the left, with no breath sounds on the right
4. Client with asthma reporting inability to "catch her breath" after exercise

7 An adolescent client newly diagnosed with asthma is being discharged from the hospital after an episode of status asthmaticus. The nurse should include which items in discharge teaching? Select all that apply.

1. Encourage client to not start smoking.
2. Relationship of symptoms to a specific trigger such as physical exercise
3. Limitations in sports that will be imposed by the illness
4. Specific instructions on use of prescribed rescue inhalers
5. Limitation to working part-time that will be imposed by the illness

8 A client with a known cardiac history is experiencing angina at night only, excessive fatigue, and according to the spouse, snores excessively. The health care provider orders a sleep apnea study with and without oxygen. The nurse explains to the client's spouse, who is also a nurse, that a pulmonary source of these symptoms is being investigated at this time for which reason?

1. Sleep apnea is an obstruction of the lower airway that impedes airflow.
2. Clients with sleep apnea have adequate amounts of REM sleep, but snoring contributes to the decrease in oxygen levels.
3. Sleep apnea causes an increase in muscle tone during REM sleep in order to make breathing possible.
4. Excess periods of apnea during sleep and severe drops in oxygen levels can contribute to the angina, which is occurring only at night.

9 The nurse anticipates that a client admitted with newly diagnosed lung cancer would exhibit which signs that are characteristic of this health problem? Select all that apply.

1. Exertional dyspnea
2. Persistent changing cough
3. Air hunger during episodes of dyspnea
4. Coughing up bloody sputum
5. Long-term pulmonary infection

10 A client is admitted to the nursing unit after being speared by a bull in the right chest wall while repairing a fence in a pasture. The client is diagnosed with a flail chest, and a chest tube is inserted. Which observation by the nurse indicates that the chest tube is working properly? Select all that apply.

1. Constant bubbles with decreased breath sounds
2. Fluctuation of the water-seal level with respirations
3. Lack of fluctuation or bubbles in the water-seal chamber after several days
4. Occasional bubbles in the water-seal chamber
5. Collection chamber completely filled with fluid from the pleural space

➤ *See pages 29–30 for Answers and Rationales.*

I. RISK FACTORS ASSOCIATED WITH RESPIRATORY HEALTH PROBLEMS

A. ***Obstructive pulmonary disorders*** such as asthma, chronic obstructive pulmonary disease (COPD), cystic fibrosis, bronchitis

1. Asthma: allergies, genetic disposition
2. COPD: primarily smoking, exposure to lung irritants, immunological factors
3. Cystic fibrosis: genetic transmission
4. Bronchitis: smoking, air pollution, or exposure to pulmonary irritants or infectious diseases

    B. ***Restrictive pulmonary disorders*** such as atelectasis, acute respiratory distress syndrome (ARDS), flail chest, pulmonary contusion, and sleep apnea
        1. Atelectasis: surgery, trauma, pneumonia or other respiratory disorders (COPD), prolonged bed rest, mechanical ventilation
        2. ARDS: shock, trauma, smoke inhalation, any cardiac or respiratory event, often unknown; see also Chapter 17
        3. Sleep apnea: obesity, COPD, smoking, aging process
    C. **Pneumonia:** aging process, compromised respiratory conditions, debilitating diseases, lack of vaccine in at-risk persons
    D. **Tuberculosis:** persons positive for human immunodeficiency virus (HIV), immigrants and disadvantaged groups, environment (overcrowding, poor ventilation, etc.)
    E. **Pleural effusion:** surgery, trauma, inflammation, malignancy, or other respiratory disorder
    F. **Pleuritis:** none: usually secondary to other respiratory conditions
    G. **Pneumothorax:** smoking, trauma, men (tall, young, thin chest), family history, underlying respiratory diseases (COPD, ARDS, cystic fibrosis, asthma)
    H. **Pulmonary embolism:** deep vein thrombosis (DVT) or other blood clots, chronic bedrest, hypercoagulability, surgery, heart conditions (congestive heart failure [CHF], myocardial infarction [MI]), obesity, and oral estrogen
    I. **Pulmonary hypertension:** young women in their 30s to 40s (primary); smoking, chronic lung disease, sleep apnea, obesity, neuromuscular disease, heart conditions leading to hypoxemia (secondary)
    J. **Lung cancer:** smoking, lung irritants, family history, air pollution
    K. **Respiratory failure:** other respiratory conditions or respiratory dysfunction (COPD, pneumonia, ARDS)

II. OBSTRUCTIVE PULMONARY DISORDERS

    A. **Overview**
        1. Defined as disorders that obstruct airflow out of lung, primarily impeding expiration, including asthma, emphysema, cystic fibrosis, and bronchiectasis
        2. Causes include infection, air pollutants, allergies, smoke inhalation, or genetics
    B. **Pathophysiology**
        1. **Asthma** is a chronic inflammatory airway disorder resulting in reversible broncho-constriction and air hunger in response to triggers from a variety of sources
            a. Primarily affects bronchial airways and causes mucosal edema, secretion of mucus, and inflammation of airway
            b. When exposed to a trigger, hyperactivity of medium-sized bronchi causes release of leukotrienes, histamine, and other substances from mast cells; these agents intensify inflammatory process and cause bronchospasm
            c. *Extrinsic asthma* is triggered by factors such as cold air, high altitude, strong odors, emotional stress, hormone changes, allergens, cigarette smoke, and exercise
            d. *Intrinsic asthma* is usually from an unknown cause; affects clients usually after age 40
            e. **Status asthmaticus** is an emergency situation when an asthma attack is prolonged and not responding to usual medications or when client has one asthma attack after another; prompt treatment is needed to avoid respiratory failure
        2. **Chronic obstructive pulmonary disease (COPD)** is a group of pulmonary diseases of a chronic nature characterized by increased resistance to airflow; consists of emphysema and bronchitis
            a. **Emphysema** is a breakdown of elastin and collagen fiber network of alveoli whereby alveoli enlarge or walls are destroyed; leads to formation of larger than normal air spaces
                1) Loss of elastic recoil from destruction of elastin and collagen fibers causes air trapping in lungs and airway collapse
                2) Air trapping results in hyper-inflated lungs, causing a barrel chest appearance

3) Client maintains arterial blood gases (ABGs) by hyperventilating and has a pink appearance to skin, thus known as a "pink puffer" early in disease; cyanosis may develop in late stages

b. Chronic **bronchitis** is an inflammatory response in small and large airways leading to vasodilation, congestion, mucosal edema, and bronchospasm; a chronic cough and productive sputum are present for a minimum of 3 months in one year

  1) Bronchial mucosal glands hypertrophy and there is an increase in number and size of goblet cells accompanied by inflammatory cell infiltration and edema of bronchial mucosa

  2) As bronchial walls thicken, airflow is impeded

  3) Unlike emphysema, a client with bronchitis cannot increase breathing efforts to maintain ABGs

  4) Presence of cyanosis and edema gives a client with bronchitis a description of "blue bloater"

  5) With severe chronic hypoxia, kidneys increase production of red blood cells (RBCs) in an attempt to bring more oxygenated blood to body cells, thus causing polycythemia, increased blood viscosity, and a higher risk for blood clots

c. Hypercapnia is typical of a client with COPD along with hypoxemia

  1) ABGs reflect a high carbon dioxide (CO_2) level and a low oxygen (O_2) level

  2) Hypoxia becomes main stimulus to breathe instead of the normal increase in CO_2

  3) A client with COPD cannot tolerate high levels of O_2

  4) Hypoxia alone is usually indicated by a partial pressure of arterial O_2 (PaO_2) less than 80 mmHg combined with a low O_2 saturation (SaO_2) (see Box 1-1)

d. Nail beds demonstrate clubbing (an angle greater than 160°) or a more flattened, yellow appearance because of chronic hypoxia

3. Cystic fibrosis (CF) is an autosomal-recessive disorder resulting in excessive production of mucus with chronic obstructive lung disease in early childhood

  a. Lack of a necessary protein needed to transport chloride results in excess absorption of water and sodium

  b. Absence of this protein in lungs also leads to thick viscous mucus and deficiency in transporting chloride

  c. Because of sodium reabsorption, sweat has high levels of sodium and chloride

  d. Excess mucus leads to atelectasis, infection, bronchiectasis, and eventually pulmonary hypertension, and **cor pulmonale** (right-sided heart failure due to pulmonary causes)

  e. In older children, pancreatic dysfunction leads to difficulty digesting foods and malabsorption because of a lack of pancreatic enzymes

4. Bronchiectasis is a permanent enlargement of large bronchi, often associated with respiratory infection

  a. A combination of infection and airway obstruction from this disorder leads to atelectasis, abscesses, destruction, and necrosis of bronchial wall

  b. Usually associated with CF, but can be related to tumors, foreign bodies, tuberculosis, or exposure to lung irritants

  c. Manifested by permanently deformed and dilated distal airways, damage to cartilage and elastic tissue supporting the airways, and fibrosis

Box 1-1		
Normal Adult Arterial Blood Gas Values	pH	7.35–7.45
	$PaCO_2$	35–45 mmHg
	PaO_2	80–100 mmHg
	HCO_3^-	21–28 mEq/L
	O_2 saturation (SaO_2)	95–100%

C. Nursing assessment
    1. Asthma

        a. Assessment includes client reports of air hunger, chest tightness, anxiety, use of accessory muscles, tachypnea (increased respiratory rate), tachycardia (increased heart rate), and altered lung sounds (wheezing, long expiratory effort, diminished breath sounds in lower airways)

        b. Diagnostic tests

            1) Pulmonary function studies (PFSs) show decreased expiratory flow of air; forced expiratory volume (FEV_1) shows amount of expired air (should be about 80% of client's potential and less than 20% variation over time)

            2) Peak expiratory flow rate (PEFR) can be measured at home using a peak flow meter (PFM) to assess amount of expired air before and after treatment

            3) Skin testing is often done to determine problems with allergies and a challenge test is performed using an inhaled histamine or by giving methacholine, followed by a breathing treatment

            4) Laboratory test for allergies may reveal high IgE and serum eosinophils

    2. COPD

        a. Assessment includes a productive cough in bronchitis and a dry cough in emphysema, dyspnea, pursed-lip breathing, use of accessory muscles, orthopnea, nasal flaring, cachectic appearance, adventitious breath sounds (wheezing, rhonchi, or crackles), increased anterior–posterior diameter (barrel chest), prolonged expiration, skin color (pink if emphysema in early stage; cyanotic if later stage or with chronic bronchitis); emphysemic client may have quiet, distant breath sounds, air hunger, fever, chest pain, and tachypnea; symptoms of right-sided heart failure (cor pulmonale) may occur later in disease process

        b. Diagnostic tests: ABGs usually show hypercapnia and hypoxemia, FEV_1 is decreased, CXR shows flattening of diaphragm, complete blood count (CBC) shows polycythemia

    3. Cystic fibrosis

        a. Assessment includes a complete history of child with particular attention to whether symptoms have changed with maturity

            1) Frequent symptoms include delayed growth and development, frequent respiratory problems (pneumonia, cough with excess mucus production, inability to exercise), clubbing of finger- and toenail beds, barrel chest, crackles, and possibly symptoms of cor pulmonale

            2) Gastrointestinal (GI) symptoms include steatorrhea (excess fat in stools), greasy foul-smelling stools, impaired digestion, and abdominal pain

            3) Diabetes mellitus and vitamin K deficiency (from malabsorption) may ensue

        b. Diagnostic tests: sweat chloride test indicates elevated sodium and chloride concentrations; ABG shows hypoxemia with reduced O_2 saturation; PFS shows reduced air flow and FEV_1; CXR may show atelectasis or hyperinflation; stool specimen shows steatorrhea

    4. Bronchiectasis

        a. Assessment includes chronic productive cough with foul-smelling, purulent sputum, wheezing or crackles, hemoptysis (blood in sputum), dyspnea, weight loss, recurrent respiratory infections, and often cor pulmonale

        b. Diagnostic tests: CXR shows enlarged airways; ABGs often show hypoxemia; PFS are similar to bronchitis; computerized tomography (CT) scan may be used to determine extent of damage

D. Nursing management
    1. Asthma

        a. Medications

            1) Bronchodilators to maintain patency in bronchi

Practice to Pass

A 7-year-old child with asthma is placed on beclomethasone (Vanceril) as a maintenance inhaler. What is the major concern for a child taking this medication?

   a) Beta adrenergic drug: metaproterenol (Alupent)
   b) Adrenergic stimulants: albuterol (Proventil, Ventolin), salmeterol (Serevent), terbutaline sulfate (Brethine), isoetharine HCL (Bronkosol), tiotropium (Spiriva)
   c) Anticholinergics: ipratropium bromide (Atrovent), ipratropium with albuterol (Combivent)
   d) Anti-inflammatory: cromolyn (Intal), nedocromil (Tilade)—do not use for acute asthmatic attacks
   e) Methylxanthine: theophylline (Theo-Dur, Slophyllin, Slo-bid) may be used as adjunct treatment; is no longer a primary treatment
   2) Steroids such as beclomethasone (Beclovent, Vanceril), dexamethasone (Decadron), fluticasone (Flonase), budesonide (Rhinocort), and fluticasone propionate (Advair) may be used on short-term basis when exacerbation of attacks occur or as a maintenance inhaler to suppress inflammatory process
   3) In children, nonsteroidal drugs are often used as maintenance inhalers
   4) Leukotriene modifiers: zafirlukast (Accolate), montelukast (Singulair)
 b. Explain differences between rescue inhalers and maintenance inhalers
   1) Rescue inhalers are used for an acute attack and include drugs such as epinephrine (Adrenalin), isoetharine inhalation (Bronkosol), albuterol (Ventolin, Proventil), and metaproterenol (Alupent)
   2) Maintenance drugs or inhalers are used to prevent an attack and include ipratropium (Atrovent), leukotriene antagonists, salmeterol (Serevent), xanthine derivatives, cromolyn (Intal), nedocromil (Tilade), and fluticasone propionate (Advair)
 c. Include in client teaching drug actions, side effects and how to use metered dose inhalers and dry powder inhalers (see Box 1-2)

Box 1-2	
Using Dry Dose Inhalers	**Purpose:** To deliver a specific dose of dry powder medication to be inhaled into the lungs for a local effect. **Rationale:** Inhaled medications are easily deposited on the oral mucosa membranes without reaching the lungs if a dry dose powder inhaler is not used properly. **Expected Outcome:** The client will correctly use an administration technique that results in medication reaching the lungs.

Client Instructions—Diskus (see Figure 1-2)
1) Open the diskus.
2) Snap the mouthpiece into position.
3) Breathe out fully, away from the mouthpiece.
4) Place the mouthpiece to the lips and take a steady, deep breath through the mouth.
5) After inhaling, the breath should be held for about 10 seconds.
6) Close the diskus and the counter will count down, showing the number of doses left in the diskus.
7) The diskus should be kept dry at all times.

Client Instructions—Capsule container (see Figure 1-3)
1) Open the container and expose the area to insert the capsule, which should come individually wrapped.
2) After placing the capsule into the appropriate area of the container, close the mouthpiece.
3) Puncture the capsule using the button attached to a needle.
4) Place the mouthpiece to the lips and inhale slowly using a deep breath through the mouth.
5) After inhaling, the breath should be held for about 10 seconds.
6) Open the mouthpiece and discard the used capsule.
7) Close the container until the next use.
8) Keep the container dry at all times.

1) Metered dose inhalers (MDIs) require attaching a canister to mouthpiece, delivering one or two "puffs," and rinsing mouth after use (see Figure 1-1); dry powder inhalers such as fluticasone propionate (Advair) require snapping mouthpiece into position and inhaling (see Figure 1-2); dry powder inhalers such as tiotropium bromide (Spiriva) require placing a capsule into canister and punching a hole in capsule using button on apparatus to release powder (see Figure 1-3)

Figure 1-1

One method for using a metered-dose inhaler

Figure 1-2

Diskus inhaler for dry powder dose

Figure 1-3

Spiriva applicator

1. dust cap
2. mouthpiece
3. base
4. piercing button
5. center chamber
6. Air intake vents

> **2)** Use steroid inhalers before brushing teeth to avoid oral infections; a spacer may be required to ensure complete dose is received, decrease bad taste of spray, and prevent thrush if a steroid is used

> **3)** Steroids can stunt growth of children, especially under age 12, and can have many side effects if used on a long-term basis

> **4)** Theophylline preparations can reach toxic levels; monitor drug levels and report tremors or jitters to provider

    d. Teach client how to identify what triggers an attack and how to avoid triggers; influenza vaccines are recommended yearly

    e. Explain disease process and how to avoid anxiety during an attack; client should seek immediate attention if rescue inhaler does not work or status asthmaticus occurs; home portable nebulizers can be purchased

    f. Teach client to carry rescue inhaler at all times; if an attack occurs and an inhaler is not available, drinking 2 regular carbonated beverages with caffeine may help until drugs are available

    g. Teach client to check inhalers frequently for fullness and expiration date, and to clean inhaler mouthpiece with tepid water (no soap) and air dry overnight (to decrease infections to mouth, such as thrush)

    h. Monitor vital signs (VS) and breath sounds, offering comfort until drugs take effect during an acute attack

    i. Monitor peak flow readings (PFRs), especially during allergy seasons

      1) These may decrease as much as 24 hours before an attack

      2) Drugs used during an attack can be evaluated as effective if PFR after drug use is 80% of client's personal best

2. COPD

    a. Medications

      1) Bronchodilators to maintain patent airways: anticholinergic agents, sympathomimetics, and methylxanthines

      2) Newer bronchodilator (inhaled) is tiotropium bromide (Spiriva)

      3) Combination drugs with glucocorticoid and beta-2 agonists: fluticasone propionate (Flonase)

      4) Steroids or anti-inflammatory drugs as needed during exacerbations; oral prednisone or inhalers similar to client with asthma; monitor for side effects, especially fluid and sodium retention

      5) Antibiotics as prescribed during acute infectious periods or prophylactically

      6) Expectorants to help loosen mucus

    b. Instruct clients to stay up to date with pneumonia and influenza vaccines

    c. Educate client about the following: smoking cessation, adequate hydration, breathing exercises (pursed-lip breathing to keep airways open by maintaining positive pressure; abdominal breathing to expand lungs), adequate nutrition, and avoiding people with respiratory infections

    d. Pulmonary hygiene measures may be needed if secretions are thick: percussion (rhythmic clapping on chest to loosen secretions), postural drainage, suctioning, and respiratory treatments

    e. Use of low flow O_2 to prevent depression of respiratory drive

    f. Evaluation of a low-profile exercise program

    g. Maintain adequate fluid intake of at least 2 liters per day

3. Cystic fibrosis

    a. Medications

      1) Bronchodilators if airway obstruction is problematic

      2) Antibiotics if an infection is present

Practice to Pass

An older client with chronic obstructive pulmonary disease (COPD) also has a history of congestive heart failure (CHF). What is the major concern for placing this client on an oral dose of a steroid such as prednisone?

3) Dornase alfa recombinant: this drug hydrolyzes DNA in sputum of clients with CF; as a result, pulmonary function is improved and number of respiratory infections is lessened

4) Mucolytics to liquefy secretions as needed

b. Maintain adequate fluid and electrolytes, diet (high in protein, fat, and calories), and adherence to pancreatic enzyme drug therapy

c. Monitor closely for signs and symptoms of infection

d. Oxygen therapy may be needed if hypoxemia is present

e. Pulmonary hygiene measures to clear airways: postural drainage, positioning, suctioning, percussion, vibration, "huff" cough technique (a valved mask is used for 20 inhalations, followed by 3 to 4 huffs)

f. Education includes respiratory care techniques, avoidance of respiratory irritants, medication administration, and dietary needs

4. Bronchiectasis: basically same as for a client with COPD

a. Medications include antibiotics for infection and bronchodilators

b. Pulmonary hygiene measures: suctioning as needed, O_2 therapy if hypoxic, percussion, and postural drainage

III. RESTRICTIVE PULMONARY DISORDERS

A. Overview

1. **Restrictive pulmonary disorders** are defined as disorders that limit ability of lungs to expand normally in a respiratory cycle

2. This category includes many disorders

   a. Disorders discussed in this section: atelectasis, flail chest, pulmonary contusion, sleep apnea

   b. Disorders discussed separately: pneumonia, pulmonary tuberculosis, pleural effusion, and pneumothorax

   c. Other disorders: Pickwickian syndrome (obesity hypoventilation syndrome), pulmonary fibrosis ("stiffening" of lung tissue from damage or scarring), pulmonary edema (fluid in alveoli caused by increased pressure in pulmonary blood vessels, often due to heart failure)

3. Causes include changes in hydrostatic or oncotic forces resulting in fluid accumulation in pleural spaces, trauma to chest wall, fractured ribs, pneumothorax, bacterial or viral pathogens, reduced lung compliance, scarring and fibrosis of lung parenchyma, musculoskeletal disorders, and neuromuscular disorders

B. Pathophysiology

1. **Atelectasis** is collapse of alveoli in lung(s)

   a. Perfusion occurs without ventilation because collapsed alveoli do not participate in air exchange

   b. Without O_2 little if any surfactant (a lipoprotein substance lining alveoli) is produced; surfactant is needed to lower surface tension, which lowers resistance to expansion on inspiration and prevents collapse of alveoli on expiration

   c. Blood flow is not interrupted, but blood travels through airless alveoli; if a large enough area of lung is affected, hypoxemia results

   d. *Primary atelectasis* is often associated with infants who are born with collapsed alveoli at birth; in premature births, a lack of surfactant may cause atelectasis

   e. *Secondary atelectasis* is a collapse of alveoli that were previously expanded and is sub-classified as 3 types

   1) *Compression atelectasis* is a result of crowding of lung tissue resulting in collapse; may be caused by fluid, tumor, puncture wound, or abdominal distention

2) *Resorption atelectasis* is a result of blockage to alveoli and can result from mucus buildup, pneumonia, CF, and surgery; alveoli distal to obstructed bronchus resorb air and cause collapse of alveolar walls

3) *Contraction atelectasis* is a result of fibrosis of lung or pleura; it results in inadequate lung expansion

2. Flail chest and pulmonary contusion (bruising of lung tissue) are acute injuries to chest wall usually caused by blunt trauma or penetrating objects; rib fractures and motor vehicle crashes are common causes of chest wall injuries

a. In flail chest, injury results in instability of chest wall

b. Negative pressure created within lung cavity upon inspiration causes chest wall section to collapse

c. Upon expiration, positive pressure causes chest wall section to expand outward

d. Penetrating objects also affect pressure within lungs, which leads to collapse of portions or an entire lung

e. Lack of proper lung expansion causes increased breathing effort, impaired gas exchange, reduced lung compliance, and pain

3. Sleep apnea is a lack of airflow in upper airways for 10 seconds or more; 3 different forms exist:

a. *Obstructive sleep apnea* is most common and is caused by an obstruction to airflow while ventilatory efforts continue

1) As many as 30 apnea periods per hour may occur while sleeping

2) Normal pharyngeal muscle tone is lost, thus allowing pharynx to collapse during inspiration

3) Further obstruction occurs when tongue falls against posterior pharyngeal wall

4) Client attempts to breathe, but each effort shortens until obstructive forces are reduced by movement or position change

b. *Central apnea* is when respiratory center of brain is affected and drive to breathe is inhibited

1) There is no effort to breathe during a period of apnea

2) This is thought to occur in sudden infant death syndrome (SIDS)

c. *Mixed apnea* is a combination of both central and obstructive types of apnea

C. Nursing assessment

1. Atelectasis

a. Assessment includes lung sounds (diminished, crackles or gurgles), tachypnea, depth and regularity of breathing, dyspnea, tachycardia, abnormal ABGs (hypoxia), temperature (if infection is suspected as a cause), and coughing

b. Diagnostic tests: CXR will usually reveal an area of collapsed lung, and ABGs show hypoxemia from reduced oxygenation in collapsed segment

2. Flail chest and pulmonary contusion

a. Assessment of flail chest includes asymmetry of chest expansion and paradoxical chest movement (affected portion of chest may sink in upon inspiration), pain upon inspiration, dyspnea, tachypnea, abnormal lung sounds (diminished, crackles, rhonchi), palpable crepitus (sound of crackling cellophane when skin is touched), and tachycardia

b. Specific symptoms for pulmonary contusion include symptoms noted above (except for paradoxical chest movement, which is unique to flail chest) plus copious (often blood-tinged) sputum, restlessness, and apprehension

c. Diagnostic tests: CXR, ABGs

3. Sleep apnea

a. Assessment includes changes in behavior and performance (irritability, daytime drowsiness, decreased ability to function, forgetfulness, lethargy), reports of feeling tired or listless, dark circles under eyes, frequent yawning, changes in posture, loud snoring, cardiac dysrhythmias, angina at night, headaches due to hypercapnia, periods of apnea during sleep, impotence, and respiratory depression (related to certain medications used)

    b. Diagnostic tests: electroencephalography (EEG) to identify stages of sleep, electrocardiogram (ECG) to identify dysrhythmias, polysomnography (overnight sleep study—with and without O_2), CBC to assess for possible erythrocytosis (or polycythemia) from reduced oxygenation, and a thyroid function study to rule out hypothyroidism

D. Nursing management

  1. Atelectasis

    a. Medications include antibiotics if an infection is suspected, bronchodilators, and analgesics as necessary

    b. Administer O_2 to enhance oxygenation at alveolar level and monitor O_2 saturation

    c. Elevate head of bed

    d. Encourage turning, coughing, and deep breathing as often as every 1–2 hours and use of incentive spirometer every 1–2 hours

    e. Encourage adequate fluid intake unless otherwise contraindicated

    f. Encourage ambulation as ordered

  2. Flail chest and pulmonary contusion

    a. Medications

      1) Analgesics for pain control, initially on a *scheduled dosing pattern* rather than as needed; continuous epidural analgesia or even intercostal nerve blocks may be recommended forms of analgesia

      2) Sedatives or neuromuscular blockers to control agitation while on mechanical ventilation

      3) Bronchodilators

      4) Antibiotics (possibly) as a preventive measure

    b. Administer O_2 as ordered

    c. Internal or external fixation of flail area may be necessary

      1) Use of a sandbag for flail chest may help to stabilize area by external fixation

      2) Endotracheal intubation and mechanical ventilation with positive end-expiratory pressure (PEEP) may support ventilation and provide internal fixation

    d. Maintain adequate hydration while avoiding overhydration

    e. Turn, cough, and deep breathe every 2 hours, yet restrict overall activity to reduce O_2 needs and plan for adequate rest periods

    f. Oral or nasal suctioning as needed

    g. Teach client how to use a pillow to splint area during coughing

    h. Maintain bed with head in an elevated position

    i. Monitor VS, O_2 saturation, and level of consciousness (LOC)

    j. Chest tube may be inserted for chest contusions if hemothorax or pneumothorax results

      1) For chest tubes, assess respiratory status every 2–4 hours; maintain a closed system; milk chest tubes only if protocol present, because this increases pleural pressure; check water seal frequently (water level should fluctuate with inspiration and have only periodic air bubbles), assess amount, color, consistency of drainage every 4–8 hours, and assess water level

      2) Continuous air bubbles usually indicate an air leak; lack of fluctuation indicates inadequate function of system or full reinflation of lung

  3. Sleep apnea

    a. Medications

      1) Medroxyprogesterone (Depo-Provera, Provera): stimulates respirations in obese clients who hypoventilate

    2) Theophylline: relaxes smooth muscle of bronchi

    3) Protriptyline (Vivactil) or fluoxetine hydrochloride (Prozac): antidepressants

    4) Clonazepam (Klonopin): an antiepileptic

    5) Acetazolamide (Diamox): carbonic anhydrase inhibitor for central sleep apnea

    6) Hypnotics, sedatives, androgens, and alcohol should be completely avoided because of their effects on respiratory system

  b. Implementation of weight reduction plan

  c. Continuous positive airway pressure (CPAP) therapy is most commonly prescribed treatment to force air into back of throat using a compressor to reduce airway occlusion in sleep apnea

  d. Nosebleeds and nasal congestion may occur while using O_2 and CPAP secondary to dryness; a humidifier is often recommended to offset this

  e. O_2 supplementation may be recommended

  f. Maintain adequate fluid intake of at least 2 liters per day

  g. Surgery may be recommended including tonsillectomy, adenoidectomy, and uvulopalatopharyngoplasty (removal of tissue contributing to obstruction from soft palate, uvula, and posterior pharyngeal wall)

  h. Oral or dental applications have been tried to reposition mandible with success in some clients

IV. PNEUMONIA

A. Overview

1. Pneumonia is defined as inflammation of bronchioles, alveoli, interstitial tissues, and on occasion pleura as a result of infection

2. Pneumonia may be described by cause, location, or contributing factors

  a. Cause: bacteria, viruses, fungi, protozoa, or parasites

    1) Common bacteria include *Streptococcus pneumonia* (most common), *Staphylococcus*, *Haemophilus influenzae*, and *Pseudomonas* (Gram-negative)

    2) Fungi include *Aspergillus fumigatus*, *Candida albicans*, and *Pneumocystis jiroveci* (formerly *carinii*)

  b. Location: lobular pneumonia involves 1 lobe, lobar pneumonia involves an entire lung, and bronchopneumonia involves lobes adjacent to bronchi

  c. Contributing factors: aspiration pneumonia often occurs with tube feedings; postoperative pneumonia occurs after a surgical procedure; and hospital-acquired pneumonia occurs after admittance to hospital

3. Atypical pneumonia is a type of pneumonia that does not present with usual symptoms or evolve in usual pattern; 2 examples are pneumocystosis, caused by *Pneumocystis jiroveci* in immunosuppressed clients or by *Legionella pneumophila*, known as Legionnaires' disease

  a. Pneumocystosis is a type of pneumococcal pneumonia caused by the parasite *Pneumocystis jiroveci*; most prominent in clients with AIDS or immunosuppressed or debilitated clients; symptoms include fever, cough, and dyspnea; has a high mortality rate and is difficult to diagnose; is treated with pentamidine isoethionate (Pentam 300)

  b. Legionnaires' disease is an acute bacterial pneumonia; symptoms are flu-like symptoms followed by fever, chills, headache, and muscle aches; usually self-limiting and not highly contagious; treated with erythromycin

4. Organisms may enter lung through accidental inhalation, close contact with an infected person, an outside means such as suctioning or intubation, or via blood; environmental reservoirs may be responsible for Legionnaires' disease

B. Pathophysiology

1. Although normal flora contains many bacteria, which are pathogens by nature, these organisms cause pneumonia when they invade lower respiratory tract

2. Organisms such as *Escherichia coli* or *Pseudomonas aeruginosa* are common in enteric flora but are not a part of upper respiratory tract; they can contaminate lungs via circulatory system

3. Inflammation within lung is similar to inflammatory process anywhere within body
   a. Introduction of bacteria promotes an antigen–antibody response and endotoxins are released
   b. Air spaces of alveoli become engorged with fluid and RBCs and exudate forms
   c. Infiltration of lymphocytes, neutrophils, RBCs, and fibrin leads to cellular infiltration and massive congestion
   d. Alveoli become airless because of exudate; perfusion accompanied by poor ventilation results
   e. Consolidation of lung tissue results and presents on CXR as white "patchy" infiltrate
   f. Damage may occur to bronchial and alveolar mucous membranes

4. Signs and symptoms of pneumonia include coughing, fatigue, pleuritic pain, dyspnea, chills, fever, elevated white blood cells (WBC), sputum production (rust-colored or purulent), lung crackles, pleural rub, and tachypnea; older adults may present with less dramatic symptoms and may experience changes in mental status or be easily agitated

C. Nursing assessment

1. Assessment
   a. Respiratory symptoms: cough (note productive or nonproductive; if productive, note color, amount, and odor; effectiveness of cough); pain with inspiration, deep breath, or cough
   b. General symptoms: fever and fatigue
   c. Inspect for dyspnea and tachycardia
   d. Auscultate lung sounds (crackles, rhonchi)

2. Diagnostic tests: CXR (consolidation in affected lobe), CBC (elevated WBC with a shift to left), and culture and sensitivity (C&S) of sputum, possible gram stain, ABGs (PaO_2 less than 75 mmHg), O_2 saturation (95% or lower), and blood cultures

D. Nursing management

1. Medications
   a. Antibiotic therapy as indicated by C&S within 4 hours of diagnosis or admission; may begin with a broad-spectrum antibiotic such as penicillin, erythromycin, or a cephalosporin until C&S results are available (see Chapter 13)
   b. Antipyretics
   c. Bronchodilators such as sympathomimetics or methylxanthines
   d. Drugs used to liquefy mucus, such as guaifenesin (Mucinex) or acetylcysteine (Mucomyst)

2. Increase fluid intake to 2,500–3,000 mL per day to help liquefy secretions unless contraindicated because of cardiac or renal condition

3. Administer O_2 therapy as prescribed with monitoring of O_2 saturation
   a. Nasal cannula for delivering 24–45% O_2 concentration
   b. Face mask for delivering 40–60% O_2 concentration
   c. Nonrebreather mask for delivering up to 100% O_2 concentration
   d. Venturi mask for precise measurement of air flow

4. Chest physiotherapy (CPT) including postural draining and percussion; lung sounds may worsen initially and cough may become more productive after CPT if congestion is consolidated and treatment is effective in loosening secretions

5. Endotracheal suctioning if necessary

6. Monitor respiratory rate, depth, and use of accessory muscles

Practice to Pass

A client with pneumonia continues to run a temperature of 102 to 103°F even after taking an antibiotic for 3 days. What could account for this and what should be done?

7. Instruct client how to splint chest wall with a pillow to cough more effectively
8. Monitor for intolerance to exercise or need for assistance with activities of daily living (ADLs)
9. Encourage client to turn, cough, and deep breathe
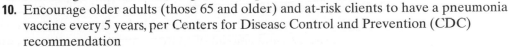
10. Encourage older adults (those 65 and older) and at-risk clients to have a pneumonia vaccine every 5 years, per Centers for Disease Control and Prevention (CDC) recommendation

V. PULMONARY TUBERCULOSIS (TB)

A. Overview

Practice to Pass

A female client visits the emergency department because of symptoms of gonorrhea. She admits that she practices prostitution and has never been tested for human immunodeficiency virus (HIV). Why would a tuberculosis (TB) skin test be an appropriate order as part of the diagnostic workup?

1. **Tuberculosis (TB)** is a type of pneumonia caused by *Mycobacterium tuberculosis*, an acid-fast bacillus
2. TB is becoming less well controlled; TB in immunosuppressed clients who do not receive health care has enhanced development of resistant strains
3. Primary defense mechanism against these bacilli is a cell-mediated immune response instead of an acute inflammatory reaction
4. Two types exist: *primary infection*, which develops in someone who has not been previously exposed and *secondary tuberculosis*, which means reactivation of dormant bacilli has occurred
5. Although organisms are contracted by airborne droplets from a person with an active form of disease, it can lie dormant for many years and be reactivated in lungs as well as invade other parts of body

B. Pathophysiology

1. Organisms carried by airborne droplets enter lungs and multiply in pulmonary alveoli
2. As organisms multiply, they enter lymphatic system and bloodstream, stimulating a cell-mediated response
3. Neutrophils and macrophages are immediately released to lungs to assist in attacking bacilli
4. Bacilli cannot be destroyed, but can be isolated; as macrophages attack organisms, a granuloma (or tubercle) is formed with inner areas of necrosis; lymphocytes and macrophages form a giant cell known as Langerhans
5. If arrested, these granulomas scar or calcify (called Gohn complex) and can be identified on a CXR; symptoms of disease may not be present if organisms are arrested early
6. If body's cell-mediated response fails, organisms within a calcified granuloma can be reactivated; if immune system is deficient or if number of organisms is extremely large, damage to lung tissue may occur
7. *M. tuberculosis* is a rod-shaped bacteria that has a waxy capsule; the waxy capsule requires Gram-staining in order to turn the organism red, and is therefore called an acid-fast bacillus
8. Major complications include poorer diffusion of O_2 and CO_2 leading to decreased gas exchange, decreased surface area available for gas diffusion, abnormal ventilation-perfusion ratio, hypoxia, and pulmonary hypertension
9. Other complications
   a. Tuberculosis pneumonia, a massive lobular or lobar pneumonia
   b. Pleuritis
   c. Extrapulmonary tuberculosis (often seen in clients with HIV)
      1) Swallowed bacilli may cause TB in small intestines of GI tract
      2) Miliary tuberculosis, spreading of tubercle into bloodstream (resemble millet seeds) and then to brain, meninges in cerebrospinal fluid (CSF), liver, kidneys, bone, and joints
   d. Sepsis and respiratory failure

10. Signs and symptoms of TB include coughing (usually dry in initial stage, productive in active stage), fever in afternoon or night (maybe low-grade), malaise, night sweats, anorexia, weight loss, chest pain, hemoptysis (later sign), dyspnea, crackles, and enlarged, often painful lymph nodes

C. Nursing assessment

1. Assessment includes: symptom analysis of type and progression of symptoms; color, consistency, and amount of sputum; knowledge of disease; weight pattern; VS; description of any pain; palpable lymph nodes; breath sounds; and activity tolerance

2. Diagnostic tests
   a. CXR shows dense lesions in upper lobes, enlarged lymph nodes, and formation of large cavities
   b. CBC shows presence of leukocytosis
   c. Fiberoptic bronchoscopy and bronchial washing is done to obtain culture specimens
   d. Tuberculin skin test should be measured and recorded in millimeters (mm) and not as positive or negative; CDC guidelines suggest these classifications to determine whether a reaction is negative or positive:
      1) Induration of greater than or equal to 5 mm is considered positive in people who are HIV positive, have recent contact with someone with TB, or have fibrotic changes in CXR consistent with prior TB; organ transplant recipients; immunosuppressed clients receiving corticosteroids (such as prednisone at dose higher than 10 mg per day)
      2) Induration of greater than or equal to 10 mm is considered positive in recent immigrants less than 5 years of age from countries with high prevalence of TB; drug users of injectable drugs; those living or working in high-risk settings such as prisons, jails, long-term care facilities, and homeless shelters; personnel working in mycobacteriology laboratories; clients with clinical conditions (such as diabetes, renal failure, hematologic disorders, malignancies) that make them high risk; children less than 4 years of age; infants through adolescents exposed to high-risk areas
      3) Induration of greater than or equal to 15 mm is considered positive in persons with no known risk factors for TB or exposure
      4) Negative results would be 0 mm or readings below levels identified in previous categories
   e. Clients who immigrated to United States may have had Bacille Calmette-Guérin (BCG) vaccine; if so, they will always have a positive skin test and need CXR evaluation
   f. Three early morning sputum collections for acid-fast staining, C&S positive for *M. tuberculosis;* results may take up to 10 days

D. Nursing management

1. Medications include *single dose* treatment for prevention or exposure and *at least 2* antibacterial medications for active case of disease or resistant strains
   a. Prevention of TB requires taking BCG vaccine once for TB or medication for 6–12 months for exposure and at least 9 months for clients with HIV; clients should be less than 40 years of age
   b. For resistant strains, 3 or more agents may be combined according to sensitivity report
   c. Medications may be prescribed prophylactically even though symptoms are not present if a positive TB result was obtained
   d. Recommended anti-infective agents: isoniazid (INH), rifampin (Rifadin), ethambutol (EMB), streptomycin (SM), pyrazinamide (PZA)
   e. Secondary agents: para-aminosalicylic acid (PAS), cycloserine (Seromycin), capreomycin (Capastat), ethionamide (Trecator-SC)

2. Hepatotoxicity is a common adverse effect for many drugs; monitor client closely

3. Teach client need for compliance with drug treatment; this is a common problem because of longer length of therapy
4. Inform clients of color changes in urine with some agents such as rifampin (Rifadin), which causes red-orange urine
5. Once a client has a positive purified protein derivative (PPD) result, it will remain positive and should not be repeated; a CXR may be prescribed to verify exposure versus active disease process
6. Monitor VS, noting a pattern of late afternoon low-grade fever
7. Assist client to turn, cough, and deep breathe and suction as needed for productive cough
8. Maintain adequate hydration and nutritional status; a high-protein, high-carbohydrate diet recommended
9. Monitor weight daily for loss
10. Place clients with active cases on airborne precautions: use private, negative-pressure room; use N-95 respiratory masks; keep door to room closed, etc.
11. Initiate screening for all family members or close contacts
12. Monitor breath sounds every 4 hours
13. Encourage frequent rest periods

VI. PLEURAL EFFUSION

A. Overview

1. **Pleural effusion** is defined as an excessive amount of fluid in pleural space between visceral and parietal layers of pleura (tends to accumulate at bases because of effects of gravity)
2. Usually considered a secondary rather than a primary disorder
3. Causes of pleural effusion are either systemic or local
   a. Systemic diseases
      1) Hydrothorax: heart failure, renal failure, liver failure
      2) Empyema (pus in pleural cavity): infections, malignancies, connective tissue disorders
   b. Local diseases
      1) Hemothorax (blood in pleural cavity): chest wall injuries, surgery to chest
      2) Chylothorax: trauma, inflammation (pneumonia, tuberculosis), or malignancy

B. Pathophysiology

1. A pleural effusion results from the following:
   a. An increase in hydrostatic pressure in pleural capillaries or decreased colloid osmotic pressure in blood vessels (known as transudative)
   b. An increased capillary permeability as a result of inflammation, infection, or malignancy (known as exudative)
2. Regardless of cause, excess pressure exerted by fluid in pleural space compresses lung and limits its ability to expand, thus compromising gas exchange
3. Amount of fluid in pleural space can become so large as to displace lung tissue and result in a compression atelectasis
4. Decreased lung volume on affected side results in diminished or absent breath sounds
5. Signs and symptoms include dyspnea, diminished or absent breath sounds on affected side, pain, limited chest wall movement, and dull or flat sounds on percussion

C. Nursing assessment

1. Assessment includes symptom analysis of any pain, dyspnea, coughing, VS (elevated temperature), respiratory rate and status (shallow respirations, asymmetry), lung sounds (diminished), and percussion for flat or dull sound over area
2. Diagnostic tests: CXR ("white out"—opaque densities of area involved); thoracentesis (aspiration of fluid from pleural space); C&S and cytological exam of any fluid removed; a CT scan and ultrasonography can determine pleural effusions if needed

D. Nursing management
1. Medications
   a. Antipyretics if fever or pain is present
   b. Antibiotics, parenterally or instillation into pleural space for repeated effusions
2. Goal of treatment should be to resolve underlying disease process and prevent complications such as atelectasis or pneumothorax
3. Assist with thoracentesis if procedure is done to remove fluid; surgical decortication may be done if recurrent
4. Monitor VS, especially respiratory rate, rhythm, and use of accessory muscles
5. Monitor lung sounds and reports of dyspnea
6. Manage pain if necessary along with bed rest

7. Monitor for signs of changing status: tachycardia, hypotension, increasing shortness of breath

VII. PLEURITIS (PLEURISY)

A. Overview
1. **Pleuritis** (pleurisy) is an inflammation of pleura, often accompanied by abrupt onset of pain
2. Classifications
   a. Primary or secondary; secondary type usually results from another respiratory illness such as pneumonia, pleural effusion, or trauma to lung
   b. Unilateral, bilateral, or local; unilateral is most typical
   c. Acute or chronic; acute is most common
   d. Fibrinous or adhesive: fibrinous is typically characterized by severe pain without any fluid return upon aspiration; adhesive occurs when parietal pleura adhere to visceral pleura (complete obliteration of pleural space can occur)
   e. May be dry or with effusion (pleural effusion); dry is more painful and usually accompanies pneumonia; adhesions may form

B. Pathophysiology
1. Inner visceral layer (adjacent to lung) and outer parietal layer (adjacent to chest wall) form a cavity (called pleural cavity) with a thin layer of serous fluid; pressure in pleural cavity is negative compared to alveolar pressure in order to keep lungs from collapsing
2. Infection such as pneumonia or viral respiratory disease can extend to pleura and cause inflammation in pleural cavity
3. Signs and symptoms of pleuritis
   a. Abrupt pain that is often unilateral and localized to a specific area of chest; pain is sharp, stabbing, and may radiate to neck or shoulder; pressure changes from breathing, movement, or coughing intensify pain
   b. Other symptoms may include fever, cough (dry, hacking), localized tenderness, diminished breath sounds, tachypnea, and pleural friction rub

C. Nursing assessment
1. Assessment includes symptom analysis of pain, VS, percussion, lung sounds, and visual inspection for symmetry of chest wall during respirations
2. Diagnostic tests: CXR (only to rule out other pulmonary disorders) and ABGs

D. Nursing management
1. Medications include analgesics or nonsteroidal anti-inflammatory drugs (NSAIDs) for pain and fever; antibiotics; cough suppressant such as codeine for nighttime cough (this should be avoided, however, if a productive cough is present)
2. Encourage bedrest
3. Monitor VS, noting fever and respiratory rate
4. Assess respiratory status, percussion, and auscultation of lung sounds
5. Encourage deep breathing and coughing every 1–2 hours and splinting of chest wall when coughing

VIII. PNEUMOTHORAX/HEMOTHORAX

A. Overview

1. **Pneumothorax** is entrance of air into pleural cavity, resulting in a complete or partial collapse of affected lung

   a. *Spontaneous pneumothorax* is a sudden collapse of a lung due to leakage of air into pleural cavity from within lung or from an unknown cause; may occur in tall, thin, healthy young men or secondary to smoking or other disease processes such as COPD, asthma, tuberculosis, emphysema, and CF; client may have family history of congenital blebs

   b. *Traumatic pneumothorax* is usually caused by a traumatic injury to chest wall causing blunt or penetrating trauma; usually results from stab or gunshot wound, rib fracture, motor vehicle crash, or a severe fall; may be open or termed a "sucking chest wound" and can be fatal due to severe hypoventilation that occurs from collapse of lung

   c. *Tension pneumothorax* is a dangerous complication and a medical emergency where entering air cannot escape by same route and pressure within pleural cavity increases, resulting in complete lung collapse; a mediastinal shift of trachea to unaffected side and a downward displacement of diaphragm can be observed

   d. *Iatrogenic pneumothorax* results from medical intervention, for example, placement of a catheter, biopsy procedures, cardiopulmonary resuscitation (CPR), mechanical ventilation, or anesthesia

2. **Hemothorax** is defined as presence of blood in pleural cavity

3. Symptoms, diagnosis, and treatment for all types of pneumothorax are similar; client symptoms will vary with severity, type, and size of pneumothorax

B. Pathophysiology

1. Pleural cavity surrounding lungs maintains an airtight seal and has less pressure than within lungs (known as "negative" pressure), enabling lungs to remain expanded; if negative pressure is lost due to any opening in pleural cavity, lung collapses because of natural contraction of elastic lung tissue; rupture of pleural cavity allows air to flow in and out of space, thus affecting expansion and recoil of lung (see Figure 1-4)

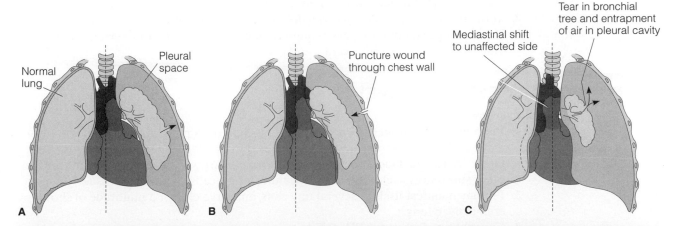

Figure 1-4

Pneumothorax. A. A spontaneous pneumothorax with an air leak from the lung into the pleural space, B. A traumatic or open pneumothorax (sucking chest wound) in which air enters the pleural space through a wound in the chest wall, C. A tension pneumothorax in which air enters the pleural space during inspiration but is unable to exit during expiration, resulting in rapid lung collapse and a shift of mediastinal structures toward the unaffected side.

    2. In a tension pneumothorax, an added complication hinders lungs even further

        a. Air enters the pleural space on inspiration as seen with a pneumothorax

        b. On expiration, rising pressure in the pleural space causes a tear or rupture and air is trapped

        c. Each consecutive breath forces more air into pleural cavity and lung collapses completely due to force of pressure being exerted

        d. Pressure is exerted on opposite lung and venous return to heart is affected; this condition can be fatal if not treated promptly (refer again to Figure 1-4)

    3. Signs and symptoms of a pneumothorax or hemothorax are severe shortness of breath, sharp, intense pain on affected side that may worsen on inspiration, tympanic resonance, absence of breath sounds on affected side, distention on one side of chest, tachypnea, distended neck veins due to pressure in thorax, subcutaneous emphysema (crepitus), hypoxemia, cyanosis, anxiety, and diaphoresis; a shift of mediastinum to unaffected side may be visibly seen in a tension pneumothorax

C. Nursing assessment

    1. Assessment includes description of pain and onset, visual inspection (asymmetry of lungs, shift of trachea, and use of accessory muscles), percussion over affected area, auscultation of lung sounds bilaterally, VS (tachycardia, hypotension, tachypnea), signs of hypoxemia (ABGs, decreased O_2 saturation, poorer color)

    2. Diagnostic tests: CXR (asymmetry of lung expansion, shift in diaphragm or mediastinum, air in pleural cavity), ABGs (decreased PaO_2, decreased pH, increased $PaCO_2$), pulse oximetry (O_2 saturation of 92% or lower), and CBC if hemothorax suspected; thoracentesis may be indicated to assess for and remove fluid in pleural cavity

D. Nursing management

    1. Medications include analgesics and antibiotics (if fluid is present and chest tube is inserted)

    2. Administer O_2 as indicated, monitoring pulse oximetry

    3. Assist with insertion and maintenance of chest tube, noting fluid drainage, color, consistency, and amount; monitor that water seal is maintained and that tubing is not obstructed; monitor insertion site for signs of infection

    4. Administer blood transfusion if indicated

    5. Assist with thoracentesis (insertion of a needle to withdraw air) as needed

    6. Monitor lung sounds and VS

    7. Maintain high-Fowler's position for ease in breathing

    8. Turn and ambulate client, allowing for frequent rest periods

    9. Recurrent pneumothorax may require thoracotomy to excise or oversew blebs; provide routine postoperative care

IX. PULMONARY EMBOLISM (PE)

A. Overview

    1. **Pulmonary embolism (PE)** is defined as blockage of a pulmonary artery (PA) by an embolus (often a blood clot that has traveled from a leg vein in DVT)

    2. Other sources include thromboembolism from heart wall in atrial fibrillation, or other substances such as air, amniotic fluid, tumor cells, or pieces of tissue

    3. PE may manifest itself as several tiny clots, one large clot, or a multitude of showered clots in lung

    4. Contributing factors for PE include venous stasis often associated with prolonged bedrest or surgery, hypercoagulability, obesity, childbirth, use of birth control pills, cardiac diseases, cardioversion in atrial fibrillation, and trauma

B. Pathophysiology

    1. A portion of a thrombus dislodges and travels (as an embolus) through venous circulation to right side of heart and enters PA, typically lodging there

2. A blocked PA causes decreased blood flow to lungs and can result in infarction to lung tissue
   a. Note that lung has 2 other sources of O_2 to compensate: air from bronchi and O_2 from blood flow from bronchial artery arising from descending aorta
   b. Death can occur if infarcted section of lung is large enough
3. Embolus may block entire main PA (*saddle embolus,* which is lethal) or may block smaller branches of pulmonary circulation, causing pulmonary infarcts (can be asymptomatic or cause pleuritic pain from irritation of pleura); the fibrinolytic mechanism in body often destroys smaller clots
4. PE leads to ventilation without perfusion, which decreases oxygenation of body tissues; with PE, alveolar dead space (alveoli not participating in gas exchange) is increased
5. As a result of PA blockage, right side of heart is unable to pump blood sufficiently and distends along with proximal portion of PA (area before the obstruction)
6. Decreased oxygenation of blood and reduced blood flow to left side of heart leads to decreased oxygenation of brain and other vital organs
7. Complications of PE include pulmonary edema, atelectasis, severe hypoxia, shock, and elevated pulmonary circulation pressures
8. Signs and symptoms include tachypnea, tachycardia, hypotension, sudden acute dyspnea with extreme anxiety, chest or pleuritic pain (sharp, localized), abnormal lung sounds (wheezing, decreased breath sounds or crackles), hypoxemia, respiratory alkalosis, friction rub, diaphoresis, and coughing; petechiae may develop with fat emboli; large clots may cause pulmonary hypertension, shock, right heart failure, or sudden respiratory arrest
9. Suspect PE whenever a client presents with *sudden onset* of pleuritic pain, SOB, and extreme anxiety while recovering from a lower extremity surgery, childbirth, major surgery, DVT, or on prolonged bed rest; anxiety is often described as a feeling of doom, impending death, and is associated with fear of suffocating

C. Nursing assessment

1. Assessment includes analysis of type of pain (increased with inspiration), anxiety level, color (cyanosis), LOC, respiratory status, VS, symptoms of thrombophlebitis (warmth, tenderness, swelling or lower leg or calf), and auscultation of lung sounds
2. Diagnostic tests
   a. CXR: wedge-shaped density (infarcted area), elevated diaphragms, atelectasis, or pleural effusions
   b. ABGs: decreased PaO_2, $PaCO_2$, and elevated pH—respiratory alkalosis
   c. Electrocardiogram (ECG): ST-T wave changes, right axis deviation; performed also to rule out MI
   d. Ventilation-perfusion lung scan or radioisotope lung scan: injection of radioisotope show no blood flow in peripherally blocked areas; does not actually diagnose an embolus
   e. Pulmonary angiography: allows direct visualization of PA and branches for a definite diagnosis
   f. Ultrasound of legs to locate source of emboli
   g. CT scan
   h. Lab work: decreased partial thromboplastin time (PTT) or prothrombin time (PT), elevated bilirubin, elevated lactic dehydrogenase (LDH), elevated fibrin degradation tests
   i. PTT is used to monitor heparin therapy once started and should be 1.5–2.5 times the control value for a therapeutic level; an international normalized ratio (INR) may be used to monitor oral anticoagulant therapy (value of 2–3 is therapeutic), follow protocol orders for these drugs; monitor client closely for signs of bleeding

D. Nursing management
1. Medications
   a. Anticoagulants: heparin followed by sodium warfarin (Coumadin) for confirmed PE
   b. Low molecular weight heparins (LMWH) such as enoxaparin (Lovenox), dalteparin (Fragmin), and tinzaparin (Innohep) for prevention of DVT and subsequent PE after surgery, particularly hip surgery
   c. Thrombolytic therapy if clot is excessively large or needs to be dissolved immediately
   d. Analgesics for discomfort or anxiety
   e. Vasopressors if needed for hypotension
2. Administer parenteral fluids as indicated
3. Avoid prolonged bed rest or sitting; limited ambulation may be allowed depending on clot location and size
4. Client should be reassured often to reduce anxiety
5. Administer O_2 as ordered
6. Apply antiembolism stockings, plexi-pulses or sequential compression devices; these aid in prevention as well as treatment
7. Prevention also includes early ambulation after surgery and leg exercises
8. Monitor ECG for cardiac dysrhythmias
9. Monitor PA wedge pressures and cardiac output
10. Monitor VS, respiratory assessment, LOC, skin color, and mental status
11. Auscultate heart and lung sounds
12. Monitor lab values and assess for bleeding if on anticoagulant therapy (hematuria, oozing from venipuncture sites or an intravenous [IV] lines, bleeding from gums or incisions, excessive bruising)
13. Daily PT or PTT values are not recommended during LMWH therapy

X. PULMONARY HYPERTENSION

A. Overview
1. **Pulmonary hypertension** is defined as elevated pressures in PA, usually resulting from pulmonary or cardiac disease
2. PA mean pressure is normally 12–15 mmHg (25 systolic/8 diastolic), a resting mean pressure greater than 20 mmHg constitutes an elevation
3. Usually classified as primary or secondary
   a. *Primary pulmonary hypertension* (PPH) is unrelated to any known cause, has a higher incidence in young women 20–30 years of age, is highly uncommon, and can lead to death in 3–5 years
   b. *Secondary pulmonary hypertension* is caused by a pulmonary or cardiac disease process such hypoxia, congenital cardiac disease, emboli, COPD, sleep apnea, mitral stenosis, left ventricular failure, and PE
   c. Cor pulmonale, right ventricular hypertrophy and failure result from long-term pulmonary hypertension

B. Pathophysiology
1. Narrowing of pulmonary vascular bed from major cardiac or pulmonary diseases is a common cause; blood vessel destruction, vasoconstriction, or obstruction may all contribute to narrowing of pulmonary vascular bed
2. The medial (muscular) layer of blood vessels thicken and extensive intimal fibrosis may occur in severe cases
3. The pulmonary vascular system usually has low pressure, high blood flow, and low resistance
4. Pulmonary hypertension can be caused by any condition that results in an exaggerated blood flow in pulmonary bed, a higher resistance to blood flow, or a blockage of blood flow

5. Complications include cor pulmonale or pulmonary edema due to inability of pressures in pulmonary artery to be lowered

6. Signs and symptoms may not be detected until a significant rise in PA pressure occurs and is reflected in a rise in systolic pressure

7. Clinical manifestations may include fatigue, angina, dyspnea (on exertion and at rest), tachypnea, abnormal breath sounds (distant, decreased, crackles), cyanosis, and dizziness especially upon exertion; in addition, there may be signs of an underlying condition that can mask symptoms of pulmonary hypertension

C. Nursing assessment

1. Assessment includes symptom analysis of any physical complaints, skin color, edema, VS, use of accessory respiratory muscles, breath sounds, and heart sounds

2. Diagnostic tests: CBC (may show polycythemia), ABGs (hypoxemia), CXR (enlarged right ventricle, dilated pulmonary arteries), ECG (right ventricular hypertrophy, right axis deviation, right bundle branch block), echocardiogram (enlarged right atrium, decreased wall motion), cardiac catheterization (elevated PA pressures, decreased cardiac output)

D. Nursing management

1. Medications
   a. Calcium channel blockers: nifedipine (Procardia) or diltiazem (Cardizem) to lower pulmonary vascular resistance
   b. Direct vasodilators: adenosine (Adenocard), inhaled nitric oxide, hydralazine (Apresoline) to decrease afterload
   c. Angiotensin converting enzyme (ACE) inhibitors
   d. Diuretics and digoxin if cor pulmonale occurs

2. Secondary pulmonary hypertension is aimed at treating underlying disease

3. Administer O_2 as ordered to assist in treating hypoxemia

4. Phlebotomy is recommended if polycythemia is present

5. Treatment of cor pulmonale includes fluid restriction, limited salt, and diuretics

6. Monitor activity if intolerance to physical exertion is severe, plan rest periods, and assist with ADLs

7. Monitor VS, lung sounds, and heart sounds

8. Assist client in high-Fowler's position if needed; encourage coughing and deep breathing

9. Teach client and family signs of cor pulmonale and pulmonary edema

XI. LUNG CANCER

A. Overview

1. Lung cancer is termed *bronchogenic carcinoma* because tumor usually stems from bronchial mucosa and is defined as cancer of epithelial lining of lung or lung parenchyma

2. Is a frequently occurring cancer of an internal organ, closely linked to cigarette smoking, and carries a poor prognosis

3. Classification of lung cancer
   a. Non–small-cell lung cancer (NSCLC): squamous cell carcinomas, large cell carcinomas, adenocarcinoma
   b. Small-cell lung cancer (SCLC): oat cell carcinoma
   c. Asbestos lung cancer: caused by exposure to asbestos
   d. Mesothelioma: cancer of lining of lung, also often caused by asbestos

B. Pathophysiology

1. Various chemicals and irritants (such as asbestos) act as carcinogens in lung, but those in tobacco smoke are a primary cause

2. Polycyclic hydrocarbons in cigarette smoke are mutagenic and can transform normal cells into malignant ones; the direct effect of carcinogens on cellular DNA may explain why some smokers get lung cancer and others do not

3. Combined action of several carcinogens in tobacco may account for the rapid neoplasia that can occur

4. Another theory is that bronchial epithelium undergoes metaplasia (a reversible state initially); in presence of carcinogenic stimuli, metaplasia progresses to carcinoma

5. Some lung cancer tumors are highly invasive and may extend into mediastinum or pleural cavity; because lungs are highly vascular, invasion into lymphatic system occurs early, contributing to metastasis; distant metastasis may occur in liver, brain, bones, kidneys, and adrenal glands

6. Complications include pneumonia, pleural effusions, Cushing's disease, hypercalcemia, anemia, disseminated intravascular coagulopathy (DIC), syndrome of inappropriate antidiuretic hormone (SIADH), and airway obstruction

7. Signs and symptoms may not occur until tumor is large enough to interfere with airway function; at that time cancer may be well advanced

8. Clinical manifestations include a persistent productive cough, hemoptysis, frequent lower respiratory tract infections, abnormal breath sounds (wheezing), angina, pleuritic pain (if pleura is involved), hoarseness and dysphagia (due to pressure from tumor)

9. In advanced stages with metastasis, weight loss, extreme dyspnea, fatigue, bone pain, and various endocrine, neurological, and cardiovascular symptoms are usually present

C. Nursing assessment

1. Assessment includes symptom analysis of any pain being experienced, changes in respiratory function or illnesses, lung sounds, sputum assessment (red or rust color), palpation of lymph nodes or enlarged liver, and analysis of weight loss

2. A persistent cough that changes in character is common with lung cancer

3. Diagnostic tests: CXR, magnetic resonance imaging (MRI), CT scan of lung, brain or bone, bronchoscopy, sputum cytology, and lab tests (CBC, liver function, electrolytes, and coagulation studies)

D. Nursing management

1. Medications
   a. Combination chemotherapy: alkylating agents such as mechlorethamine (Mustargen), antitumor antibiotics such as doxorubicin (Adriamycin) or other drugs such as cisplatin (Platinol)
   b. Bronchodilators
   c. Antibiotics if an infection is present
   d. Analgesics: nonopioids, NSAIDs, opioids

2. Radiation (use of high-energy radioactive particles) to decrease tumor size before surgery or for palliative treatment)

3. Surgical procedures may include lobectomy (removal of a lobe) or pneumonectomy (removal of entire lung); thoracotomy refers to incision of chest wall as an approach to a specific surgical procedure

4. Photodynamic therapy (PDT) is a type of laser therapy that involves injecting a special chemical into bloodstream that remains only in cancer cells; a laser light activates chemical and kills affected cancer cells; often used to treat small tumors or reduce symptoms

5. Administer oxygen therapy as ordered

6. Assess respiratory status and VS; auscultate lung and heart sounds

7. Manage pain (around the clock) and teach family how to treat pain, especially if client is being discharged; palliative care is essential especially in end-stage of disease

8. Assist client to turn, cough, and deep breathe; placing bed in a high-Fowler's position may be helpful

9. Provide CPT with percussion and postural drainage, suctioning as needed

10. Plan rest periods, especially immediately following an analgesic

11. Assist client and family with grieving process

XII. RESPIRATORY FAILURE

A. Overview

1. Respiratory failure is an inability of lungs to maintain adequate oxygenation and is usually manifested by hypoxemia, hypercapnia, and respiratory acidosis

2. ABGs reveal a PaO_2 less than 60 mmHg, $PaCO_2$ greater than 50 mmHg and pH less than 7.35; it is not a primary disease process, but is a secondary event that signals severe respiratory system dysfunction

3. In a client with COPD, a drop of 10–15 mmHg O_2 from *previous levels* indicates respiratory failure

4. Classification

   a. *Acute* (ARF): develops suddenly and can be life threatening; causes can be pulmonary diseases, cardiac diseases, or non-pulmonary disorders (infections, injuries); ARF can develop in individuals with normal lungs

   b. *Chronic* (CRF): develops slowly or more gradually and is usually a result of chronic bronchitis or emphysema

5. Can also be classified by whether there is impairment of ventilation or diffusion

   a. Impaired ventilation can be caused by airway obstruction (laryngospasm, foreign body aspiration, laryngeal or tracheal edema), respiratory diseases (asthma, COPD), neurologic disorders (spinal cord injury, stroke, neuromuscular diseases), or chest trauma (pneumothorax, flail chest)

   b. Impaired diffusion can be caused by disorders affecting alveoli (pneumonitis, pneumonia), pulmonary edema (near-drowning, ARDS, cardiac failure), or ventilation-perfusion mismatch (pulmonary embolus)

6. Types include Type I (hypoxemia only), Type II (hypoxemia with hypercapnia), or Type III (hypercapnia caused by hypoventilation)

B. Pathophysiology

1. Lungs are unable to remove CO_2 and there is inadequate O_2 inhalation; severe hypoventilation of lungs causes a rise in CO_2 and respiratory acidosis

2. In chronic respiratory disorders such as emphysema and COPD, breathing becomes more labored, respiratory muscles weaken, and airway resistance is increased

3. Client becomes exhausted and loses energy to breathe; ventilation, diffusion, or perfusion problems may result in respiratory failure (see Figure 1-5)

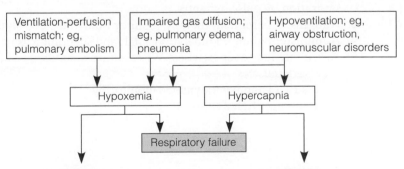

Figure 1-5

Causes of respiratory failure include ventilation, perfusion, or diffusion problems leading to hypoxemia and/or hypercapnia

4. Respiratory failure is a cycle that can end in death; as breathing difficulty increases, less O_2 is brought to alveoli, resulting in decreased production of surfactant and increased resistance to expansion

5. If client is hyperventilating, pCO_2 may be low; if client is hypoxic only, pH will be less than 7.35 and pCO_2 will be normal; if bicarbonate levels are low, metabolic acidosis can occur

6. Complications include ARDS, cardiac dysrhythmias, and cardiac failure

7. Signs and symptoms include those of underlying disease process along with hypoxemia, hypercapnia, dyspnea, neurological changes (restlessness, apprehension, impaired judgment and motor skills), cyanosis, diaphoresis, cool skin, and initial VS changes (tachycardia, hypertension, tachypnea)

8. As fatigue develops and hypoxemia worsens, cardiac output decreases, cardiac dysrhythmias may develop, and VS decrease (bradycardia, bradypnea, and hypotension)

C. Nursing assessment

1. Assessment includes: LOC, neurovascular assessment, skin color, VS, use of accessory respiratory muscles, breath sounds, and ECG pattern

2. Diagnostic tests: ABGs (mild hypoxia with PaO_2 of less than 80 mmHg, moderate hypoxia with PaO_2 of less than 60 mmHg, or severe hypoxia with PaO_2 less than 40 mmHg), CXR (shows underlying disease process), ECG (dysrhythmias), hemodynamic monitoring, sputum for C&S

D. Nursing management

1. Medications
   a. Bronchodilators: methylxanthines or inhaled sympathomimetics or anticholinergics
   b. Corticosteroids
   c. Antibiotics if an infection exists
   d. Analgesia as indicated while on mechanical ventilation
   e. Benzodiazepines: diazepam (Valium), lorazepam (Ativan), or midazolam (Versed) to decrease respiratory drive or achieve sedation
   f. Neuromuscular blocking agents: pancuronium bromide (Pavulon) or vecuronium (Norcuron) to suppress respiratory effort while on ventilator

2. Administer O_2 therapy as ordered (usually low levels) or maintain mechanical ventilation with PEEP; high O_2 levels may cause hypoventilation; monitor O_2 saturation by pulse oximetry

3. Administer parenteral therapy, monitor fluid and electrolyte status

4. Administer nebulized inhalation, CPT, and suctioning as needed

5. Auscultate lung sounds; assess VS, respiratory status, nasal flaring, and use of accessory muscles

6. Assess ECG and hemodynamic monitoring

7. Maintain nutritional support

Case Study

A 10-year-old child has just been diagnosed with asthma related to allergies. The clinic nurse is responsible for discharging the child on montelukast (Singulair) 1 tablet every day, albuterol (Ventolin) inhaler as needed for an asthma attack, nedocromil (Tilade) inhaler once a day, and albuterol (Ventolin) drops with saline for use with a nebulizer in the event the rescue inhaler does not work.

1. What discharge instructions should the nurse give the mother about the child's medications?

2. What explanation should the nurse give the mother about asthma?

3. What instructions should the nurse give the mother about when to seek immediate medical attention?

4. What should the child know about an asthma attack?

5. What are triggers and how do they affect asthma?

For suggested responses, see page 461.

POSTTEST

1 A client, who was not wearing a seat belt, was involved in a motor vehicle crash (MVC). The client now exhibits crepitus and decreased breath sounds on the left, reports shortness of breath, and has a respiratory rate of 34/min. Which assessment findings are of most concern to the nurse?

1. Temperature of 102°F and a productive cough
2. Arterial blood gases (ABGs) with a PaO_2 of 92 and $PaCO_2$ of 40 mmHg
3. Trachea deviating to the right
4. Barrel-chested appearance

2 A nurse is teaching a client newly diagnosed with emphysema about the disease process. Which statement that best explains the problems associated with emphysema could the nurse adapt for use in client education?

1. "Hyperactivity of the medium-sized bronchi caused by an inflammatory response leads to wheezing and tightness in the chest."
2. "Larger than normal air spaces and loss of elastic recoil cause air to be trapped in the lung and collapse airways."
3. "Vasodilation, congestion, and mucosal edema cause a chronic cough and sputum production."
4. "Chloride is not being transported properly, producing excess absorption of water and sodium and thick, viscous mucus."

3 A sweat test is ordered for a child with respiratory symptoms suggestive of cystic fibrosis (CF). The nurse concludes that which chloride result is consistent with this diagnosis?

1. 45 mEq/L
2. 25 mEq/L
3. 35 mEq/L
4. 65 mEq/L

4 A client who underwent a hysterectomy experiences shortness of breath when walking. She has never had shortness of breath before. Upon auscultation, no breath sounds are heard in the left lower lobe. All other findings and breath sounds are normal. Which etiology should the nurse consider as a contributing factor?

1. Pleurisy
2. Pneumonia
3. Atelectasis
4. Pulmonary embolism

5 A client admitted to the hospital with classic symptoms of tuberculosis (TB) tests positive on a purified protein derivative (PPD) skin test. Several months later, the nurse who cared for the client also tests positive on an annual TB skin test. What would be the most likely course of treatment if the nurse's chest x-ray (CXR) is negative?

1. Repeat a tuberculosis (TB) skin test in 6 months.
2. Treat the nurse with an anti-infective agent for 6 months.
3. Monitor for signs and symptoms within the next year.
4. Follow up every six months with a repeat chest x-ray (CXR).

6 The nurse instructs a client with severe sleep apnea to plan frequent rest periods and activities around how well the client feels. When asked by the client how this is will help, the nurse further explains that energy conservation techniques may minimize which of the following?

Select all that apply.
1. Cardiac dysrhythmias
2. Daytime fatigue and sleepiness
3. Jaw pain
4. Memory loss
5. Personality changes and depression

7 A client who smokes cigarettes and has a known history of cardiac problems enters the clinic reporting the sudden onset of sharp, stabbing pain that intensifies with a deep breath. The pain occurs on only one side and can be isolated upon general assessment. The nurse concludes that the client's pain is consistent with which of the following?

1. Pleurisy
2. Pleural effusion
3. Atelectasis
4. Tuberculosis

8 The nurse is delivering postmortem care to a client who died from a large pulmonary embolus (PE). While reflecting on the client's death, the nurse considers that it was most likely caused by which of the following?

1. Decreased blood flow
2. Decreased alveolar dead space
3. Inefficiency of the heart to pump adequately
4. Infarction of the lung tissue

9 An older adult client recuperating from major abdominal surgery will be in bed for much of the immediate postoperative period. The nurse anticipates that the client will most likely be placed on which medication to prevent a pulmonary embolism (PE)?

1. Tissue plasminogen activator (t-PA)
2. Warfarin (Coumadin)
3. Enoxaparin (Lovenox)
4. Heparin

10 A 50-year-old client with chronic obstructive pulmonary disease (COPD) who smokes 2 packs of cigarettes per day is admitted to the intensive care unit for acute exacerbation of COPD. Which client data should alert the nurse that pulmonary hypertension may have developed? Select all that apply.

1. Pulmonary artery mean pressure of 30 mmHg
2. Fatigue and syncope with exertion
3. Thick, viscous mucus
4. Absent breath sounds
5. Progressive dyspnea

➤ *See pages 30–32 for Answers and Rationales.*

ANSWERS & RATIONALES

Pretest

1 **Answer: 1** **Rationale:** Clients with COPD tend to have low oxygen (O_2) and high carbon dioxide (CO_2) levels. They cannot tolerate high levels of O_2 because hypoxia becomes the main stimulus for ventilation in persons with chronic hypercapnia. Increasing the level of oxygen would decrease the stimulus to breathe. It is unlikely that the CO_2 levels will ever be low. High O_2 levels do not directly cause acidemia; rather, acidemia tends to result from retained CO_2 and possibly from metabolic alterations caused by hypoxia. **Cognitive Level:** Applying **Client Need:** Basic Care and Comfort **Integrated Process:** Teaching and Learning **Content Area:** Adult Health **Strategy:** Note the critical word *chronic* in the stem of the question. Consider the stimulus for ventilation in clients with COPD and use the process of elimination to select the option that reflects the pathophysiology of COPD. **Reference:** Huether, S. E., & McCance, K. L. (2012). *Understanding pathophysiology* (5th ed.). St. Louis, MO: Mosby, Inc., p. 689.

2 **Answer: 4** **Rationale:** A combined low PO_2 and low SaO_2 represent hypoxia. The pH, PCO_2, and HCO_3 are normal. ABGs will not necessarily be altered in TB or pleural effusion. Initially, in pneumonia, both the PO_2 and PCO_2 are usually low because the hypoxia caused by the infection leads to hyperventilation. **Cognitive Level:** Analyzing **Client Need:** Reduction of Risk Potential **Integrated Process:** Nursing Process: Diagnosis **Content Area:** Adult Health **Strategy:** First view the pH, noting that the pH is on the acidotic end of normal. Note the critical word *best* in the question, indicating that more than one option may be plausible but one is better than the others. Choose the option that fits the client's clinical picture regardless of the exact underlying etiology. **Reference:** Huether, S. E., & McCance, K. L. (2012). *Understanding pathophysiology* (5th ed.). St. Louis, MO: Mosby, Inc., p. 680.

3 **Answer: 2, 3, 4** **Rationale:** An individual with pulmonary emboli usually presents with the sudden onset of pleuritic chest pain, dyspnea, tachypnea, tachycardia, and unexplained anxiety. Warm, dry skin is a normal finding and bradycardia is an opposite finding. **Cognitive Level:** Applying **Client Need:** Physiological Adaptation **Integrated Process:** Nursing Process: Assessment **Content Area:** Adult Health **Strategy:** Note the critical words *impaired oxygen perfusion with pulmonary emboli* in the stem of the question. Recall symptoms of pulmonary emboli, which will enable you to select options that indicate a late compensatory response. **Reference:** Huether, S. E., & McCance, K. L. (2012). *Understanding pathophysiology* (5th ed.). St. Louis, MO: Mosby, Inc., p. 698.

4 **Answer: 2** **Rationale:** Shortness of breath, increased respiratory rate, and slightly labored respirations could be caused by any of the conditions listed. The distinguishing symptom is the lack of breath sounds in the right lung base when a portion of the lung has collapsed. Atelectasis causes diminished or absent breath sounds since the lung is not expanding with inspiration when a portion of the lower lung has collapsed. Atelectasis tends to develop after surgery and is estimated to occur in more than 90% of individuals administered a general anesthesia. Pulmonary embolus, cardiac tamponade, and cor pulmonale are not distinguished by absent breath sounds. **Cognitive Level:** Analyzing **Client Need:** Physiological Adaptation **Integrated Process:** Nursing Process: Diagnosis **Content Area:** Adult Health **Strategy:** Consider the physiological response to and possible etiologies of impaired gas exchange in the lungs. Also note that the client is one day postoperative. Recall the risks of surgery and associated respiratory manifestations to choose correctly. **Reference:** Huether, S. E., & McCance, K. L. (2012). *Understanding pathophysiology* (5th ed.). St. Louis, MO: Mosby, Inc., p. 685, 700.

5 **Answer: 1, 4, 5** **Rationale:** The respiratory treatment should loosen congestion and cause bronchodilation, thus improving lung sounds and producing a more productive cough. When pneumonia resolves, the lungs should begin to clear and the cough should diminish. The expected effects of treatment are decreased airway resistance and decreased viscosity of mucoprotein strands, helping to liquefy mucus, producing more sputum and less congestion. Wheezing should lessen with bronchodilation. Symptoms of poor gas exchange, such as anxiety and confusion, should improve. The cough will remain productive in the acute stage. Absent breath sounds would suggest a worsening of the condition. **Cognitive Level:** Analyzing **Client Need:** Physiological Adaptation **Integrated Process:** Nursing Process: Evaluation **Content Area:** Adult Health **Strategy:** Notice that the question asks about an *acute case*; be careful to note the situation in the stem. Watch for opposites in the answer options. **Reference:** LeMone, P., Burke, K., & Bauldoff, G. (2012). *Medical-surgical nursing: Critical thinking in patient care* (5th ed.). Upper Saddle River, NJ: Pearson Education, pp. 1180–1182.

6 **Answer: 3** **Rationale:** A shift on the trachea to the left with no breath sounds on the right are consistent with a tension pneumothorax, which is considered a medical emergency. The lung on the affected side collapses, and pressure shifts mediastinal structures to the unaffected side of the chest, compromising venous return to the heart and placing pressure on the opposite lung as well. Sharp pain outlines symptoms of pleurisy, which is not an emergency situation. A client exhibiting yellow productive sputum, low-grade fever, and crackles presents symptoms of bronchitis, not an emergency. A client with asthma should expect difficulty breathing after exercise; this client may need immediate attention if the rescue inhaler is ineffective. **Cognitive Level:** Analyzing **Client Need:** Management of Care **Integrated Process:** Nursing Process: Planning **Content Area:** Adult Health **Strategy:** The critical word in the stem of the question is *immediate*. Use nursing knowledge and the process of elimination to select tension pneumothorax as the emergency situation. **Reference:** LeMone, P., Burke, K., & Bauldoff, G. (2012). *Medical-surgical nursing: Critical thinking in patient care* (5th ed.). Upper Saddle River, NJ: Pearson Education, pp. 1207–1209.

7 **Answer: 1, 2, 4** **Rationale:** A young person needs to know the triggers of asthma. Physical exercise in school and life will be ever-present, and prevention of an attack before exercise is essential at this time in the client's life. Living a productive, normal life should be stressed. Sports do not have to be limited in all asthmatic people. The client may have to use preventive medications before a sport of choice. The fear associated with asthma is common and may take a while to overcome. Instructions on identifying triggers and use of rescue inhalers need to be taught and the fear will eventually subside. Encourage all patients to not start smoking, and if they do smoke, to quit. **Cognitive Level:** Applying **Client Need:** Physiological Adaptation **Integrated Process:** Teaching and Learning **Content Area:** Adult Health **Strategy:** Consider the developmental stage of the client and the clue words *newly diagnosed*. With these in mind, use nursing knowledge and the process of elimination to make a selection **Reference:** LeMone, P., Burke, K., & Bauldoff, G. (2012). *Medical-surgical nursing: Critical thinking in patient care* (5th ed.). Upper Saddle River, NJ: Pearson Education, p. 1237.

8 **Answer: 4** **Rationale:** Clients who have sleep apnea do not get adequate amounts of REM sleep and are often awakened frequently during the night in order to make breathing possible. Sleep apnea is related to decreased muscle tone of upper airways. Upper airflow obstruction occurs, the CO_2 rises, and cardiac dysrhythmias and angina can occur because of the lack of oxygenated blood supply to the heart. **Cognitive Level:** Analyzing **Client Need:** Physiological Adaptation **Integrated Process:** Teaching and Learning **Content Area:** Adult Health **Strategy:** Recall that progressive asphyxia causes many brief arousals during sleep with resulting physiological effects. Note also that the angina is being experienced only at night. Use this information and knowledge of pathophysiology of sleep apnea to make a selection. **Reference:** LeMone, P., Burke, K., & Bauldoff, G. (2012). *Medical-surgical nursing: Critical thinking in patient care* (5th ed.). Upper Saddle River, NJ: Pearson Education, pp. 1162–1163.

9 **Answer: 2, 4, 5** **Rationale:** Common signs of cancer of the lung include a persistent cough that changes, chronic dyspnea, bloody sputum, and long-term pulmonary infection. Exertional dyspnea is common with chronic obstructive pulmonary disease (COPD). Air hunger that is associated with dyspnea commonly occurs with asthma. **Cognitive Level:** Applying **Client Need:** Physiological Adaptation **Integrated Process:** Nursing Process: Assessment **Content Area:** Adult Health **Strategy:** Consider that manifestations are related to the location of the lesion and its possible metastasis. Then eliminate the findings commonly seen with other conditions. **Reference:** LeMone, P., Burke, K., & Bauldoff, G. (2012). *Medical-surgical nursing: Critical thinking in patient care* (5th ed.). Upper Saddle River, NJ: Pearson Education, pp. 1218–1220.

10 **Answer: 2, 3, 4** **Rationale:** Chest tubes are inserted and attached to a closed drainage system to allow lung reexpansion while preventing air from entering the pleural space. Periodic bubbles are normal and indicate that the air is being removed from the chest. Fluctuation of the water level in the tube with respiration indicates the system is intact. Fluctuations and bubbles will cease when the lung is expanded. Continuous bubbles may indicate an air leak in the system that could result in collapse of the lung. Drainage in excess of 70 mL per hour may indicate hemorrhage or infection, depending on the drainage characteristics. A system that is full needs to be replaced. **Cognitive Level:** Applying **Client Need:** Physiological Adaptation **Integrated Process:** Nursing Process: Evaluation **Content Area:** Adult Health **Strategy:** Consider principles in working with a closed drainage system. Read carefully for clarifying terms in the options. **Reference:** LeMone, P., Burke, K., & Bauldoff, G. (2012). *Medical-surgical nursing: Critical thinking in patient care* (5th ed.). Upper Saddle River, NJ: Pearson Education, pp. 1218–1220.

Posttest

1 **Answer: 3** **Rationale:** Since the client was involved in a motor vehicle crash (MVC), assessment would be targeted at acute traumatic injuries to the lungs, heart, or chest wall, such as tracheal deviation from tension pneumothorax. An elevated temperature and productive cough are common with pneumonia, ABG values with PaO_2 of 92 and $PaCO_2$ of 40 mmHg are not alarming, and a barrel-chested appearance is typical of someone with chronic obstructive pulmonary disease (COPD). **Cognitive Level:** Analyzing **Client Need:** Physiological Adaptation **Integrated Process:** Nursing Process: Assessment **Content Area:** Adult Health **Strategy:** Look for the most life threatening condition. Read all the options before making a selection. **Reference:** LeMone, P., Burke, K., & Bauldoff, G. (2012). *Medical-surgical nursing: Critical thinking in patient care* (5th ed.). Upper Saddle River, NJ: Pearson Education, Inc., pp. 1207–1209.

2 **Answer: 2** **Rationale:** Emphysema is characterized by destruction of the walls of the alveoli, with resulting enlargement of abnormal air spaces; thus, these conditions best describe the pathophysiology behind emphysema. Asthma is characterized by hyperactivity of the medium-sized bronchi leading to wheezing and tightness in the chest. Bronchitis is characterized by vasodilation, congestion, and mucosal edema, which cause a chronic cough and sputum production. Cystic fibrosis is characterized by chloride not being transported properly, producing excess absorption of water and sodium. **Cognitive Level:** Applying **Client Need:** Physiological Adaptation **Integrated Process:** Communication and Documentation **Content Area:** Adult Health **Strategy:** Choose the option that describes the pathophysiology of emphysema. Recall that even a true statement is not the correct option unless it answers the question asked. **Reference:** LeMone, P., Burke, K., & Bauldoff, G. (2012). *Medical-surgical nursing: Critical thinking in patient care* (5th ed.). Upper Saddle River, NJ: Pearson Education, Inc., p. 1239.

3 **Answer: 4** **Rationale:** Cystic fibrosis is diagnosed by a high chloride level on the sweat test. The normal chloride level on this test is less than 50 mEq/L in a child. The only correct answer is the one with a chloride level above 50 mEq/L. **Cognitive Level:** Applying **Client Need:** Reduction of Risk Potential **Integrated Process:** Nursing Process: Diagnosis **Content Area:** Child Health **Strategy:** Recall that parents of children with cystic fibrosis often report that the child tastes "salty" when kissed. Use this to reason that the chloride level (part of salt) would be high, and choose a high value from the options available. **Reference:** Kee, J. L. (2010). *Laboratory and diagnostic tests with nursing implications* (7th ed.). Upper Saddle River, NJ: Pearson/Prentice Hall, p. 125.

4 **Answer: 3** **Rationale:** Resorption atelectasis can occur after surgery resulting from removal of air from obstructed or hypoventilated alveoli or from inhalation of concentrated oxygen or anesthetic agents. This is a common complication and is manifested by decreased or absent breath sounds in the affected lobe. Pleurisy would also be accompanied by pain upon inspiration. Pneumonia is common after surgery but would have additional symptoms. Pulmonary embolism would also accompanied by chest pain, acute dyspnea, and severe air hunger with anxiety. **Cognitive Level:** Analyzing **Client Need:** Reduction of Risk Potential **Integrated Process:** Nursing Process: Assessment **Content Area:** Adult Health **Strategy:** Which option stands out from the others and fits the findings described in the stem? **Reference:** Huether, S. E., & McCance, K. L. (2012). *Understanding pathophysiology* (5th ed.). St. Louis, MO: Elsevier Inc., p. 685.

5 **Answer: 2** **Rationale:** Exposure with a positive tuberculosis (TB) skin test usually requires 6 months of prophylactic treatment unless contraindicated. The TB skin test should not be repeated; the results will always be positive. Monitoring will not prevent TB, and the nurse has been exposed. Appropriate therapy is needed to control the spread of TB. A chest x-ray (CXR) is usually not required annually in the event that the skin test was positive; however, many health care employers require a CXR every 3–5 years for employees to verify that the disease has not reactivated. **Cognitive Level:** Applying **Client Need:** Physiological Adaptation **Integrated Process:** Nursing Process: Implementation **Content Area:** Adult Health **Strategy:** A positive purified protein derivative (PPD) is a cell-mediated immune response that indicates that the person has mounted an immune response. It does not mean that the disease is active. **Reference:** LeMone, P., Burke, K., & Bauldoff, G. (2012). *Medical-surgical nursing: Critical thinking in patient care* (5th ed.). Upper Saddle River, NJ: Pearson Education, pp. 1191–1194.

6 **Answer: 1, 2, 4, 5** **Rationale:** Recurrent nocturnal asphyxia due to airway obstruction increases the workload of the heart and may cause cardiac symptoms such as bradycardia or tachycardia. Clients with coronary heart disease may develop ischemia or angina. The deprivation of oxygen during the night and lack of REM sleep often leaves individuals with fatigue or sleepiness during the day. Jaw pain may be a symptom of myocardial infarction or temporomandibular joint disease (TMJ). Neither of these is directly related to sleep apnea. Recurrent apnea and loss of slow-wave sleep contribute to neurological and behavioral symptoms, such as memory loss, personality changes and depression. **Cognitive Level:** Applying **Client Need:** Physiological Adaptation **Integrated Process:** Teaching and Learning **Content Area:** Adult Health **Strategy:** Which option fits a daytime symptom for a nighttime problem? What ongoing physiologic effects can recurrent apnea and arousal during sleep cause? **Reference:** LeMone, P., Burke, K., & Bauldoff, G. (2012). *Medical-surgical nursing: Critical thinking in patient care* (5th ed.). Upper Saddle River, NJ: Pearson Education, pp. 1162–1163.

7 **Answer: 1** **Rationale:** Pleuritic pain is typically sharp and stabbing, and typically abrupt. Pleurisy is common in smokers. Pleural effusion can cause pain but usually has other symptoms such as dyspnea and diminished or absent breath sounds. Atelectasis can cause pain but it usually has other symptoms such as dyspnea and diminished or absent breath sounds. Tuberculosis causes chest pain and may cause pleuritis along with other symptoms; however, this is not the first problem suspected when a client presents with the pain described. **Cognitive Level:** Analyzing **Client Need:** Physiological Adaptation **Integrated Process:** Nursing Process: Diagnosis **Content Area:** Adult Health **Strategy:** Rule out the options that are not manifested by the type of pain described in the stem. **Reference:** LeMone, P., Burke, K., & Bauldoff, G. (2012). Medical-surgical nursing: Critical thinking in patient care (5th ed.). Upper Saddle River, NJ: Pearson Education, p. 1205.

ANSWERS & RATIONALES

8 **Answer: 4** **Rationale:** If the blockage is large enough and blood flow is hindered to the lung, the tissue will die. This usually occurs when a large clot blocks the entire main pulmonary artery. Decreased blood flow is rather vague statement because blood flow is decreased to the heart, lung, brain, and other vital organs due to the blockage but the amount of decrease can be variable. Dead space is increased with pulmonary embolism (PE). Inefficiency of the heart to pump adequately is correct in pulmonary embolism but is not usually the cause of death. **Cognitive Level:** Applying **Client Need:** Physiological Adaptation **Integrated Process:** Nursing Process: Diagnosis **Content Area:** Adult Health **Strategy:** Eliminate the options known to be wrong. Select the best answer from the remaining choices. Read all the options before choosing the answer. **Reference:** LeMone, P., Burke, K., & Bauldoff, G. (2012). *Medical-surgical nursing: Critical thinking in patient care* (5th ed.). Upper Saddle River, NJ: Pearson Education, pp. 1255–1257.

9 **Answer: 3** **Rationale:** Without any evidence of a blood clot or pulmonary embolism (PE), a low molecular weight heparin (LMWH) such as enoxaparin is usually used for prevention purposes, especially since the client is elderly and will be in bed for a period of time. Heparin and warfarin (anticoagulants) are used when a confirmed clot exists. Thrombolytics such as tissue plasminogen activator (t-PA) are used when a clot needs to be immediately dissolved. **Cognitive Level:** Applying **Client Need:** Pharmacological and Parenteral Therapies **Integrated Process:** Nursing Process: Implementation **Content Area:** Adult Health **Strategy:** Consider the etiology of pulmonary embolism (PE). Which drugs are therapeutic and which are prophylactic? This situation asks for prevention. **Reference:** LeMone, P., Burke, K., & Bauldoff, G. (2012). *Medical-surgical nursing: Critical thinking in patient care* (5th ed.). Upper Saddle River, NJ: Pearson Education, pp. 1257–1258.

10 **Answer: 1, 2, 5** **Rationale:** A sustained elevation in the resting mean pressure above 20 mmHg from a pulmonary artery is defined as pulmonary hypertension, which could be caused by chronic obstructive pulmonary disease (COPD). Manifestations of pulmonary hypertension are progressive dyspnea, fatigue, angina, and syncope upon exertion. Thick, viscous mucus is not a manifestation of pulmonary hypertension. Absent breath sounds can occur in various pulmonary disorders, such as pneumonia and pneumothorax, but not in pulmonary hypertension. **Cognitive Level:** Analyzing **Client Need:** Physiological Adaptation **Integrated Process:** Nursing Process: Assessment **Content Area:** Adult Health **Strategy:** Consider the known history of chronic obstructive pulmonary disease (COPD) for a pathophysiologic hint. Note that the critical word *hypertension* in the stem may link to a related word in the correct option (pressure). **Reference:** LeMone, P., Burke, K., & Bauldoff, G. (2012). *Medical-surgical nursing: Critical thinking in patient care* (5th ed.). Upper Saddle River, NJ: Pearson Education, pp. 1260–1261.

References

Advair Diskus (2011). GlaxoSmith-Kline. *Important safety information about Advair Diskus.* Retrieved from http://www.advair.com/

Centers for Disease Control and Prevention (2011). *Tuberculin Skin Testing.* Retrieved from http://www.cdc.gov/tb/publications/factsheets/testing/skintesting.htm.

Kee, J. L. (2010). *Laboratory and diagnostic test with nursing implications* (8th ed.). Upper Saddle River, NJ: Pearson Education.

Kee, J., Hayes, E., & McCuistion, L. (2012), *Pharmacology: A nursing process approach* (7th ed.). St. Louis, MO: Elsevier, pp. 587–614.

LeMone, P., Burke, K., and Bauldoff, G. (2011). *Medical-surgical nursing: Critical thinking in patient care* (5th ed.). Upper Saddle River, NJ: Pearson Education, pp. 1123–1283.

McCance, K., & Huether, S. (2010). *Pathophysiology: The biologic basis for disease in adults and children* (6th ed.). St. Louis, MO: Elsevier.

Mesothelioma Treatment Options. Retrieved from http://www.mesothelioma-lung-cancer.org/mesothelioma-treatments.html.

Porth, C. (2011). *Essentials of pathophysiology* (3rd ed.). Philadelphia: Lippincott Williams & Wilkins pp. 513–599.

Spiriva Handihaler, (2011). Boehringer Ingelheim Pharmaceuticals, *How to use SPIRIVA handihaler.* Retrieved from http://www.spiriva.com/about-spiriva/using-spiriva.html.

Venes, D., Thomas, C. L., & Taber, C. (2009). *Taber's cyclopedic medical dictionary* (21st ed.). Philadelphia: F. A. Davis.

Wilson, B., Shannon, M., & Shields, K. (2012). *Nurse's drug guide 2012.* Upper Saddle River, NJ: Pearson Education.

ANSWERS & RATIONALES

Cardiac Health Problems

2

Chapter Outline

Risk Factors Associated with Cardiac Health Problems
Coronary Heart Disease (CHD)
Angina Pectoris

Myocardial Infarction (MI)
Congestive Heart Failure (CHF)
Cardiac Dysrhythmias

Inflammatory Diseases of Heart
Valvular Heart Disease

Objectives

➤ Define key terms associated with cardiac health problems.
➤ Identify risk factors associated with the development of cardiac health problems.
➤ Explain the common etiologies of cardiac health problems.
➤ Describe the pathophysiologic processes associated with specific cardiac health problems.
➤ Distinguish between normal and abnormal cardiac findings obtained from nursing assessment.
➤ Prioritize nursing interventions associated with specific cardiac health problems.

NCLEX-RN® Test Prep

Use the accompanying online resource, NursingReviewsandRationales, to test yourself with hundreds of NCLEX®-style practice questions.

Review at a Glance

afterload pressure against which heart must pump

angina pectoris chest pain associated with anaerobic metabolism from decreased oxygen supply to myocardium

automaticity ability of a cardiac muscle cell to contract independently, without stimulation

cardiac output amount of blood pumped out of left ventricle each minute; determined by HR × stroke volume

collateral circulation additional outgrowth of tiny vessels that supply heart muscle with oxygenated blood

congestive heart failure (CHF) inability of heart to pump sufficient blood to maintain adequate oxygen and nutrients to tissues

coronary heart disease (CHD) atherosclerotic plaque deposits lining walls of coronary arteries and narrowing these vessels, causing decreased oxygen supply to myocardium

electrocardiogram (ECG or EKG) graphic representation of electrical activity of heart

intermittent claudication cramping in lower extremities, especially when walking or with exercise

ischemia insufficient blood flow leading to decreased oxygen supply to tissues causing anaerobic cellular metabolism rather than aerobic metabolism

mitral valve prolapse mitral valve opens backward toward atrium causing regurgitation of blood from ventricle to atrium

myocardial infarction (MI) death of tissue of myocardium caused by lack of oxygen supply

myocarditis an inflammatory disorder of heart muscle that is unrelated to coronary artery disease or myocardial infarction

pericarditis inflammation of pericardium and/or pericardial sac surrounding heart

preload volume of blood returning to heart, creating "stretch" or tension of myocardial fibers at end diastole

reentry phenomenon blockage of an impulse through a bundle branch, causing impulse to retrograde backwards, reenter other side and cause a premature contraction

regurgitation a condition in which blood flows backward through a valve that should be closed but cannot close completely because of damage or disease

stenosis a condition in which valves of heart become hardened and blood does not flow through them adequately

stroke volume amount of blood ejected from left ventricle with each heartbeat

ventricular fibrillation chaotic, irregular quivering of ventricles; a lethal dysrhythmia requiring immediate defibrillation

PRETEST

1 The client experiences chest pain after mowing the lawn. The emergency department nurse who receives a telephone call from the client's significant other considers that the pain is most likely the result of which of the following?

1. Pericardial effusion of fluid
2. Pulmonary edema
3. Myocardial ischemia
4. Pulmonary emboli

2 The client who has peripheral edema during the day states he is awakened at night with difficulty breathing. The nurse concludes that the client's symptoms are consistent with which health problem?

1. Angina pectoris
2. Orthopnea
3. A sinus infection
4. Sleep apnea

3 The client reports onset of shortness of breath, productive cough, tachycardia, and orthopnea. The nurse concludes that these manifestations are frequently consistent with which health problem?

1. Hypertension (HTN)
2. Left ventricular failure
3. Coronary heart disease (CHD)
4. Peripheral vascular disease (PVD)

4 The client has S-T segment depression on the 12-lead electrocardiogram (ECG). The nurse concludes that this ECG finding is consistent with which of the following changes?

1. Necrosis
2. Injury
3. Ischemia
4. Bradycardia

5 The nurse anticipates that left ventricular failure can result in which of the following problems in the client? Select all that apply.

1. Right ventricular failure
2. Diminished left atrial pressure
3. Higher pulmonary pressures
4. Pulmonary edema
5. Decreased peripheral circulation and perfusion to the brain

6 A client undergoing cardiac monitoring by telemetry has sinus rhythm with a heart rate of 54 beats per minute. The nurse appropriately documents which cardiac rhythm?

1. Sinus bradycardia
2. Sinus tachycardia
3. Sinus arrhythmia
4. Accelerated nodal rhythm

7 A client with a history of unstable angina is being assessed in the emergency department. The client demonstrates significant Q waves on the electrocardiogram (ECG) compared with an ECG taken 1 week ago. The nurse notifies the health care provider because this is indicative of which problem?

1. Gangrene
2. Ischemia
3. Infection
4. Infarction

8 The client in the emergency department who is diagnosed with acute myocardial infarction (MI) asks the nurse to explain what this is. The nurse responds that an MI usually occurs because of which of the following?

1. Obstruction of a coronary artery with death of tissue distal to the blockage
2. Spasm of a coronary artery causing temporary decreased blood supply
3. A slow heart rate leading to decreased blood supply to myocardium
4. Dilation of the ventricular wall causing decreased blood supply

9 The nurse is teaching a client about risk factors for the development of atherosclerosis. The nurse should place highest priority on addressing which risk factor when conducting client teaching?

1. Being female age 59
2. Total cholesterol level of 199 mg/dL
3. Use of chewing tobacco
4. Sedentary lifestyle and obesity

10 The client comes to the clinic for a repeat visit following new onset of stable angina. When teaching the client about precipitating causes of angina, such as exercise and stress, what should the nurse include as a way to manage the precipitating causes?

1. Avoid these activities.
2. Perform such activities anyway.
3. Lead a sedentary lifestyle.
4. Use a nitroglycerin (NTG) tablet before the activity.

➤ *See pages 64–65 for Answers and Rationales.*

I. RISK FACTORS ASSOCIATED WITH CARDIAC HEALTH PROBLEMS

- **A. Coronary heart disease (CHD), angina, and myocardial infarction (MI)**: smoking, alcohol intake, obesity, sedentary lifestyle, diabetes mellitus (DM), hypercholesterolemia (total cholesterol over 200 mg/dL), hyperlipidemia (LDL over 160 mg/dL); nonmodifiable risk factors include age (over 45 years for male and over 55 years for female), male gender, family history (genetics), hypertension, stress, race, personality type, elevated triglycerides
- **B. Congestive heart failure (CHF)**: anyone with cardiac conditions such as CHD, MI, hypertension (HTN), DM, pericarditis; clients with pulmonary conditions such as chronic obstructive pulmonary disease (COPD), pulmonary HTN, post–coronary bypass clients
- **C. Cardiac dysrhythmias**: clients with known cardiac diseases (CHD, MI, CHF); older adults; electrolyte disturbances; any condition that creates stress on body (fever, hypoxia, etc.)
- **D. Inflammatory disease**: environmental and economic factors, damp weather, crowded living conditions, malnutrition, immunodeficiency, decreased access to health care, other illnesses such as streptococcal infections or severe stress/trauma to heart; may have genetic tendency; risk factor for myocarditis can be alcohol use, stress, age, and ionizing radiation
- **E. Valvular heart disease**: aging process, diseases such as MI, congenital heart defects
- **F. Control of risk factors** by effective screening and public education can reduce cardiac morbidity and mortality

II. CORONARY HEART DISEASE (CHD)

- **A. Overview**
    1. **Coronary heart disease (CHD)** is defined as a narrowing of coronary arteries resulting in narrowed lumen and decreased blood flow through those arteries
    2. Coronary atherosclerosis is most common cause of CHD
        a. Defined as narrowing of vessel wall by atherosclerotic plaques
        b. These factors speed development of plaque, which in turn impedes blood flow to myocardium, thereby decreasing oxygen (O_2) availability to tissue
            1) Elevated cholesterol and triglyceride levels
            2) Elevated blood pressure (BP) by damaging lining
            3) Infection that initiates inflammatory response
            4) Elevated iron levels carry free radicals that cause damage to lining
            5) Elevated homocysteine levels (clients often have vascular disease also)
- **B. Pathophysiology**
    1. Injury to lining of artery occurs, resulting in increased permeability of endothelial cells, allowing components of plasma to enter
    2. An inflammatory reaction occurs, bringing macrophages and platelets to area of injury

3. Hemorrhage into plaque produces thrombi; thrombus formation within arterial lumen is initiated by platelet aggregation
4. Embolization of a thrombus or plaque fragment can occur
5. Cholesterol, fat, and thrombi develop into a plaque formation
6. Progressive narrowing of lumen by plaque enlargement results in **ischemia** (insufficient blood flow leading to decreased O_2 supply to myocardium) due to narrowing of artery lumen
   a. ECG changes (inverted T wave; depressed S-T segment) occur during an acute or severe episode of ischemia (Figure 2-1)
   b. Chest pain or angina pectoris occurs
7. Cholesterol and triglycerides circulate in blood as lipoproteins
   a. High-density lipoprotein (HDL), known as "good cholesterol" is protective against coronary heart disease (CHD) by taking fats away for breakdown
   b. Low-density lipoprotein (LDL) and very low-density lipoprotein (VLDL) helps fat remain in cells, known as "bad cholesterol"
8. Signs and symptoms include chest pain, hypertension, increased pulse, increased respirations, pallor of skin, diminished peripheral pulses occasionally; a comparable symptom of atherosclerosis in legs is called **intermittent claudication** (cramping in lower extremities, especially when walking or with exercise)

C. Nursing assessment
1. Assessment
   a. Pain
      1) Location: midsternal, arms, jaw, abdomen, back
      2) Description: heaviness, tightness
      3) Duration: more than 3 minutes
      4) Intensity: rating of 1 to 10 on a verbal rating scale (VRS) or visual analog scale (VAS)
   b. Other: assess vital signs, heart sounds, exercise tolerance, peripheral pulses, skin color

Figure 2-1

S-T depression suggesting ischemia

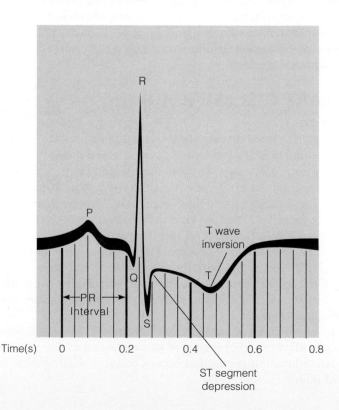

2. Potentiating factors: exercise, stress, cold temperature, anemia, substance abuse, thyrotoxicosis, hyperthyroidism
3. Relieving factors: rest, removal of stressors
4. Diagnostic tests: cholesterol level (HDL [highest], VLDL [lowest], LDL [lower than HDL]), triglyceride level, radiographic studies of arteries (arteriogram, angiogram), ECG

D. Nursing management
1. Medications
    a. Antihyperlipidemic agents and those that lower triglycerides: nicotinic acid (niacin) and HMG-CoA reductase inhibitors (also called *statins*) such as atorvastatin (Lipitor), simvastatin (Zocor) and others
    b. Antiplatelets: acetylsalicylic acid (aspirin)
    c. Antihypertensives if necessary
    d. Antianginals: nitroglycerine (Nitrostat; NTG)
    e. Antimicrobials if indicated
2. Teach risk factor management: low-fat diet, regular exercise, regular check-ups, cessation of smoking, stress management
3. Teach client to recognize signs and symptoms of CHD: shortness of breath, chest pain, and dyspnea on exertion; females may have atypical signs
4. Teach client to stop and rest at onset of discomfort

Practice to Pass

A client who is diagnosed with coronary heart disease (CHD) states that she did not know she had experienced a heart attack. What should the nurse's response be?

III. ANGINA PECTORIS

A. Overview
1. **Angina pectoris** is defined as chest pain caused by myocardial ischemia from reduced blood flow or reduced myocardial O_2 supply compared to demand; cause may be temporary or reversible
2. Classified as stable, unstable, or Prinzmetal's angina
3. Causes include CHD, coronary blood vessel spasms, thrombi, or any condition that creates an imbalance between myocardial O_2 supply and demand

B. Pathophysiology
1. When there is decreased blood flow (O_2 supply) to myocardium (ischemia) and/or increased demand for O_2 that cannot be met, angina occurs; angina is a forewarning that a myocardial infarction (MI) or heart attack may occur
    a. *Reduced O_2 supply* causes a switch from aerobic metabolism to anaerobic metabolism
        1) Anaerobic metabolism causes lactic acid buildup
        2) Anaerobic metabolism affects cell membrane permeability releasing histamine, bradykinins, and specific enzymes that stimulate terminal nerve fibers in myocardium, sending pain impulses to central nervous system (CNS)
        3) Congestive heart failure, congenital heart defects, pulmonary hypertension, left ventricular hypertrophy, and cardiomyopathy also may cause decreased O_2 supply to myocardium
        4) Silent ischemia: caused by decreased O_2 supply, just without warning signs of pain
        5) Coronary artery spasm: another form of occlusion and cause of ischemia; occurs from an unknown etiology; causes temporary narrowing of coronary arteries and angina
    b. *Increased O_2 demand* of myocardium results in angina and can be caused by anemia, exercise, thyrotoxicosis, substance abuse (cocaine), hyperthyroidism, and emotional stress
2. Types of angina
    a. Stable angina (most common type): is caused by specific amount of activity and is rather predictable; is relieved with rest and nitrates; there is no change in cause, amount, or duration of pain over time

  b. Unstable angina (more concerning)
     1) Pain occurring with increasing frequency, severity, and duration over time; is unpredictable and occurs with decreasing levels of activity or stress; may occur at rest
     2) High risk for myocardial infarction
  c. Prinzmetal's (variant) angina
     1) Atypical form occurring without identified precipitating cause; may occur at same time each day or awaken client from sleep
     2) May intensify or worsen over years but does not carry same concern as unstable angina
     3) Usual cause is coronary artery spasm, therefore making it difficult to control
  3. Signs and symptoms include pressure or heaviness in chest, which client may describe using other terms; may be accompanied by sweating, light-headedness, hypotension, pulse changes (low or high), or indigestion; pain may radiate to arms, jaw, abdomen, or back; depressed S-T segment on electrocardiogram

C. Nursing assessment
  1. Assessment includes symptom analysis of pain (location, duration, precipitating factors and relieving factors); vital signs; dyspnea; respiratory pattern; color (pallor); anxiety; heart sounds
  2. Diagnostic tests: **electrocardiogram (ECG or EKG)** graphic representation of electrical activity of heart, stress test (with or without contrast), radiographic study (angiogram), MUGA scan, troponin T or troponin I, creatinine phosphokinase (CK or CPK) and lactic dehydrogenase (LDH) (with isoenzymes), myoglobin to rule out MI, possible tests for gastric esophageal reflux disease (GERD) to rule out gastric causes

D. Nursing management
  1. Medications
     a. Antianginals: nitroglycerin (Nitrostat, NTG)
     b. Antiplatelet agents
     c. Beta blockers
     d. Calcium channel blockers to decrease **afterload** (pressure against which heart must pump) and spasms
     e. Analgesics for headache (common side effect of NTG)
     f. Thrombolytic therapy if thrombi identified as cause; glycoprotein IIb/IIIa inhibitors
     g. Stool softeners
     h. Class I-A (sodium channel blockers) or I-B or class III (potassium channel blockers; amiodarone) antidysrhythmics may be given prophylactically if premature ventricular contractions (PVCs) occur
  2. Goal is to reduce O_2 demand and improve blood and O_2 supply; primary nursing care is related to client education
     a. Signs and symptoms of angina pectoris
     b. Use of NTG: take 1 tablet or one spray every 5 minutes for 3 doses in 15 minutes; report to health care provider if no relief
     c. NTG can be used prior to activities that may cause angina (such as sexual activity, work-related activities that cannot be modified, etc.)
  3. Administer O_2 as needed
  4. Treatment may consist of percutaneous coronary revascularization
     a. Percutaneous transluminal coronary angioplasty (PTCA), including balloon angioplasty and stent placement
     b. Coronary artery bypass grafting (CABG)
     c. Minimally invasive coronary artery surgery: port access coronary artery bypass or minimally invasive coronary artery bypass
     d. Transmyocardial laser revascularization (TMLR)

Practice to Pass

The client presents with history of stable angina and asks the nurse, "Does this mean I will have a heart attack?" How should the nurse respond?

5. Monitor vital signs (VS); heart sounds
6. Monitor EKG pattern; heart rate (HR) may increase as sympathetic nervous system (SNS) response if blood pressure (BP) drops
7. Instruct client not to strain for bowel movement (BM) or create excess pressure by bending; administer stool softener as needed
8. Help client identify known stressors
9. Begin cardiac exercise program
10. Measure pulse before beta blocker administration and withhold dose if pulse is less than 60 beats per minute; also assess BP as hypotension can occur
11. Check BP before each NTG tablet and record since NTG can cause drastic hypotension; morphine sulfate (MS) may be administered in small doses if BP is below 100 systolic
12. Carefully assess BP during administration of calcium channel blockers

IV. MYOCARDIAL INFARCTION (MI)

A. Overview

1. **Myocardial infarction (MI)** is defined as death of cells in myocardium, usually related to prolonged or severe ischemia to that area
2. Many MIs are caused by sudden onset of ventricular fibrillation
3. Other causes include embolus, thrombosis, atherosclerotic occlusion, prolonged vasospasm

B. Pathophysiology

1. Cellular injury occurs because of a lack of O_2 over time (ischemia); prolonged (20–45 minutes) ischemia can lead to cell death (necrosis)
2. Coronary artery occlusion results in cell death distal to occlusion
3. Scar replaces muscle, but does not contract or conduct an impulse
4. Damage begins at subendocardial layer and progresses to epicardium within 1–6 hours
5. Damaged cells cause a decrease in myocardial contractility resulting in:
   a. Decreased **stroke volume** (volume of blood ejected by left ventricle with each heartbeat)
   b. Decreased **cardiac output** (CO), which is volume of blood ejected from left ventricle each minute; usually 4–8 liters/min in adults, leading to decreased BP and decreased tissue perfusion
6. Myocardial ischemia that reoccurs over time may initiate development of **collateral circulation** (additional outgrowth of tiny vessels), which provides for delivery of O_2 and nutrients to area of ischemia
7. MIs are described by:
   a. Location
      1) Anterior: usually occurring in area supplied by left anterior descending artery (LAD)
      2) Posterior: usually occurring in area supplied by the right coronary artery (RCA)
      3) Lateral: occurring in area supplied by left circumflex artery
   b. Myocardial surface
      1) Transmural infarct: endocardium to epicardium
      2) Subendocardial: endocardial surface into myocardial muscle
      3) Intramural infarction: patchy areas of myocardium
8. Signs and symptoms associated with MI
   a. Pain (typical): midsternal, radiating to jaw, arms, abdomen, or shoulder; tightness, crushing feeling; lasting 15–20 minutes; not relieved with NTG and rest; may be pain free (silent MI)
   b. Duration of pain important in distinguishing from angina pectoris

ST segment
elevation

Time(s)   0   0.2   0.4   0.6   0.8
A

Time(s)   0   0.2   0.4   0.6   0.8
B   Q wave

    c. Sudden onset of pain, usually not associated with activity, may awaken in middle of night

    d. Tachycardia related to pain and increased need of tissue for O_2

    e. Diaphoresis, nausea or vomiting

    f. Tachypnea, dyspnea

    g. Change in LOC, anxiety, feelings of impending doom

    h. ECG changes: depressed or *elevated S-T segment* (most common), inverted T wave, formation of Q waves (Figure 2-2)

    i. Elevated cardiac markers: enzymes are normally present in muscle fibers and are not elevated in serum unless injury occurs; when any muscle is injured, enzymes are released into blood stream as a response to injury; isoenzymes are a breakdown of total enzyme level and indicate (when elevated) which particular type of muscle has been damaged

        1) Cardiac muscle troponins: proteins are released during a myocardial infarction; cardiac-specific troponin T (cT_nT) and cardiac-specific troponin I (cT_nI) are specific to cardiac muscle necrosis and are sensitive in detecting small MIs (Table 2-1)

        2) Myoglobin: first cardiac marker to be detectable in blood after MI; is released quickly after symptoms occur but has limited usefulness because it is not cardiac specific

        3) Creatinine phosphokinase (CK or CPK): isoenzymes are CPK I (BB) present in brain tissue and smooth muscle; CPK II (MB) present in heart tissue; and CPK III (MM) present in muscle tissue; when total CPK level is elevated, assess for an elevated CPK II or MB isoenzyme to determine if an MI has occurred

        4) Lactic dehydrogenase (LDH): isoenzymes are LDH_1 present in cardiac muscle; LDH_2 present in reticuloendothelial system; LDH_3 present in lungs and other tissue; LDH_4 present in placenta, kidneys, and pancreas; and LDH_5 present in liver and striated muscle; normally LDH_1 is less than LDH_2, however in an MI, LDH_1 is greater than LDH_2 (termed a "flipped ratio"); when total LDH level is elevated, assess for an elevated LDH_1 isoenzyme to determine if an MI has occurred; this enzyme is less useful because it elevates later than other cardiac markers already listed

    j. Elevated temperature

    k. Leukocytosis

Table 2-1	Enzyme Markers in MI					
Marker	Normal Level	Primary Tissue Location	Significance of Elevation	Appears	Peaks	Duration
CK (CPK)	Male: 12–80 units/L Female: 10–70 units/L	Cardiac muscle, skeletal muscle, brain	Injury to muscle cells	3–6 hours	12–24 hours	24–48 hours
CK-MB	0–3% of total CK	Cardiac muscle	MI, cardiac ischemia, myocarditis, cardiac contusion, defibrillation	4–8 hours	18–24 hours	72 hours
cT_nT	< 0.2 mcg/L	Cardiac muscle	Acute MI, unstable angina	2–4 hours	18–24 hours	10–14 days
cT_nI	< 3.1 mcg/L	Cardiac muscle	Acute MI, unstable angina	2–4 hours	18–24 hours	7–10 days

Source: LeMone, Priscilla; Burke, Karen M.; Bauldoff, Gerene, *Medical-Surgical Nursing: Critical Thinking in Patient Care*, 5th Edition, © 2011. Printed and Electronically reproduced by permission of Pearson Education, Inc., Upper Saddle River, New Jersey.

l. Cardiac dysrhythmias: premature ventricular contractions (PVCs), ventricular tachycardia caused by irritability

 9. The most common reaction to an MI is to deny symptoms and delay health care

C. Nursing assessment

 1. Assessment includes symptom analysis of chest pain (location, duration, radiation, quality); associated symptomatology (diaphoresis, nausea/vomiting); vital signs; heart sounds (murmur, friction rub, gallop [S_3 or S_4]); cardiac rhythm; nonverbal cues of discomfort

2. Diagnostic tests: CPK (and possibly LDH) with isoenzymes, troponin level, 12-lead ECG, chest x-ray (CXR), angiogram, echocardiogram, stress tests, MUGA scan, arterial blood gases (ABGs), electrolytes, complete blood count (CBC), use pulse oximetry for quick reference of oxygen saturation

D. Nursing management

 1. Medications

a. Antianginals: nitroglycerin (Nitrostat, NTG) for vasodilation; anticipate use of sublingual/topical spray, Nitrol drip, and/or Nitrol paste or patch

b. Analgesics as needed for pain relief; morphine sulfate if BP too low or pain unrelieved by nitroglycerin; note that morphine may lower BP also

c. Stool softener

d. Electrolyte replacement as necessary

e. Antihypertensives such as angiotensin converting enzyme (ACE) inhibitors, calcium channel blockers, or beta blockers

f. Anticoagulants such as heparin, warfarin (Coumadin) or low molecular weight heparin (LMWH) such as enoxaparin (Lovenox)

g. Antidysrhythmics may be given prophylactically

1) Amiodarone hydrochloride (Cordarone): ventricular antidysrhythmics such as PVCs

2) Atropine: treatment of bradydysrhythmias

3) Short-acting beta blockers: treatment of tachydysrhythmias

h. Thrombolytics such as streptokinase (Streptase) as indicated

 2. Supplement O_2 via nasal cannula at 2 to 5 L/min

3. Elevate head of bed for respiratory comfort

4. Maintain intravenous (IV) access site

5. Monitor bowel movements, encourage client not to strain, and offer stool softener as needed

6. Provide for physical and psychological rest

7. Provide emotional support for client and family

Practice to Pass

The client arrives in the emergency department with complaints of midsternal chest pain, diaphoresis, and nausea. The client states, "I'm dying." How should the nurse respond?

8. Reassess client frequently for pain relief or continued pain; use pain scale to assess quality of pain
9. Teach client and family when they are ready to listen and absorb information
10. Monitor VS and record with administration of nitrates, beta blockers, and calcium channel blockers: withhold dose if pulse is less than 60 beats per minute or BP is less than 100 systolic
11. Begin cardiac rehabilitation program for education and exercise as ordered
12. Monitor for major side effects of medications: hypotension, bradycardia, bleeding, constipation, and depression

V. CONGESTIVE HEART FAILURE (CHF)

A. Overview

1. **Congestive heart failure (CHF)** is defined as heart's inability to pump sufficiently to meet body's metabolic needs, causing decreased tissue perfusion as a result of decreased CO
2. May be acute (pulmonary edema or cardiogenic shock) or chronic (heart failure); left sided, right sided, or both
3. Causes include diseases such as MI, hypertension, CHD, or kidney failure; cardiomyopathies; valve disorders; inflammatory conditions; water intoxication; and side effects of medications such as corticosteroids (Table 2-2)
4. Prognosis is determined by effectiveness of therapeutic regimen

B. Pathophysiology

1. Heart pumps blood to both pulmonary and systemic vascular systems; an adequate blood supply to heart is needed to produce a sufficient CO
2. Demand for CO is regulated by metabolic needs of body
3. Damage to pump (heart) regardless of cause leads to decreased CO and decreased tissue perfusion
4. Two dysfunctions that contribute to CHF
   a. *Diastolic dysfunction*: occurs when ventricle pumps against an extremely high afterload as in primary hypertension; this leads to a decrease in ventricles' ability to comply, decreases **preload** (volume of blood returning to heart creating "stretch" or tension of myocardial fibers at end of diastole), which leads to decreased stroke volume (SV); hypotension can result
   b. *Systolic dysfunction*: occurs when ventricle experiences damage as in MI and ventricle cannot contract effectively; SV decreases, leading to an increased preload and ventricle becomes distended; signs of decreased CO can result

Table 2-2	Causes of Heart Failure				
Excess Volume Load	**Excess Pressure Load**	**Increased Metabolic Demand**	**Acute Conditions**	**Altered Function**	**Filling Disorders**
Volume overload	Hypertension	Anemias	Acute hypertensive crisis	Cardiomyopathy	Valve stenosis (mitral or tricuspid)
Valve regurgitation	Aortic stenosis	Thyrotoxicosis		Myocarditis	
Left-to-right shunts	Hypertrophic cardiomyopathy	Pregnancy Infection	Aortic valve rupture	Rheumatic fever Infective endocarditis	Cardiac tamponade Restrictive pericarditis
	Coarctation of aorta	Fever	Massive pulmonary embolism	Coronary heart disease	
		Physical, emotional, or environmental stressors		Dysrhythmias Toxic disorders	

   5. Compensatory mechanisms for heart failure (HF) (Table 2-3)
      a. Frank-Starling mechanism: force of contraction determined by amount of stretch
      b. Neuroendocrine responses
         1) Sympathetic nervous system (SNS) activation: increase in HR
         2) Renin: angiotensin-aldosterone mechanism activation to retain sodium and water
      c. Ventricular hypertrophy
   6. Decreased CO stimulates aortic baroreceptors, causing release of norepinephrine to increase HR and contractility; this causes vasoconstriction, thereby increasing blood return to heart and increasing CO
   7. Decreased CO leads to decreased renal perfusion; remember that kidneys need blood in order to function properly
      a. Decreased renal perfusion leads to release of renin from juxtoglomerular cells
      b. Activation of renin-angiotensin-aldosterone mechanism
         1) Causes vasoconstriction
         2) Stimulates adrenal cortex to produce aldosterone and antidiuretic hormone (ADH) from posterior pituitary gland
            a) Aldosterone causes sodium reabsorption and water retention, thus increasing BP
            b) ADH inhibits water excretion in distal tubules and causes vasoconstriction, thus increasing vascular volume and raising BP
   8. Vasoconstriction causes increased blood return to heart (preload), causing greater stretch (Frank-Starling law), and therefore increases CO

Table 2-3   Compensatory Mechanisms Activated in Heart Failure

Mechanism	Physiology	Effect on Body Systems	Complications
Frank-Starling mechanism	Greater stretch of cardiac muscle fibers leads to greater force of contraction.	↑ contractile force leading to ↑ CO	↑ myocardial O_2 demand Limited by overstretching
Neuroendocrine response	↓ CO causes sympathetic nervous system stimulation and catecholamine release.	↑ HR, BP, contractility ↑ vascular resistance ↑ venous return	Tachycardia with decreased filling time and decreased CO ↑ vascular resistance ↑ myocardial work and O_2 demand
	↓ CO and ↑ renal perfusion stimulate renin angiotensin system.	Vasoconstriction and ↑ BP	↑ myocardial work Renal vasoconstriction and ↓ renal perfusion
	Angiotensin stimulates aldosterone release from adrenal cortex.	Salt and water retention by kidneys ↑ vascular volume	↑ preload and afterload Pulmonary congestion
	ADH is released from posterior pituitary	Water excretion inhibited ↑ sodium excretion Diuresis	Fluid retention and ↑ preload and afterload
	Atrial natriuretic factor is released.	↑ sodium excretion Diuresis	
	Blood flow is redistributed to vital organs (heart and brain).	↓ perfusion of other organ systems ↓ perfusion of skin and muscles	Renal failure Anaerobic metabolism and lactic acidosis
Ventricular hypertrophy	↑ cardiac workload causes myocardial muscle to hypertrophy and ventricles to dilate.	↑ contractile force to maintain CO	↑ myocardial O_2 demand Cellular enlargement

Source: LeMone, Priscilla; Burke, Karen M.; Bauldoff, Gerene, *Medical-Surgical Nursing: Critical Thinking in Patient Care*, 5th Edition, © 2011. Printed and Electronically reproduced by permission of Pearson Education, Inc., Upper Saddle River, New Jersey.

9. Atrial stretch stimulates release of atrial natriuretic factor (ANF) or atriopeptin that balances effects of renin and aldosterone, promotes sodium and water excretion and inhibits norepinephrine, renin, and ADH

10. Ventricular hypertrophy results from excess fluid volume and pressure causing cells to enlarge, stiffen, thereby decreasing force of contraction

11. Compensatory mechanisms hasten deterioration of cardiac function and onset of HF
    a. Increased HR decreases diastolic filling time, compromises coronary artery perfusion, and increases myocardial O_2 demand; the resulting ischemia leads to decreased CO
    b. Beta receptors in heart become less sensitive to SNS stimulation, thereby decreasing HR and contractility
    c. Alpha receptors on peripheral blood vessels are increased in sensitivity, which promotes vasoconstriction, thereby increasing afterload and therefore cardiac workload

12. Chronic ventricular dilation leads to ventricular wall thinning, degeneration, and loss of effective contractility

13. Chronic atrial dilation leads to depletion of ANF leaving renin, aldosterone, and norepinephrine to continue unabated; causes increased preload, afterload, and further deterioration in HF, thereby decreasing O_2 supply to tissues, leading to further ischemia and tissue death (infarction)

14. Left-sided HF (see Figure 2-3)
    a. Left side affected more often than right side
    b. Results from left ventricular wall damage or dilatation

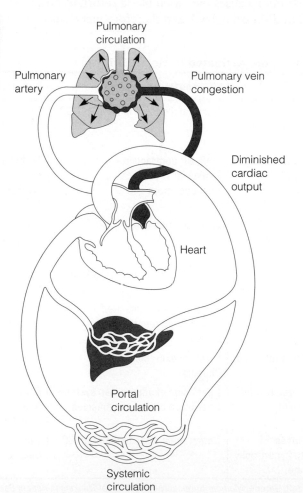

Figure 2-3

Pathophysiology of left-sided heart failure

    c. Left ventricular and atrial end-diastolic pressures increase and CO decreases

    d. Impaired left ventricular filling results in congestion and increased pulmonary artery (PA) pressures; remember "**L**"eft and "**L**"ung, the fluid "backs up" to lungs

        1) Increased PA pressure causes shifting of fluid interstitially, leading to alveolar congestion and pulmonary edema

        2) Increased PA pressures as measured by a PA catheter (normal PA pressure 25/10 mmHg)

    e. Signs and symptoms of left HF: fatigue, activity intolerance, dizziness, syncope, dyspnea, shortness of breath, cough, orthopnea, pulmonary crackles on auscultation, S_3 heart sound, tachycardia with possible atrial dysrhythmia, and decreased urine output

15. Right-sided HF (see Figure 2-4)

    a. Right-sided HF caused by pulmonary hypertension (cor pulmonale) and left HF

    b. Right ventricular infarction can cause right-sided HF

    c. Pulmonary hypertension causes increased pressure that right ventricle must pump against, so right ventricle cannot empty; hypertrophy and dilation result

    d. Right ventricular distention leads to blood accumulation in systemic veins; remember "**R**"ight and "**R**"est of body, the fluid "backs up" to rest of body

    e. Increased venous pressure causes abdominal organ congestion and peripheral edema

        1) Lower extremity edema occurs in client who is ambulatory

        2) A bedridden client will experience sacral and/or scrotal edema

Figure 2-4

Pathophysiology of right-sided heart failure

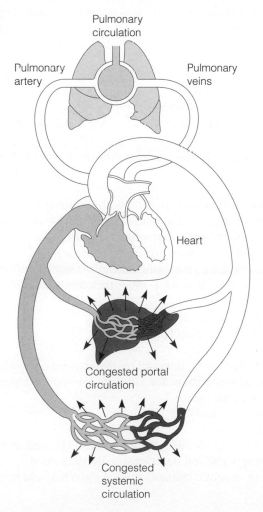

3) Liver engorgement will lead to right upper quadrant pain

4) Anorexia and nausea occur with gastrointestinal (GI) venous congestion

   f. Jugular venous distention occurs

16. Biventricular failure; both ventricles fail

   a. Client experiences signs and symptoms of both left and right failure

   b. Paroxysmal nocturnal dyspnea (PND) occurs as peripheral edema is reabsorbed into circulation when client goes to bed and feet are elevated, causing fluid overload and pulmonary congestion

   c. Severe HF predisposes client to dyspnea at rest

   d. S_3 and S_4 heart sounds may be heard

   e. Hepatomegaly and splenomegaly result from abdominal engorgement or congestion: increased abdominal pressure, ascites, GI problems (anorexia, nausea, and vomiting), decreased digestion and absorption of nutrients

   f. Dysrhythmias may develop from myocardial distention, causing interference with conduction and lowering CO

   g. Cardiogenic shock or acute pulmonary edema may develop as cardiac function deteriorates

C. Nursing assessment

1. Assessment includes VS; cardiac monitor; heart rhythm; pulse quality (full, bounding, thready); respiratory status (dyspnea, shortness of breath, tachypnea); lung sounds (crackles, rhonchi, wheezes); heart sounds (S_3 or S_4, murmur or rub); jugular neck vein distention; abdominal assessment (palpation, distention, ascites); edema; activity tolerance

2. Diagnostic tests

   a. Electrocardiogram

     1) Signs of ischemia: depressed S-T segment, inverted T wave

     2) Signs of injury: elevated S-T segment, Q wave development

   b. Atrial natriuretic factor (ANF) or B-type natriuretic peptide (BNP): increase in CHF

   c. Other: electrolytes, liver function tests, ABG analysis, chest x-ray, echocardiogram, O_2 saturation

   d. Tests to rule out an MI may be done if client is having chest pain also

D. Nursing management

1. Medications

   a. Diuretics: often with a loop diuretic such as furosemide (Lasix)

   b. Positive inotropic agents: dopamine (Inotropin)— increases urinary output, systemic vasoconstrictor; dobutamine (Dobutex)

   c. Phosphodiesterase inhibitor: amrinone (Inocor)

   d. Analgesics to decrease stress and discomfort and allow decreased O_2 needs

   e. Antihypertensives such as ACE inhibitors, direct vasodilators, or beta adrenergic blockers

   f. Antidysrhythmics as needed

   g. Cardiac glycosides: digoxin (Lanoxin)

   h. Nitrates

2. Primary goal is to reduce O_2 demand on myocardium: physical and psychological rest

3. Manage prescribed medications for reducing cardiac workload, improving contractility, and management of symptoms

4. Management of decreased CO

   a. Monitor and record VS

     1) Decreased CO stimulates SNS to increase HR and increase diastolic BP; as heart's pumping action deteriorates, BP decreases

     2) Assessment of subtle changes in vital signs may aid in early intervention

    b. Auscultate heart and lung sounds

       1) S_1 and S_2 may be diminished as cardiac function fails

       2) S_3 is an early sign of HF (ventricular gallop)

       3) S_4 may also be present (atrial gallop)

       4) Basilar crackles may be heard

       5) Increasing crackles and dyspnea mean worsening of condition

    c. Note level of consciousness (LOC)

       1) Mental status changes occur as blood flow to brain decreases

       2) Reduction in oxygen saturation may also lead to decreased LOC

    d. Note urine output (UO)

       1) Decreased blood flow to kidneys leads to decreased UO

       2) Assessing UO assists in evaluating effectiveness of some medications used to treat HF, such as diuretics and positive inotropic agents

    e. Note skin color and temperature

       1) Cool, clammy skin frequently present in acute phase of HF

       2) Pale and then cyanotic color is seen in later stages as cardiac pumping action deteriorates

    f. Monitor client for cardiac dysrhythmias

       1) Sinus tachycardia is usually present

       2) Atrial dysrhythmias are frequently seen in HF: atrial fibrillation, atrial flutter, premature atrial contractions (PACs), and atrial tachycardia

       3) Ventricular dysrhythmias will be seen as ventricular hypertrophy and dilation occurs

    g. Supplemental O_2 is given to decrease effects of hypoxia and ischemia

    h. Place client at rest with head of bed elevated to improve respiratory function and reduce cardiac workload

       1) Assist with personal care needs

       2) Use bedside commode to reduce effort and metabolic energy that would be necessary if bed pan is used

       3) Instruct client to avoid performing Valsalva maneuver

       4) Avoid isometric exercises

    i. Promote psychological rest and minimize anxiety to reduce O_2 consumption and improve cardiac function: maintain quiet environment, allow expression of fear, and explain procedures to client's satisfaction

  5. Management of fluid volume excess

    a. Assess respiratory status; declining respiratory status indicates worsening left HF—shortness of breath, dyspnea, cough, orthopnea, paroxysmal nocturnal dyspnea

    b. Acute pulmonary edema can develop rapidly

       1) Air hunger develops and client needs to sit straight up in bed

       2) Client begins to panic with overwhelming sense of impending doom

       3) Tachypnea develops quickly

       4) Productive cough with large amounts of pink, frothy sputum occurs

    c. Monitor UO closely

       1) Notify provider if UO is equal to or less than 30 mL/hr

       2) Use of diuretics reduces circulating volume, producing hypovolemia even in presence of peripheral edema

       3) Decreased UO could indicate decreased CO and renal ischemia

    d. Weigh client daily at same time, on same scale, and in same clothing

       1) Weight provides objective measure of fluid status

       2) 1 liter of fluid is equal to 2.2 pounds of weight

    e. Assess and record abdominal girth every shift; measure at level of umbilicus; mark area measured for consistency among measurements

1) Venous congestion leads to development of ascites and may produce GI complaints: nausea, loss of appetite, abdominal discomfort

2) Increasing girth means increased ascites production (third-spacing)

f. Keep client on bedrest with head of bed elevated 45 degrees to improve lung expansion and reduce cardiac workload

g. Assess for signs of deteriorating condition

h. Monitor hemodynamics (if PA catheter in place), including PA pressures (normal 25/10 mmHg), pulmonary capillary wedge pressure, right atrial pressure (CVP), CO, cardiac index, and systemic vascular resistance

i. Restrict fluids if ordered to decrease fluid overload

6. Management of activity intolerance: minimal or no cardiac reserve for increased activity leads to self-care deficits

a. Allow adequate rest periods prior to activity

b. Assess for signs of decreasing activity tolerance

c. Assist with activities of daily living (ADLs) allowing client to do as much as possible to provide some control to client and reduce feelings of helplessness

d. Provide passive and active range-of-motion (ROM) to progressively promote improved cardiac function

e. Teach client about discharge instructions

1) Low-sodium diet

2) Perform activities as independently as possible

3) Space meals and activities, allowing time for rest and relaxation

4) Stop any activity that causes chest pain or shortness of breath

5) Avoid straining

6) Begin slowly progressive exercise program

7. Closely monitor and record drug therapy

a. Monitor apical pulse for 1 minute prior to administering digoxin (Lanoxin); withhold dose and notify prescriber if pulse is less than 60 beats per minute

b. Monitor VS and intake and output (I&O) carefully while administering dopamine (Intropin)

1) Low doses: renal perfusion

2) Moderate to high doses: elevate BP

c. Close monitoring of I & O with diuretics, avoid giving furosemide (Lasix) by IV push (IVP) at rate greater than 4 mg/min—ototoxicity can occur

Practice to Pass

The client is being discharged tomorrow after a 6-day hospitalization for heart failure. The client asks when he can return to work. How should the nurse explain the recovery phase?

VI. CARDIAC DYSRHYTHMIAS

A. Overview

1. Electrical stimulation of normal heart causes depolarization of myocardium, producing a synchronized, rhythmic contraction of myocardium (a heartbeat), and propelling blood through arteries and capillaries

2. Cardiac dysrhythmias are defined as alterations in this stimulation, which interrupt synchronized pattern of contractions and may reduce cardiac efficiency

3. Normal sinus rhythm conduction progresses from sinoatrial (SA) node → atrioventricular (AV) node → bundle of His → bundle branches (right and left) simultaneously → Purkinje fibers, causing contraction of atria and ventricles

4. Cardiac dysrhythmias

a. May be benign or lethal

b. Caused by many factors (see Table 2-4)

c. Any dysrhythmia can affect cardiac function, regardless of cause

d. Client's response to rhythm determines urgency of treatment

5. Dysrhythmias originate as sinus, atrial, junctional, ventricular, or heart blocks

Table 2-4   **Causes of Cardiac Dysrhythmias**

Dysrhythmia	Common Causes
Sinus arrhythmia	Increase in vagal tone, digoxin toxicity, or morphine administration
Sinus tachycardia (ST)	Normal response to any condition that increases body's need for more O_2 and nutrients: fever, stress, exercise, hypoxia, anemia, hypovolemia, hyperthyroidism, MI, HF, cardiogenic shock
Sinus bradycardia (SB)	Increased vagal tone; depressed automaticity; may be normal in athletic heart syndrome or during sleep; other causes include pain, increased intracranial pressure, sinus node disease, MI, hypothermia, acidosis, certain drugs such as digoxin (Lanoxin), beta blockers, calcium channel blockers
Sick sinus syndrome (SSS)	Injury during surgery, myocardial ischemia, MI, fibrosis of conduction fibers associated with aging, drugs such as digoxin (Lanoxin), beta blockers, and calcium channel blockers
Premature atrial contractions (PAC)	Strong emotions, excessive alcohol intake, tobacco, adrenergic stimulants (caffeine), MI, HF, pericarditis, valvular disorders, hypoxemia, pulmonary embolism, digoxin toxicity, hypokalemia, hypomagnesemia, metabolic alkalosis
Atrial tachycardia (AT) or paroxysmal supraventricular tachycardia (PSVT)	Sympathetic nervous system stimulation, fever, sepsis, hyperthyroidism, heart disease, MI, rheumatic heart disease, myocarditis, acute pericarditis
Atrial flutter	Sympathetic nervous system stimulation, anxiety, caffeine, alcohol intake, thyrotoxicosis, CHD, MI, pulmonary embolism, abnormal conduction syndromes, older adults with rheumatic heart disease or valvular disease
Atrial fibrillation (A-fib)	CHF, mitral valve disease, rheumatic heart disease, CHD, hypertension, hyperthyroidism, thyrotoxicosis
Junctional rhythm	Digoxin toxicity, quinidine reaction, overdose of beta blockers or calcium channel blockers, hypoxemia, hyperkalemia, increased vagal tone, damage to the AV node, MI, CHF
Premature ventricular contractions (PVC)	Anxiety or stress, tobacco, alcohol, caffeine use, hypoxia, acidosis, electrolyte imbalances, sympathomimetic drugs, ischemic heart disease, CHD, MI, CHF, mechanical stimulation of heart, reperfusion after thrombolytic therapy
Ventricular tachycardia	Myocardial ischemia, MI, valvular disease, rheumatic heart disease, cardiomyopathy, anorexia nervosa, metabolic disorders, drug toxicity
Ventricular fibrillation	Myocardial ischemia or MI
First-degree heart block	MI, digoxin toxicity, complications from cardiac surgery, chronic heart disease, effects of certain drugs
Second-degree heart block, type I, Wenckebach	MI, electrolyte imbalance, acute rheumatic infections, myocarditis, drug toxicity: digoxin (Lanoxin), procainamide (Procan), quinidine sulfate (Quinidine), propranolol (Inderal), verapamil (Isoptin)
Second-degree heart block, type II, Classical	MI, electrolyte imbalance, acute rheumatic infections, myocarditis, progressive from Type I heart block, drug toxicity from digoxin (Lanoxin), procainamide (Procan), quinidine sulfate (Quinidine), propranolol (Inderal), verapamil (Isoptin)
Third-degree or complete heart block	Ischemia or damage to AV node, frequently associated with inferior or anteroseptal MI, degenerative conduction system disease, damage to conduction system during surgery, acute myocarditis, increased vagal tone, digoxin (Lanoxin) or propranolol (Inderal) toxicity, electrolyte imbalance, progression from Type II heart block

B. Pathophysiology
   1. Altered electrical activity may cause alterations in cardiac function
   2. Dysrhythmias may result from internal or external forces
      a. Internal forces include hypoxia, electrolyte disturbances, acidosis, diseases of myocardium, and atherosclerotic processes
      b. External forces include stress, exercise, pain, anemia, and hypovolemia

3. Cardiac muscle cells have capability of **automaticity** (ability to fire without stimulation), allowing cell to serve as a pacemaker or cause premature beats
4. Each heartbeat creates distinctive wave forms: P, QRS, and T (see Table 2-5); each QRS should correspond to a pulse
5. An action potential is the electrical activity that occurs in a cell by movement of ions across cell membranes
   a. During resting state, cell is *polarized*, with positive and negative ions equal on either side of cell membrane; maintained by the sodium (Na^+)-potassium (K^+) pump
   b. Depolarization (contraction) requires a change from a negative to positive state; Na^+ ions enter rapidly, opening the Na^+ channels; calcium (Ca^{++}) is allowed in, K^+ is not allowed to cross
   c. A threshold potential is reached when cell becomes less negative, creating an action potential that depolarizes cardiac muscle cells; Ca^{++} enters cell and causes contraction of cardiac muscle

Table 2-5 | **Wave Formations on an EKG**

Configuration	Wave Form	Characteristics
	P wave	First upright, positive wave; normally smooth, round configuration; one should proceed each QRS; demonstrates atrial contraction
	QRS—Q wave	First negative deflection
	QRS—R wave	First positive deflection after Q
	QRS—S wave	Next negative deflection after R wave; called QRS regardless of presence of all 3 waveforms; demonstrates ventricular contraction
	T wave	Large wave form after QRS, upright, positive, round; demonstrates ventricular relaxation
	P-R interval	From beginning of P wave to beginning of Q wave; length of time it takes impulse to travel from SA node through bundle of His; normally 0.12–0.20 sec
	QRS interval	Beginning of Q wave to end of S wave; length of time it takes impulse to travel from bundle of His to Purkinje fibers; ventricular contraction (depolarization) and beginning of repolarization (resting); normally 0.04–0.10 sec
	S-T segment	Should be a straight line between S wave and beginning of T wave (isoelectric); demonstrates beginning and end of ventricular repolarization

    d. Repolarization then occurs to return cell to a polarized state, Na^+ channels close and cell begins to gain negative charge; the Na^+-K^+ pump restores ions to proper concentration

    e. Sequence is repeated for each heartbeat

6. A refractory period is a stage in conduction cycle where there is resistance to stimulation

    a. *Absolute refractory period*: from beginning of Q to middle of T wave; no stimulus of any size can cause another impulse to occur

    b. *Relative refractory period*: from middle of T to end of T wave; a stimulus larger than one usually needed to create an impulse can cause muscle cells to contract; an example is when a PVC occurs at same time as a T wave, resulting in ventricular tachycardia or ventricular fibrillation

7. Two major categories of dysrhythmias

    a. Alteration in impulse formation

        1) Rate: tachycardia or bradycardia

        2) Rhythm: regular or irregular

        3) Ectopic beats (extra impulse): premature atrial contractions (PAC), premature junctional contractions (PJC), junctional escape rhythm, premature ventricular contractions (PVC)

    b. Alteration in conductivity

        1) Heart blocks

        2) Reentry phenomenon is blockage of an impulse through a bundle branch, causing impulse to retrograde backwards, reentering other bundle branch and causing a premature beat

8. Cardiac rhythms are classified according to site of impulse formation or site and degree of conduction block (see Table 2-6)

    a. Sinus rhythms

        1) Normal sinus rhythm (NSR): impulse originates at SA node; waveform is normal, smooth, and upright

        2) Sinus dysrhythmia: sinus rhythm that varies in rate during inspiration (faster) and expiration (slower); common in very young and very old

        3) Sinus tachycardia (ST)

            a) Same configuration as NSR except rate is greater than 100 beats per minute

            b) Can be an early warning sign of cardiac dysfunction, such as HF, or may represent other physiologic stressor, such as illness or injury

            c) Client may be asymptomatic; symptoms experienced may be "racing" feeling, syncope, dyspnea

            d) Treatment is to find and treat cause

        4) Sinus bradycardia (SB)

            a) Same configuration as NSR except rate is less than 60 beats per minute

            b) Clients may be asymptomatic; if not tolerating low rate, may experience decreased LOC, syncope, and hypotension; may be treated with atropine if symptomatic

        5) Sinus arrest or sinus block

            a) All configurations are normal but one or more complexes is dropped

            b) Sinus block: measurement of R-R interval (beginning of one QRS to beginning of next QRS) will be exact, even with missing complex

            c) Sinus arrest: measurement of R-R will not be exact with missing complex

            d) Symptoms may not be present unless pause is great enough to decrease CO; client will experience same symptoms as bradycardia

Table 2-6	Characteristics of Selected Cardiac Rhythms and Dysrhythmias	
Rhythm/ECG Appearance	**ECG Characteristics**	**Management**
Supraventricular Rhythms		
Normal sinus rhythm (NSR)	Rate: 60–100 beats per minute Rhythm: Regular P:QRS: 1:1 PR interval: 0.12–0.20 sec QRS complex: 0.06–0.10 sec	None; normal heart rhythm.
Sinus arrhythmia	Rate: 60–100 beats per minute Rhythm: Irregular, varying with respirations P:QRS: 1:1 PR interval: 0.12–0.20 sec QRS complex: 0.04–0.10 sec	Generally none; considered a normal rhythm in very young and very old.
Sinus tachycardia	Rate: 101–150 beats per minute Rhythm: Regular P:QRS: 1:1 (with very fast rates, P wave may be hidden in preceding T wave) PR interval: 0.12–0.20 sec QRS complex: 0.04–0.10 sec	Treated only if client is symptomatic or at risk for myocardial damage. Treat underlying cause (e.g., hypovolemia, fever, pain). Beta blockers or verapamil may be used.
Sinus bradycardia	Rate: < 60 beats per minute Rhythm: Regular P:QRS: 1:1 PR interval: 0.12–0.20 sec QRS complex: 0.04–0.10 sec	Treated only if client is symptomatic with IV atropine and/or pacemaker therapy.
Premature atrial contractions (PAC)	Rate: Variable Rhythm: Irregular, with normal rhythm interrupted by early beats arising in atria P:QRS: 1:1 PR interval: 0.12–0.20 sec, but may be prolonged QRS complex: 0.4–0.10 sec	Usually require no treatment. Advise client to reduce alcohol and caffeine intake, reduce stress, and stop smoking.
Paroxysmal supraventricular tachycardia (PSVT)	Rate: 100–280 beats per minute (usually 150–200 beats per minute) Rhythm: Regular P:QRS: P waves often not identifiable PR interval: Not measured QRS complex: 0.04–0.10 sec	Treat if client is symptomatic: vagal maneuvers (Valsalva, carotid sinus massage); O_2 therapy; adenosine, verapamil, procainamide, propranolol, and esmolol; and synchronized cardioversion.

Rhythm/ECG Appearance	ECG Characteristics	Management
Atrial flutter	Rate: Atrial 240–360 beats per minute; ventricular rate depends on degree of AV block and usually is < 150 beats per minute Rhythm: Atrial regular, ventricular usually regular P:QRS: 2:1, 4:1, 6:1; may vary PR interval: Not measured QRS complex: 0.04–0.10 sec	Synchronized cardioversion; drugs to slow ventricular response such as a beta blocker or calcium channel blocker (verapamil), followed by quinidine, procainamide, flecainide, or amiodarone.
Atrial fibrillation	Rate: Atrial 300–600 beats per minute (too rapid to count); ventricular 100–180 beats per minute in untreated clients Rhythm: Irregularly irregular P:QRS: Variable PR interval: Not measured QRS complex: 0.04–0.10 sec	Synchronized cardioversion; drugs to reduce ventricular response rate: verapamil, propranolol, digoxin, anticoagulant therapy to reduce risk of clot formation and stroke.
Junctional escape rhythm	Rate: 40–60 beats per minute; junctional tachycardia 60–140 beats per minute Rhythm: Regular P:QRS: P waves may be absent, inverted and immediately preceding or succeeding QRS complex, or hidden in QRS complex PR interval: < 0.10 sec if P wave is prior to QRS complex QRS complex: 0.04–0.10 sec	Treat cause if client is experiencing symptoms.

Ventricular Rhythms

Premature ventricular contractions (PVC)	Rate: Variable Rhythm: Irregular, with PVC interrupting underlying rhythm and followed by a compensatory pause P:QRS: No P wave noted before PVC PR interval: Absent with PVC QRS complex: Wide (> 0.12 sec) and bizarre in appearance; differs from normal QRS complex	Treat if client is experiencing symptoms. Advise against stimulant use (caffeine, nicotine). Drug therapy includes IV lidocaine, procainamide, quinidine, propranolol, phenytoin, bretylium.
Ventricular tachycardia (VT or V tach)	Rate: 100–250 beats per minute Rhythm: Regular P:QRS: P waves usually not identifiable PR interval: Not measured QRS complex: 0.12 sec or greater; bizarre shape	Treat if sustained or if client is symptomatic using IV procainamide or lidocaine IV and/or immediate defibrillation if client is unconscious or unstable.

Rhythm/ECG Appearance	ECG Characteristics	Management
Ventricular fibrillation (VF, V fib)	Rate: Too rapid to count Rhythm: Grossly irregular P:QRS: No identifiable P waves PR interval: None QRS: Bizarre, varying in shape and direction	Immediate defibrillation.
Atrioventricular Conduction Blocks		
First-degree AV block	Rate: Usually 60–100 beats per minute Rhythm: Regular P:QRS: 1:1 PR interval: > 0.20 sec QRS complex: 0.04–0.10 sec	None required.
Second-degree AV block, type I (Mobitz I, Wenckebach)	Rate: 60–100 beats per minute Rhythm: Atrial regular; ventricular irregular P:QRS: 1:1 until P wave blocked with no subsequent QRS complex PR interval: Progressively lengthens in a regular pattern QRS complex: 0.04–0.10 sec; sudden absence of QRS complex	Monitoring and observation; atropine or isoproterenol if client is symptomatic.
Second-degree AV block, type II (Mobitz II)	Rate: Atrial 60–100 beats per minute; ventricular < 60 beats per minute Rhythm: Atrial regular; ventricular irregular P:QRS: Typically 2:1, may vary PR interval: Constant PR interval for each QRS conducted QRS complex: 0.04–0.10 sec	Atropine or isoproterenol; pacemaker therapy.
Third-degree AV block (Complete heart block)	Rate: Atrial 60–100 beats per minute; ventricular 15–60 beats per minute Rhythm: Atrial regular; ventricular regular P:QRS: No relationship between P waves and QRS complexes; independent rhythms PR interval: Not measured QRS complex: 0.04–0.10 sec if junctional escape rhythm; > 0.12 sec if ventricular escape rhythm	Immediate pacemaker therapy.

6) Sick sinus syndrome (SSS)
   a) A dysfunction that causes problems with formation, transmission, or conduction of impulses; results from diseases that affect SA node; often found in older clients

b) ECG characteristics of SSS are changes in type of rhythm, pacemaker site and/or rate; client may alternate between: sinus bradycardia or sinus arrhythmia; sinus pauses or sinus arrest; atrial tachydysrhythmias such as atrial fibrillation, atrial flutter, or atrial tachycardia; brady-tachy syndrome (alternating periods of bradycardia and tachycardia)

c) Signs and symptoms of SSS: dizziness, light-headedness, syncope, fatigue or other signs of decreased CO

b. Atrial dysrhythmias

1) Impulse originates in atrial tissue (ectopic) outside normal conduction system (SA node)

2) Premature atrial contraction (PAC): ectopic beat that comes early in cycle with same configuration as normal beats; usually asymptomatic and benign

3) Atrial tachycardia (AT) or paroxysmal supraventricular tachycardia (PSVT)

a) Fast rate with unidentifiable P wave, normal P wave or P wave with a different configuration

b) Has sudden onset and sudden termination; usually related to reentry mechanism around AV node; seen more often in females

c) Signs and symptoms: palpitations, "racing" heart, anxiety, dizziness, dyspnea, angina pain, diaphoresis, extreme fatigue, polyuria

4) Atrial flutter

a) Usually regular rhythm (but may be irregular) with saw-toothed flutter or F waves instead of P waves; thought to result from intra-atrial reentry mechanism

b) Signs and symptoms: asymptomatic, palpitations or "fluttering" in chest; if rapid ventricular response is present, signs of decreased CO occur because of loss of "atrial kick" and decreased ventricular filling time

5) Atrial fibrillation (A-fib)

a) Chaotic atrial electrical activity causing atria to quiver instead of contract normally; may be intermittent or chronic

b) Rapid impulses firing from atrial wall bombard AV node, resulting in a wavy baseline between QRS complexes (no P waves), and an irregular ventricular response

c) Clinical signs and symptoms depend on ventricular response: signs and symptoms of decreased CO, hypotension, shortness of breath, fatigue, angina, syncope, HF; peripheral pulses will be irregular and variable in quality

d) High risk for thromboemboli formation due to pooling of blood in atria and absence of "atrial kick"; should be managed aggressively

c. Ventricular dysrhythmias

1) All originate in ventricles; denoted by wide and bizarre QRS complexes longer than 0.12 second in duration with increased amplitude, abnormal S-T segment, and a T wave that has an opposite deflection from QRS complex; P waves have no relationship to QRS complexes

2) Premature ventricular contraction (PVC)

a) Most common dysrhythmia; occurs early in cardiac cycle; common and usually clinically insignificant in older adults

b) Incidence is greatest following myocardial ischemia, MI, hypertrophy, or infection

c) May be unifocal (coming from one site) or multifocal (coming from different sites in ventricular wall)

d) May come in patterns: bigeminy—every other beat is a PVC; trigeminy—every third beat is PVC; couplets—2 beats together

e) Danger signs include PVCs that are frequent (greater than 6/min, multifocal, occurring in couplets or pairs, and R on T (PVC occurs on T wave of preceding beat); these indicate myocardial irritability and may precipitate lethal dys-rhythmias

    f) Signs and symptoms: may be asymptomatic; client may feel "skipped beats," chest discomfort, dyspnea, or dizziness; hypotension can occur

3) Ventricular tachycardia (V tach or VT)

    a) Defined as 3 or more consecutive PVCs; can be short burst or sustained rhythm; usually regular with a rate greater than 100 beats per minute

    b) Reentry mechanism is usual cause

    c) Signs and symptoms: fluttering in chest, palpitations, shortness of breath, signs of decreased CO, hypotension, loss of consciousness, no palpable pulses, may soon deteriorate into lethal rhythm

4) Ventricular fibrillation (VF, V-fib)

    a) Rapid chaotic ventricular rhythm causing ventricles to quiver; heart does not pump; cardiac arrest occurs and leads to death without effective treatment

    b) Effective treatment: defibrillation and cardiopulmonary resuscitation (CPR)

    c) ECG shows chaotic irregular wavy lines with no discernable rate or rhythm

5) Idioventricular rhythm

    a) Normal complexes are not present; P waves, if present, are not associated with QRS; QRS wide and bizarre like a PVC; overall rate slow (20–40 beats per minute)

    b) Lethal dysrhythmia; may follow defibrillation, V-fib or V tach

    c) Signs and symptoms: decreased CO, usually unconscious

d. Atrioventricular conduction blocks (heart blocks)

    1) Conduction defects that delay or block transmission of sinus impulse through AV node; may be from injured or diseased SA node or AV node or because of increased vagal tone; may be benign or severe but should be monitored for progression to a more severe level of block

    2) First-degree AV block

        a) Benign condition and is not considered a true block

        b) Prolonged but constant PR interval (greater than 0.20 sec) in duration, otherwise normal sinus rhythm (see Table 2-7)

        c) Usually asymptomatic; can progress to higher level block

    3) Second-degree AV block: Mobitz Type I (Wenckebach)

        a) Tip to remember: "W"enckebach and "w"eird pattern

        b) Cyclic pattern of complexes with a progressively prolonging PR interval until one QRS is totally blocked or dropped (see Table 2-7)

        c) Signs and symptoms: asymptomatic; if rate drops, then signs and symptoms of decreased CO would occur

    4) Second-degree AV block: Mobitz Type II or classical

        a) Usually seen in CHD and anterior wall MI

        b) Nonconducted impulses usually occurring in a regular manner; must have more P waves than QRS complexes (can have several Ps to each QRS)

        c) PR interval is constant (see Table 2-7)

        d) Signs and symptoms depend on ventricular rate

Table 2-7   **Determining the Type of Heart Block**

PR Interval Is Constant	PR Interval Is NOT Constant
First-degree heart block—PR interval > 0.20	Second-degree heart block—Type I, Mobitz I, Wenckebach
Second-degree heart block—Type II, Mobitz II, Classical	Third-degree heart block

        5) Third-degree AV block (complete heart block)

          a) SA node fires, P waves are regular but do not conduct through AV node; ventricular rhythm (QRS) will be regular but QRS is unrelated to P wave; may or may not have more Ps than QRSs; PR interval constantly varies (see Table 2-7)

          b) Signs and symptoms associated with bradycardia and decreased CO: light-headedness, confusion, syncope

          c) Requires intervention, can be life-threatening

C. Artificial pacemaker rhythms (following pacemaker insertion)

    1. Pacemaker can be atrial (paces atrium), ventricular (paces ventricle) or A-V sequential (paces dual atrial and ventricular chambers)

    2. Demand pacemaker: set at a rate that is individualized for each client; should begin to fire when client's own HR drops to or below set rate

    3. Types

        a. Atrial pacemaker: spike occurs before each P wave while in demand mode

        b. Ventricular pacemaker: spike occurs before each QRS wave while in demand mode

        c. A-V sequential: 2 spikes occur while in demand mode; 1 before P wave and 1 before QRS

    4. Problems encountered

        a. Failure to sense or undersensing: pacemaker does not sense client's own rhythm and continues to send an impulse; ECG will show spike at regular intervals throughout client's regular rhythm

        b. Failure to pace or oversensing: pacemaker fails to begin firing when HR drops below set rate; ECG may show whatever baseline rhythm caused need for pacemaker insertion

        c. Noncapture (pacemaker fires in a regular pattern but ventricle does not depolarize); ECG shows pacemaker spikes with no QRS following spike

D. Nursing assessment

    1. Nursing assessment includes VS, symptoms of decreased CO; analysis of monitor pattern for rate, rhythm, assessment of P wave morphology, calculation of intervals; assessment of S-T segment, determination of rhythm

    2. Diagnostic tests: 12-lead ECG; single-lead telemetry (usually lead II); electrophysiologic studies

        a. No specific laboratory test for cardiac dysrhythmias

        b. Laboratory tests may be helpful in determining cause of dysrhythmia, such as hypoxia, electrolyte imbalances, acid-base imbalances, or drug levels

E. Nursing management

    1. Medications: antidysrhythmic drugs (see Table 2-8); magnesium if level is low

    2. Recognize NSR as well as knowledge of dysrhythmias

    3. Observe monitoring system and use rapid decision making process

    4. Engage in collaborative care with health care provider; standing orders are needed for lethal dysrhythmias

    5. Administer O_2 as necessary

    6. Countershock

        a. Used to interrupt cardiac rhythms that compromise CO; causes simultaneous depolarization of all cardiac cells, obliterating dysrhythmia and allowing SA node to resume normal rhythm

        b. Two types of countershock

          1) Defibrillation: emergency treatment for ventricular fibrillation; the quicker the delivery of shock, the higher the survival rate; place paddles or pads at base and apex of heart

Practice to Pass

The client is on telemetry monitoring showing a normal sinus rhythm with a rate of 82 beats per minute. The alarm sounds and the monitor shows chaotic activity on the screen. What should the nurse's actions include?

Table 2-8 Antidysrhythmic Drug Classifications

Class	Group	Action	Common Drugs
I	Sodium channel blockers Class I-A	Prolong action potential, reduce automaticity	Quinidine sulfate (Quinidine), quinidine polygalacturonate (Cardioquin), procainamide (Pronestyl), disopyramide (Norpace)
	Class I-B	↓ refractory period, slow conduction velocity	Lidocaine (Xylocaine), mexiletine (Mexitil), tocainide (Tonocard), phenytoin (Dilantin)
	Class I-C	↓ automaticity and conduction through AV node	Flecainide (Tambocor), propafenone (Rythmol)
II	Beta blockers	↓ automaticity and conduction through AV node, lower BP	Esmolol (Brevibloc), propranolol (Inderal), acebutolol (Sectral)
III	Potassium channel blockers	Prolong repolarization and refractory period; ↓ intraventricular conduction	Sotalol (Betapace), amiodarone (Cordarone), dofetilide (Tikosyn)
IV	Calcium channel blockers	Block calcium influx across myocardial cell; negative dromotropic effect, lower BP and HR	Verapamil hydrochloride (Isoptin), nifedipine (Procardia), diltiazem (Cardizem)
V	Miscellaneous antidysrhythmics	↓ automaticity, slow conduction through AV node	Adenosine (Adenocard), digoxin (Lanoxin), ibutilide (Corvert)

2) Synchronized cardioversion: countershock synchronized with R wave so that heart is totally depolarized at same time (allows all cells to repolarize at same time) and SA node can resume sinus rhythm; also used as an electrical procedure to treat tachydysrhythmias (atrial fibrillation, atrial flutter, supraventricular tachycardia, stable ventricular tachycardia)

7. Implantable cardioverter-defibrillator (ICD) can be surgically implanted to detect life-threatening changes in rhythm; device will automatically deliver an electric shock to convert rhythm; ICDs are useful in preventing sudden death due to ventricular fibrillation

8. Pacemakers

a. Temporary pacemakers are used after surgery (particularly CABG) or during a code situation for emergency pacing; an external pulse generator is used

b. Permanent pacemakers are surgically implanted to treat acute and chronic conduction defects; these are primarily used for bradydysrhythmias, but are available for use with tachyarrhythmias

VI. INFLAMMATORY DISEASES OF HEART

A. Overview

1. Inflammatory diseases of heart are defined as inflammation of any layer of cardiac tissue (endocardium, myocardium, pericardium) that can damage valves, muscle, or pericardial lining

2. Conditions include rheumatic heart disease, endocarditis, myocarditis, and pericarditis

3. Causes

a. Rheumatic heart disease: *Beta-hemolytic streptococcus* bacteria

b. Infective endocarditis: bacterial infection or abnormal immunological reaction

c. Myocarditis: viral, bacterial, or fungal infection, often *Coxsackie virus*

d. Pericarditis: cardiac trauma, MI, infection, neoplasm, kidney disease, rheumatic fever

B. Pathophysiology

1. Rheumatic heart disease (RHD)

a. A chronic condition characterized by valvular deformity that slowly progresses; follows an acute or repeated episode of rheumatic fever (inflammatory disease from a *Beta-hemolytic streptococcus*)

b. In acute stage, valves become red, swollen, and inflamed with lesions developing on leaflets

   c. In chronic stage, scar tissue develops, leaflets become rigid and deformed; stenosis or regurgitation may develop
   d. Left heart valves are affected more often; mitral valve most often
   e. Signs and symptoms of RHD: precordial chest discomfort, tachycardia, cardiomegaly, evidence of HF, pericardial friction rub (leathery, grating sound), pericardial effusion, S_3 (atrial gallop) or S_4 (ventricular gallop), possible murmur from mitral or aortic regurgitation

2. Infective endocarditis
   a. Defined as inflammation of lining of heart; involves any part of endothelial lining of heart, most often mitral valve
   b. *Staphylococcus aureus* is usual infective organism
   c. Acute and subacute classifications exist
   d. Begins with platelet—fibrin vegetation on healthy valves (acute) and on damaged valves or endocardial tissue (subacute)
   e. Signs and symptoms of infective endocarditis: murmur, cough, shortness of breath, anorexia, abdominal pain, anemia, splenomegaly, fever (greater than 101.5°F), chills, night sweats, flulike symptoms, joint pain, and petechiae

3. **Myocarditis**
   a. Defined as an inflammatory disorder of heart muscle that is unrelated to CHD or MI
   b. Infection can be caused by viruses, bacteria, or protozoa; immunologic response can be due to effects of radiation, chemical poisons, drugs, burns, or *Coxsackie B enterovirus* (most common in United States)
   c. Inflammatory process causes local or diffuse swelling and damage to myocardial cells, abscesses in interstitial tissue from infectious agents; pinpoint hemorrhage in layers of heart
   d. If condition deteriorates, could lead to dilated cardiomyopathy
   e. Results in weakening of heart muscle and decreased contractility
   f. Signs and symptoms depend on degree of cardiac damage
      1) May be asymptomatic at first
      2) Signs of inflammation: fever, chills, fatigue, malaise, dyspnea, palpitations, arthralgias
      3) Signs of HF: tachycardia, dysrhythmias, S_3 or S_4 gallop, systolic murmur, transient pericardial friction rub, cardiomegaly, and ECG abnormalities

4. **Pericarditis**
   a. Defined as an inflammation of pericardium (fluid-filled sac surrounding heart)
   b. May be primary or secondary to other disease processes; usually viral; affects more men than women
   c. Frequent complication of end stage renal failure; frequently seen after MI or following cardiac surgery
   d. When inflammatory mediators are released, vasodilation occurs, causing hyperemia (increased blood flow) and edema
   e. Increased capillary permeability allows plasma proteins and fibrinogen to gather in pericardial space
   f. Exudate is formed that may contain RBCs or be purulent if infective
   g. Fibrosis and scarring may restrict heart's ability to function effectively; pericardial effusions may develop
   h. Chest pain occurs due to inflammation of nerve fibers in pericardium
   i. Acute pericarditis lasts 2 to 6 weeks
   j. Signs and symptoms
      1) Sharp chest pain (rapid onset) worsening with deep breath, cough or change in position; pain improves if elevated or sits up
      2) Dyspnea and dry cough

   3) Fever (low grade)

   4) Pericardial friction rub heard most commonly on expiration

   k. Complications include cardiac tamponade or pericardial effusions

C. Nursing assessment

1. Assessment

   a. Rheumatic fever: VS, lung sounds, heart sounds, apical pulse, symptom analysis of any chest discomfort

   b. Infective endocarditis: VS, symptom analysis of complaints, nutritional status, palpate spleen, skin assessment for bleeding; heart sounds, peripheral pulses, capillary refill

   c. Myocarditis: VS, symptom analysis of complaints and pain, ECG pattern, heart sounds

   d. Pericarditis: VS, symptom analysis of pain and what worsens or relieves it, lung sounds, respiratory status

2. Diagnostic tests

   a. Rheumatic fever: CBC, C-reactive protein (show inflammation), erythrocyte sedimentation rate (ESR), antistreptolysin (ASO) titer

   b. Infective endocarditis: CBC, immune testing, blood cultures, urine (increased creatinine, protein, and hematuria), ECG

   c. Myocarditis: ESR, CBC, antiviral antibodies, ECG, heart catheterization with biopsy of heart muscle, serum immunoglobulins, cultures

   d. Pericarditis: ESR, ECG, echocardiogram, hemodynamic monitoring, CXR, CT scan, and MRI

D. Nursing management

1. Medications

   a. Rheumatic fever: antibiotics, salicylates (aspirin), or corticosteroids for inflammation and joint pain

   b. Infective endocarditis: antibiotics (may use multiple drugs), antipyretics, anti-inflammatory agents

   c. Myocarditis: antipyretics, antidysrhythmics, anticoagulants, digoxin (Lanoxin) if HF occurs, corticosteroids or immunosuppressive drugs, antimicrobial agents

   d. Pericarditis: non-narcotic analgesics, NSAIDs, antipyretics, corticosteroids

2. Provide supportive care, emotional rest

3. Prevent complications and future recurrences; IV therapy if indicated

4. Monitor VS, heart sounds, ECG pattern, respiratory status

5. Priorities of nursing care

   a. Assess and treat pain

   b. Assist with ADLs; allow rest periods

   c. Provide diversional activity

   d. Monitor for signs of infection

   e. Monitor for signs of decreased CO

   f. Teach client importance of compliance and taking antibiotics until completed

   g. Teach client effective coping mechanisms

6. With myocarditis, client needs to decrease workload and increase O_2 supply to heart

7. Pericarditis may require a pericardiocentesis (removal of fluid) or surgery

8. Administer O_2 as needed

VII. VALVULAR HEART DISEASE

A. Overview

1. Valvular heart disease is defined as diseases or conditions that interfere with unidirectional blood flow in heart

2. Can be acquired from either acute (endocarditis or calcium deposits) or chronic (rheumatic heart disease) conditions

3. Occurs as **stenosis** (inability of leaflets to open and close properly) or **regurgitation** (backflow of blood through a valve that cannot close properly due to damage or disease)
4. Other causes include MI and congenital heart defects

B. **Pathophysiology**
   1. Stenosis
      a. Involves fusion of valve leaflets producing a narrow opening and rigidity
      b. Fusion may result from scarring of valves caused by endocarditis, MI, or calcification
      c. Blood flow is impeded resulting in decreased CO and impaired ventricular filling, ejection fraction, and stroke volume
      d. Can affect mitral, tricuspid, aortic, or pulmonary valve
   2. Regurgitation
      a. Caused by insufficient or incompetent valves causing incomplete closure, allowing backflow of blood
      b. Result from deformity or erosion of valve by vegetative lesions of bacterial endocarditis; scarring or tearing from MI; cardiac dilation—as heart enlarges, valves stretch; leaflets no longer meet, causing regurgitation

   3. Hemodynamic changes occur
      a. Blood volume and pressure are reduced in front of affected valve
      b. Volume and pressure increase behind affected valve
   4. Chambers behind affected valve hypertrophy due to increased pressure; CO falls as compensatory mechanisms become ineffective; heart begins to fail
      a. Increased muscle size leads to increased O_2 demand
      b. Decreased blood supply to enlarged muscle leads to HF
      c. Infarction occurs and loss of functional muscle
   5. Affects aortic and mitral valve; **mitral valve prolapse** occurs when mitral valve prolapses back into atrium causing regurgitation of blood from ventricle to atrium
   6. Signs and symptoms
      a. Stenosis: pulmonary congestion, dyspnea, pulmonary hypertension, dizziness, fatigue, tachycardia, murmur or rub, S_3 or S_4 heart sound, angina; pulmonary stenosis may cause venous distention and swelling of ankles
      b. Regurgitation
         1) Mitral: dyspnea, pulmonary hypertension, decreased CO, dizziness and fatigue, tachycardia, angina, murmur or rub, S_3 or S_4 heart sound
         2) Aortic: wide pulse pressure, hyperkinetic (strong, bounding) peripheral pulses, signs and symptoms of CHF, angina

C. **Nursing assessment**
   1. Assessment includes: VS, heart sounds, lung sounds, symptom analysis of complaints and pain, respiratory status, exercise tolerance, presence of edema, peripheral pulses
   2. Diagnostic tests: ECG, echocardiogram, CXR, cardiac catheterization

D. **Nursing management**
   1. Medications include digoxin (Lanoxin), diuretics, Class I or III antidysrhythmics, prophylactic antibiotics before invasive procedures
   2. Close observation for progression of disease, angina that might occur
   3. Monitor prophylactic therapy to prevent infection of diseased valves
   4. Observe for signs and symptoms of CHF; treat as necessary
   5. Teach client not to abruptly stop taking beta blockers or symptoms may return
   6. Prepare client for and monitor following percutaneous balloon valvuloplasty, if indicated
   7. Provide pre- and postoperative teaching if medical treatment no longer effective and surgical intervention is necessary

Practice to Pass

The client has been diagnosed with mitral prolapse. What should the nurse teach the client regarding treatment plans?

Case Study

M. J. presents to the emergency department with complaints of substernal crushing chest pain radiating to his left arm. He is a 58-year-old executive. He was having dinner with a client when the pain began. He states the pain started 2 hours ago and has been increasing in intensity since that time.

1. What type of assessment should the nurse do?

2. What parts of his past medical history would be important?

3. What diagnostic studies should the nurse anticipate the health care provider ordering?

4. What medications should the nurse anticipate being ordered for his chest pain?

5. What ECG changes should the nurse look for?

For suggested responses, see pages 461–462.

POSTTEST

1 The client on a telemetry unit exhibits cardiac rhythm strip complexes of normal duration and a heart rate of 82 beats/min. In assessing the client, the nurse notes that for each complex there is a corresponding palpable pulse. What conclusion should the nurse draw?

1. Ventricles are contracting regularly.
2. Ventricles are in fibrillation.
3. Client has ventricular tachycardia.
4. Atria are not contracting.

2 The client arrives in the emergency department with a heart rate of 130. The client appears anxious and is tachypneic. The nurse interprets that what physiological mechanism is most likely responsible for the increased heart rate?

1. Parasympathetic nervous system (PNS) activity
2. Sympathetic nervous system (SNS) activity
3. Increase in circulating acetylcholine
4. Decrease in circulating catecholamines

3 The client arrives in the emergency department with a diagnosis of right-sided heart failure. What clinical manifestations should the nurse expect to assess in this client? Select all that apply.

1. Distended neck veins
2. Pitting edema in the feet and ankles
3. Crackles in the lungs
4. Abdominal ascites
5. Reflex bradycardia with activity

4 A client with a history of angina pectoris is given nitroglycerin (NTG) 0.4 mg by the sublingual route for chest pain. Prior to the NTG dose, the blood pressure was 110/78. After 5 minutes, the client says the chest pain is better but not gone. The nurse should anticipate performing which nursing actions? Select all that apply.

1. Giving another nitroglycerin (NTG) tablet.
2. Checking the pulse rate.
3. Checking for a prescription to administer morphine sulfate.
4. Checking the blood pressure (BP).
5. Comparing pre- and post-nitroglycerin (NTG) BP.

POSTTEST

5 A client with congestive heart failure has digoxin (Lanoxin) ordered every day. Prior to giving the medication, the nurse assesses that the digoxin level is 1.2 ng/mL and auscultates a 1-minute apical pulse rate of 62. What action should the nurse take?

1. Withhold the digoxin.
2. Withhold the dose and request an order for a potassium level.
3. Notify the health care provider.
4. Give the digoxin as ordered.

6 Which of the following clients is at high risk for developing coronary heart disease (CHD) that may not be responsive to diet and exercise alone? Select all that apply.

1. A client who has diabetes mellitus
2. A client who has a strong family history of cardiovascular disease
3. A client who is overweight
4. A client who had a hemorrhagic stroke at age 40
5. A client who is 73 years old

7 The client presents to the emergency department with substernal chest pain and is diagnosed with a subendocardial myocardial infarction (MI). The client asks the nurse what that means. What information should the nurse include when responding to the client about the myocardial damage?

1. It is located on the anterior wall of the left ventricle.
2. It is located on the posterior wall of the left ventricle.
3. It involves the full thickness of the wall.
4. It involves the inner layer of the heart.

8 The client is admitted to the coronary care unit (CCU) with a diagnosis of left-sided heart failure. When listening to lung sounds, the nurse hears crackles bilaterally. The nurse concludes that this is an expected finding because left-ventricular failure leads to which of the following?

1. Increased coronary artery perfusion
2. Pulmonary emboli
3. Increased peripheral resistance
4. Pulmonary congestion

9 The client with a diagnosis of anterior wall myocardial infarction (MI) begins to show dysrhythmias on the cardiac monitor. The nurse anticipates that the client is most at risk for which dysrhythmias based on the location of the MI? Select all that apply.

1. Ventricular fibrillation
2. Atrioventricular (AV) block
3. Atrial fibrillation
4. Premature ventricular contractions (PVCs)
5. Sinus bradycardia

10 The client who experienced a myocardial infarction (MI) is being discharged from the hospital. What important self-care measures should the nurse teach the client to reduce the risk of reinfarction? Select all that apply.

1. Comply with ongoing thrombolytic therapy.
2. Increase exercise to include activities like high-intensity aerobics.
3. Consume a low-fat, low-sodium diet.
4. Use resources provided to attempt smoking cessation.
5. Eliminate all alcohol intake.

➤ *See pages 65–67 for Answers and Rationales.*

POSTTEST

ANSWERS & RATIONALES

Pretest

1 **Answer: 3** **Rationale:** Angina pectoris is a term used to describe chest pain or pressure that is intermittent and associated with myocardial ischemia. The presence of ischemia and subsequent angina are exacerbated with increased cardiac workload such as exercise. Discomfort and pain from pericardial effusion is not caused by activity. Acute onset of dyspnea would result from pulmonary edema; pain may or may not be present. Pain related to a pulmonary embolus is sudden and not necessarily related to activity. **Cognitive Level:** Applying **Client Need:** Physiological Adaptation **Integrated Process:** Nursing Process: Assessment **Content Area:** Adult Health **Strategy:** Consider the activity of the client at the time of the pain. Narrow the choices by eliminating some of the options in which pain is not associated with exertion. **Reference:** Braun, C.A., & Anderson, C. M. (2010). *Pathophysiology: A clinical approach.* Baltimore, MD: Lippincott Williams & Wilkins, p. 579.

2 **Answer: 2** **Rationale:** Orthopnea is dyspnea that occurs when an individual lies flat and is common in clients with peripheral edema. Lying down redistributes body water, causes abdominal contents to exert pressure on the diaphragm and significantly decreases the efficiency of respiratory muscles. The client may have beginning signs of congestive heart failure and should be checked. Sleep apnea may cause orthopnea but not edema; angina pectoris does not necessarily cause edema, but chest pain would be a hallmark of this health problem. Sinus infections do not cause edema. **Cognitive Level:** Analyzing **Client Need:** Physiological Adaptation **Integrated Process:** Nursing Process: Diagnosis **Content Area:** Adult Health **Strategy:** Note the critical word *edema* and use knowledge of concepts of fluid movement and cardiovascular system to answer this question. Note that the question focuses on respiratory manifestations. Consider the interrelationship between the cardiovascular and respiratory systems to aid in making a selection. **Reference:** Huether, S.E., & McCance, K. L. (2012). *Understanding pathophysiology* (5th ed.). St. Louis, MO: Elsevier, Inc., p. 679.

3 **Answer: 2** **Rationale:** Left ventricular failure impedes the flow of blood from pulmonary vessels into the left side of the heart. This leads to pulmonary congestion and increases cardiac workload as the right side of the heart must pump against higher pulmonary pressures. Signs of left ventricular failure include dyspnea, orthopnea, cough or frothy sputum, fatigue, decreased urine output

and edema. Hypertension is often silent. Coronary artery disease (CAD) often manifests with chest pain called angina pectoris. Peripheral vascular disease (PVD) is characterized by leg pain while ambulating. **Cognitive Level:** Analyzing **Client Need:** Physiological Adaptation **Integrated Process:** Nursing Process: Assessment **Content Area:** Adult Health **Strategy:** Remember Left and Lung—the two Ls go together; two of the symptoms deal with respiratory symptoms and none of the other answers are related to a diagnosis affecting the lungs. **Reference:** Huether, S.E., & McCance, K. L. (2012). *Understanding pathophysiology* (5th. ed.). St. Louis, MO: Elsevier, Inc., pp. 623–625.

4 **Answer: 3** **Rationale:** Electrocardiography is a critical tool for the diagnosis of myocardial ischemia. Depressed S-T segments and inverted T waves represent myocardial ischemia in the leads that correspond with the area of the heart affected. Necrosis results from pathological Q waves. An S-T segment elevation represents injury. Bradycardia is characterized by a heart rate less than 60 beats per minute. **Cognitive Level:** Applying **Client Need:** Physiological Adaptation **Integrated Process:** Nursing Process: Diagnosis **Content Area:** Adult Health **Strategy:** Read the question carefully, noting the critical words *S-T segment depression.* Apply principles of electrocardiography to determine the etiology. **Reference:** Huether, S.E., & McCance, K. L. (2012). *Understanding pathophysiology* (5th ed.). St. Louis, MO: Elsevier Inc., pp. 602–603.

5 **Answers: 1, 3, 4, 5** **Rationale:** The initial failure originates on the left side, but right heart failure is a long term result when an increase in left ventricular filling pressure is reflected back into the pulmonary circulation. The right ventricle is not prepared to compensate for the increased afterload and fails as a result, and pressure rises in the venous circulation, resulting in increased peripheral edema. The effect of heart failure leads to a decrease in peripheral blood flow and perfusion. **Cognitive Level:** Analyzing **Client Need:** Physiological Adaptation **Integrated Process:** Nursing Process: Diagnosis **Content Area:** Adult Health **Strategy:** Consider the pathophysiology of left-sided heart failure. When the blood does not move from the left side, what is the chain of events? **Reference:** Huether, S.E., & McCance, K. L. (2012). *Understanding pathophysiology* (5th ed.). St. Louis, MO: Elsevier, Inc., pp. 626–627.

6 **Answer: 1** **Rationale:** Normal sinus rhythm (NSR) is a normal heart rhythm in which impulses originate in the sinoatrial node and has a rate of 60–100 beats/min. in an adult. Sinus bradycardia is a regular rhythm with a rate under 60 beats/min. Sinus tachycardia is a regular rhythm with a rate of 101 to 150 beats/min. Sinus arrhythmia is an irregular rhythm varying with respiration, with a rate of 60 to 100 beats/min. Accelerated nodal rhythm is an increase of a nodal rate ranging from 60 to 100 beats/min. **Cognitive Level:** Applying **Client Need:** Physiological Adaptation **Integrated Process:** Communication and Documentation **Content Area:** Adult Health **Strategy:** Consider the features of each rhythm represented in the options and make an association between the critical data *54 beats/min* and the word *bradycardia* in the correct option. **Reference:** LeMone, P., Burke, K., & Bauldoff, G. (2012). *Medical-surgical nursing: Critical thinking in patient care* (5th ed.). Upper Saddle River, NJ: Pearson Education, pp. 946–947.

7 **Answer: 4** **Rationale:** Myocardial Infarction (MI) results when there is prolonged ischemia causing irreversible damage to the heart muscle. Clients who suffer unstable angina are at risk for myocardial infarction. Development of pathologic Q waves is seen in the electrocardiogram (ECG), therefore immediate focused attention is needed for this client. Gangrene and infection would not be seen on ECG. Ischemia would reflect an inverted T wave in the affected area of the heart on the ECG. **Cognitive Level:** Analyzing **Client Need:** Reduction of Risk Potential **Integrated Process:** Nursing Process: Assessment **Content Area:** Adult Health **Strategy:** Review electrocardiogram (ECG) and physiological changes following acute myocardial infarction (MI). One option best fits the pathophysiology of MI even if the ECG changes are unfamiliar. **Reference:** Huether, S.E., & McCance, K. L. (2012). *Understanding pathophysiology* (5th ed.). St. Louis, MO: Elsevier Inc., pp. 606–608.

8 **Answer: 1** **Rationale:** A myocardial infarction (MI) is caused by an occlusion of a coronary artery which blocks the coronary blood flow and prevents oxygen from reaching the myocardium. Spasm of a coronary artery with a temporary decrease in blood supply is characteristic of Prinzmetal (variant) angina. A slow heart rate leading to a decreased blood supply to the myocardium describes either bradycardia or atrioventricular (AV) heart block. Dilation of the ventricular wall can occur with ventricular hypertrophy. **Cognitive Level:** Applying **Client Need:** Physiological Adaptation **Integrated Process:** Nursing Process: Implementation **Content Area:** Adult Health **Strategy:** Only 1 option describes the pathophysiology of myocardial infarction (MI). Use knowledge of this pathophysiology and the process of elimination to make a selection. **Reference:** LeMone, P. Burke, K., & Bauldoff, G. (2012). *Medical-surgical nursing: Critical thinking in patient care* (5th ed.). Upper Saddle River,

NJ: Pearson Education, Inc., pp. 946–950. Huether, S.E., & McCance, K. L. (2012). *Understanding pathophysiology* (5th ed.). St. Louis, MO: Elsevier, Inc., pp. 604–605.

9 **Answer: 4** **Rationale:** Sedentary lifestyle and obesity are modifiable risk factors that are associated with atherosclerosis. Therefore, they would have high priority when the nurse is conducting client teaching. Age and gender are nonmodifiable risk factors; cannot be changed, therefore are the lowest priority when the nurse is conducting client teaching. Hyperlipidemia (total cholesterol over 200 mg/dL) may be changed by modifying behavior, but a value of 199 is just within normal range. Use of chewing tobacco is associated with increased risk of oral cancer. **Cognitive Level:** Analyzing **Client Need:** Health Promotion and Maintenance **Integrated Process:** Nursing Process: Planning **Content Area:** Adult Health **Strategy:** Note the presence of the critical words *highest priority* in the stem, which means the correct option is one that is either the most significant option or is able to be changed. Use this information and the process of elimination to make a selection. **Reference:** LeMone, P. Burke, K., & Bauldoff, G. (2012). *Medical-surgical nursing: Critical thinking in patient care* (5th ed.). Upper Saddle River, NJ: Pearson Education, Inc., pp. 912–913.

10 **Answer: 4** **Rationale:** A prophylactic dose of nitroglycerin before engaging in activities that precipitate angina (such as climbing stairs, sexual intercourse) helps maintain cardiac perfusion when increased work is anticipated, preventing ischemia and chest pain. Performing activities despite angina is dangerous. Avoiding activities and leading a sedentary lifestyle should not be a recommendation. **Cognitive Level:** Applying **Client Need:** Physiological Adaptation **Integrated Process:** Nursing Process: Planning **Content Area:** Adult Health **Strategy:** Choose a client-centered answer that allows the client to manage the disease. **Reference:** LeMone, P. Burke, K., & Bauldoff, G. (2012). *Medical-surgical nursing: Critical thinking in patient care* (5th ed.). Upper Saddle River, NJ: Pearson Education, Inc., pp. 924–925.

Posttest

1 **Answer: 1** **Rationale:** Depolarization of the myocardium results in contraction (systole) and that produces the palpable pulse and the corresponding QRS complex on the cardiac rhythm strip. This heart is beating regularly at 82 beats per minute. Ventricular fibrillation does not produce a pulse. Ventricular tachycardia is characterized by a rate greater than 100 beats/min. Atrial activity cannot be assessed from the information given. **Cognitive Level:** Applying **Client Need:** Reduction of Risk Potential **Integrated Process:** Nursing Process: Diagnosis **Content Area:**

Adult Health **Strategy:** Identify equally plausible options and eliminate them because the correct answer must be an option that is better than the others. **Reference:** LeMone, P. Burke, K., & Bauldoff, G. (2012). *Medical-surgical nursing: Critical thinking in patient care* (5th ed.). Upper Saddle River, NJ: Pearson Education, Inc., pp. 891–892, 947–949.

2 **Answer: 2** **Rationale:** Stimulation of the sympathetic nervous system (SNS) increases heart rate, blood pressure, and respiratory rate. The SNS is mediated by epinephrine and norepinephrine, which are catecholamines. The parasympathetic nervous system (PNS) is mediated by acetylcholine and decreases the heart rate. **Cognitive Level:** Applying **Client Need:** Physiological Adaptation **Integrated Process:** Nursing Process: Diagnosis **Content Area:** Adult Health **Strategy:** Note that the client has both rapid breathing (tachypnea) and rapid pulse (tachycardia). Remember the fight-or-flight response is mediated by the sympathetic nervous system and this increases the heart rate. **Reference:** LeMone, P., Burke, K., & Bauldoff, G. (2012). *Medical-surgical nursing: Critical thinking in patient care* (5th ed.). Upper Saddle River, NJ: Pearson Education, Inc., pp. 479, 1019.

3 **Answers: 1, 2, 4** **Rationale:** Right-sided heart failure leads to backward venous congestion, resulting in jugular vein distention, peripheral edema, and portal hypertension leading to abdominal venous congestion and ascites. Crackles are found in left-sided heart failure. Reflex bradycardia with activity does not occur with either left or right heart failure; instead, the heart rate would increase with activity because of increased myocardial demand. **Cognitive Level:** Applying **Client Need:** Physiological Adaptation **Integrated Process:** Nursing Process: Assessment **Content Area:** Adult Health **Strategy:** Remember "R"ight means "R"est of the body, whereas "L"eft means "L"ung in identifying where fluids stagnate. **Reference:** LeMone, P., Burke, K., & Bauldoff, G. (2012). *Medical-surgical nursing: Critical thinking in patient care* (5th ed.). Upper Saddle River, NJ: Pearson Education, Inc., pp. 974–975.

4 **Answers: 1, 4, 5** **Rationale:** The client needs another dose of nitroglycerin (NTG) if the chest pain is still present; however, a BP should be assessed *first*. Vasodilation may lower the BP; however, this client's BP started at 140/78. The nurse should measure BP before and 5 minutes after giving NTG doses and withhold drug if BP is less than 90 or 100 systolic, according to protocol order. If systolic BP is greater than the stated parameter, another NTG can be given. If systolic BP is less than the parameter, the provider should be consulted. The heart rate is not necessarily changed by the NTG. Administration of morphine sulfate should be anticipated only if NTG is not effective after 3 doses. **Cognitive Level:** Analyzing **Client Need:** Pharmacological and Parenteral Therapies

Integrated Process: Nursing Process: Implementation **Content Area:** Adult Health **Strategy:** Note the initial blood pressure and the clue word *first*. The wording of the question indicates that more than one option may be correct. **Reference:** Adams, M., Holland, L., & Urban, C., (2011). *Pharmacology for nurses: A pathophysiologic approach* (3rd ed.). Upper Saddle River, NJ: Pearson Education, Inc., p. 345.

5 **Answer: 4** **Rationale:** The therapeutic serum range for digoxin is 0.5–2 ng/mL. The dose should be given as ordered since the apical pulse rate is greater than 60 per minute. The dose of digoxin should be withheld for a pulse rate less than 60, unless a different specific parameter is ordered by the prescriber. It is not necessary to notify the health care provider or to request an order for a potassium level with the information in the question. **Cognitive Level:** Applying **Client Need:** Pharmacological and Parenteral Therapies **Integrated Process:** Nursing Process: Implementation **Content Area:** Adult Health **Strategy:** Apply nursing standards for administering medications. Compare the heart rate and digoxin level in the stem of the question to normal parameters. **Reference:** Adams, M., Holland, L., & Urban, C., (2011). *Pharmacology for nurses: A pathophysiologic approach* (3rd ed.). Upper Saddle River, NJ: Pearson Education, Inc., p. 331. LeMone, P., Burke, K., & Bauldoff, G. (2012). *Medical-surgical nursing: Critical thinking in patient care* (5th ed.). Upper Saddle River, NJ: Pearson Education, p. 982.

6 **Answers: 2, 5** **Rationale:** Family history (genetics) and age are nonmodifiable risk factors. Although proper diet and exercise are encouraged, these may not be sufficient to lower cholesterol and prevent CHD. Diabetes mellitus or overweight status may relate to risk of CHD but these risks may be more amenable to reduction with diet and exercise. A hemorrhagic stroke can occur because of hypertension, neurological factors such as intracranial aneurysm or arteriovenous malformation, and may not relate to development of CHD. **Cognitive Level:** Analyzing **Client Need:** Physiological Adaptation **Integrated Process:** Nursing Process: Diagnosis **Content Area:** Adult Health **Strategy:** The core issue of the question is identification of the client whose risk factors for CHD may not easily be reduced. Interpret the information in the question to indicate that the answer is a nonmodifiable risk factor. **Reference:** LeMone, P., Burke, K., & Bauldoff, G. (2012). *Medical-surgical nursing: Critical thinking in patient care* (5th ed.). Upper Saddle River, NJ: Pearson Education, pp. 912–914, 924.

7 **Answer: 4** **Rationale:** The inner layer of the heart is referred to as the endocardium, and thus a myocardial infarction (MI) that affects this layer is termed an endocardial MI. An anterior MI would affect the anterior wall of the left ventricle, while a posterior MI would affect the posterior wall of the left ventricle. An MI that affects the full thickness of the myocardial wall is called a transmural MI. **Cognitive Level:** Applying **Client Need:** Physiological Adaptation **Integrated Process:** Nursing Process: Diagnosis **Content Area:** Adult Health **Strategy:** Use knowledge of anatomy and physiology and look for a clue word that indicates the area of the heart involved. **Reference:** LeMone, P., Burke, K., & Bauldoff, G. (2012). *Medicalsurgical nursing: Critical thinking in patient care* (5th ed.). Upper Saddle River, NJ: Pearson Education, pp. 934–935.

8 **Answer: 4** **Rationale:** Left-ventricular failure leads to pulmonary congestion. When the left ventricle fails and has inadequate emptying, congestion occurs in the lungs because blood from the lungs cannot flow freely into the left atrium and ventricle. Coronary perfusion would be decreased rather than increased. Pulmonary emboli typically arise from thrombi in the legs (most common), fat from a bone fracture, air, or amniotic fluid. Increased peripheral vascular resistance may be associated with increased blood pressure. **Cognitive Level:** Applying **Client Need:** Physiological Adaptation **Integrated Process:** Nursing Process: Diagnosis **Content Area:** Adult Health **Strategy:** The question asks for a response to left congestive heart failure (CHF), not an etiology. Distinguish between CHF and pathophysiology because of respiratory or other conditions. **Reference:** LeMone, P., Burke, K., & Bauldoff, G. (2012). *Medical-surgical nursing: Critical thinking in patient care* (5th ed.). Upper Saddle River, NJ: Pearson Education, pp. 974–975.

9 **Answers: 1, 4, 5** **Rationale:** The ischemia causing the myocardial infarction (MI) can also cause the cardiac muscle cells to become irritable and fire early, causing ventricular dysrhythmias. Premature ventricular contractions (PVCs) are common when the anterior wall is affected, and ventricular fibrillation is a dangerous complication (not atrial fibrillation). Sinus bradycardia may occur because of ischemia to the sinoatrial (SA) node. Atrioventricular (AV) block is more likely to

occur when there is ischemia to the AV node, which is more common in clients with an inferior wall MI, with blockage of the right coronary artery that also supplies the AV node in most people. **Cognitive Level:** Applying **Client Need:** Physiological Adaptation **Integrated Process:** Nursing Process: Assessment **Content Area:** Adult Health **Strategy:** Recall the pathophysiology of myocardial infarction (MI) and link this to the underlying anatomy to determine which cardiac dysrhythmias are most likely to occur with an anterior wall MI. **Reference:** LeMone, P., Burke, K., & Bauldoff, G. (2012). *Medicalsurgical nursing: Critical thinking in patient care* (5th ed.). Upper Saddle River, NJ: Pearson Education, pp. 950–953.

10 **Answers: 3, 4** **Rationale:** Anticoagulant therapy with aspirin, not thrombolytic therapy may be recommended. Exercise slows the atherosclerotic process and helps develop collateral circulation to the heart muscle. Smoking cessation reduces further risk for reinfarction. A low-fat, low-sodium diet aids in the reduction of cholesterol and/ or triglycerides that can cause atherosclerosis resulting in development of a myocardial infarction (MI). In middle-aged and older adults, limited alcohol intake may reduce risk for coronary heart disease (CHD). Consumption of no more than 2 drinks per day for men and 1 drink per day for women is recommended. Alcohol intake should be discussed with the health care provider. **Cognitive Level:** Applying **Client Need:** Physiological Adaptation **Integrated Process:** Nursing Process: Implementation **Content Area:** Adult Health **Strategy:** Read the question carefully and note critical words that modify or change the meaning of an option (such as *thrombolytic, highintensity,* and *decrease*). Use knowledge of self-care after discharge and the process of elimination to make your selections. **Reference:** LeMone, P., Burke, K., & Bauldoff, G. (2012). *Medical-surgical nursing: Critical thinking in patient care* (5th ed.). Upper Saddle River, NJ: Pearson Education, pp. 916–917, 924, 945.

References

Adams, M., Josephson, O., & Holland, L. (2011). *Pharmacology for nurses: A pathophysiologic approach* (3rd ed.). Upper Saddle River, NJ: Pearson Education, pp. 282–366.

Ignatavicius, D., & Workman, L. (2012). *Medical surgical nursing: Patient-centered collaborative care* (7th ed.). Philadelphia, PA: W. B. Saunders.

Lewis, S., Heitkemper, M., Dirksen, S., Bucher, L., & Camera, I. (2011). *Medical surgical nursing: Assessment and management of clinical problems* (8th ed.). St. Louis, MO: Elsevier.

McCance, K., & Huether, S. (2009). *Pathophysiology: The biologic basis for disease in adults and children* (6th ed.). St. Louis, MO: Elsevier.

LeMone, P., Burke, K. M., & Bauldoff, G. (2011). *Medical-surgical nursing: Critical thinking in patient care* (5th ed.). Upper Saddle River, NJ: Pearson Education.

Porth, C., & Matfin, G. (2010) *Pathophysiology: Concepts of altered health states* (8th ed.). Philadelphia, PA: Lippincott Williams & Wilkins.

Venes, D., & Thomas, C. (2009). *Taber's cyclopedic medical dictionary* (21st ed.). Philadelphia, PA: F. A. Davis.

Walraven, G. (2010). *Basic arrhythmias* (7th ed.). Upper Saddle River, NJ: Pearson Education.

Wilson, B.A., Shannon, M.T., & Shields, K.M. (2012). *Pearson nurse's drug guide 2012.* Upper Saddle River, NJ: Pearson Education.

ANSWERS & RATIONALES

3 Vascular Health Problems

Chapter Outline

Risk Factors Associated with
  Vascular Health Problems
Hypertension
Peripheral Vascular Disease

Aneurysms
Thrombophlebitis
Varicose Veins

Arteriospastic Disease
  (Raynaud's Disease)
Thromboangiitis Obliterans
  (Buerger's Disease)

NCLEX-RN® Test Prep

Use the accompanying online resource,
NursingReviewsandRationales, to test
yourself with hundreds of NCLEX®-style
practice questions.

Objectives

➤ Define key terms associated with vascular problems.
➤ Identify risk factors associated with development of a vascular
  health problem.
➤ Explain the common etiologies of vascular health problems.
➤ Describe pathophysiologic responses associated with specific
  vascular health problems.
➤ Distinguish between abnormal and normal vascular findings
  obtained from nursing assessment.
➤ Prioritize nursing interventions associated with specific vascular
  health problems.

Review at a Glance

aneurysm a dilatation or an outpouching of a wall of an artery or vein
that can occur anywhere in body
arterial steal a phenomenon that
occurs when arterioles are maximally
dilated because of hypoxia; in order to
meet metabolic needs of tissues, these
arterioles steal from cutaneous and
peripheral vessels, causing client to
be aware of a "pins and needles"
sensation in affected area(s)
chronic venous insufficiency
chronic failure of venous valves to
function, resulting in interference with
venous blood return to heart and production of generalized systemic edema
diastolic pressure of blood against
arterial walls when ventricles of heart
are at rest
embolus a foreign object such as a
piece of a thrombus floating in bloodstream until such time as it becomes
trapped in a vessel

hemodynamics a study of
movement of blood within body
hypertension a blood pressure that
is greater than normal, usually greater
than 140 systolic and 90 diastolic
ischemia a deficiency in supply of
oxygenated blood caused by a circulatory
obstruction to a body part; client experiences considerable pain in affected part
orthostatic hypotension
syncope or dizziness with sudden
position changes, usually from supine to
upright position, because of a drop
in blood pressure
**peripheral vascular resistance
(PVR)** sum of all resistances that body
has within vascular system
pheochromocytoma a tumor that
originates in neural crest cells of sympathetic nervous system and is responsible
for about 0.1–2.0% of cases of hypertension; tumor cells release catecholamines
that cause episodic and sustained heart

palpitations, sweating, headaches, faint-
ing, and hypertensive emergencies
primary hypertension
an elevated blood pressure from unknown
causes that occurs in about 95% of diagnosed hypertensive clients; also known
as idiopathic hypertension or essential
hypertension
primary varicose veins
dilated superficial veins; seldom involves
communicating veins; if valvular
breakdown occurs, it is caused by
hereditary factors
pulse pressure difference between
systolic and diastolic blood pressures;
range of difference is usually 30 to 40 mmHg
secondary hypertension an
elevated blood pressure associated with
pulmonary, circulatory, endocrine, and
renal diseases such as hyperaldosteronism,
pheochromocytoma, Cushing's disease,
diabetes mellitus, coarctation of aorta,
and hyperthyroidism

secondary varicose veins veins that are characterized by venous stasis and chronic venous insufficiency; occurs in deep and communicating veins

systolic pressure of blood against arterial walls when ventricles of heart are contracted

thrombophlebitis inflammation of a vein with clot formation within that vein

thrombus a collection of fibrin, platelets, clotting factors, and cellular elements of blood that attach to interior wall of artery or vein; sometimes, it will occlude a vessel

varicose veins dilated, tortuous leg veins

vasospasm spasm or constriction of a blood vessel

white coat phenomenon hypertension that occurs in a normotensive client when a health care professional measures blood pressure; differentiation between white coat hypertension and secondary hypertension is essential for effective therapy to begin

PRETEST

1 A client at the local health clinic has a blood pressure (BP) of 164/98. The nurse tells the client that which factors are associated with primary hypertension? Select all that apply.

1. An increase in the heart's electrical activity, causing hypertrophy of the left ventricle
2. Glucose intolerance (insulin resistance and diabetes mellitus)
3. Use of some over-the-counter medications
4. Genetic predisposition to hypertension
5. Low dietary intake of potassium, calcium, and magnesium

2 The nurse makes it a priority to measure blood pressure (BP) as part of the administration of which drug to an assigned client at 9:00 a.m.?

1. Sulfinpyrazone (Anturane)
2. Propranolol (Inderal)
3. Glucagon (GlucaGen)
4. Calcitonin (Calcimar)

3 The nurse should discuss which of the following as nonmodifiable risk factors influencing hypertension?

1. Ethnicity and stress
2. Obesity and substance abuse
3. Nutrition and occupation
4. Family history and gender

4 When examining an adult client with a possible diagnosis of hypertension, the nurse should gather data using which of the following methods? Select all that apply.

1. Person is seated and the arm is supported at heart level.
2. Person should not have smoked or ingested any caffeine in the previous 30 minutes.
3. Assessing 2 consecutive readings, 1 immediately after the other.
4. Cuff and Doppler blood pressure in both arms
5. The person must be at rest for 5 minutes.

5 The nurse is teaching a client with Buerger's disease. Which measure in managing the disease is of highest priority for the nurse to include in discussions with this client?

1. Wear gloves if the air is cool to prevent chilling.
2. Avoid wearing flat-heeled shoes.
3. Report severe pain that may require opioid analgesics.
4. Cease smoking.

6 A hypertensive client exhibits nonadherence to the care regimen after hospital discharge. The home care nurse considers that this client's behavior is likely to be influenced by which of the following factors? Select all that apply.

1. Medication not working as indicated by the client statement, "I don't feel any different."
2. Antihypertensive drug causes unpleasant side effects.
3. Many lifestyle changes needed in diet, exercise, and smoking patterns seem overwhelming.
4. Client has helped in planning goals and treatment.
5. Client often does not feel symptoms of high blood pressure and does not know pressure is elevated.

7 Which of the following clients has the greatest risk of developing a thromboembolism?

1. 20-year-old client
2. Client with a cardiac disease
3. Female client
4. Client with known kidney disease

8 The nurse anticipates that the management of deep vein thrombosis (DVT) in an assigned client will include which of the following? Select all that apply.

1. Orders for anticoagulant therapy to inhibit clotting factors
2. Keeping the client's legs in any position of comfort
3. Using low molecular weight heparin (LMWH) once confirmed diagnosis exists
4. Elevating head of the bed 6 inches on wooden blocks
5. Ensure that the affected area is not rubbed or massaged.

9 A 68-year-old client enters the emergency department with reports of back pain and fatigue. His blood pressure is 200/110, pulse is 120, and hematocrit and hemoglobin are both low. The abdomen is soft and nontender, but the nurse notes a pulsating mass and auscultates an abdominal bruit. The nurse concludes that the client's manifestations are compatible with which health problem?

1. Secondary hypertension
2. Aortic aneurysm
3. Congestive heart failure (CHF)
4. Buerger's disease

10 The nurse is caring for a client with Raynaud's disease. Which of the following outcomes concerning the medication regimen should be considered priorities? Select all that apply.

1. Relaxing smooth muscle to avoid vasospasms
2. Relieving the pain if vasospasms occur
3. Avoiding lesions on the feet
4. Preventing major disabilities that may occur
5. Discontinuing medication as soon as symptoms disappear

➤ *See pages 86–88 for Answers and Rationales.*

I. RISK FACTORS ASSOCIATED WITH VASCULAR HEALTH PROBLEMS

A. Hypertension (HTN)

1. Risk factors that cannot be modified
   a. Family history: multifactorial and multiple genes may be involved; may have elevated intracellular sodium levels with an associated lower potassium-sodium ratio; clients who have parent(s) with HTN are at higher risk at a younger age
   b. Age
      1) Primary HTN: usually appears between ages 30–50 years
      2) Clients over age 50 years have a higher incidence and clients over age 60 years of age have a 50–60% chance of HTN
      3) Blood pressure (BP) readings are a good predictor for potential stroke, coronary heart disease, heart failure (HF), and renal disease
   c. Mortality from HTN by ethnicity indicates a higher risk of mortality in blacks than whites, especially black females
   d. Gender: men have a higher incidence of HTN until about age 55; men and women are approximately equal between ages of 55 and 74; women are at greater risk for HTN
2. Factors responding to physiological modification

   a. Stress: can include environmental stressors (noise, heat, and cold), personality characteristics (responses to life events and/or life-changing events) and physiological events (such as pain, decreased blood O_2 concentration, drugs, and obesity)

      b. Food choices

        1) High sodium intake may induce release of high amounts of atrial natriuretic peptide (ANP) hormone, suggesting a possible link to increasing BP

        2) Low intake of potassium, calcium, and magnesium

        3) Being overweight and distribution of fat, particularly to upper body

        4) High consumption of alcohol, legal and illegal drugs

        5) Smoking: nicotine from cigarette smoking immediately raises BP

        6) Caffeine consumption: coffee, soda with caffeine, and chocolate are stimulants that can raise BP

B. Peripheral vascular disease

  1. Arterial

      a. Diseases such as atherosclerosis, autoimmunity

      b. Clotting problems: **embolus** (a foreign object such as part of thrombus floating in bloodstream), **thrombus** (collection of fibrin, platelets, clotting factors, and cellular elements of blood that attach to interior wall of an artery or vein)

      c. Trauma, inflammation

      d. Vasospasm (spasm or constriction of blood vessel)

      e. Obesity

  2. Venous

      a. Over 40 years of age

      b. Surgery longer than 30 minutes using general anesthesia, spinal anesthesia, or epidural anesthesia

      c. Venous stasis caused by prolonged travel, bed rest, cerebrovascular accident (CVA or stroke)

      d. History of previous deep vein thrombosis (DVT), family history of blood clotting disorder

      e. Cardiac disease such as HF, myocardial infarction (MI), cardiomyopathy, malignancy

      f. Pregnancy, estrogen therapy, and oral contraceptives

      g. Obesity

C. Aneurysms: clients with HTN and/or atherosclerosis

D. *Thrombophlebitis*: diseases causing venous stasis, surgery, oral contraceptives, varicose veins, obesity, pregnancy, prolonged immobility

E. Raynaud's disease: gender (female, 18 to 40); heredity

F. Buerger's disease: smoking, gender (males), Asian or Eastern European descent

II. HYPERTENSION

A. Overview

  1. Hypertension (HTN) is defined as a sustained BP that is 140 mmHg or higher **systolic** (pressure of blood against arterial walls when ventricles of heart contract) and 90 mmHg or higher **diastolic** (pressure of blood against arterial walls when ventricles of heart are at rest); however, age specifics need to be considered

  2. Two types

      a. Primary hypertension, also known as *idiopathic HTN* or *essential HTN* (elevated BP from unknown causes; occurs in about 95% of diagnosed clients)

      b. Secondary hypertension (elevated BP associated with a disease process or abnormality; cause can usually be identified: pulmonary, circulatory, renal diseases, endocrine (hyperaldosteronism, **pheochromocytoma**—a tumor that releases catecholamines and causes hypertensive emergencies, Cushing's disease, diabetes mellitus, hyperthyroidism), medicines such as volume expanders, and increased sodium (Na^+) intake

3. **White coat phenomenon**: client is normotensive except when BP is measured by a health professional
4. Isolated systolic HTN: a systolic BP greater than 140 mmHg and a diastolic BP less than 90 mmHg; has a higher incidence with advancing age
5. Labile HTN is extreme elevation of BP at one time with a normal BP later without other noted causes; limited physiological changes; changes do occur over time in heart, brain, and kidneys; should be closely monitored
6. Pregnancy-induced HTN: a complication of pregnancy now called preeclampsia
   a. Diagnosed when BP increases 30 mmHg systolic and 15 mmHg diastolic over baseline BP on 2 assessments at least 6 hours apart, as well as confirmed presence of proteinuria and edema
   b. Occurs most often in third trimester of pregnancy; must be treated promptly to avoid progression to eclampsia, a dangerous condition
7. Malignant HTN is a progressive, rapidly developing HTN that causes vascular damage and possibly death; persistent severe diastolic HTN of over 110–120 mmHg; often occurs after anesthetic drugs are given
8. HTN is called a "silent killer" because many clients do not have symptoms
9. Diagnosis should be made after 3 or more consistent BP readings are taken after a 5-minute period of rest (BP can vary from day to day, within different periods of same day, and because of many factors)

B. **Pathophysiology**
   1. Regulation of BP
      a. Is continually influenced by cardiac output (CO) and **peripheral vascular resistance (PVR)** (sum of all resistances within vascular system)
      b. Regulated also by arterioles, venules, heart, and kidneys
      c. Blood Pressure = Cardiac Output × Peripheral Vascular Resistance ($BP = CO \times PVR$)
      d. Regulation of CO occurs through autonomic nervous system (NS), heart rate (HR) and stroke volume (SV) and fluid volume (influenced by mineralocorticoids, sodium, and water)
      e. Peripheral resistance
         1) A narrowing diameter of vessel will increase PVR, causing BP to rise; a widened diameter decreases PVR and BP falls
         2) Increases in PVR may be caused by increased activity of sympathetic NS, angiotensin and catecholamines, and thickening of blood vessel walls from atherosclerosis
      f. Neurohormonal mediators
         1) Baroreceptors are located in carotid sinuses and wall of left ventricle; these monitor arterial BP and counteract rising pressure by vasodilation through stimulation of vagus nerve
         2) Chemoreceptors are located in medulla and carotid and aortic bodies
            a) Sensitive to changes in blood pH produced by variations in concentrations of carbon dioxide (CO_2), oxygen (O_2), and hydrogen ions
            b) A major reflex response occurs with changes in body's O_2 saturation, but to a lesser extent changes in blood pH and CO_2 concentration
      g. Body fluid volume
         1) Excess concentration of Na^+ and water: as systemic fluid volume increases, BP and kidney glomerular filtration pressure rise, causing diuresis

    2) BP is altered through loss of salt and water and an over-production of sodium-retaining hormone

  h. Increased activity of renin/angiotensin/aldosterone (RAA) system

    1) Renin is released under control of central neural influence, leading to reduced blood flow to kidneys, a fall in BP, and decreased concentration of tubular Na^+

    2) Angiotensin I combines with renin to form a nonpressor form of angiotensin I, which is converted in lungs to angiotensin II (a potent vasoconstrictor) by angiotensin converting enzyme; angiotensin II causes release of aldosterone, leading to reabsorption of Na^+ and water, further increasing BP

    3) Additional contributing factors to HTN

      a) Inability of kidneys to excrete more Na^+ in response to an elevated systolic BP

      b) Failure of normal sodium-potassium or sodium-calcium transport mechanism within intracellular space

  i. Vascular autoregulation

    1) Blood viscosity: resistance to blood flow increases as blood becomes thicker, and resistance decreases as viscosity decreases

    2) Autoregulation is aided through kinins by arteriolar smooth muscle, which increases capillary permeability and constriction of venules

    3) Prostaglandins may lead to either vasoconstriction or vasodilation

2. Primary HTN

  a. Primarily caused by an increased PVR, resulting from vasoconstriction or narrowed peripheral blood vessels

  b. In HTN, left ventricle must work harder to overcome resistance met when emptying (afterload); a constant increased workload and more pressure within left ventricle leads to hypertrophy (known as left ventricular hypertrophy or LVH)

  c. Initially, LVH is a compensatory mechanism by heart to regulate BP; later LVH is a complication because more O_2 and blood flow is needed for muscle to meet workload demands

  d. Initially, arterioles increase resistance to blood flow, leading to increased PVR and HTN

  e. Later, kidneys become involved by activating RAA system

3. Secondary HTN

  a. Multiple system involvement with direct or indirect impact on renal system

  b. Aldosterone, cortisol, and catecholamines are produced in excess

  c. Chronic stress: prolonged excess of catecholamines

4. Signs and symptoms

  a. May be asymptomatic but headache is most common if any symptom is felt

  b. Severe HTN: dizziness, nausea, vomiting, confusion (can signify encephalopathy), visual disturbances, renal insufficiency, aortic dissection, hypertensive crisis

5. Complications include stroke, HF, ventricular hypertrophy, damage to retina, renal insufficiency, aortic dissection, and hypertensive crisis

C. Nursing assessment

1. Health history and physical exam

  a. Complete health, nutritional, medication, and social history

  b. Assess for associated symptoms

    1) Occipital headache (HA) in morning and length of time HA occurs

    2) Periods of dizziness: frequency, when it occurs, its duration, and relationship to any activity

    3) Tinnitus: characteristics, if this phenomenon occurs

        4) Pounding in chest: frequency, duration, and last occurrence

   c. Assess client's BP: obtain BP in each arm using 3 positions—lying down, sitting, standing (orthostatic BP), with 1–2 minutes between readings; have client sit with arm supported at heart level; record findings, identifying position for each reading; note **pulse pressure** (difference between systolic and diastolic BP; range of difference is 30–40 mmHg)

   d. Conduct physical examination, with emphasis on cardiovascular and associated systems

        1) Abdominal masses: may pulsate, describe location and size

        2) Bruits: where found and whether bilateral or unilateral

        3) Adrenal disease: characteristics of Cushing's disease or signs of pheochromocytoma

        4) Funduscopic eye examination

        5) Cardiac, vascular, and extremity examination

        6) Pulmonary examination

 2. Diagnostic tests

   a. Urinalysis and tests for renin, cortisol, urine catecholamines; 24-hr urine collection

   b. Blood chemistries (potassium [K^+], Na^+, fasting glucose, complete blood count [CBC], blood urea nitrogen [BUN], creatinine, and lipid profile), serum calcium (Ca^{++}), and magnesium (Mg^{++})

   c. Other: electrocardiogram (ECG), echocardiogram, and possible vascular studies to determine end-organ damage

   d. Measurement of BP with appropriate cuff size for a week

D. Nursing management

 1. A change in lifestyle is always recommended *first*: diet control, weight loss, increased activity, and decreasing stress

 2. Medications include diuretics (combination, loop and potassium-sparing), beta blockers, calcium channel blockers, and ACE inhibitors

   a. Clients are usually started on diuretics or beta blockers initially; if managed on 1 drug, no further action is taken

   b. Clients not responding to 1 drug may have another added; ACE inhibitors are combined with many drugs successfully

   c. Management of HTN follows guidelines of Joint National Committee on Prevention, Detection, Evaluation, and Treatment of High Blood Pressure (JNC–7); see Table 3-1

 3. Discuss client's nutritional needs

   a. Assess amount of Na^+ consumption and recommend no more than 2–6 grams daily

   b. Serum cholesterol of less than 200 mg/dL; note breakdown

        1) LDL: 60–160 mg/dL normal; risk for CHD is high if greater than 160 mg/dL, moderate if 130–159 mg/dL, and low if less than 130 mg/dL; a value 100 mg/dL is desirable

        2) HDL: 29–77 mg/dL normal; risk for CHD is high if less than 35 mg/dL, moderate if 35–45 mg/dL, and low if 46–59 mg/dL

   c. Reduction of calories and weight: body mass index (BMI) should be 24.9 or lower

 4. Monitor vital signs (VS) and intake and output (I & O); test for edema

 5. Monitor weight daily at same time, in same amount of clothing, on same scale, preferably upon arising from sleep and after voiding

 6. Emphasize compliance with food, medications, and risk involved in not keeping BP in appropriate range; factors to be considered include:

   a. High cost of medication(s), unpleasant side effects, interference with lifestyle, and lack of understanding need to take medications when feeling well; also males may have sexual side effects

		Initial Antihypertensive Therapy	
Blood Pressure Classification	**Systolic/Diastolic Blood Pressure (mmHg)**	**Without Compelling Indication***	**With Compelling Indication***
Normal	119/79 or less		
Prehypertension	120–139/80–89	Lifestyle modification; no antihypertensive indicated	Drugs may be used for compelling indications
Stage 1 hypertension	140–159/90–99	Thiazide-type diuretic for most; may consider ACEI, ARB, BB, CCB, or combination.	Drugs may be used for compelling indications. Other antihypertensive drugs: diuretics, ACEI, ARB, BB, CCB, as needed.
Stage 2 hypertension	160 or higher/100 or higher	Two-drug combination	

Table 3-1   **Management of Hypertension**

*Compelling indications include heart failure, post-MI, high risk for coronary artery disease, diabetes, chronic kidney disease, and recurrent stroke prevention.

Drug abbreviations: ACEI, angiotensin converting enzyme inhibitor; ARB, angiotensin receptor blocker; BB, beta blocker; CCB, calcium channel blocker.

Source: The Seventh Report of the Joint National Committee on Prevention, Detection, Evaluation, and Treatment of High Blood Pressure, National Heart, Lung, and Blood Institute.

      b. Underestimation of HTN as serious disease because asymptomatic

      c. Some lifestyle changes prescribed for client are difficult to accept and implement; support groups may be of assistance

7. Teach client how to check own BP at home, plan a realistic schedule for measuring and recording BP, and teach client and significant others when to call provider (an unusually high or low reading)

8. Monitor HR and BP before administering antihypertensives

      a. Withhold dose if systolic BP less than 100 mmHg and HR less than 50–60 beats/min. as determined by provider

      b. Always check HR and BP before taking beta blockers

      c. Monitor for **orthostatic hypotension** (syncope or dizziness with sudden position changes because of a drop in BP)

9. Discuss importance of medical follow-up for a lifetime

10. Discuss over-the-counter (OTC) medications that client is taking; educate about avoiding cold remedies that can increase BP

11. Health maintenance program should include an individualized aerobic exercise program, monitored via a self-reporting system or within an organized club

      a. Elements to monitor are HR during exercise, perceived reduction in physical and emotional stress, and reduction in systemic BP

      b. Guidelines for aerobic exercise are 20–30 minutes, 5–6 times per week, but these depend on client age and physical condition

      c. Maximal heart rate (MHR) is determined by subtracting client's age from 220

      d. Prior to beginning rehabilitation, an exercise physiologist must conduct a detailed performance evaluation

12. Avoid smoking cigarettes or cigars, or using chewing tobacco or alcohol

13. Monitor drug effectiveness, especially in older adults who may experience fluid shifts, which can change distribution

Practice to Pass

A client was diagnosed 3 months ago with essential hypertension. The client states to the nurse, "It doesn't matter if I forget to take my medicine. I just take the make-up dose at the next medication time." How should the nurse answer?

III. PERIPHERAL VASCULAR DISEASE

A. Overview

1. Peripheral vascular disease (PVD) is defined as those conditions that interfere with blood flow to or from extremities
2. Can be arterial or venous in origin (Table 3-2)
   a. Peripheral arterial occlusive disorders: partial stenosis or complete occlusion
   b. Venous disorders: can be acute (such as thromboembolism) or chronic (such as **varicose veins** [dilated, tortuous leg veins] and **chronic venous insufficiency** [chronic failure of venous valves to function]) which interfere with venous blood return to heart
3. Causes include cardiovascular disease, thrombi, prolonged immobility, excess standing, and pulmonary diseases

B. Pathophysiology

1. Arterial
   a. Any reduction in blood supply compromises O_2 supply
   b. Prolonged change in blood flow or decreased perfusion to large areas will start a sequence of vasodilation; this will promote development of collateral arterial pathways, and shift to anaerobic metabolism to meet cellular O_2 demands
   c. Vasodilation has a limited effect, as arteries deprived of O_2 become maximally dilated and **arterial steal** occurs (when maximally dilated because of hypoxia, arterioles steal from cutaneous and peripheral vessels, causing "pins and needles" sensation in affected area)
   d. Of concern is risk for tissue acidosis, which occurs when large amounts of lactic acid and pyruvic acid build up quickly; these acids are very toxic to body

   e. If compensatory mechanisms are inadequate, client experiences pain called intermittent claudication (lower extremities)
   f. Lower limbs are most susceptible to arterial occlusive disorders and atherosclerosis because of limitation in collateral circulation
   g. Signs and symptoms
      1) Intermittent claudication

      2) Dusky, purplish discoloration when feet are dependent and white, pale color when legs are elevated
      3) Trophic changes: thickened toenails; hair loss; and thin, shiny skin in affected area (from tissue malnutrition)
      4) Ulcers on legs (see Table 3-2)
      5) Venous refilling when foot is dependent
      6) Decreased or absent pedal pulse
      7) Numbness and cold, tingling feeling in extremity

Table 3-2	Comparison of Arterial and Venous Insufficiency	
	Arterial	**Venous**
Description of pain	Intermittent claudication, relieved by dependent position	Aching, cramping, relieved by elevation
Pulse assessment	Diminished or absent	Present
Ulcer characteristics	Deep, pale; located on toes, feet, or other area of skin	Superficial, pink; over inner or outer ankle
Skin characteristics	Dependent rubor; pallor upon elevation; dry, shiny skin; cool or cold temperature; edema mild if present at all	Thick and tough; brawny (brown) pigment; skin normal temperature; may have edema
Complications	Gangrene	Poor healing

      h. Progression of symptoms from onset is slow, beginning from age 20–40 years; some clients have associated CHD and symptoms are influenced by body's use and speed of O_2 consumption in legs

  2. Venous

      a. Blockage within venous system may occur in system of superficial veins or deep veins

      b. Causes of thrombus formation

         1) Venous stasis from immobility, prolonged travel, obesity, pregnancy, and heart disease

         2) Hypercoagulability from conditions causing dehydration and blood dyscrasias may cause platelet counts to rise, decrease fibrolysis, increase clotting factors, thus changing blood viscosity; in addition, oral contraceptives and hematologic disorders may increase blood coagulability

         3) Injury to vessel wall may be caused by trauma of an intravenous infusion, fractures, contusions, chemical injury from sclerosing agents, and from Buerger's disease (thromboangiitis obliterans)

           a) Injury to venous wall attracts platelets and debris gathers

           b) With low blood flow, a hypercoagulable state occurs and thrombus forms

      c. Signs and symptoms: discoloration of lower extremities, edema over tibia, ulcers (see Table 3-2), tenderness in legs, and calf pain on dorsiflexion of foot (Homan sign; is nonspecific; can occur in any painful condition of calf)

C. Nursing assessment

  1. Assessment

      a. Arterial

         1) Symptom analysis of reason for seeking medical help

         2) Activity tolerance and presence of pain

         3) Palpation of arterial pulses; use a Doppler if necessary to detect them and document whether each is palpated or auscultated

         4) Other circulatory assessments: capillary refill, skin color and temperature, presence of venous refilling, and edema

         5) Observe sitting position of client for crossing of legs at knees or ankles, use of garters or knee stockings

      b. Venous

         1) Identify clients who are at high risk for thrombophlebitis

         2) Assess client's legs for discoloration, edema, and tenderness

         3) Measure and record leg circumference

         4) Determine amount of discomfort client is experiencing by asking about location, intensity, and duration

         5) Inquire about Homan sign

  2. Diagnostic tests: cholesterol and lipid panel, arteriogram, Doppler ultrasonic flow study to identify blood flow through arteries, digital subtraction angiography (to identify arteries in specific areas), oscillometry (determine pulse volume), stress testing, and coagulation studies, including partial thromboplastin time (PTT) for heparin, and prothrombin time (PT) or INR for warfarin (Coumadin)

D. Nursing management

  1. Medication: pentoxifylline (Trental) to decrease blood viscosity and increase microcirculation, vasodilator (prostaglandins), anticoagulant or thrombolytic therapy (for thrombus), and antiplatelet drugs, such as cilostazol (Pletal)

  2. Risk reduction through weight loss for overweight clients using a low-fat, low-cholesterol diet with fruits and vegetables

  3. Risk reduction through physical exercise: encourage clients to walk 30–60 minutes each day if skin is intact; clients should have individualized physical exercise program

Practice to Pass

A client with a peripheral vascular disease (PVD) asks the nurse why it is essential to follow the health care provider's plan of care to reduce his cardiovascular risk. What should the nurse tell this client?

4. Educate on smoking cessation and harmful effects of nicotine; refer client to a support group

5. If client has hyperlipidemia, evaluate need to reduce total calorie intake, and fat and cholesterol intake; when genetics are a major risk factor, management requires drug therapy

6. Explain reasons to avoid standing in one spot for prolonged time; if intermittent claudication occurs, stop, rest and then continue activity; avoid long car trips or air travel (if necessary, use frequent rest stops or position changes)

7. Recommend that client wear light warm clothing in order to prevent vasoconstriction of vessels of lower legs

8. Inform client to avoid crossing legs or ankles, which decreases perfusion, and to elevate legs when sitting in a chair or when in bed

IV. ANEURYSMS

A. Overview

1. An **aneurysm** is a permanent dilatation of an artery or an outpouching of an arterial wall

2. Most aortic aneurysms are located below level of renal arteries; other sites are at bifurcation of aorta or within structure of an artery or vein anywhere in body

3. Classified as true or false aneurysm

   a. *True aneurysm*: results from weakening of vessel wall over time and is usually a result of high BP or atherosclerosis

   b. *False aneurysm*: usually results from a traumatic break in vascular wall instead of a weakening seen in true form

4. Aneurysms vary in pathophysiology, clinical findings, and treatment depending on where aneurysm is located; they may occur in either an artery or vein

5. Causes of include HTN, trauma, atherosclerosis, or infections

B. Pathophysiology

1. Morphology (shape)

   a. Fusiform: cylindrical and involves entire circumference of vessel

   b. Saccular: outpouching of a sac on vessel; example: berry aneurysm

   c. Pseudoaneurysm: wall of aneurysm is not original wall of aorta; mass is made up of connective tissue and structures surrounding extravasated blood

2. Etiology: aneurysms may be classified according to cause, including atherosclerotic, mycotic (bacterial infection) and luetic (syphilis)

3. Location: type of aneurysm is determined by its location

   a. Thoracic aorta: progresses rapidly and often ruptures; symptoms include pain in back, neck and substernal areas; respiratory problems (stridor, dyspnea, cough); hoarseness

   b. Superior vena cava: signs are distended neck veins, facial edema

   c. Abdominal aorta

      1) Most develop below level of renal arteries; are most frequent

      2) Often asymptomatic with audible pulsation in abdomen or pulsating mass in abdomen

      3) Other symptoms can include mild to severe abdominal and back pain, cool extremities, and claudication

4. A dissecting aneurysm is a medical emergency

   a. Hemorrhage occurs because of a tear in aorta intima, often in high pressure areas such as ascending aorta

   b. Symptoms include pain (abrupt, severe), elevated BP, undetectable pulses, syncope, and HF

Figure 3-1

Surgical repair of aneurysm.
A. Clamping of aorta and
visualization of clot within the
vessel, B. Graft within the
vessel used for repair.

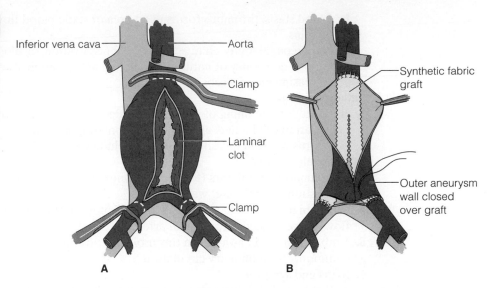

Inferior vena cava — Aorta — Clamp — Laminar clot — Clamp — Synthetic fabric graft — Outer aneurysm wall closed over graft

A   B

Practice to Pass

A 70-year-old client
with an abdominal
aortic aneurysm needs
an MRI every 6 months.
The aneurysm currently
measures 4.5 cm. The
physician tells the
family surgery is usu-
ally not done until it is
greater than 5 cm, as
long as there is no
evidence of growth or
hemorrhage. The
family asks the nurse
why surgery can't be
performed now. How
should the nurse
respond?

5. An aneurysm of 5 cm may be palpable in a nonobese client
6. Treatment of an abdominal aneurysm is surgery (Figure 3-1)

C. **Nursing assessment**
1. Assessment includes characteristics of client's pain (intense pain in abdomen, back, flank, and scrotum); auscultation of abdomen; palpation (rigid because of accumulation of blood); VS; signs of hemorrhagic shock
2. Diagnostic tests: ultrasonography, CT scan or MRI, chest x-ray (CXR), and renal function studies

D. **Nursing management**
1. Medications: includes antihypertensives, beta-adrenergic blockers, anticoagulants, as well as antibiotics and analgesics postsurgery
2. Monitor for complications following a major surgical procedure
   a. Postoperative atelectasis and exacerbation of chronic obstructive pulmonary disease (COPD)
   b. Decreased toleration of changes in **hemodynamics** (movement of blood within body) such as low blood volume and fluid shifts
   c. Underlying coronary heart disease (CHD) leading to MI
   d. Kidney function: reflects integrity of cardiovascular system
   e. Emboli
3. Postoperative care
   a. Monitor for fluid volume deficit from insufficient intravenous fluids or hemorrhage
   b. Monitor client for increasing HR, decreasing BP, clammy skin, anxiety, changing level of consciousness, oliguria, pallor, and thirst as signs of shock from reduced circulating volume
4. Educate client about compliance with measures to control HTN

V. THROMBOPHLEBITIS

A. **Overview**
1. An inflammation of vein with a clot formation made up of various elements in blood supply trapped in a fibrin mesh
2. Causes are usually associated with Virchow's triad
   a. Injury to vessel wall: mechanical trauma, thermal injury, septic states, or an autoimmune problem

b. Blood stasis: thrombus forms in an area of static blood flow and in valve cusps of veins

c. Hypercoagulability, change in blood concentration, or blood coagulation factors; deficiency of naturally occurring antithrombins; and factors that assist in increasing blood viscosity

B. Pathophysiology

1. Injury to intimal lining of vein causes a decrease in circulation and stimulates aggregation of platelets and other inflammatory mediators

2. A protrusion from this site begins to occlude vessel and may partially or completely block blood flow

3. Inflammatory mediators (leukocytes, lymphocytes, and fibroblasts) gather, causing congestion within vessel wall

4. Thrombi may occur in any vessel, but are more prominent in veins because blood flow is more sluggish than in an artery

5. Emboli can break away from thrombi and travel to different parts of body, most commonly to pulmonary circulation

6. Signs and symptoms

   a. Small- and medium-sized veins may produce no symptoms

   b. Larger vessels: temperature (102°F)

   c. Superficial veins: redness, pain, tenderness, and swelling

   d. DVT: calf pain, tenderness in calf muscle, positive Homan sign (is nonspecific)

   e. Iliofemoral vein: thigh and/or groin pain, edema (may be pitting), cyanotic appearance to leg, fever, tachycardia; brawny edema (skin is thick, hard, has "orange-peel" appearance, and edema)

C. Nursing assessment

1. Assessment includes neurovascular status of affected part (capillary refill, temperature, pulses, sensation, color of skin); VS; symptom analysis of pain; positive Homan sign

2. Diagnostic tests: blood cultures and CBC, phlebography (assess location of clot using a contrast medium), Doppler ultrasound, venous pressure measurement, plethysmography (measures changes in fluid volume passing through a vessel)

D. Nursing management

1. Medications: anticoagulants, low-molecular weight heparin (LMWH), antiplatelets, anti-inflammatory agents, thrombolytics, and antibiotics

2. Elevate foot of bed 6–8 inches on blocks or elevate affected part

3. Maintain client on bedrest initially; later encourage client to rest affected part

4. Administer moist heat to involved extremity; if warm moist soaks are prescribed, they are usually every 4–6 hours for 30 minutes; an aquathermia pad may be applied over a moist towel

5. Listen to client's concerns; use community referrals as needed

6. Monitor intravenous infusions carefully

7. Monitor effect of medications and treatments used; teach client about effects of medications and potential side effects

VI. VARICOSE VEINS

A. Overview

1. A superficial vein that is twisted and enlarged and causes incompetence of vein valves; may involve any part of body but occur most often in lower extremities and esophagus

2. Types: **primary varicose veins** (involving superficial veins and not communicating veins and **secondary varicose veins** (involving deep communicating veins)

    3. Causes
       a. Primary varicose veins: are frequently familial
       b. Secondary: occur with trauma, DVT, and inflamed or damaged valves

B. Pathophysiology
    1. Chronic venous insufficiency results from incompetent valves that decrease venous return and increase venous pressure and stasis
    2. Excessive dilation of vein causes spreading of valve cusps
    3. This causes valvular incompetency and produces a reflux of blood from superficial veins to enter deep veins by muscular pump
    4. Signs and symptoms appear after veins have been chronically engorged and tortuous
       a. Distended veins that may be bluish in color and bulging
       b. Pain in feet and ankles; heaviness or feeling of heat in legs
       c. Swelling of lower extremities
       d. Stasis ulcers
       e. Itching of skin over affected extremity

C. Nursing assessment
    1. Assessment includes inspection of lower extremities for edema, discoloration, tenderness or discomfort (location and intensity), positive Homan sign, signs of pulmonary embolism (anxiety, dyspnea, increased respiratory rate, "air hunger," tachycardia, diaphoresis, chest pain); bowel habits for constipation
    2. Diagnostic tests: tourniquet tests (determine location of incompetent valves), Doppler ultrasonic flow tests, angiographic studies, and plethysmography

D. Nursing management
    1. Medications are not recommended unless OTC analgesics are needed
    2. Discuss smoking cessation as needed; may refer client to a support group
    3. Encourage client to walk daily for 30–60 minutes; stop and rest if intermittent claudication occurs
    4. A referral to Bureau of Vocational Rehabilitation may be helpful if client's position cannot be accommodated by employer
    5. Suggest that light warm clothing is essential to prevent vasoconstriction of blood vessels in lower extremities
    6. Instruct not to stand in one position for long periods of time, avoid crossing legs or ankles when sitting, and elevate legs when supine
    7. Prevent constipation or straining

VII. ARTERIOSPASTIC DISEASE: RAYNAUD'S DISEASE

A. Overview
    1. Arteriospastic disease: Raynaud's disease is a condition of small arteries and arterioles of fingers and skin that constrict in response to cold, vibration, or emotional upsets (Table 3-3); primarily affects young women
    2. Raynaud's disease occurs when symptoms persist for 3 years with intermittent attacks
    3. May be associated with autoimmune disorders, such as systemic lupus erythematosus, genetic tendency, or unknown cause

B. Pathophysiology
    1. Raynaud's disease causes color changes in hands when hands are exposed to causative stimuli
    2. Digital arteries go into spasm, and hands change color, becoming very pale
    3. Tissue hypoxia occurs, causing arteries to dilate slightly
    4. Fingers appear bluish because of deoxygenated blood; this may occur in one or both hands
    5. A rubor (redness) will occur when arterial spasms have stopped

Table 3-3	Comparison of Raynaud's Disease and Buerger's Disease	
	Raynaud's Disease	**Buerger's Disease**
Definition	Condition of small arteries and arterioles of the fingers and skin; constriction in response to cold or emotional upsets	An inflammatory occlusive vascular disease involving the medium-sized arteries and veins
Causative factors	Autoimmune disorders such as systemic lupus erythematosus; genetic tendency; unknown etiology	Genetic disposition; smoking; tobacco allergy; autoimmune response
Population affected	Primarily affects young women	Primarily men of Asian and Jewish or Eastern European descent, under age 40, history of heavy smoking
Pathophysiology	Causative stimuli leads to color changes in hands; digital artery spasm; tissue hypoxia causes arteries to dilate; rubor occurs when spasms cease	Thrombi develop; vessel is blocked; lesion becomes fibrotic; vasospasms obstruct flow of blood
Signs and symptoms	Red-white-blue syndrome of digits; pallor or cyanosis that is bilateral or unilateral; normal pulse; sensory changes in extremities; pain	Pain at rest; intermittent claudication; decreased or absent pulses; rubor and cyanosis of extremities; signs of decreased circulation
Characteristics	Triggers include exercise, long-term exposure to cold, stress; lesions can progress to gangrene	Triggered by smoking, cold, and emotional stress; most commonly affects hands and feet; upper extremities may be affected also; has periods of exacerbations and remissions; gangrene is a complication

6. One digit may demonstrate severe **ischemia** (deficiency in supply of oxygenated blood) with other digits demonstrating good blood flow

7. Stenosis may cause an absence of pulse and a localized bruit

8. Stimuli triggering an attack include exercise, long-term exposure to cold, and stress

9. Signs and symptoms

   a. Known as blue-white-red disease because digits turn blue, then white, then red as spasm resolves

   b. Other: pallor or cyanosis that is bilateral or unilateral; normal pulse; sensory changes (tingling, stiffness, pain, decreased sensation)

   c. Long-term: fingertips thicken because of lack of O_2 and nails become brittle (trophic change); gangrene is a serious complication

C. **Nursing assessment**

   1. Assessment

      a. Obtain a careful history from client presenting with hand(s) that have discomfort and are demonstrating changes in color

      b. Palpate distal pulses bilaterally noting rate and volume

      c. Assess pain levels, noting frequency of pain, its duration, intensity, location and current pain treatment; determine if present medication management is sufficient to control pain

      d. Assess all extremities for edema, lesions, and gangrene

      e. If lesions are present, measure circumference of each extremity; measure and document location of any lesion

      f. Assess client's use of medications

      g. Assess if client is continuing to smoke

   2. Diagnostic tests: diagnosis is determined by symptoms and ruling out other causes of decreased circulation

D. Nursing management

1. Medications include: vasodilators; a low-dose calcium channel blocker such as nifedipine (Procardia); nitrates (transdermal nitroglycerine or long-acting oral forms); analgesics for pain
2. Discuss smoking cessation as needed; may refer client to a support group or to provider for nicotine patches or other medications
3. Encourage use of loose and warm clothing to aid maintenance of circulation: warm gloves, wool or heavy socks, comfortable supportive shoes, and a warm hat
4. Teach relaxation techniques to reduce effects of stress

VIII. THROMBOANGIITIS OBLITERANS: BUERGER'S DISEASE

A. Overview

1. Buerger's disease is defined as an inflammatory occlusive vascular disease involving medium-sized arteries and veins (see Table 3-3)
2. Primary clients are men (Asian and Eastern European) who are less than 40 years of age and have a history of heavy smoking
3. Commonly affects legs and feet, but may affect upper extremities
4. Known for periods of exacerbations and remissions; long-term effects include more intense and longer episodes with ulcerations and gangrene as complications
5. Causes include genetic disposition; smoking (primary); tobacco allergy; autoimmune response

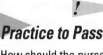

Practice to Pass

How should the nurse explain to a client the difference between Raynaud's disease and Buerger's disease?

B. Pathophysiology

1. Characteristic problems in this disease are development of panarteritis (inflammation of coats of one or more arteries) and panphlebitis (inflammation of veins)
2. Thrombi develop on vessel wall, which subsequently block vessel, and lesion becomes fibrotic; arteriosclerosis is not noted in lesion
3. Vasospasms occur commonly and may obstruct blood flow
4. Primary result is arterial occlusion but veins may become involved
5. Signs and symptoms
   a. Pain (most common) at rest or intermittent claudication; may be triggered by smoking, cold, emotional stress
   b. Decreased pulses (even absent), cool or cold temperature in feet with intolerance to cold
   c. Rubor and cyanosis of extremities
   d. Trophic changes: loss of hair, thin, shiny skin and thick nails in extremities
   e. Signs of decreased circulation in extremities; changes with position changes

C. Nursing assessment

1. Symptom analysis of pain including toes and forefoot when client is at rest
2. Assess lower extremities and foot muscles for claudication
3. Assess for migratory thrombophlebitis in a variety of veins
4. Assess foot for fulminating digital ischemia (temperature, capillary refill, pulses) and development of gangrene in foot

D. Nursing management

1. Medications: calcium channel blockers, antiplatelet agent, and if needed, antibiotics, corticosteroids, vasodilators, and anticoagulants
2. Discuss smoking cessation as needed; may refer client to a support group or to provider for medication
3. Surgical treatment consists of amputation of affected limb
4. Use a bedcradle to relieve pressure from linens if necessary

5. Instruct client to avoid drugs that decrease circulation, triggers, extreme temperature changes, tight or restrictive clothing or shoes, and standing in one position for prolonged amount of time

6. Instruct client to inspect feet frequently; keep clean and dry and use soft padding if necessary

Case Study

A 65-year-old female has been diagnosed with essential hypertension. She attends the local Council on Aging (COA) and sees a different health care provider (HCP) at a local clinic when necessary. Her blood pressure (BP) is monitored at the COA monthly by a volunteer nurse. She takes a beta blocker and a diuretic, and her BP ranges from 130–140/70–90. She adheres to her diet, doesn't smoke, and watches her weight. During the autumn, she has a few colds and begins to experience an increase in BP, ranging from 190–210/100–120. The COA arranges for her BP to be checked more often, and she is referred to her HCP. The doses of her beta blocker and diuretic are increased, and she continues to have high BP readings. Concerned about risk of stroke, her family is notified and a copy of the last month's BP readings is given to the family. She is again referred by the nurse to her HCP, who prescribes an ACE inhibitor.

1. What information should the HCP gather about the client's present state of health and history data?

2. What education does the family need?

3. What is the essential information for clients to know about self-administration of their pharmacological regime?

4. What are the nursing priorities of care for this client? What is the plan for the implementation of this client's care?

5. How should the nurse explain the diagnosis of essential hypertension to the client and family?

For suggested responses, see page 462.

POSTTEST

1 In teaching a group of middle-aged men concerned about hypertension, the nurse should emphasize which items of information? Select all that apply.

1. Eat a diet rich in fruits and vegetables, and low in salt and saturated fat.
2. Alcohol consumption should not exceed 5 ounces per day.
3. Smoking contributes to high blood pressure.
4. Remain active with activities like walking several days a week.
5. A sedentary lifestyle is best to keep the blood pressure lower.

2 The nurse is teaching a pregnant female who has been diagnosed with hypertension. Which statement about secondary hypertension would be most useful for this client?

1. "Hypertension in pregnancy is expected and is not a cause for alarm."
2. "The renin-angiotensin system raises the blood pressure when the blood volume is increased."
3. "Hypertension in pregnancy needs to be controlled to reduce the health risks to you and the baby."
4. "White coat hypertension is a secondary hypertension because the cause has been identified."

POSTTEST

3 The nurse suggests a dietary sodium reduction to help lower blood pressure in an obese sedentary client. What rationale should the nurse share for reducing sodium intake?

1. "A low-sodium diet has been shown to reduce the systolic and diastolic blood pressure."
2. "The blood volume will be decreased after a high intake of sodium."
3. "Reduced salt makes food taste less appealing so you will lose weight."
4. "Salt intake and smoking go together so reducing one helps with the other."

4 The nurse reviews the results of which laboratory tests that are helpful in evaluating the etiology of hypertension in a newly diagnosed client? Select all that apply.

1. International normalized ratio (INR)
2. Hematocrit
3. Cholesterol level
4. Serum creatinine
5. Troponin

5 Which client is at highest risk for developing a deep vein thrombosis (DVT)?

1. 25-year-old male who is a smoker with hypertension
2. 67-year-old overweight female recovering from a hip replacement (1st day postop)
3. 22-year-old female with a history of Raynaud's disease in the family
4. 72-year-old male with a history of arthritis and bypass surgery

6 A male client reports right leg pain while walking. The right foot is dusky purple when the client sits up at the side of the stretcher. The right dorsalis pedis pulse is palpable but diminished, and he states his foot "tingles on occasion." After the clinic nurse has him lie supine on the stretcher with the foot elevated for about 10 minutes, the foot shows pallor. The nurse concludes these manifestations are consistent with which disorder?

1. Varicose veins
2. Thrombophlebitis
3. Raynaud's disease
4. Arterial insufficiency

7 The home care nurse notes that a client with intermittent claudication of the left leg has developed tissue breakdown of the left foot. The nurse explains to the client that the plan of care should include which activity level at this time?

1. Increased exercise to stimulate blood flow
2. Bed rest to minimize tissue oxygen demands
3. Active range of motion exercises to maintain joint flexibility
4. Walking in comfortable light slippers to minimize impact on fragile tissue

8 The nurse is answering questions from a client who has been diagnosed with a thrombus in the popliteal vein. When asked what causes deep vein thrombosis (DVT), the nurse would include which factors in a response?

1. Arterial stasis, hypercoagulability, and arterial wall injury
2. Myocardial infarction, stroke, and prolonged sitting
3. Venous stasis, hypercoagulability, and injury to blood vessel wall
4. Motor vehicle crash and prolonged bed rest

POSTTEST

9 The nurse would expect to document which signs and symptoms in a client with thrombophlebitis of the left lower leg? Select all that apply.

1. Positive Homan sign
2. Negative Homan sign
3. Toe to knee pain
4. Positive stretch reflex
5. Warmth or redness in the affected leg

10 The nurse evaluates that teaching for a client with Raynaud's disease is effective when the client makes which statements? Select all that apply.

1. "I will decrease my smoking to 6 cigarettes per day."
2. "I will try to learn to relax and avoid emotional upsets."
3. "I will wear gloves in cool weather and socks to bed at night."
4. "I will try to eat a healthier diet."
5. "I will avoid caffeine and drugs with vasoconstrictive effects."

➤ *See pages 88–89 for Answers and Rationales.*

ANSWERS & RATIONALES

Pretest

1 **Answers: 2, 3, 4, 5** **Rationale:** An increase in the heart's electrical activity would not necessarily lead to hypertension, although it would increase the pulse rate. Hypertension may occur after the use of over-the-counter (OTC) cold remedies containing an adrenergic drug, such as a decongestant. Genetic predisposition to hypertension is believed to be polygenic. The inherited defects are associated with renal sodium excretion, insulin, and insulin activity. Low dietary intake of potassium, calcium, and magnesium are associated with a decrease of cell membrane sodium or calcium transport. **Cognitive Level:** Applying **Client Need:** Physiological Adaptation **Integrated Process:** Teaching and Learning **Content Area:** Adult Health **Strategy:** Consider the etiology or risk factors for hypertension and eliminate the incorrect options. **Reference:** Huether, S. E., & McCance, K. L. (2012). *Understanding pathophysiology* (5th ed.). St. Louis, MO: Elsevier Inc., pp. 586–587.

2 **Answer: 2** **Rationale:** Propranolol is a beta blocker used to treat hypertension and tachycardia. The drug should not be given if the apical pulse is below 60 beats per/min, there is a significant drop in the BP, or if systolic BP is below 100 mmHg. Sulfinpyrazone (Anturane) is a medication used to manage long-term gout. Glucagon (GlucaGen) is used to manage hypoglycemia when oral glucose is not appropriate. Calcitonin (Calcimar) is used in the treatment of Paget's disease by decreasing the rate of bone destruction. **Cognitive Level:** Applying **Client Need:** Pharmacological and Parenteral Therapies **Integrated Process:** Nursing Process: Implementation **Content Area:** Adult Health **Strategy:** Recall that both parts of a multiple part option must be correct to be the right answer. Eliminate any option where one part is wrong.

Reference: LeMone, P., Burke, K., & Bauldoff, G. (2012). *Medical-surgical nursing: Critical thinking in patient care* (5th ed.). Upper Saddle River, NJ: Pearson Education, pp. 522, 1023–1026.

3 **Answer: 4** **Rationale:** Family history and gender cannot be modified as risk factors in any form of hypertension. Current research suggests there are several genes influencing the development of hypertension. Ethnicity is a nonmodifiable risk factor; however, stress can be modified if the interruption of the stressor is undertaken. Obesity and substance abuse are risk factors that may be managed through behavioral modification and support groups. Nutrition and occupation are both modifiable with assistance. **Cognitive Level:** Applying **Client Need:** Health Promotion and Maintenance **Integrated Process:** Nursing Process: Implementation **Content Area:** Adult Health **Strategy:** The critical word in the question is *nonmodifiable.* Focus on answers that refer to factors that cannot be changed and use the process of elimination to make a selection where both parts of the option are correct. **Reference:** LeMone, P., Burke, K., & Bauldoff, G. (2012). *Medical-surgical nursing: Critical thinking in patient care* (5th ed.). Upper Saddle River, NJ: Pearson Education, pp. 911–914.

4 **Answers: 1, 2, 5** **Rationale:** A single elevated blood pressure reading does not mean that a person has hypertension. Diagnosis requires the measurement of blood pressure on at least 2 separate occasions, averaging the 2 readings, at least 2 minutes apart with the following conditions: the person is seated, the arm is supported at the heart level, the person must be at rest for at least 5 minutes, and the person should not have smoked or ingested caffeine in the previous 30 minutes. Using a cuff and Doppler device to measure blood pressure in both arms does not provide enough information.

Cognitive Level: Applying **Client Need:** Physiological Adaptation **Integrated Process:** Nursing Process: Assessment **Content Area:** Adult Health **Strategy:** Evaluate each option as a true or false statement and choose the options where the conclusion is "true." **Reference:** Huether, S. E., & McCance, K. L. (2012). *Understanding pathophysiology* (5th ed.). St. Louis, MO: Elsevier Inc., p. 590.

5 **Answer: 4** **Rationale:** Smoking is the primary etiological factor identified with clients diagnosed with Buerger's disease. Emphasis should be placed on cessation of smoking. Wearing gloves to prevent chilling is an appropriate measure but is not of highest priority for this disorder. Shoes are not the highest priority, although the client should choose those that are well fitted and comfortable. Although pain is present, the use of opioids analgesics is usually not indicated. **Cognitive Level:** Analyzing **Client Need:** Health Promotion and Maintenance **Integrated Process:** Nursing Process: Implementation **Content Area:** Adult Health **Strategy:** Recall that cigarette smoking is the single most significant cause of Buerger's disease and relates directly to the pathophysiology. **Reference:** LeMone, P., Burke, K., & Bauldoff, G. (2012). *Medical-surgical nursing: Critical thinking in patient care* (5th ed.). Upper Saddle River, NJ: Pearson Education, p. 1045.

6 **Answers: 2, 3, 5** **Rationale:** Frequently, clients perceive themselves as helpless when confronted with multiple lifestyle changes. The health care team and the client need to determine the most significant lifestyle modification needed and begin to work with this one. Many times the therapeutic action of the medication will not cause the client to feel or perceive any difference in his or her well-being. Client education, a concern for the nurse, can help to enlighten a client about the need for lifelong therapy. Antihypertensive drugs may cause unpleasant side effects while the disease often has no symptoms. If the client is a partner in the plan, it has a better chance of compliance. **Cognitive Level:** Applying **Client Need:** Health Promotion and Maintenance **Integrated Process:** Nursing Process: Implementation **Content Area:** Adult Health **Strategy:** Note that the wording of the question indicates that the correct answer is one that promotes poor adherence to therapy. With this in mind, eliminate any answer that aids in the client's compliance. **Reference:** LeMone, P., Burke, K., & Bauldoff, G. (2012). *Medical-surgical nursing: Critical thinking in patient care* (5th ed.). Upper Saddle River, NJ: Pearson Education, pp. 917–919.

7 **Answer: 2** **Rationale:** Cardiac diseases such as congestive heart failure, myocardial infarction, and cardiomyopathy are conditions that coexist with thromboembolism. Each of these conditions creates the possibility of thrombus occurring because of ineffective emptying of the heart during its pumping action. Thromboembolism generally occurs in clients over the age of 40. Gender usually does not play a role in thromboembolism.

Kidney disease has not been identified as a cause of thromboembolism. **Cognitive Level:** Analyzing **Client Need:** Health Promotion and Maintenance **Integrated Process:** Nursing Process: Assessment **Content Area:** Adult Health **Strategy:** Recall that thromboembolism is most likely to occur when blood flow is sluggish from inadequate cardiac pumping action or when blood is viscous. Use this information and the process of elimination to make a selection. **Reference:** LeMone, P., Burke, K., & Bauldoff, G. (2012). *Medical-surgical nursing: Critical thinking in patient care* (5th ed.). Upper Saddle River, NJ: Pearson Education, pp. 1047–1048.

8 **Answers: 1, 3, 5** **Rationale:** Part of the medical regime will include anticoagulant therapy to prevent development or extension of thrombi by either inhibiting synthesis of clotting factors or deactivating the mechanism. The client's legs need to remain in an elevated position for comfort and to facilitate venous circulation to prevent the development of emboli and thrombi in the lower extremities. Low molecular weight heparins are increasingly used to prevent and treat venous thrombosis. The head of the bed may be elevated for activities such as eating and bathing but not continually. **Cognitive Level:** Applying **Client Need:** Physiological Adaptation **Integrated Process:** Nursing Process: Planning **Content Area:** Adult Health **Strategy:** Recall care of a client with a DVT and use knowledge to decide what care is needed. **Reference:** Lemone, P., Burke, K., & Bauldoff, G. (2012). *Medical-surgical nursing: Critical thinking in patient care* (5th ed.). Upper Saddle River, NJ: Pearson Education, pp. 1952–1953.

9 **Answer: 2** **Rationale:** Most abdominal aortic aneurysms are found in adults over age 65. Most abdominal aneurysms are asymptomatic, but a pulsating mass in the mid and upper abdomen and a bruit over the mass are found on exam. There isn't enough information to determine if the hypertension is secondary or essential. There is no evidence of congestive heart failure (CHF) in the client. Signs of Buerger's disease involve the extremities. **Cognitive Level:** Analyzing **Client Need:** Physiological Adaptation **Integrated Process:** Nursing Process: Diagnosis **Content Area:** Adult Health **Strategy:** Analyze the abdominal assessment findings and use the process of elimination to make a selection. **Reference:** LeMone, P., Burke, K., & Bauldoff, G. (2012). *Medical-surgical nursing: Critical thinking in patient care* (5th ed.). Upper Saddle River, NJ: Pearson Education, pp. 1034–1036.

10 **Answers: 1, 2** **Rationale:** The major task of the health care team is to medicate the client with drugs that produce smooth muscle relaxation, which will decrease the vasospasm and thus increase arterial flow to the affected area. The drugs used are calcium antagonists. Frequently, the client will be medicated during the cold months when vasoconstriction is a physiological response to the environmental temperature. Relieving pain is also a concern. If the medications work, pain will be reduced and blood flow maintained

ANSWERS & RATIONALES

(thus lesions are prevented). Raynaud's disease does not usually cause major disabilities. A client may develop gangrene of the skin of the tips of the digits, but these are in the upper extremities. **Cognitive Level:** Analyzing **Client Need:** Physiological Adaptation **Integrated Process:** Nursing Process: Planning **Content Area:** Adult Health **Strategy:** Note the diagnosis in the question and recall that this is caused by inadequate circulation to the upper extremities and is often accompanied by vasospasm. **Reference:** LeMone, P., Burke, K., & Bauldoff, G. (2012). *Medical-surgical nursing: Critical thinking in patient care* (5th ed.). Upper Saddle River, NJ: Pearson Education, pp. 1046–1047.

Posttest

1 Answers: 1, 3, 4 Rationale: The nurse must emphasize that the client eat a diet high in magnesium, calcium, and potassium, which are contained in fruits and vegetables. The consumption of alcohol is limited to 1 ounce per day; however, with some anti-hypertensive medications, the recommendation is that the client should not consume any alcohol. Aerobic exercise, such as walking, 3 to 5 days a week reduces stress and blood pressure. Smoking and being sedentary are not part of a healthy lifestyle. **Cognitive Level:** Analyzing **Client Need:** Health Promotion and Maintenance **Integrated Process:** Nursing Process: Implementation **Content Area:** Adult Health **Strategy:** Consider healthy lifestyle recommendations for middle-aged men and choose these options since the wording of the question indicates the correct answer(s) will be true statements. **Reference:** LeMone, P. Burke, K., & Bauldoff, G. (2012). *Medical-surgical nursing: Critical thinking in patient care* (5th ed.). Upper Saddle River, NJ: Pearson Education, Inc., pp. 917, 1021–1022.

2 Answer: 3 Rationale: Secondary hypertension has an underlying physiological cause. Gestational hypertension exists when transient elevation of BP occurs for the first time after mid pregnancy without proteinuria or other signs of preeclampsia. Hypertension occurs in 6–8% of pregnancies, which increases risk to both fetus and mother. Pregnancy raises peripheral vascular resistance and cardiac output. The kidneys signal the renin-angiotensin system, which is triggered by low blood volume. A client with white coat syndrome has an otherwise normal BP except when measured by a health care provider. **Cognitive Level:** Applying **Client Need:** Physiological Adaptation **Integrated Process:** Communication and Documentation **Content Area:** Adult Health **Strategy:** The wording of the question indicates the correct option is a true statement. Evaluate each option as to its accuracy and use the process of elimination. **Reference:** Davidson, M., London, M., & Ladewig, P. (2012). *Olds' maternal-newborn nursing & women's health across the lifespan* (9th ed.). Upper Saddle River, NJ: Pearson Education, pp. 476–477. Huether, S. E., & McCance, K. L. (2012). *Understanding pathophysiology* (5th ed.). St. Louis, MO: Elsevier Inc., pp. 587–589.

3 Answer: 1 Rationale: Increased salt intake has been suspected as an etiology in hypertension. Results from using the low-sodium DASH (Dietary Approaches to Stop Hypertension) diet have shown reduced blood pressure. More fluid is retained to balance a high sodium intake so the blood pressure is not lowered. There is no known link between smoking and salt intake or salt intake and anorexia. **Cognitive Level:** Applying **Client Need:** Health Promotion and Maintenance **Integrated Process:** Communication and Documentation **Content Area:** Adult Health **Strategy:** Do not be fooled by distracting information in the stem. Look for a physiologic rationale. **Reference:** Huether, S. E., & McCance, K. L. (2012). *Understanding pathophysiology* (5th ed.). St. Louis, MO: Elsevier Inc., pp. 586–589.

4 Answers: 2, 3, 4 Rationale: International normalized ratio (INR) does not give data information related to hypertension. An elevated cholesterol level would be used as an indicator of atherosclerosis and coronary artery disease. A lowered hematocrit could indicate fluid volume overload, which is useful data related to hypertension. Creatinine is the most specific indicator of kidney function, a cause of hypertension. Troponin levels do not give data related to hypertension. **Cognitive Level:** Analyzing **Client Need:** Reduction of Risk Potential **Integrated Process:** Nursing Process: Diagnosis **Content Area:** Adult Health **Strategy:** Recall the contributing factors that lead to elevation of the blood pressure and consider which of these is evidenced in the laboratory tests listed. **Reference:** Kee, J. L. (2010). *Laboratory and diagnostic test with nursing implications* (8th ed.). Upper Saddle River, NJ: Pearson Education, pp. 83, 358–360.

5 Answer: 2 Rationale: An overweight client on bed rest from a hip surgery is at higher risk because of the two risk factors (obesity and immobility). Even though the client will be ambulated and progressively increase weight bearing, the potential exists because of the immobility. Hypertension does not increase the risk, nor does smoking. Raynaud's disease is not a factor; a history of arthritis and bypass surgery is vague about the cardiac history and further information is needed. **Cognitive Level:** Analyzing **Client Need:** Physiological Adaptation **Integrated Process:** Nursing Process: Assessment **Content Area:** Adult Health **Strategy:** Look for the situation that has the highest risk. In this question each option contains two parts, so the correct answer is the one in which both elements represent a risk for deep vein thrombosis. **Reference:** LeMone, P., Burke, K., & Bauldoff, G. (2012). *Medical-surgical nursing: Critical thinking in patient care* (5th ed.). Upper Saddle River, NJ: Pearson Education, pp. 1050–1053.

6 Answer: 4 Rationale: Clinical manifestations of arterial insufficiency include the "6 Ps"—pain, pallor, polar, paralysis, pulselessness, and paresthesia. The client's signs and symptoms are consistent with arterial insufficiency. The diagnosis is supported by the pallor when the feet are elevated for 10 minutes. The pulse is diminished because this is an arterial occlusion and not venous. Discomfort and itching are usually felt with varicose veins. Thrombophlebitis is associated with redness, warmth, and swelling of an extremity. Raynaud's is more involved with the digits of the hands rather than the feet. **Cognitive Level:** Analyzing **Client Need:** Physiological Adaptation **Integrated Process:** Nursing Process: Assessment **Content Area:** Adult Health **Strategy:** Recall that gravity affects blood flow to extremities. Evaluate the described findings in terms of how gravity influences blood flow and eliminate the options that do not fit the expected findings. **Reference:** Lewis, S., Dirksen, S., Heitkemper, M., Bucher, L., & Camera, I. (2011). *Medical-surgical nursing: Assessment and management of clinical problems* (8th ed.). St. Louis, MO: Elsevier, pp. 880–881.

7 **Answer: 2** **Rationale:** Whenever there is tissue breakdown associated with intermittent claudication, the client will be confined to bed so the body can meet the oxygen requirements for the damaged tissues. Activity in any form raises the amount of oxygen required to sustain both healthy and diseased tissues to a point where deficits will occur and healing will be delayed. When the client is ready to resume ambulation, the shoe of choice is a supportive, comfortable shoe. **Cognitive Level:** Applying **Client Need:** Physiological Adaptation **Integrated Process:** Nursing Process: Implementation **Content Area:** Adult Health **Strategy:** Recall that options that are similar cannot be correct. The option that is different is the one that does not involve activity and increased tissue demand for oxygen. **Reference:** LeMone, P., Burke, K., & Bauldoff, G. (2012). *Medical-surgical nursing: Critical thinking in patient care* (5th ed.). Upper Saddle River, NJ: Pearson Education, pp. 874–875.

8 **Answer: 3** **Rationale:** Venous thrombosis is involves the formation of a thrombus in association with inflammation of a vein, not an artery. Deep vein thrombosis is a disorder involving a thrombus in a deep vein, most commonly the iliac and femoral veins. Venous stasis, hypercoagulability, and venous wall injury are known as Virchow's triad and are the most commonly associated reasons for a thrombosis. Myocardial infarction and prolonged sitting contribute to venous stasis; however, not a stroke. Injury such as a motor vehicle crash may or may not cause thrombi; however, continued bed rest can contribute. **Cognitive Level:** Applying

Client Need: Physiological Adaptation **Integrated Process:** Nursing Process: Assessment **Content Area:** Adult Health **Strategy:** Recall that when there are multiple parts to an option, all the parts of that option must be correct for the option to be the correct answer. **Reference:** LeMone, P., Burke, K., & Bauldoff, G. (2012). *Medical-surgical nursing: Critical thinking in patient care* (5th ed.). Upper Saddle River, NJ: Pearson Education, pp. 882–883.

9 **Answers: 1, 5** **Rationale:** The client with thrombophlebitis of the leg could have unilateral leg edema, extremity pain, a sense of fullness in the thigh or calf, paresthesia, warm skin, erythema, and a systemic temperature greater than 100.4. A positive Homan sign (pain on dorsiflexion of the foot) is a classic but nonspecific sign. If the client feels nothing or just feels like the calf muscle is stretching, that is a normal finding (negative Homan sign). Toe to knee pain is not descriptive of venous thrombosis. There is no positive stretch reflex. **Cognitive Level:** Applying **Client Need:** Physiological Adaptation **Integrated Process:** Nursing Process: Assessment **Content Area:** Adult Health **Strategy:** Recall signs and symptoms of venous thrombosis. **Reference:** Lewis, S., Dirksen, S., Heitkemper, M., Bucher, L., & Camera, I. (2011). *Medical-surgical nursing: Assessment and management of clinical problems* (8th ed.). St. Louis, MO: Elsevier, pp. 884–885.

10 **Answers: 2, 3, 5** **Rationale:** The primary focus of nursing management of Raynaud's disease is client teaching. Instructions should focus on preventing recurrent episodes. Clients should wear loose warm clothing, including gloves, when using a refrigerator or freezer or when handling cold objects. The client should stop using all tobacco products and avoid caffeine and other drugs that have vasoconstrictive effects. Exposure to cold, emotional upsets, caffeine use, and stress usually precipitate symptoms. **Cognitive Level:** Analyzing **Client Need:** Health Promotion and Maintenance **Integrated Process:** Nursing Process: Evaluation **Content Area:** Adult Health **Strategy:** The wording of the question tells you that the correct option also contains a true statement. Which client statement follows the treatment regime for Raynaud's disease? **Reference:** Lewis, S., Dirksen, S., Heitkemper, M., Bucher, L., & Camera, I. (2011). *Medical-surgical nursing: Assessment and management of clinical problems* (8th ed.). St. Louis, MO: Elsevier, pp. 881–882.

References

Adams, M., Josephson, D., & Holland, L. (2011). *Pharmacology for nurses: A pathophysiologic approach.* (3rd ed.) Upper Saddle River, NJ: Pearson Education, pp. 297–322.

Berman, A. J., & Snyder, S. (2012). *Kozier & Erb's fundamentals of nursing: Concepts, process, and practice* (9th ed.). Upper Saddle River, NJ: Pearson Education.

Davidson, M., London, M., & Ladewig, P. (2012). *Olds' maternal-newborn nursing & women's health across the lifespan* (9th ed.). Upper Saddle River, NJ: Pearson Education.

ANSWERS & RATIONALES

Guyton, A., & Hall, J. E. (2011). *Textbook of medical physiology* (12th ed.). Philadelphia, PA: W. B. Saunders.

Huether, S. E., & McCance, K. L. (2012). *Understanding pathophysiology* (5th ed.). St. Louis, MO: Elsevier.

Ignatavicius, D., & Workman, L. (2012). *Medical surgical nursing: Patient-centered collaborative care* (7th ed.). Philadelphia, PA: W. B. Saunders.

JNC–7 Express: The Seventh Report of Joint National Committee on Prevention, Detection, Evaluation, and Treatment of High Blood Pressure. National High Blood Pressure Education Program, National Heart, Lung, & Blood Institute (2003). Retrieved from http://www.nhlbi.nih.gov.

Kee, J. (2009). *Laboratory and diagnostic tests with nursing implications* (8th ed.). Upper Saddle River, NJ: Pearson Education, Inc.

LeMone, P., & Burke, K. M., & Bauldoff, G. (2011). *Medical surgical nursing: Critical thinking in patient care* (5th ed.). Upper Saddle River, NJ: Prentice Hall.

Lewis, S., Heitkemper, M., Dirksen, S., Bucher, L., & Camera, I. (2011). *Medical surgical nursing: Assessment and management of clinical problems* (8th ed.). St. Louis, MO: Elsevier Science.

McCance, K., & Huether, K. (2010) *Understanding pathophysiology: The biologic basis for disease in adults and children* (6th ed.) St. Louis, MO: Elsevier.

Porth, C., & Matfin, G. (2010) *Pathophysiology: Concepts of altered health states* (8th ed.). Philadelphia, PA: Lippincott Williams & Wilkins.

Smith, S., Duell, D., & Martin, B. (2012). *Clinical nursing skills: Basic to advanced skills* (8th ed.). Upper Saddle River, NJ: Pearson Education.

Neurological Health Problems

4

Chapter Outline

Risk Factors Associated with Neurological Health Problems

Increased Intracranial Pressure (ICP)

Intracranial Hematomas

Cerebrovascular Accident (CVA)/Stroke

Spinal Cord Injuries

Encephalitis

Meningitis

Seizures

Guillain-Barré Syndrome

Myasthenia Gravis

Parkinson's Disease

Multiple Sclerosis (MS)

Amyotrophic Lateral Sclerosis (ALS)

Pain

Alzheimer's Disease

Objectives

➤ Define key terms associated with neurological health problems.

➤ Identify risk factors associated with the development of neurological health problems.

➤ Explain the common etiologies of neurological health problems.

➤ Describe the pathophysiological processes associated with specific neurological health problems.

➤ Distinguish between normal and abnormal neurological findings obtained from nursing assessment.

➤ Prioritize nursing interventions associated with specific neurological health problems.

➤ Describe the pathophysiology of pain.

➤ Prioritize nursing interventions used to treat pain.

Test Yourself

Are you ready for the NCLEX-RN® or course exams? Use the practice tests on the companion website to check.

Review at a Glance

anterior cord syndrome complete paralysis and hyperaesthesia below level of lesion; hypalgesia below level of lesion; preservation of touch, position, pressure, and vibration

automatism automatic action or behavior without conscious knowledge; repetitive, semi-purposeful, patterned movement such as lip smacking

autonomic hyperreflexia a life-threatening involuntary response of sympathetic nervous system to a noxious stimulus when there is injury above T6

Brown-Séquard syndrome hemi-section of spinal cord; ipsilateral motor loss below level of lesion; ipsilateral

loss of position and vibration sense below level of lesion; contralateral loss of pain and temperature sensation below level of lesion

Brudzinski sign neck pain and hip and knee flexion that occur when neck is flexed

bulbocavernous reflex contraction of bulbocavernosis muscle upon percussion of dorsum of penis

central cord syndrome greatest percentage of incomplete injuries; motor loss in upper extremities greater than loss in lower extremities; spasticity in lower extremities; variable degrees of sensory loss and bladder dysfunction

cogwheel rigidity manual manipulation of body parts may take on feel of a cogwheel

decerebrate extensor posturing indicating brainstem injury

decorticate flexor posturing indicating corticospinal tract lesions

diplopia double vision

equianalgesic chart shows pain relief obtained with different drugs, doses, and routes

hematomyelia hemorrhage within spinal cord

hydrocephalus brain substance expanded into a watery sac protruding through a cleft in cranium

Kernig sign flexion of hip and knee and then extension of leg causes hamstring pain

lead-pipe rigidity cataleptic condition during which limbs remain in any position in which placed; smooth, stiff movement

Monro-Kellie hypothesis as volume of one brain component increases, volume of another decreases, to a limit

nuchal rigidity muscle contraction in nape of neck

neurogenic pulmonary edema an extremely rapid discharge of nerve impulses from a cerebral injury disrupting vascular permeability

paresthesia localized sensation of numbness, tingling, and heightened sensitivity

phantom pain sensation that pain exists in a removed part

spinal shock a neurophysiologic cessation of all or nearly all reflexes below level of injury

status epilepticus intense, repetitive seizures with very short periods of calm between them

PRETEST

1 Which of the following items would be a high priority for the nurse who is preparing the room for a client to be admitted with a new C7 level spinal cord injury?

1. Special kinetic bed
2. Halo brace device
3. Ventilator on stand-by
4. Catheterization tray

2 Upon return from the radiology department after a CT scan, a client with closed head injury is positioned on the side with the head of bed elevated 30 degrees and with a towel roll placed vertically under the pillow. The nurse explains to the client that this unique positioning facilitates which of the following?

1. Prevention of pulmonary embolism
2. Venous drainage from the brain
3. Airway management
4. Intracranial pressure (ICP) readings

3 After regaining consciousness, a male client reports a tremendous headache as he was taken by ambulance from the site of a motorcycle accident. The wife is unprepared when arriving at the hospital to find he had become comatose. The nurse explains the cause as which of the following?

1. Expanding epidural hematoma
2. Reticular activating system concussion
3. Diffuse axonal injury
4. Expanding pericardial hematoma

4 Following a grand mal seizure, the client is unconscious and unresponsive when the nurse tries to awaken the client. The nurse implements which of the following actions?

1. Calls the rapid response team
2. Notifies the health care provider
3. Administers the next dose of phenytoin (Dilantin) IV instead of by mouth
4. Allows gradual awakening

5 The nurse assesses the client's understanding of discharge needs and goals after experiencing a cerebrovascular accident (CVA). Which client statement indicates further information and teaching will be necessary? Select all that apply.

1. "I'm getting at least a year's supply of adult disposable briefs."
2. "I will never have another stroke."
3. "I've got to find a walking buddy."
4. "I'm getting a rail installed in my tub."
5. "I'll be glad to get home and have a cigarette."

6 When developing a plan of care for a client newly hospitalized with meningitis, the nurse determines that which of the following areas should be the major focus of nursing care?

1. Enhancing coping skills
2. Providing cognitive stimulation
3. Assessing risk for injury and preventing complications
4. Increasing cardiac output

7 The client comes to the emergency department with weakness that has been progressing upward in both legs for 2 days. The nurse, suspecting Guillain-Barré syndrome (GBS), begins care by doing which of the following? Select all that apply.

1. Taking medical history, noting recent viral influenza
2. Giving the client orange juice for fatigue and low blood glucose
3. Assessing neurological and respiratory function
4. Evaluating for petit mal seizures
5. Assessing vital signs

8 Which of the following items would be of priority for the nurse to include in a teaching plan for a client with myasthenia gravis?

1. Exercise to increase peripheral circulation.
2. Plan important activities for late afternoon.
3. Identify signs of and action during crisis.
4. Eat 3 well-balanced meals a day.

9 The client with Parkinson's disease tells the nurse that the resting tremor present in the right hand is very frustrating. The nurse advises the client to do which of the following?

1. Practice deep breathing for relaxation.
2. Take a warm bath to aid microcirculation to the extremities.
3. Hold an object in that hand to control hand movements.
4. Take diazepam (Valium) as needed for relaxation of muscles.

10 A first-day postoperative client who rates his pain as 9 on a scale of 0 (no pain) to 10 (worst pain) is laughing and talking with visitors. The care plan indicates that the client has identified a pain level of 5 as his comfort level goal and he has a prescription for analgesics every 3 hours. His last dose was three hours ago with no untoward effects. Which actions should the nurse take at this time? Select all that apply.

1. Record his pain level at 5.
2. Administer a dose of the analgesic.
3. Telephone the surgeon for an order for patient-controlled analgesia.
4. Reassess the pain 30 minutes after analgesic is administered.
5. Ask client if he can wait a while longer for medication since his behavior does not reflect acute pain.

➤ *See pages 128–129 for Answers and Rationales.*

I. RISK FACTORS ASSOCIATED WITH NEUROLOGICAL HEALTH PROBLEMS

A. **Increased intracranial pressure**: stroke, tumor, head trauma, inflammation, and neurological conditions such as meningitis

B. **Intracranial hematomas**: males (adolescent to young adulthood), injury, radiation, jobs or incidents where electrocution is a possibility, outside employment where weather can be severe or falls are a high probability

C. **Stroke**: diseases (hypertension [HTN], sickle cell anemia, polycythemia, atherosclerosis, cardiac valvular disease, diabetes), valve and organ replacement, anticoagulant therapy, atrial fibrillation, cardioversion, oral contraceptives, drug abuse, smoking, high salt or alcohol intake, sedentary lifestyle

D. **Spinal cord injury (SCI)**: athletes, drug and/or alcohol abuse, employment where falls are a high probability, diseases such as tumors, syringomyelia, and degenerative diseases

E. **Encephalitis**: living close to an abundance of mosquitoes, especially if cattle and horses are nearby; drinking goat's milk; exposure to ticks; metal poisonings; recent immunizations and illnesses such as German measles or chickenpox

F. **Meningitis**: impaired immune function as in very old or very young clients or those with HIV or on chemotherapy, those with otitis media, sinusitis, basal skull fracture, neurosurgery, systemic sepsis, or crowded living conditions (college dorms, military institutions, and prisons)

G. **Seizures**: brain tumors, family history, head injury, or neurological disorders

H. **Guillain-Barré Syndrome**: viral infections, recent immunizations

I. **Myasthenia gravis (MG)**: family or previous history of autoimmune diseases

J. **Parkinson's disease (proposed theories only)**: cerebral anoxia, advancing age, genetic factors, and factors toxic to dopaminergic cells

K. **Multiple sclerosis (MS)**: living in colder climates; genetic or family history of MS or autoimmune illnesses; age

L. **Amyotrophic lateral sclerosis (ALS)**: possibly genetics

M. **Pain**: work requiring strenuous lifting or bending, individuals with poor posture, stage of life factors, chronic diseases, arterial or ischemic wounds

N. **Alzheimer's disease**: aging, head trauma, family history, trauma, presence of risk gene (APO–E4)

II. INCREASED INTRACRANIAL PRESSURE (ICP)

A. **Overview**
1. A rise in pressure of cerebrospinal fluid (CSF) that maintains subarachnoid space between skull and brain; a balance among volumes of content of cranial vault usually exists (brain 80%, blood 10%, CSF 10%)
2. Increased ICP is an ICP greater than 15 mmHg; a significant increase is termed intracranial hypertension
3. Causes
    a. Increases in tissue volume, such as occur with neoplasm; cerebral edema (interstitial); tumor or trauma (vasogenic); or ischemic injury, infarction, infection or other disease state (hypoxic)
    b. Increases in blood volume: hemorrhage and hematoma formation, increased arterial inflow, and decreased venous return
    c. Increases in CSF volume from: obstruction of CSF pathways leading to **hydrocephalus** (brain substance expanded into a watery sac), deficient CSF absorption (often from blockage of arachnoid villi or idiopathic as in normal pressure hydrocephalus postbleed), or overproduction of CSF
    d. Other causes: congenital or developmental, metabolic, or pseudotumor cerebri (benign intracranial hypertension), abscess

B. **Pathophysiology**
1. **Monro-Kellie hypothesis**: as volume of 1 component (brain tissue, blood, CSF) increases, volume of another decreases, to a limit
    a. Controlled by autoregulation: cerebral arterioles change diameter to maintain blood flow when ICP increases
    b. Brain tissue unable to compensate (decrease volume)
2. Maximal compensation occurs after volume increases; ICP begins to increase
3. ICP values
    a. ICP value alone is not a reliable measure of brain's compliance: ICP may be in normal range (less than 15 mmHg), but client may still be in danger of herniation because of poor compliance
    b. Changes in ICP in response to stimuli may be predictive of compliance; decreased compliance is indicated by sustained increases in ICP in response to stimuli or large increases in response to non-noxious stimuli

4. Cerebral blood flow (CBF): normally 750 mL/min
   a. Hypercarbia: $PaCO_2$ greater than 45 mmHg produces vasodilation; increases ICP by increasing volume
   b. Hypocarbia: $PaCO_2$ less than 25 mmHg produces rebound cerebral vasodilation, loss of autoregulation
5. Cerebral perfusion pressure (CPP): normally 60–100 mmHg; determines CBF
   a. Hyperperfusion and increased ICP occur with CPP above 100 mmHg
   b. Reduction in CPP leads to hypoperfusion and cerebral ischemia (CPP 40–60 mmHg), irreversible ischemia and infarction (CPP less than 40 mmHg), and brain death (CPP 0–40 mmHg)
6. Compensatory mechanisms
   a. Activated when increase in ICP occurs to balance volumes within cranial vault to protect brain; rapid increases in ICP prevent activation
   b. Compensatory mechanisms involve CSF changes, which include normal shunting of CSF into spinal subarachnoid space to reduce pressure (most common), increased absorption of CSF, or decreased secretion of CSF
   c. Venous blood may also be shunted to allow more room for expansion
7. Failure of compensatory mechanisms causes ischemia, hypoxia, herniation, and brain death
8. Signs and symptoms
   a. Gastrointestinal: ulceration and bleeding
   b. Cardiovascular: elevation or depression of S-T segments; large positive or negative U waves; prolonged Q-T or Q-U intervals; Q waves in both standard and precordial leads; deeply inverted or tall spiky upright T waves; dysrhythmias
   c. Cushing's triad or response
      1) Involves 3 classic signs: widening pulse pressure, elevated systolic BP, and bradycardia; respirations may become irregular
      2) Brainstem reflects final effort to maintain cerebral perfusion
      3) Caused by rapidly expanding lesions such as epidural hematoma or lesion in posterior fossa
      4) Seen when ICP is greater than 45 mmHg or when ICP approaches systemic diastolic BP
      5) Pressure on brainstem causes ischemia of vasomotor center of medulla
      6) Systolic BP increases while diastolic remains the same causing widened pulse pressure
      7) Increased BP: sensed in baroreceptors of carotid arteries and aortic arch; causes vagal response of bradycardia
   d. **Neurogenic pulmonary edema** is an extremely rapid discharge of nerve impulses from an injured brain disrupting vascular permeability
   e. Intracranial effects
      1) Increase in ICP decreases microvascular CBF leading to tissue hypoxia and causing respiratory center dysfunction
      2) Hypoventilation leads to increased $PaCO_2$ and decreased blood pH
      3) Hypercarbia causes cerebral vessel vasodilation and edema
      4) Increased ICP results in herniation, cerebral ischemia, and brain death
9. Herniation syndromes occur, which are displacement of a portion of brain through or around linings of brain or openings within intracranial cavity
   a. Mechanism is categorized as supratentorial, infratentorial, or extracranial
      1) Caused by increased pressure in 1 or more compartments; usually occurs when a pressure difference exists between supratentorial and infratentorial (posterior fossa) compartments

        2) Supratentorial herniation syndromes: herniation of structures normally lying above tentorium cerebelli; include cingulated herniation; uncal herniation; and transtentorial or central herniation

        3) Infratentorial herniation syndrome: herniation of structures lying below tentorium cerebelli; include upward transtentorial herniation and downward cerebellar or tonsillar herniation

        4) Extracranial herniation syndrome: occurs when opening in skull allows intracranial contents under pressure to herniate outward; may occur through open wound, surgical incision, ICP monitor site or through fractures of ear or nose; resulting decrease in volume lowers ICP and possibly prevents intracranial herniation

    b. Results: compression, laceration, distortion, or necrosis of brain structures; vascular compromise; blocked flow of CSF; brain compression and death

C. Nursing assessment of increased ICP

    1. Assessment

        a. Airway patency and breathing patterns: central nervous system (CNS) dysfunction is associated with decreased level of consciousness (LOC), hypercapnia, and potential for pulmonary edema

        b. Pupillary dysfunction (early sign): compression of oculomotor nerve (CN III) results in dilation of ipsilateral pupil, sluggish or no response to light, inability to move eye upward, and ptosis (drooping) of eyelid; note that a nonreactive, dilated pupil is a late sign and a neurological emergency heralding transtentorial brain herniation

        c. Changes in vital signs (late sign): Cushing's triad of increased systolic BP, widening pulse pressure, bradycardia, and possible irregular respiratory pattern is seen with sustained and elevated ICP; fever is possible as compensatory measures fail

        d. Visual abnormalities: impaired or blurred vision or decreased extraocular movements

        e. Papilledema: swelling of optic disc, as seen with an ophthalmoscope; indicative of long-standing increased ICP

        f. Motor function: contralateral hemiparesis or hemiplegia may be seen; no movement or flaccidity is worst sign; localization to a painful stimulus may result in an effort to produce movement

            1) Decorticate: flexor posturing indicating corticospinal tract lesions (see Figure 4-1a)

            2) Decerebrate: extensor posturing indicating brainstem injury (see Figure 4-1b)

Figure 4-1

Abnormal posturing seen in head injuries.
A. Decorticate,
B. Decerebrate.

A

B

       g. Headache: unusual, seen with slowly increasing ICP, worse with straining and position changes, especially on awakening

       h. Emesis: projectile vomiting without nausea

   2. Diagnostic tests: arterial blood gases (ABGs), complete blood count (CBC), CSF cultures, computed tomography (CT) scan, and serum osmolality

D. Nursing management

   1. Medications include stool softener, diuretic (osmotic, loop), the corticosteroid dexamethasone (Decadron), antipyretic such as acetaminophen (Tylenol), H_2 receptor antagonist, and antiepileptics (if seizures occur)

   2. Secure airway patency and clearance

       a. Hyperventilate and oxygenate with 100% O_2 using sigh mode on ventilator prior to suctioning; avoid suctioning for longer than 10 seconds

       b. Auscultate lungs and clear any secretions

       c. Position client side to side to decrease aspiration risk in case of emesis

       d. Promote normal breathing pattern: monitor arterial carbon dioxide pressure ($PaCO_2$) to remain 25–30 mmHg, avoiding cerebral vasodilation

   3. Optimize cerebral perfusion

       a. Position client to avoid extreme rotation or flexion of neck, which increases jugular venous pressure and ICP; a neutral or midline position aids cerebral venous drainage

       b. Avoid or greatly reduce extreme hip flexion, which causes an increase in intra-abdominal and intrathoracic pressure, producing increased ICP

       c. Provide high-fiber diet to decrease use of Valsalva maneuver; assist with bowel movements using bedpan

       d. Avoid physiological and environmental stimuli

       e. Monitor nursing care to keep ICP below 25 mmHg and to promote return to baseline levels within 5 minutes

       f. Prevent fluid overload

   4. Monitor for symptoms of rising ICP prior to herniation

       a. Report and treat per protocol signs of acutely increasing ICP: decreasing Glasgow Coma Scale (GCS) score, behavioral changes, disorientation, difficulty in following simple commands, speech changes, less purposeful response to painful stimuli, posturing movements, loss of or abnormal (i.e., positive Babinski) reflexes

       b. Notify health care provider and follow unit protocol for pupil and eye changes: blurred vision, **diplopia** (double vision), extraocular movement (EOM) abnormalities, and nystagmus

   5. Prevent infection

       a. Adhere to protocols for care of client with an intracranial pressure monitoring device

       b. Monitor indicators of infection: white blood cell (WBC) counts, positive cultures, fever, chills, nuchal rigidity, and changes in vital signs

       c. Inspect ICP monitoring site and connections for leaking CSF or drainage

   6. Avoid administration of drugs such as narcotics that can mimic signs of increased ICP

   7. Support family: encourage family to visit client; provide information to optimize decision making when clients are unable to make treatment choices; anticipate grieving and identify sources of community support

III. INTRACRANIAL HEMATOMAS

A. Overview

   1. Defined as a break in a blood vessel within cranium or skull that leads to swelling caused by hemorrhage

2. Peak occurrence during evening and night hours on weekends
3. Pathological mechanisms
   a. Direct impact
      1) Acceleration: rapidly moving object strikes relatively stationary head
      2) Deceleration: coming to a sudden, abrupt stop, as when head strikes an immobile object/static surface (more severe damage because of effects on brain stem)
      3) Rotation: lateral blow rotates brain, contusing brain stem and disrupting white matter
   b. Indirect stresses: trauma not to head but involves brain; rotational displacement of head on extreme motion of neck causes shear, tensile strains and compressive forces transmitted to brain; landing on buttocks or feet from a height transmits force through spinal column to base of brain
   c. Systemic: chronic alcoholism, cerebral atrophy, anticoagulants, long history of hypertension
4. Mechanisms of injury: blunt (closed, non-penetrating); penetrating (open); and compression: skull compressed between two forces causing a crush effect on brain
5. Types of injury include scalp injuries, skull fractures, or dural integrity injury (closed such as with simple linear fracture, or open with dura torn by laceration, such as with compound or depressed fractures, or penetrating objects)
6. Intracranial hemorrhage classified as epidural, subdural, or intracerebral
7. Common causes: vehicular crashes (automobiles, motorcycles), falls, violence, sports-related injuries, ingestion of alcohol and/or drugs, other (intrauterine and birth injury, radiation, electrocution, heat stroke, lightning)

B. **Pathophysiology**
1. *Epidural* hematoma: cerebral artery bleed above dura mater; usually in middle fossa caused by laceration of middle meningeal artery; constitutes 2–6% of head injuries
   a. Signs of brain stem compression usually occur within 24 hours
   b. Signs and symptoms
      1) Short period of unconsciousness followed by a lucid interval
      2) Lucid interval followed by progressive depression of consciousness
      3) Focal signs: ipsilateral pupil dilation, weakness of contralateral extremities
2. *Subdural* hematoma: bleeding into subdural space of brain with disruption of cortical veins; most often over parietal areas; 29% of head injuries
   a. Acute: symptomatic within 24–72 hours
      1) Most clients deteriorate quickly, become deeply comatose, with brain unable to compensate from rapid compression; often associated with severe brain trauma and high mortality; may mimic epidural hematoma
      2) Signs and symptoms include depressed LOC, usually from time of injury; ipsilateral pupil dilation and contralateral weakness
   b. Subacute: symptomatic within 2–10 days
      1) Better prognosis than acute, still 25–35% mortality
      2) Signs and symptoms include headaches; decreased LOC and focal signs of compression; failure to show improvement
   c. Chronic: symptoms occur after 10 days (elusive, nonspecific, and fluctuating)
      1) Gradual clot formation allows brain time to accommodate; traumatic etiology may be unclear, minor, or forgotten; prognosis good; may reaccumulate
      2) Signs and symptoms include slowly progressive change in behavior (apathy) or personality, headaches; variable LOC; lethargy, confusion, motor weakness with loss of upward gaze, dysphasia, urinary or bowel incontinence
3. *Intracerebral* hematoma: bleeding from small arteries or veins in subcortical white matter
   a. Lucid interval followed by decreased LOC

      b. Focal signs based on location

      c. Signs and symptoms include possible headache, hemiplegia, ipsilateral pupil dilation, progressing ICP with potential for herniation; petechiae common, usually seen with contusion, edema; majority occur in frontal and temporal lobes; signs and symptoms according to location

  4. Subarachnoid hemorrhage

      a. Bleeding between pia mater of covering of brain and spinal cord and arachnoid membrane

      b. Signs and symptoms include severe headache and restlessness; **nuchal rigidity** (muscle contraction to nape of neck), fever, and a positive **Kernig sign** (flexion of hip and knee and then extension of leg causes hamstring pain), (see Figure 4-2); positive **Brudzinski sign** (flexion of neck causes flexion at hip; see Figure 4-3); positive Babinski reflex (dorsiflexion of great toe upon stimulating sole of feet)

C. Nursing assessment

  1. Assessment

      a. Airway and breathing pattern

      b. Assess vital signs (VS), LOC, pupils, and motor responses; document baseline and monitor for subtle, sudden changes

      c. Observe for clinical indications of expanding lesions

         1) Localized/focal signs: hemiplegia, visual field defect, eye deviation, cerebellar signs, cranial nerve signs

         2) Generalized signs of increased ICP: headache, restlessness, irritability

      d. Gather data about traumatic event from family, witnesses including: details and time of injury; change in consciousness (lucid period, duration of unresponsiveness); and seizure activity

      e. Assess signs and symptoms of increased ICP, which may occur suddenly, resulting in tentorial herniation and sudden respiratory arrest

  2. Diagnostic tests: CT scan, magnetic resonance imaging (MRI), ABGs, CBC

Figure 4-2
Kernig sign

Figure 4-3
Brudzinski sign

D. Nursing management
1. Surgery is recommended treatment; there is no specific medication therapy

2. Maintain adequate airway and cerebral perfusion: monitor respiratory pattern, breath sounds, cyanosis, restlessness, and use of accessory muscles; monitor ICP readings; prepare for O_2 administration, intubation or tracheostomy; prepare for possible cranial surgery if inadequate perfusion
3. Advocate for client rest periods between frequent VS and neuro checks
4. Provide seizure precautions because of risk for seizures secondary to increased ICP (when dura interrupted)
5. Support client and family in understanding condition and treatment

IV. CEREBROVASCULAR ACCIDENT (CVA)/STROKE

A. Overview
1. Defined as an abrupt loss of consciousness with resulting paralysis that may be temporary or permanent
2. Often preceded by transient ischemic attacks (TIAs), which mimic a stroke without permanent paralysis; cause of TIA is a temporary interference in cerebral blood flow causing neurological deficits from focal or retinal ischemia (clinical symptoms typically last less than 1 hour with no evidence of an acute infarction)
3. Causes of stroke include thrombus (most common), embolus, and hemorrhage

B. Pathophysiology
1. Cellular level changes begin 4–5 minutes after blood flow and oxygenation of neurons are reduced
2. The sodium pump and neurotransmitters fail because of anaerobic glycolysis, resulting in cerebral edema as sodium (Na^+) draws water into brain
3. Cerebral blood vessel walls swell, circulation is compromised, and vasospasm combined with blood viscosity reduces cerebral perfusion
4. Outcomes of decreased cerebral perfusion: cerebral anoxia caused by interrupted blood supply; cerebral infarction (irreversible damage) if anoxia lasts longer than 10 minutes; cerebral edema causing secondary damage; contralateral deficits when stroke is in cerebral hemisphere; permanent deficits reflecting locality of stroke
5. Signs and symptoms: decreased LOC or unconsciousness, stertorous breathing, unequal pupils (larger pupil noted on same side as stroke), paralysis of one side, perspiration, aphasia (abnormal or absent speech), blank stare, dysphagia, inability to make decisions, loss of memory, and gait instability

C. Nursing assessment
1. Assessment
   a. Nursing history: interview client and family; history of risk factors; client and family's understanding of illness
   b. Assessment: airway obstruction and hypoxia if decreased LOC; neurological deficits; vital signs; urine output; fluid and caloric needs; visual impairment (corneal abrasions, eye discomfort, diplopia); loss of sensation and functional ability of mouth, face and swallowing ability; bowel and bladder function; immobility issues; communication; perceptual deficits; psychosocial needs; and understanding of treatment
2. Diagnostic tests: electrolytes, CT scan, MRI, ABGs, arteriography, ultrasound of carotid arteries, lumbar puncture, coagulation studies such as prothrombin time (PT), partial thromboplastin time (PTT), international normalized ratio (INR)

D. Nursing management
1. Medications include stool softeners, anticoagulants or thrombolytics, antiplatelet agents, calcium channel blockers, diuretics (if increased ICP exists), antiepileptics if seizures occur; monitor effects of drugs

2. Monitor neurological status
   a. Hyperthermia: maintain temperature within normal limits
   b. Neglect syndrome: provide care around perceptual deficits
   c. Seizures: promote safety and cerebral perfusion
   d. Agnosia: support recognition of previously known subject
   e. Communication deficits: consult with speech therapist, use communication board
   f. Visual: provide care with recognition of hemianopia, diplopia, or decreased acuity; placing a patch over one eye reduces double vision
   g. Cognitive changes: create plan of care with health care team to address memory loss, poor attention span, distractibility, judgment, problem solving difficulty, and disorientation
   h. Behavioral changes: educate family as to causes and approaches to use with labiality, loss of inhibitions, fear, anger, and depression
   i. Increased ICP: monitor closely for any changes in LOC
3. Respiratory status
   a. Airway obstruction: suction per assessment, after oxygenating and with goal of preventing increased ICP; monitor ABGs
   b. Poor cough and gag reflexes: intermittent positive pressure breathing (IPPB) therapy and position client on side to decrease risk of aspirating own secretions
   c. Pulmonary emboli: mobilize client as soon as tolerated; administer anticoagulant therapy, monitoring appropriate lab values
4. Monitor gastrointestinal system
   a. Dysphagia (difficulty swallowing): provide swallow evaluation before instituting feeding
   b. Constipation: provide stool softeners and bowel routine
   c. Stool impaction: encourage roughage, high fiber, and mobility to prevent impaction; increase fluid intake; remove any fecal impaction and document
5. Monitor genitourinary system
   a. Incontinence: evaluate behavioral, pharmacological, and supportive devices to assist client for long-term maintenance but discourage dependency on adult disposable briefs early in stroke
   b. Urgency: offer bedpan, urinal, or commode use every 2 hours; avoid caffeine
   c. Retention: avoid in-dwelling urinary catheters because of risk for infection; develop intermittent catheterization schedule; use bladder scan device or straight catheterization to detect postvoid residuals
   d. Renal calculi: keep urine dilute (at least 2,000 mL per day), prevent urinary stasis and infection; teach clients a prevention diet that is low in oxalate-rich foods and purines; monitor fluid and nutritional status
6. Monitor musculoskeletal system
   a. Hemiplegia: apply pneumatic compression device or elastic hose to reduce deep vein thrombosis; instruct family on range of motion (ROM) exercises of joints from shoulder to ankle; initiate physical therapy for gait training
   b. Contractures: create positioning schedule of 2 hours on unaffected side, 30 minutes on affected side, 30 minutes prone; indicate schedule in charting; use high top tennis shoes or therapeutic boots to prevent foot drop
   c. Atrophy: begin ROM exercises early, combined with stretching at least 4 times a day, instructing family as able
   d. Dysarthria (difficulty and defective speech caused by impairment of tongue or other muscles essential to speech): use communication board, avoid frustration; keep communication simple; consult with speech pathology for motor relearning plan
   e. Osteoporosis: facilitate weight-bearing activity, screen for progression

Practice to Pass

A client who had a stroke is preparing for transfer to a rehabilitation setting. What would support the client and family's transition?

    f. Sensory deprivation: create plan to optimize balance in sensory stimulation; provide appropriate repetition for learning

    g. Self-image: provide positive feedback; encourage grooming and street attire; begin rehabilitation as soon as tolerated

    h. Sexual dysfunction: encourage open communication among partners; inform client and partner of options; introduce topic before discharge from acute care

7. Monitor safety: explore what life will be like in home setting with new deficits; provide safety assessment for home setting, identifying areas to modify based on fall risk; create plan with client and family to optimize return to community, identify support services, and recognize warning signs of another stroke event

V. SPINAL CORD INJURIES

    A. Overview

        1. SCI is defined as a fracture or injury (twisting, compression, pulling) of bones of spinal column; damage may involve part of or all of spinal cord

        2. Incidence is more prominent in young males (18–30 years); is increasing in young females; increases with use of alcohol and/or drugs

        3. Types of injury

            a. Level of injury: cervical (most common site); thoracic (least common site); and lumbar

            b. Upper and lower motor neuron damage (see Table 4-1)

                1) Upper motor neurons (UMN) drive voluntary movement; UMNs originate in cerebral cortex and end at anterior horn cell of cord resulting in spastic paralysis and reflexes

Table 4-1 Degrees of Motor and Sensory Loss in Spinal Cord Injury	
Level of Lesion	**Degree of Motor and/or Sensory Loss**
Central cord syndrome, greatest percentage of incomplete injuries	Motor loss in upper extremities greater than loss in lower extremities; spasticity of lower extremities Variable degree of sensory loss Variable degree of bladder dysfunction Associated with hyperextension injuries of cervical spine, especially in osteoarthritis of spine
Anterior cord syndrome, associated with flexion injuries of cervical spine	Complete paralysis below level of lesion Hyperesthesia below level of lesion Hypalgesia below level of lesion Preservation of touch, position, pressure, and vibration **Paresthesia** (localized sensation of numbness, tingling, and heightened sensitivity) may be present
Brown-Séquard syndrome, (hemi-section of the cord) associated with open penetrating wounds to the cord	Ipsilateral motor loss below level of lesion Ipsilateral loss of position and vibration sense below level of lesion Contralateral loss of pain and temperature senses below level of lesion
Posterior cord syndrome (rare)	Loss of light touch and proprioception below level of lesion Motor function of extremities, pain, and temperature remain intact Associated with cervical hyperextension
Sacral sparing	Preservation of sensation in genitals and saddle area (S_3–S_5) Can occur in presence of profound motor and sensory loss Characteristic of central and anterior cord syndromes
Cauda equina lesions	Sparing of function unpredictable: unilateral or bilateral, motor, sensory, or both Indirect trauma to peripheral nerves associated with fractures Potential for regrowth and recovery

2) Lower motor neuron (LMN) begins at anterior horn cell; LMNs become part of peripheral nerve to muscle, motor side of reflex arc; usually present in cauda equina injuries; areflexia results in flaccid paralysis; these neurons are responsible for innervation and contraction of skeletal muscles

4. Forces leading to injury: hyperflexion (usually with rotation), hyperextension (usually with rotation), vertical compression (axial loading), cord contusion without vertebral disruption (fracture, dislocation), and penetrating wounds (see Figure 4-4)

Figure 4-4

Forces leading to spinal cord injury. A. Hyperflexion, B. Hyperextension, C. Axial loading as one type of compression.

   5. Types of vertebral injury
   a. Fractures: spinous, lateral and/or articular processes, body, pedicles
      1) Odontoid fractures: Types I, II, III
      2) Hangman's fracture: bilateral arches of axis, with or without dislocation of axis on C3
      3) Jefferson: burst fracture of atlas
      4) Occiput-atlanto dislocation
   b. Dislocation: unilateral or bilateral facets, vertebral body
   c. Subluxation: facets
   d. Compression: burst or wedge fractures
   e. Fracture: dislocation
   6. Common causes: motor vehicle crashes; falls and falling objects; athletics (diving, football, skiing, boating); penetrating wounds: gunshot, stabbing
B. Pathophysiology
   1. Influencing factors
   a. Spinal cord is located in a relatively small space
   b. Canal space varies; is wider in children (fewer children with traumatic cervical injuries become quadriplegic; wide canal allows cord more space to move without compression) and narrower with congenital anomalies, cervical spondylosis, age, and osteoarthritic changes
   c. Variability of vascular supply
   d. Presence of osteophytes (bony spurs)
   2. Mechanisms
   a. Concussion: pressure waves are propagated through cord, resulting in transient loss of function with immediate flaccid paralysis and complete recovery in minutes to hours
   b. Compression: bone, ligaments, extruded disc material and hematoma
   c. Contusion: results in edema, petechial hemorrhages, neuronal changes, inflammation
   d. Hematomyelia: hemorrhage within cord
   e. Transection: actual (rare) or functional
   f. Overstretching: causing disruption of tissue
   g. Edema: further impairs capillary circulation and venous return
   h. Ischemia: interruption of anterior or posterior arterial blood flow by compression
   3. Necrosis of spinal cord substance
   a. Vascular pathology: ischemia is implicated as causing reduction or interruption of blood supply, leading to necrosis
      1) SCI increases permeability of blood vessels (BV), which leads to edema formation and decreases blood flow to area
      2) Further ischemia leads to necrosis with vascular stasis, causing thrombosis, which further reduces blood flow and a vicious cycle ensues, leading eventually to necrosis of gray matter (in 4–48 hours)
   b. Neuronal pathology
      1) Injury alters electrophysiology of affected neurons, causing sodium leakage into cells, creating a negative resting potential
      2) This results in spinal shock stage, where there is a neurophysiologic cessation of all or nearly all reflexes below level of injury
   c. Biochemical pathology
      1) Accumulated vasoactive amines (norepinephrine, serotonin, dopamine, histamine) are released or transported to wounded tissue after injury
      2) Induces maximal toxic vasospasm, impedes microcirculation, diminishes local oxygenation, and produces necrosis of BVs and neurons

     d. Disintegration of myelin sheath and axis cylinder

     e. Spinal cord may liquefy in severe disruption

4. Hematomyelia and cord edema may ascend above level of initial injury; syringomyelia (progressive, chronic spinal cord disease) may result

5. Degree of functional impairment of spinal cord

     a. Complete: total sensory/motor loss and autonomic disruption below level of lesion, reflecting irreversible spinal cord damage

          1) Tetraplegia or quadriplegia: occurs in cervical region; loss of leg function with variable loss of arm function depending on level of injury

          2) Paraplegia: occurs in thoracic region and lumbar 1 and 2 region; loss of leg function

     b. Incomplete and variable degrees of motor and/or sensory loss below level of lesion, reflecting sparing of certain tracts

6. Horner syndrome

     a. Incomplete cord transection involving cervical sympathetic nerves

     b. Ipsilateral ptosis of eyelid, constricted pupil, and lack of facial sweating (anhidrosis)

7. Spinal cord segmental level: functional loss depends on degree of spinal cord damage, may not correspond to vertebral level, particularly in thoracolumbar and sacral level (see Table 4-2)

8. **Spinal shock**: loss of all reflex activity below level of injury

     a. Duration: 2 days to several months

     b. Associated with hypotension and bradycardia

     c. **Bulbocavernous reflex** (contraction of bulbocavernous muscle on percussing dorsum of penis) is an early sign of resolving spinal shock: absence of this spinal reflex arc implies there is no physiological continuity between lower spinal cord and supraspinal centers

     d. Appearance of involuntary spastic movement and positive deep tendon reflexes below level of injury indicate spinal shock has resolved

Table 4-2	**Functional Loss According to Spinal Cord Segmental Level**	
Spinal Column	**Vertebrae**	**Functional Loss**
Cervical	C 1–2	Total tetraplegia and respiratory paralysis
	C 3–4	Total tetraplegia, weak diaphragm, absent intercostals
	C 5–6	Tetraplegia with gross arm movements; diaphragm may be impaired initially
	C 6–7	Tetraplegia with biceps and deltoid function; no triceps
	C 7–8	Tetraplegia with triceps function; no intrinsic hand function
Thoracic	T 1–5	Paraplegia often with diaphragmatic breathing; arm function intact; loss of leg function, bladder, bowels; sensation present down to nipple line
	T 6–12	Paraplegia with no abdominal reflexes present at T12; usually spastic paralysis of lower limbs; at level of T12, sensation is present down to groin area
Below T12	Conus medullaris	Bowel and bladder sphincter dysfunction; may have lower leg weakness; sacral dermatome hyperaesthesia or anesthesia, back pain
	Cauda equina	Asymmetric, atrophic, areflexic paralysis (lower motor neuron); sensory root loss; outer aspect legs, ankles, posterior lower limbs, and saddle area; sphincter dysfunction
Sacral	S 1–5	Loss of bladder, bowel, sex function; some foot displacement may be present; no paralysis of leg muscle from S3 to S5; loss of sensation involves saddle area, scrotum, perineum, penis, anal area, and upper third of posterior aspect of thigh

9. Degree of functional loss: depends on level and amount of damage to spinal cord; myelopathy refers to cord damage; radiculopathy refers to dysfunction of nerve roots; may have some sparing or eventual return, as part of peripheral nervous system

10. Early intervention (within first few hours after injury) reduces or minimizes cellular damage leading to better prognosis for function

11. Prognosis for degree of bladder, bowel, and sexual function varies with level of lesion and is related to upper or lower motor neuron lesion; if sacral nerve roots are damaged, prognosis for reflex activity of these functions is poor

12. Late stage: spinal cord may become fibrotic, and pathological changes may extend above and below damaged segment

13. Signs and symptoms include hypotension, loss of motor control and sensation below level of injury, decreased or absent reflexes, urinary retention, stool and urinary incontinence, neurogenic bladder, impotence, muscle spasms, muscle atrophy, paraplegia, tetraplegia, decreased chest expansion, decreased cough reflex, hypercalcemia, cardiac dysrhythmias, pain (note: manifestations will depend on level of injury)

14. Complications of SCI: stress ulcers, paralytic ileus, pressure ulcers, stool impaction, decreased venous return, pathologic fractures caused by bone demineralization and joint contractions

C. Nursing assessment

1. Assessment
   a. Emergency assessment at scene or in emergency department
      1) Suspect cervical spine (C-spine) injury until proven otherwise; all head injuries are also considered spinal cord injuries until ruled out by diagnostic methods, such as C-spine x-rays
      2) Maintain airway (using chin lift/jaw thrust method), breathing, and circulation
      3) Maintain neck in neutral position, palpate cervical spine region
      4) Assess movement and sensation in extremities: if *conscious*, ask client to move toes, feet, legs, fingers, hands, arms; ask if client can feel touch on toes, feet, legs, fingers, hands, arms; test for reflex withdrawal; if *unconscious*, observe any spontaneous movements by client; use stimuli to elicit more purposeful voluntary movements or reflex withdrawal
   b. Physical examination
      1) Precise level of motor and sensory findings include sacral sparing, voluntary toe flexion
      2) Presence/absence of all deep tendon and superficial reflexes
      3) Tenderness or gaps between spinous processes
      4) Deformities, swelling, limitation of movement particularly in neck
      5) Evidence of other trauma: head, chest, abdomen, extremities
   c. Establish early, accurate baseline: motor and sensory function of all extremities; breathing pattern; presence of sweating; subjective reports of pain; bladder function, distention, voiding reflex; presence of bowel sounds, anal reflex; vital signs; neuro exam, including cognition level; and sexuality
   d. Assess abdomen for distention; ileus is common
   e. Assess for trauma to other systems; note lacerations, abrasions, etc.
   f. Collect pertinent data to assist in formulation of care plan: previous health problems, allergies; health programs (include medications, treatments); and psychosocial data (include previous hospital experience)
   g. Collect data about etiology of SCI: type of accident; speed, site of impact; symptoms at time of injury (drugs/alcohol, hypoxia, hypotension, arrest)

h. Assess for **autonomic hyperreflexia** (a life-threatening involuntary sympathetic response of CNS to a noxious stimuli) with injury above T6
        1) Occurs after spinal shock is resolved
        2) Precipitated by bowel or bladder distention or other noxious stimuli (such as temperature or pressure)
        3) Symptoms: severe and sudden hypertension, bradycardia, headache, profuse sweating above level of injury and pale, cold, dry skin below injury
  2. Diagnostic tests: include multiple spine films specific to area of suspected injury (C-spine films to rule out fracture; C7 to T1 difficult to view; may need "swimmer's" view; clients with head injury generally require C-spine films), CT scan with or without contrast, laminar tomography (useful for injuries at cervicothoracic junctions), and labs (CBC, electrolytes, ABGs)

D. Nursing management
  1. Medications include: stool softeners, H_2 antagonists or antacids, low-dose anticoagulant therapy, vasopressor drugs if hypotensive, topical antibiotics if halo brace applied, corticosteroids, antispasmodics, a nonsteroidal anti-inflammatory drug (NSAID) as analgesic, and/or antidepressants
  2. Emergency management at scene or in emergency department: secure an airway without flexing, extending or rotating neck; immobilize neck before moving client, transport supine with forehead taped to stretcher to prevent movement; administer O_2 or place on ventilator, and monitor cardiovascular stability
  3. Promote optimal breathing
    a. Observe client, consult with health care team to treat decreasing vital capacity and ABGs
    b. Suction bronchial and pharyngeal secretions with care to avoid vagal nerve irritation leading to bradycardia and potential cardiac arrest
    c. Provide percussion or appropriate chest physiotherapy for weak cough
    d. Plan routine breathing exercises with client to support accessory muscles of inspiration
    e. Hydrate client and ensure humidification to thin pulmonary secretions
    f. Create cough during exhalation by pushing in and up between umbilicus and xiphoid process
  4. Prevent and treat autonomic hyperreflexia
    a. Prevent fecal impaction, bladder distention, or other triggering stimuli
    b. Raise head of bed immediately and remove compression stockings to decrease venous return, and assess BP
    c. Catheterize immediately; remove impaction after antihypertensive medication given
    d. Continue to assess BP while medicating, until stable
    e. Assess client's knowledge of prevention and management
  5. Report any deterioration in neuro function; do not turn until treatment plan has been established; monitor LOC, pupillary reaction, possibility of head injury; note affect, reaction to information and events
  6. Check motor and sensory level hourly or as prescribed; sensory level may be marked on client's skin
  7. Monitor cardiovascular status: interruption of sympathetic function leads to wide fluctuations of BP, hypotension, and dysrhythmias
  8. Prevent hazards of immobility
    a. Maintain dorsal or supine body alignment until placement of halo brace if appropriate (cervical injuries)
    b. Reposition and turn every 2 hours, monitoring clients with mid-thoracic or higher lesions for hypotension

    c. Provide client with passive ROM exercises and instruct family members how to assist in preventing contractures and atrophy within 48–72 hours after injury

    d. Initiate deep vein thrombosis and pulmonary embolism precautions: low-dose anticoagulation therapy and pneumatic compression devices

    e. Reduce hypotensive episodes: slowly change positions, use abdominal corset if appropriate before sitting upright, thigh-high elastic stockings and vasopressor drugs

9. Maintain skin integrity: inspect skin, pad or lubricate bony prominences, and reposition every 2 hours; apply skin barrier ointment/spray to perineum before irritation begins; teach and encourage client and family to prevent pressure ulcers

10. Promote urinary elimination

    a. Involve client and family in intermittent catheterization routine addressing prevention of distention and infection

    b. Encourage client and family to track fluid intake to assure adequate fluids and to assess voiding pattern and characteristics of urine

    c. Teach client to practice trigger voiding technique prior to straight catheterization: stroking inner thigh, pulling pubic hair, tapping on abdomen over bladder, and pouring warm water over perineal area in female clients

    d. Explain that successful stimulation of parasympathetic nerve fibers causes reflex activity; this triggered voiding should be followed by catheterization for residual urine during bladder retraining; less than 80 mL of residual urine is acceptable

11. Optimize bowel function

    a. Check for residual amounts of tube feeding, and client tolerance of gastric feedings after bowel sounds resume

    b. Offer a high-calorie, high-protein, high-fiber diet, gradually increasing oral amounts as tolerated

    c. Institute a bowel retraining program; use stool softeners, rectal suppositories with digital stimulation as needed after meals

    d. Manual removal of stool on a routine timetable may be required for client with LMN injury lacking a defecation reflex

12. Halo brace care

    a. Prevent infection at pin sites by clipping hair around pins to facilitate inspection; clean with ½-strength peroxide, normal saline, and topical antibiotic ointment, or soap and water as per hospital or agency protocol

    b. Maintain integrity of halo device by inspecting pins and traction bars for tightness; report loosened parts to provider

    c. Cleanse client's skin under sheepskin liner of vest per protocol; do not use powder or allow vest to become wet

    d. Change sheepskin vest when soiled and per protocol

    e. Maintain client position so that back of head is free of pressure point, massaging gently and with care not to move neck

    f. Keep wrench with vest and know how to release if cardiopulmonary resuscitation is needed

13. Provide sexuality information: offer accurate information on sexual function; discuss alternatives to intercourse if not physically possible and strategies for initiating or maintaining a sexual relationship; secure sexual counseling for client as needed

14. Support optimal self-esteem: keep open communication lines, encourage client self-awareness; encourage decision making and progressive self-care; identify with client strategies to address goals; refer to support groups and family counseling

15. Prepare for discharge

    a. Update baseline data regarding self-care and explore mobility issues

    b. Facilitate preparation of home setting and identify community resources

   c. Plan for ongoing psychological support
   d. Evaluate client and family's knowledge of medications, activities of daily living, use of assistive devices, and caregiver respite

VI. ENCEPHALITIS

A. Overview
1. Defined as a CNS disorder with inflammation of brain tissue; if both brain and meninges are affected, it is termed meningoencephalitis
2. Viral encephalitis is more serious than meningitis; can be fatal or cause long-term neurologic disability
3. Names: Western equine encephalitis (occurs in West and in horses); Eastern equine encephalitis (occurs in East and in horses); St. Louis and California encephalitis (not limited to those geographic areas); herpes encephalitis (usually fatal); Japanese encephalitis (similar to St. Louis); Russian spring-summer encephalitis (tick-borne)
4. Outbreaks are usually in summer and fall when mosquito (vector) is most active
5. Causes include transfer of arthropod-borne virus (arbovirus) from animals (particularly horses) to humans by mosquitoes; following diseases (rabies, German measles, chickenpox, herpes virus, smallpox); postvaccination; can be caused by viruses, bacteria, rickettsia, parasites, and fungi; exposure to toxins such as lead poisoning

B. Pathophysiology
1. Organism (usually virus) enters body and makes its way to CNS through cerebral capillaries and choroid plexus, then affecting specific cells and producing a wide variety of effects
2. Damage to CNS results in invasion and lysis of cells, demyelination and selective lysis, an immune response to viral antigens; and destruction of cells without inflammation
3. Effects of viral encephalitis vary with client's age and may include general symptoms, focal impairment, movement limitations, brain stem involvement, mental and personality changes, cerebral edema, hemorrhage, and even coma

4. Signs and symptoms include cerebral edema, headache, photophobia, high fever (always present), confusion, seizures, restlessness, hemiparesis, asymmetry of reflexes, positive Babinski reflex, ataxia, difficulty in speaking or understanding, facial weakness, ocular palsies, mental deterioration, muscle stiffness, malaise, sore throat, upper respiratory tract problems, nuchal rigidity, projectile vomiting, pupil irregularities, changes in VS, ptosis, diplopia, strabismus, and abnormal sleep patterns

C. Nursing assessment
1. Assessment includes neurovascular assessment, fluid status, symptom analysis of pain or discomfort, reflexes, ambulation, coordination, VS, cranial nerves
2. Diagnostic tests: lumbar puncture for CSF (increased pressure, increased proteins, normal glucose and chloride); CBC, electrolytes, MRI, CT scan

D. Nursing management
1. Medications include antipyretics, antiviral agents, corticosteroids, antiepileptics if seizures occur, sedatives, analgesics, stool softeners
2. Monitor fluid balance, measure intake and output (I & O)
3. Monitor nutritional status, measure weight
4. Monitor for signs of increasing ICP
5. Keep environment conducive to rest and decrease stimulation (lights low, limit visitors)
6. Protect client from injury if seizures occur
7. Reposition client frequently, positioning neck for comfort and to decrease joint stiffness
8. Physical therapy should be initiated for range-of-motion (ROM) exercises
9. Offer assurance to client and family, especially if a child is involved

VII. MENINGITIS

A. Overview

1. Meningitis is defined as an inflammation of meninges (pia mater and arachnoid membrane) surrounding brain and spinal cord
2. Classifications: viral (aseptic) meningitis (usually self-limiting with complete recovery) or bacterial (septic) meningitis (may leave residual effects or lead to death)
3. Higher incidence occurs in fall, winter, and early spring with children more susceptible because they have more upper respiratory tract infections
4. Causes include bacterial or viral infection, often after an upper respiratory tract infection; fungi or toxins may also be causes
5. Preventive public education includes information on meningococcal vaccine

B. Pathophysiology

1. Infection occurs when pathogen crosses blood–brain barrier and migrates throughout CNS
   a. Bacterial meningitis is most often preceded by *Neisseria meningitis* (meningococcal), *Streptococcus pneumoniae*, or *Haemophilus influenzae*
   b. Viral meningitis often occurs after mumps or herpes zoster, herpes simplex, or cytomegalovirus (CMV) infection
2. An inflammatory response causes increased CSF, as well as pressure and purulent exudate that spreads quickly throughout brain and spinal cord in bacterial meningitis
3. Signs and symptoms
   a. Acute infection with inflammation: high fever, nausea, vomiting, chills, malaise, tachycardia
   b. Irritated meninges (nuchal rigidity and photophobia): stiff and sore neck, positive Kernig sign (refer back to Figure 4-2), and positive Brudzinski sign (refer back to Figure 4-3)
   c. Signs of increased ICP
   d. Vascular problems
      1) Thrombophlebitis of cerebral BVs may lead to infarction, seizures, and stroke
      2) Septic emboli may block small BVs of hands and feet leading to gangrene
      3) Fibrinolysis occurring in bacteremia may lead to disseminated intravascular coagulopathy (DIC), a generalized response to injury associated with septic shock with simultaneous bleeding and clotting

C. Nursing assessment

1. Assessment includes pain (especially neck); reflexes (Brudzinski or Kernig sign); LOC; VS, peripheral neurovascular status of all extremities (cool pale to cyanotic extremities with decreased pulses and sensation may indicate emboli); fluid status, respiratory status, nutritional status
2. Diagnostic tests: lumbar puncture with CSF analysis (high protein, low glucose, positive for bacteria), CT scan, MRI (swelling and sites of necrosis), blood urea nitrogen (BUN), creatinine, electrolytes, ABGs, C&S of throat, blood, urine, sputum; urine specific gravity

D. Nursing management

1. Medications include broad-spectrum antibiotics (penicillins, third-generation cephalosporins) until cultures return, analgesics, antipyretics, antiemetics if nausea occurs, antiepileptics if seizures occur, and diuretics for cerebral edema; narcotics (opioids) that further depress CNS
2. Provide careful assessment and supportive intervention as needed for acute infection, irritated meninges and increased ICP; older adult clients should receive pneumonia and flu vaccines per recommended schedules
3. Carefully monitor VS, neurological and neurovascular status for changes

Practice to Pass

A client has bacterial meningitis caused by *Streptococcus pneumoniae*. What measures should the nurse institute to protect the client, health care professionals, and others?

a. Signs of increasing ICP such as changes in LOC (early) or widening pulse pressure, bradycardia, bounding pulse (late)
b. Neurological: severe headache, seizures, or cranial nerve dysfunction
c. Signs of neurovascular compromise: cool, pale, decreased sensation, faint to absent pulses

4. Carefully monitor fluid and electrolyte status: strict I & O, daily weights, condition of mucous membranes, skin turgor, and urine specific gravity

5. Promote effective airway clearance and exchange: monitor O_2 saturation levels, ABGs; turn every 2 hours, perform chest physiotherapy; suction if needed; elevate head of bed to 30 degrees

6. Relieve hyperthermia; apply cooling blanket or tepid sponge baths as needed

7. Relieve pain: maintain a quiet, dark environment, administer analgesics, encourage gentle ROM, back rub and massage, arrange care/visitors to promote periods of rest

8. Protect from injury: have oral airway, O_2 and suction equipment available; keep side rails up, bed in low position; rails padded; record seizure: event, length, head and eye deviations, interventions, postictal state; monitor for generalized bleeding

9. Maintain adequate nutrition via nasogastric tube feeding if needed, high protein, high calorie, in small frequent feedings

10. Promote health maintenance: instruct client in all medications and take complete course of all antibiotics; instruct client to have close contacts seek exposure care (prophylactic antibiotics) for fever, headache, irritability, and neck stiffness; refer as needed for rehabilitation of residual effects

VIII. SEIZURES

A. Overview
1. Seizures are defined as uncontrolled discharge of neurons of cerebral cortex that interfere with normal function; may be associated with involuntary muscle contractions; may originate as aura or sensory experience before clinical signs are evident

2. **Status epilepticus** can develop during seizure activity; seizures become continuous with very short periods of calm between intense, repetitive seizures; the cumulative effect is life threatening

3. Epilepsy is defined as recurrent paroxysmal disorder of cerebral function characterized by sudden, brief attacks of altered consciousness, motor activity, or sensory phenomena

4. Classifications of seizures
   a. Partial (focal): simple or partial (Jacksonian), complex
   b. Generalized: tonic-clonic (grand mal) or absence (petit mal), myoclonic, atonic, tonic, or clonic

5. Causes
   a. Genetic tendency/chromosomal abnormalities
   b. Structural factors: head trauma, infections (encephalitis, meningitis, brain abscess, opportunistic lesions from AIDS); cerebrovascular disorders: hemorrhage, embolism, ischemia; space-occupying lesions: primary and metastatic tumors, neurofibromatosis, arteriovenous malformation (AVM), subdural hematoma
   c. Metabolic-nutritional factors: water imbalance, hyponatremia, hypocalcemia, hypoglycemia, hypoxia, acidosis, pyridoxine (vitamin B_6) deficiency, fat and amino acid metabolism disorder, toxins and toxic factors (heavy metals), systemic disorders (uremia and toxemia), drugs (such as "street" drugs or theophylline overdose), and withdrawal (alcohol, barbiturates, antiepileptics, benzodiazepines)
   d. Idiopathic: no known etiology, possible genetic tendency

B. Pathophysiology

1. Excessive synchronous discharge of neurons
2. Neurons in epileptogenic focus recruit other neurons to fire synchronously in adjacent and more distant areas
3. Abnormal electrical discharge may occur without clinical manifestations
4. Clinical manifestations occur when sufficient number of neurons are excited
5. Resulting clinical manifestations depend upon part of brain from which discharge originates and path of spread
6. Classification and clinical characteristics
   a. Partial seizures (involve part of brain)
      1) Simple partial seizures (consciousness not impaired), with motor symptoms: "Jacksonian" march, spread topographically (systematically); limited to one part of body
      2) Simple partial seizures, with sensory or somatosensory symptoms: may be somatic sensory phenomena only, e.g., tingling, numbness of body part; may have visual, auditory, olfactory or taste symptoms only; dizzy spells may be seizure manifestations
      3) Complex partial seizures (impaired consciousness): begin as simple partial and progress to impairment of consciousness; impairment of consciousness at onset: most commonly involves **automatisms** (automatic actions or behavior without conscious knowledge; repetitive, semi-purposeful, patterned movements such as lip smacking); may include antisocial or aggressive behavior especially if forcefully restrained
      4) Partial seizures secondarily generalized: may spread from original discharge site to other parts of brain and become generalized; generalized seizure preceded by specific aura is partial seizure that becomes generalized
   b. Generalized seizures (involving whole brain at onset) are classified as tonic-clonic, tonic, absence, myoclonic, tonic, or infantile spasms
      1) Absence—simple (petit mal): staring spell; usually lasts less than 15 seconds, during which client is unaware of surroundings; diagnosed by a 3 cycle/second (C/S) spike and wave on electroencephalogram (EEG); usually present only in children
      2) Absence—atypical: staring spell accompanied by myoclonic jerks and automatisms such as chewing and smacking of lips; atypical spike wave pattern on EEG
      3) Myoclonic—single jerk of one or more muscle groups; lasting only a second
      4) Atonic—drop attack; sometimes associated with myoclonic seizure
      5) Clonic—jerking of muscle groups
      6) Tonic—stiffening of muscle groups
      7) Tonic clonic (grand mal): starts with tonic or stiffening phase followed by clonic or jerking phase, unconsciousness, possible bowel and bladder incontinence, may have only tonic or only clonic phase, may bite tongue, reduced consciousness during postictal recovery
      8) Metabolic or toxin induced seizure activity—usually generalized; usually does not recur as long as underlying cause remains corrected
   c. Status epilepticus: continuing or immediately recurring seizures, recovery between attacks incomplete, usually lasts 30 minutes or more
7. Precipitating factors (unique for each individual)
   a. Physical: specific sensory stimuli (flashing lights and certain sounds); fever (children under 5 years of age at risk); injury; physical exhaustion; sleep deprivation; inadequate nutrition; drugs, alcohol, other addictive substances; and hyperventilation
   b. Psychosocial: family and environmental stress, coping, shock

8. Signs and symptoms include partial or complete loss of consciousness, falling, incontinence of bowel and bladder, aura before event, muscular contractions, tonic-clonic convulsions of all extremities, facial movements, tongue biting, salivation, a postictal stage (decreased LOC, decreased VS), headache, and fatigue

C. Nursing assessment

1. Assessment
   a. History: description of seizure from client or witness; antecedent events; precipitating factors and postictal events; frequency and duration; past history of illness, trauma, infection; alcohol or drug use; family history of seizures; perinatal history, growth and development
   b. Physical and neurological exam: seizure activity (length, progression of jerking, time started and other associated signs, such as incontinence), presence of oral bleeding, postictal stages, vital signs, posturing
   c. Assess client's lifestyle and factors that may trigger seizures
2. Diagnostic tests
   a. Laboratory results: hyponatremia, hypocalcemia (especially in children), hypoglycemia, BUN, and ABGs (hypoxia and acidosis)
   b. CSF analysis: infection and/or hemorrhage
   c. Drug screen: toxicity of sedatives, hypnotics, heavy metals, drug interactions, "street" drugs, theophylline, and antiepileptic drug levels
   d. EEG: may be normal between seizures
   e. Initial studies may include CT scan or MRI, or positive emission tomography (PET) scan

D. Nursing management

1. Medications
   a. Antiepileptics: phenytoin (Dilantin), carbamazepine (Tegretol), valproic acid (Depakene), ethosuximide (Zarontin), clonazepam (Klonopin), gabapentin (Neurontin)
   b. Diazepam (Valium), lorazepam (Ativan), phenytoin (Dilantin) or phenobarbital may be used for status epilepticus
2. Document details of seizure: date, time of onset, duration of seizure; activity of client at time of onset; precipitating factors, if any; aura; seizure activity (body parts involved and sequence); character of movements (tonic, clonic, head or eye deviation, behavior)
3. Monitor autonomic signs: pupil size and reactivity, respirations, cyanosis, diaphoresis, incontinence, salivation
4. Record and evaluate LOC during and after seizure: arousability, duration of reduced consciousness, awareness of and memory for event
5. Monitor postictal state (period immediately after seizure stops; usually lasts 30-90 minutes): confusion, exhaustion, sleepiness, difficulty to arouse, muscle soreness, headache, weakness, aphasia, inability to maintain airway if not arousable, partial paralysis
6. Inspect for injury (lacerations or bruises), especially to head or tongue
7. Provide safety management during seizure: protect from injury; do not force hard object between teeth; do not restrain; turn to side to keep airway open during postictal period
8. Monitor serum drug levels to determine if antiepileptic drug (AED) in therapeutic range; clarify that AED must be taken on a continuous basis; if adverse effects occur, dose is lowered or different drug is tried
9. Control precipitating factors
10. Surgery may be a treatment option: cortical resection of epileptic focus may be indicated if criteria met
11. Maintain large vein access while hospitalized to treat status epilepticus

Practice to Pass

How will the nurse prepare a client who is newly diagnosed with seizures for his first EEG?

IX. GUILLAIN-BARRÉ SYNDROME

A. Overview

1. Defined as an acute (sudden onset), rapidly progressing inflammation of peripheral motor and sensory nerves characterized by:
   a. Variable motor weakness and paralysis

   b. Paralysis that ascends symmetrically from lower extremities in most cases
   c. With excellent care has a 96% complete recovery
2. Occurs most often between ages 30–50 years, equally in both genders
3. Causes include unknown etiology, autoimmune attack; are common after viral infections, immunizations, febrile illness, injury, or surgery

B. Pathophysiology

1. A cell-mediated immune reaction is triggered by a viral illness or immunization
2. Instead of normal antibody role of preventing invading organism from causing harm, the antibody formed has a damaging effect on peripheral nerve myelin; an IgM antimyelin antibody exists, lymphocytes are sensitized and aid in damaging myelin
3. With demyelination, nerve impulses are slowed or stopped and muscles lose innervation and begin to waste without exercise
4. During recovery, remyelination occurs in descending order over a period of a few months to a couple of years

5. Signs and symptoms include weakness/paresis (partial paralysis), paralysis progressing upward from lower extremities to total paralysis requiring ventilatory support; paresthesias (numbness and tingling) and pain; muscle aches, cramping, and nighttime pain; respiratory compromise and/or failure: dyspnea, diminished vital capacity, breath sounds, decreasing O_2 saturation, abnormal blood gases; cranial nerve involvement: impaired extraocular eye movements, dysphagia, diplopia, difficulty speaking; and autonomic dysfunction: orthostatic hypotension (lowered BP and dizziness with sudden position changes), hypertension, change in heart rate (bradycardia, heart block, asystole or tachycardia), bowel and bladder dysfunction, flushing and diaphoresis

C. Nursing assessment

1. Includes onset and chronology of symptoms including any illnesses in previous 1–8 weeks; head to toe muscle strength testing (see Tables 4-3 and 4-4); head-to-toe sensory assessment; cranial nerve involvement, respiratory status, fluid balance, skin integrity, bladder and bowel control
2. Diagnostic tests: electrolytes, ABGs, nerve conduction tests, lumbar puncture for CSF (elevated protein)

Table 4-3	Muscle Strength Scale
0	No visible muscle contraction: paralysis
1	Trace: slight contraction but no movement
2	Poor: ROM with gravity eliminated
3	Fair: ROM against gravity
4	Good: ROM against gravity with some resistance
5	Normal: full ROM and full resistance

Table 4-4	Head-to-Toe Muscle Strength Testing
Ocular and lids	Close eyes tightly
Facial	Puff cheeks, stick out tongue
Neck	Bend head forward and back
Deltoid	Hold arms up
Biceps	Flex arm
Triceps	Extend arm
Wrists	Flex and extend
Finger	Grip examiner's crossed plexor and second finger
Hip	Raise straight leg from supine
Gluteal and leg	Cross legs
Ankle and foot	Flex and extend

D. Nursing management

1. Medications and treatment
   a. IV immunoglobulins: may cause low-grade fever, muscle aches, headache, acute renal failure (rare), retinal necrosis
   b. Plasmapheresis: plasma is removed and separated from whole blood and blood cells are returned without plasma to remove antibodies responsible for disease; monitor for complications (loss of clotting factors, bleeding, and fluid and electrolyte imbalance)
   c. Adrenocorticoid hormone (ACTH) and corticosteroids or antiinflammatory drugs
   d. Other: stool softeners, antacids or H_2-receptor antagonists, analgesics

2. Care is supportive with attention to function of all systems, especially respiratory and cardiac
   a. Monitor respiratory status: rate, depth, breath sounds, vital capacity, note secretions and check gag, cough, and swallowing reflexes
   b. Monitor cardiac status: heart rate, BP, dysrhythmias
3. Administer chest physiotherapy and pulmonary hygiene measures
4. Maintain adequate nutrition as appropriate: administer tube feeding, parenteral nutrition or assisted small frequent feedings of soft foods; weigh client weekly; check electrolyte status, give mouth care every 2 hours
5. Monitor bowel and bladder function: assess bowel sounds and frequency, amount, color of bowel movements; offer bed pan; check for distention and residuals in client who cannot void spontaneously; perform intermittent catheterization as needed; encourage fluid intake to 3,500 mL/day unless contraindicated by concurrent cardiac or renal disease

6. Prevent complications of immobility
   a. Encourage use of weak extremities as able; work with physical therapy to plan passive and active ROM to all extremities
   b. Protect immobile extremities with use of: air mattress or special bed and elbow and heel protectors
   c. Turn and position in good body alignment
   d. Elevate extremities to prevent dependent edema
   e. Use antiembolism compression devices/stockings

7. Provide eye care for client unable to close eyelids completely: instill artificial tears, cleanse eyes as needed, use eye shields and tape eyes closed as needed
8. Provide comfort and analgesics as needed: assess pain with VS; administer analgesics before painful activities; log roll and move client gently; use imagery, relaxation, distraction, humor, music as appropriate; pain is common, and nocturnal pain is reported as more severe

Practice to Pass

List nursing diagnoses in order of priority for the client with Guillain-Barré syndrome who is in the acute phase experiencing tetraplegia (quadriplegia).

9. Promote communication, encouragement, and support to client and family
   a. If client is on ventilator or is unable to communicate because of weak speech muscles, collaborate with speech therapist to develop a communication system
   b. Explain all care with rationale and provide information about progression of disease; encourage client and family to express feelings and participate in care as much as possible
10. Begin to plan for discharge needs upon admission to acute care setting

X. MYASTHENIA GRAVIS

A. Overview

1. Myasthenia gravis (MG) is a chronic progressive disorder of peripheral nervous system affecting transmission of nerve impulses to voluntary muscles, causing muscle weakness and fatigue that increases with exertion and improves with rest; eventually leads to fatigue without relief from rest

2. Varies from mild disturbance of ocular movement to respiratory failure from weakness of the diaphragm and muscles of respiration; 3 types exist and are labeled as ocular, bulbar, and generalized

3. Characterized by unpredictable remissions and exacerbations

4. Affects women 3 times more than men until after age 50 with onset usually between ages 20–30 years

5. Causes include family history of autoimmune disorders, tumor of thymus gland, and unknown etiology

B. **Pathophysiology**

1. An autoimmune process triggers formation of autoantibodies that decrease number of acetylcholine (Ach) receptors and widen gap between axon ending and muscle fiber in neuromuscular junction; muscle contraction is hindered because IgG autoantibodies prevent Ach from binding with receptors; destruction of receptors at neuromuscular junction occurs

2. Associated with continued production of autoantibodies by thymus gland in 75% of cases

3. Onset is usually slow but can be precipitated by emotional stress, hormonal disturbance (pregnancy, menses, autoimmune thyroid disorder), infections or vaccinations, trauma and surgery, temperature extremes, excessive exercise, drugs that block or decrease neuromuscular transmission (opioids, sedatives, barbiturates, alcohol, quinidine, anesthetics), and thymus tumor

4. Signs and symptoms: mild diplopia (double vision) and unilateral ptosis (eyelid drooping) caused by weakness in extraocular muscles; weakness may involve face, jaw, neck, and hip; complications arise when severe weakness affects muscles of swallowing, chewing, and respiration; respiratory distress manifested by tachypnea, decreased depth, abnormal ABGs, O_2 saturation less than 92%, decreased breath sounds; bowel and bladder incontinence, paresthesias, and pain in weak muscles

5. Myasthenic crisis: sudden motor weakness; risk of respiratory failure and aspiration; most often caused by not enough medication or an infection

6. Cholinergic crisis: severe muscle weakness; caused by overmedication; signs are cramps, diarrhea, bradycardia, and bronchial spasm with increased pulmonary secretions and risk of respiratory compromise

C. **Nursing assessment**

1. Assessment

   a. Progression and severity of fatigue; which body parts are affected; effect on ADLs; adequacy of coping skills

   b. Cranial nerve dysfunction

      1) Ocular: diplopia and ptosis; test for ptosis by asking client to look upward for 2 to 3 minutes; eyelid droop will increase so that eye can hardly be held open; after rest, eyes can open

      2) Facial: smile may resemble a snarl; jaw may need to be propped closed

      3) Laryngeal and pharyngeal: voice may be weak with a nasal twang, may have dysphagia (difficulty swallowing), and difficulty chewing with some choking

   c. Other muscle weakness

      1) Test all muscle groups (see Table 4-3): flexors of neck, shoulder, and hip may be affected: difficulty holding head up, difficulty climbing stairs, lifting, raising arms over head, difficulty holding, sitting, standing posture

      2) Bowel and bladder incontinence

   d. Respiratory distress from weakened diaphragm and respiratory muscles and difficulty swallowing secretions; lung sounds, respiratory rate (RR) and depth

2. Diagnostic tests: diagnosis is confirmed with Tensilon test: IV edrophonium chloride (Tensilon) is injected, which allows Ach to being with receptors and leads to voluntary muscle contraction and temporary improvement of symptoms (weakness returns after effects of Tensilon wear off); pulmonary function tests and ABGs; and electromyography (EMG), which shows decreased amplitude when motor neurons are stimulated

D. Nursing management

1. Medications and treatment
   a. Anticholinesterases: neostigmine (Prostigmin), pyridostigmine (Mestinon); give medications on time to maintain muscle strength during essential activities and eating, or else client may be too weak to swallow
   b. Immunosuppressants: corticosteroids, azathioprine (Imuran), cyclosporine (Cytoxan)
   c. Anti-inflammatory drugs
   d. Thymectomy (removal of thymus gland)
   e. Plasmapheresis: removes IgG antibodies
   f. Atropine sulfate (Atropine) for cholinergic crisis

2. Maintain effective breathing pattern and airway clearance
   a. Thoroughly assess for respiratory distress
   b. Monitor meals and teach client to bend head slightly forward while eating and drinking
   c. Teach client to avoid exposure to infections, especially respiratory
   d. Teach client effective coughing, use chest physiotherapy and incentive spirometry
   e. Have oral suction available and teach client how to use it
   f. Have intubation equipment on hand

3. Provide adequate nutrition
   a. Schedule medications 30–45 minutes before eating for peak muscle strength while eating
   b. Offer food frequently in small amounts that are easy to chew and swallow; soft or semisolid as needed
   c. Administer IV fluids and nasogastric tube feedings if unable to swallow

4. Instruct in alternative methods of communication if needed: eye blink, finger wiggle for yes or no; flash cards, communication board; teach to support lower jaw with hands to assist with speech

5. Promote improved physical mobility
   a. Provide passive and active ROM and refer to physical and/or occupational therapy
   b. Instruct client to plan rest periods and to conserve energy
      1) Plan major activities early in day
      2) Schedule activities during peak medication effect
   c. Instruct client to avoid extremes of hot and cold, exposure to infections, emotional stress and medications that may worsen or precipitate an exacerbation (alcohol, sedatives, and local anesthetics)
   d. Instruct client in signs of crisis and differences between causation of myasthenic and cholinergic crises
   e. Encourage client to wear a MedicAlert bracelet

6. Provide eye care: instill artificial tears, use a patch over one eye for double vision; wear sunglasses to protect eyes from bright lights

7. Promote positive body image and coping skills: encourage participation in treatment plan; actively listen to client and encourage expression of feelings; reinforce progress and explain all care; provide low energy diversional activities; refer to myasthenia gravis self-help group

XI. PARKINSON'S DISEASE

A. Overview

1. Defined as a progressive gradual neurological degenerative disorder of brain characterized by "resting" (nonintentional) tremors, bradykinesia (slow, sometimes frozen movement), and muscle rigidity or stiffness
2. Affects mostly older adults between age 50–60 years
3. Classified as primary (unknown cause) or secondary (caused by infection; neoplasms; encephalitis; intoxication with carbon monoxide, manganese, and mercury; use of drugs such as reserpine, methyldopa, haloperidol, phenothiazines; and hypoxia and cerebral ischemia)

B. Pathophysiology

1. Affects brain centers that control and regulate movement
2. Neurons in substantia nigra and corpus striatum in midbrain degenerate and become deficient in production and storage of neurotransmitter dopamine
3. When dopamine levels that inhibit motor activity deplete, Ach is not inhibited, allowing increased excitation that leads to motor symptoms
4. Signs and symptoms
   a. Tremors
      1) Mild "pill-rolling": nonintentional tremor of thumb and first finger as if rotating a small object
      2) May begin in 1 hand with tremor spreading to arm, then other arm, and later head
      3) Usually lessens with purposeful movement
   b. Bradykinesia and loss of automatic movement characterized by: mask-like face with staring gaze; soft, monotone voice; drooling of saliva; impaired balance and loss of righting reflex (correcting posture when changing positions); stooped posture; difficulty initiating movement; and unsteady shuffling propulsive gait
   c. Rigidity
      1) **Cogwheel rigidity**: manual manipulation of body parts may take on feel of a cogwheel; increased resistance to passive ROM with jerky catches when joint is moved
      2) **Lead-pipe rigidity**: cataleptic condition during which limbs remain in any position in which placed; smooth, stiff movement
   d. Autonomic dysfunction: insomnia, oily skin, sweating, heat intolerance, orthostatic hypotension
   e. Other symptoms include weight loss, constipation, dysphagia, depression, and dementia

C. Nursing assessment

1. Assessment includes onset and progression of disease; changes in function throughout day and in response to medication (difficulty dressing, eating, walking, writing); movement (tremors, bradykinesia, rigidity), bowel function, nutritional status, mental status (forgetfulness, long-term and short-term memory), reflexes, and memory
2. Diagnostic tests: none specific; diagnosis is based on signs and symptoms; glucose may be tested because of side effects of drugs

D. Nursing management

1. Medications
   a. Dopaminergics: levodopa (L-dopa), carbidopa–levodopa (Sinemet), amantadine (Symmetrel), pramipexole (Mirapex)
   b. Dopamine agonists: bromocriptine (Parlodel), pergolide (Permax)
   c. Anticholinergics: trihexyphenidyl (Artane), benztropine mesylate (Cogentin)
2. Monitor for symptom control and adverse reactions to medications such as anemia, dystonia (prolonged muscle contraction that may cause twisting and repetitive

movements or abnormal posture), nausea, darkened urine and sweat, orthostatic hypotension, changes in mentation and vision, tachycardia, urinary retention, dry mouth, constipation, and impaired glucose tolerance

3. Encourage mobility with daily exercise directed by physical therapy; use of assistive devices as needed
   a. Spring-loaded chair/straight-backed chair with arms and slight elevation of back legs; elevated toilet seat
   b. Slip-on shoes or Velcro-fastened shoes; Velcro fasteners on clothes
   c. Canes, splints, braces as needed
   d. Rope tied to foot of bed to assist getting to sitting position
   e. Instruct client who "freezes" to think about stepping over something
   f. Instruct client to lift legs and take big steps when walking to offset shuffling, propulsive gait
   g. Instruct client to hold an object to decrease resting tremors
   h. Instruct client to "look at horizon" when walking to prevent lowering of head that increases risk of falls

4. Provide a safe environment: remove throw rugs and excess furniture; provide grab bar in bathroom, handrails on both sides of stairs; ensure adequate lighting

5. Promote a well-balanced diet
   a. Assess client's nutritional status, ability to feed self and swallow
   b. Consult with dietician, speech and occupational therapists as needed
   c. Provide food of proper consistency to prevent aspiration as determined by swallowing function
   d. Provide stabilized dishes and utensils, flexible straw for drinking
   e. Offer small frequent meals and snacks
   f. Encourage high fiber and 3,000 mL of water intake a day under additional fluids contraindicated by concurrent renal or cardiac disease

6. Promote adequate rest
   a. Assess client's perception of adequacy of rest, sleep pattern and existing conditions, medications that might impact sleep
   b. Avoid exercise or napping close to bedtime
   c. Limit caffeine and alcohol intake; drink milk before bedtime
   d. Provide a firm mattress with a small pillow, sheepskin or air mattress
   e. Darken bedroom and decrease noise

7. Allow client to participate in own care; maintain an unhurried environment to allow sufficient time for client to attempt own ADLs

Practice to Pass

A client with Parkinson's disease has dysphagia (difficulty swallowing). What mealtime interventions should the nurse consider to prevent aspiration and ease swallowing?

XII. MULTIPLE SCLEROSIS (MS)

A. Overview

1. Defined as a chronic disorder of CNS where myelin and nerve axons in brain and spinal cord are destroyed
2. Most prominent in women and European Americans
3. Four forms based on rate of progression: benign, relapsing-remitting, primary progressive, and secondary progressive
4. Four syndromes based on which nerve tract is originally affected: corticospinal, brain stem, cerebellar, and cerebral syndromes; symptoms will usually be suggestive of 1 of these areas
5. Exacerbations can be precipitated by stress, pregnancy, illness, fever, fatigue
6. Causes: unknown etiology, possibly an autoimmune or genetic basis; childhood viral infections also suggested

B. Pathophysiology

1. Destruction of myelin and nerve axons causes a temporary, repetitive, or sustained interruption in conduction of nerve impulses

2. Plaque formation occurs throughout white matter of CNS also affects nerve impulses; disorder affects optic nerves, cervical spinal cord, and thoracic and lumbar spine

3. Inflammation occurs around plaques as well as normal tissue; astrocytes (gliosis) appear in lesions and scar tissue forms, replacing axons and leading to permanent disability

4. The immune response

   a. Helper T-cells are elevated in CSF at onset of disease

   b. T-suppressor cells are decreased in serum before and during an exacerbation of illness

   c. Immunocompetent cells are present within plaques

   d. Antibody production is evident intrathecally

5. Types (based on rate of progression of disease)

   a. *Benign*: neurological dysfunction occurs in different episodes, full recovery follows

   b. *Relapsing-remitting* (most common): neurological exacerbations occur but improvement can be seen with either complete or partial recovery

   c. *Primary progressive*: sudden loss of neurological function occurs, which may not resolve; leaves severe functional impairments; these may actually worsen over time; no remission follows

   d. *Secondary progressive*: starts similar to relapsing-remitting; changes to a primary progressive form; no remission follows

6. Signs and symptoms include visual disturbances or blindness (retrobulbar neuritis), sudden, progressive weakness of one or more limbs, spasticity of muscles, nystagmus, tremors, gait instability, fatigue, bladder dysfunction (UTIs, incontinence), depression

C. Nursing assessment

1. Assessment includes symptoms analysis of complaints, neurovascular assessment, movement, mental assessment, and eye exam

2. Diagnostic tests: lumbar puncture for CSF (clonal IgG bands present), MRI, CT scans, PET scans, muscle testing of evoked potentials

D. Nursing management

1. Medications include immunomodulators (interferon alpha and beta) and glatiramer (Copaxone), antiviral drugs, corticosteroids, antibiotics for UTIs, anticholinergic drugs, antispasmodics, immunosuppressants, and muscle relaxants (baclofen [Lioresal], dantrolene [Dantrium], and diazepam [Valium])

2. No cure is available, supportive care should be maintained; may include intrathecal baclofen (Lioresal), or dorsal rhizotomy for intractable spasms

3. Maximum support to client and family is usually needed

4. Client education should include medications, symptoms, bladder training, self-intermittent catheterization, sexual functioning, avoiding complications, and possible triggers

5. Safety should be assessed in home and work environments

XIII. AMYOTROPIC LATERAL SCLEROSIS (ALS)

A. Overview

1. Defined as a degenerative disease of upper and lower motor neurons of cerebral cortex, brain stem, and spinal cord that results in total paralysis (except for cranial nerves III, IV, and VI); also known as Lou Gehrig disease

2. More common in men during 4th or 5th decade of life; usually fatal in 3–5 years

3. Causes include unknown etiology, viral infections, metabolic disorders, and trauma; familial patterns and autoimmune responses have been implicated

B. Pathophysiology

1. Motor neurons in cortex, brain stem, and spinal cord are lost; disease is noninflammatory; axon degeneration causes demyelination
2. Effect on UMN function leads to spastic, weak muscles and increased deep tendon reflexes
3. Effect on LMN function causes muscle atrophy and flaccid paralysis
4. Only one muscle group may be affected initially; clinical symptoms vary according to muscle groups involved; loss of muscle innervation → muscle atrophy → decrease in muscle mass → increasing fatigue
5. Mentation, cognitive ability, vision, hearing, and sensation are not lost; client loses control of function without losing mental awareness
6. Signs and symptoms
   a. Musculoskeletal: weakness, fatigue, loss of fine motor control, spasticity, paresis, hyperreflexia, atrophy, paralysis; fasciculations of tongue, slurred speech and facial muscles
   b. Respiratory: dyspnea, ineffective airway clearance, upper respiratory infection (URI), respiratory failure
   c. Nutritional: dysphagia, inability to chew, malnutrition
   d. Other: depression, impotence, loss of bowel and bladder control

C. Nursing assessment

1. Assessment includes coordination, muscle stiffness and wasting, gait, signs of atrophy, dysarthria, dysphagia, dyspnea, decreased reflexes, decreased respiratory function; and changes in VS, weight, and bowel function
2. Diagnostic tests: creatinine phosphokinase (elevated), CSF (elevated protein), myelography, CT scan, muscle biopsy, EMG, nerve conduction studies

D. Nursing management

1. Medications: anticholinesterase agents, steroids, antibiotics, muscle relaxants
2. Administer O$_2$ and ventilatory support as needed; suction as needed
3. Monitor cardiac status and VS; auscultate breath sounds
4. Monitor fluid status and offer nutritional support
5. Initiate physical therapy
6. Encourage client to administer own ADLs as long as possible
7. Monitor bowel and bladder function, avoid constipation
8. Turn every 2 hours as needed; encourage ambulation; avoid strenuous exercise and plan rest periods
9. Involve client in support group; refer to ALS center to minimize cost and maximize effectiveness
10. Client education about avoiding complications, importance of ongoing outpatient care, need to maintain physical mobility, use of assistive devices
11. Encourage client and family to ventilate feelings; counseling for advance directives with decision about use of ventilator for respiratory support

XIV. PAIN

A. Overview

1. Pain is a subjective feeling, an individual response to noxious stimuli on sensory nerve endings
2. Components of pain are affective (emotional), behavioral (behavioral responses), cognitive (beliefs, attitudes), sensory (perceptual), and physiological

3. Unrelieved pain has harmful effects that slow healing; stimulation of stress response causes increased muscle tension, local vasoconstriction, increased myocardial activity and O_2 consumption

    a. Pain tolerance is the degree of pain a person can withstand; differences in affect, behavioral response, and cognitive factors vary among people

    b. Pain threshold is the point of pain recognition; it varies somewhat among people also

4. Pain can be classified according to source, speed, duration, and if "referred"

    a. Sources of pain

        1) Cutaneous: from skin and subcutaneous tissue

        2) Deep somatic: from muscles, tendons, joints

        3) Visceral/splanchnic: from abdominal organs; contractions, distention, colic

        4) Psychogenic/functional: pain of unknown physical cause

    b. Speed

        1) Fast: carried by A-delta fibers that are myelinated and carry sharp, bright, well-localized pain

        2) Slow: carried by C-fibers, which are unmyelinated and carry dull, burning, aching diffuse sensations

    c. Duration is considered either acute or chronic with different times and physiological and/or psychological responses

        1) Acute pain: lasts 6 months or less, usually sudden in onset and localized in affected area; physiological response (often see in autonomic sympathetic "flight or fight" response), psychological response (heightened emotional response with anxiety, fear)

        2) Chronic pain: lasts longer than 6 months, is poorly localized, and often diffuse; physiological response may be absent or may be a fatigued autonomic response with depressed vital signs; psychological response is characterized by attention to pain as all-consuming and may be accompanied by signs of depression (sleep disorder, anorexia or overeating, crying, flat or sad affect, and withdrawal)

    d. Referred pain is pain that is perceived at a site different from its origin

5. **Phantom pain** (pain that exists in a removed part) occurs in an amputated body part or limb, possibly caused by spontaneous firing of spinal cord neurons that have lost their normal sensory input

6. Intractable pain or malignant pain is chronic progressive pain that is unrelenting and severely debilitating

7. Causes of pain include surgery, injury, trauma, chronic diseases (cancer, arthritis, AIDS, etc.), strenuous work, hormone shifts (migraines, menstruation), pregnancy, earache, toothaches, and infections

B. Pathophysiology

1. Nociception: process of how pain is recognized consciously and can be considered in 4 steps: transduction, transmission, perception, and modulation

    a. Transduction: conversion of a stimulus to an action potential at site of tissue injury

        1) Chemicals are released with cellular damage from such things as burns, radiation, pressure, tears, and cuts

        2) These chemicals sensitize primary afferent nociceptors (PANs), fibers that carry painful stimuli; PANs are: A-delta (fast pain); C-fibers (slow pain)

        3) Analgesics that work to block transduction by interfering in production of chemicals that sensitize PANs include: corticosteroids, which block the formation of arachidonic acid and NSAIDS, which block formation of prostaglandins

   b. Transmission: a neuronal action potential is transmitted to and through CNS so that pain can be perceived
   1) Impulse is projected to spinal cord, processed in dorsal horn and transmitted to brain
   2) Analgesics that work at level of transmission stabilize membranes by inactivating sodium channels, thus inhibiting the action potential
   3) Referred pain occurs when nerve fibers from visceral areas and somatic areas that converge in same area in dorsal horn are processed so they are perceived as originating in an area of somatic sensory A-delta fibers rather than visceral C-fibers (e.g., myocardial ischemia is perceived as pain in left arm)
   4) Gate control theory of pain offers an explanation for why such interventions as TENS (transcutaneous electrical nerve stimulator), heat and cold, and massage are effective
      a) There are theoretical gates in dorsal horn
      b) Small-diameter nerve fibers carry pain impulses through a gate, but large-diameter sensory nerve fibers going through same gate can close gate and inhibit transmission
      c) Pain perception (experience of pain) occurs in cerebral cortex; may occur at a basic level in thalamus
      d) Modulation, inhibition of nociception
         1) Efferent fibers descending from brain stem modulate or alter pain; mechanisms include:
            a) Endogenous opioids (naturally occurring, morphine-like chemicals) made in CNS inhibit transmission of pain by binding to opioid receptors in CNS to block transmission of nociceptive signals (e.g., endorphin, norepinephrine, enkephalin)
            b) Endogenous analgesia center in midbrain produces profound analgesia when stimulated
         2) Many analgesics modulate pain by mimicking endogenous neuromodulators; examples include tricyclic antidepressants that block serotonin reuptake (work well for neuropathic pain that is dull, aching, burning) and synthetic opioids; variability of individual endorphin levels may explain how pain thresholds to same stimulus are different from person to person
         3) Surgical treatment of intractable pain (chronic, progressive pain that is unrelenting and severely debilitating) interrupts pain pathways; types include: nerve block (destroys nerve roots chemically with phenol or alcohol); rhizotomy (destroys sensory nerve roots at level of entry into spinal cord); and cordotomy (transects spinal pain pathway before impulses ascend spinothalamic tracts)
  2. Signs and symptoms of pain may include elevated BP, increased HR, increased RR, grimacing, crying, sweating, posturing, depression, dilated pupils, anxiety and/or agitation, hypermotility
C. Nursing assessment
   1. Assessment
      a. Sensory components of pain (location, character or quality, pattern, duration, quantity or severity)
         1) Location and radiation
         2) Character or quality (aching, burning, shooting, stinging, constant, intermittent, sharp, dull)
         3) Pattern and precipitating and alleviating factors
         4) Duration
         5) Intensity or severity (using 0 to 10 rating scale (see Figure 4-5)

A visual analog scale for rating pain intensity

        b. Affective, behavioral, and cognitive components of pain; emotion will influence pain; expression of pain and beliefs about pain will vary from culture to culture
    2. Diagnostic tests: not recommended generally; specific tests to determine cause of pain are used according to reports voiced and location of pain
  D. Nursing management
    1. Medications include OTC analgesics such as acetaminophen (Tylenol), NSAIDs such as ibuprofen (Motrin), opioid analgesics such as morphine or hydrocodone, antiepileptics for chronic pain (such as gabapentin [Neurontin]), and antiemetics
    2. General principles in nursing management of pain
        a. Establish a trusting nurse–client relationship
        b. Always listen; believe and respect client
        c. Clarify responsibilities, collaborate with client to promote control and participation: discuss client's role in reporting pain, client's acceptable level of pain and nurse's commitment when client reports pain
        d. Offer support, concern, empathy, and reassurance
        e. Explain all interventions for pain and how they work
    3. Intervene to relieve pain
        a. Administer pain medications as prescribed early in pain episode to achieve client's acceptable pain level
        b. Consider round-the-clock administration of pain medication if pain is present most of day
        c. If client has patient-controlled analgesia (PCA) (intravenous delivery of opioid by pump on demand with preset dose and frequency limits and option of preset continuous dosage):
            1) Instruct in concept and demonstrate
            2) Emphasize that client controls the device, not the family
        d. If client has an epidural catheter, assess for orthostatic hypotension and inspect insertion site for infection
        e. Assess pain with using an analgesic scale each time VS are taken, after each administration of medication and with peak effect; minimize other symptoms that aggravate pain
        f. Assess for analgesic side effects: sedation, nausea, constipation, respiratory depression, urinary retention, and hypotension
        g. Clients taking opioids should be on a bowel management program, using a stool softener or laxative
        h. Include pain management in discharge teaching
    4. Promote rest and relaxation; implement nondrug pain treatments (alternative or complementary therapies) as appropriate; these include:
        a. Cognitive strategies, such as distraction (music, TV, reading, humor), guided imagery, and positive suggestion (such as desired effect will be obtained with analgesics and alternative therapies); use words such as "episode" and "experience" instead of "attack," and "comfort" instead of "pain"
        b. Behavioral approaches such as rhythmic, slow breathing
        c. Therapeutic touch

      d. Cutaneous stimulation such as pressure, acupressure, heat and cold therapy, and massage

      e. Lower lights and reduce noise

      f. Reposition, support body parts, encourage mild activity such as gentle ROM

      g. Plan care and schedule visitors to provide uninterrupted rest periods

5. Chronic pain requires a comprehensive approach to manage it effectively; assess how pain affects client's ability to perform ADLs and consider this in developing plan of care

 6. Monitor constraints to effective pain management including these misconceptions:

      a. Use of opioids to manage acute pain can lead to addiction: research indicates that only 0.1% of persons using opioids for acute postoperative pain become addicted; addiction should *not* be confused with:

         1) Physical dependence: experience of physiological withdrawal symptoms with rapid discontinuance of opioids

         2) Tolerance: a need for increasing amounts of opioids to achieve same level of pain relief

      b. It is better to wait until pain peaks to take analgesics: less analgesic is needed and better relief is obtained when analgesic is given at onset of pain

      c. Oral analgesics do not work as well as intravenous or intramuscular routes: if an **equianalgesic chart** (same pain relief obtained with different drugs, doses, and routes) is used, the oral route is equally effective; amount of drug needed is increased because of first-pass effect of liver

7. Intervene to alter the affective and cognitive components of pain

      a. Encourage client to discuss factors that may contribute to pain experience such as sociocultural influences, economic stress, and past experiences with pain

      b. Assist client to identify previously effective coping strategies

      c. Refer as needed to health care resources for counseling and therapy such as psychologist, occupational or physical therapist, or social worker

XV. ALZHEIMER'S DISEASE

A. Overview

1. Defined as a chronic, progressive form of dementia (cognitive impairment from organic syndrome) with cerebral degeneration; etiology has been linked to genetic tendency

2. Occurs most often after age 65 (senile dementia), but can occur between 40–60 years of age (presenile dementia)

B. Pathophysiology

1. Plaques, pathological changes, and neuronal tangles occur in brain; within these plaques are dying nerve terminals and abnormal protein fragments

2. Theories as to cause:

      a. An abnormal processing of a protein known as amyloid precursor protein (APP) allows part of protein to kill cells

      b. Inheritance of a gene coding for apolipoprotein E (APO-E4), which causes neuronal cell death

3. The number of functioning neurons is decreased, which accounts for decline in cognition, memory, and thought

 4. Signs and symptoms include:

      a. Forgetfulness, decreased judgment, personality changes, behavioral changes, loss of short-term memory, and speech and language problems

      b. In terminal stages, loss of ability to perform ADLs, seizures, delusions, paranoia, depression, and inability to recognize loved ones

      c. Death usually results from complications of immobility

C. Nursing assessment

1. Assessment includes mental status, memory (short- and long-term), ability to make decisions or plans, ability to calculate, speech, energy level, mood, sleep patterns, initiative and motivation, VS, indications of gastrointestinal (GI) or urinary problems (anorexia, dysphagia, urinary or fecal incontinence), emotional status, skin assessment for trauma

2. Diagnostic tests: no specific tests are available for diagnosis, MRI, positron emission tomography (PET), and single photon emission computed tomography (SPECT) scans support diagnosis

D. Nursing management

1. Medications include acetylcholinesterase inhibitors: tacrine (Cognex), donepezil (Aricept), galantamine (Reminyl), and rivastigmine (Exelon)

2. Client education should include memory aids, diet, and safety

3. Plans should be made with family for support measures and safety issues

4. Assist with reality orientation: repeat caregivers' names on a regular basis, use written instructions and directions, large-face clocks, orient client as needed; use familiar objects and memory aids

5. Be consistent, use simple instructions, avoid rushing

6. Allow client to perform ADLs as long as possible, assisting as necessary

7. Monitor fluid and nutritional status

8. Involve family and multidisciplinary team to decide whether client can safely remain at home or when placement (such as an Alzheimer's unit) is needed

Case Study

An older adult man with newly diagnosed Parkinson's disease has just been admitted to an extended-care facility. He was admitted reluctantly by his family, who cannot care for him at home where he lived alone. The client does not feel he needs to be admitted and wants his family to leave him alone.

1. What signs and symptoms should the nurse anticipate?

2. What nursing diagnosis will be the highest priority?

3. When will be the best time to schedule his physical therapy session?

4. When it takes him a long time to get dressed in the morning, the nurse offers assistance. He becomes very upset. How should the nurse handle this?

5. What are some specific instructions the nurse should give him to assist with his mobility problems?

For suggested responses, see pages 462–463.

POSTTEST

1 A young female diagnosed with multiple sclerosis (MS) has just learned she is also pregnant. She and her husband have been trying to conceive for years and are very excited. What client education should the nurse provide to the client regarding MS and pregnancy?

1. Immediately report weakness that progresses upward in the extremities.
2. Report a change in level of consciousness, severe headache, or slow pulse.
3. Recognize that a sore or stiff neck and pain with neck flexion must be reported.
4. Immediately report spasticity, weakness, or visual changes.

2 A client has seizure activity that is continuous in nature. The seizures subside and then immediately resume and continue. The client's color is getting worse. The nurse identifies the need to use standing orders to treat which condition?

1. Anticonvulsant syndrome
2. Status epilepticus
3. Brain herniation
4. Syphilitic posturing

3 Which assessment findings in a 35-year-old client with an intracranial hematoma should be of concern to the nurse? Select all that apply.

1. Hamstring pain when the hip and knee are flexed and then extended
2. Dorsiflexion of the big toe and fanning of the other toes when stroking the bottom of the foot upward
3. Muscle aches and cramping, especially at night
4. Cogwheel and lead pipe rigidity
5. Headache, drowsiness, and confusion

4 After a client undergoes magnetic resonance imaging (MRI) to rule out an expanding brain lesion, the nurse prepares the client for a lumbar puncture. The nurse would include which information in discussion with the client?

1. Risk of paralysis because the needle is inserted through the spinal cord
2. Maintaining a full bladder in case a catheterized specimen is needed
3. Maintaining bed rest for a prescribed time after the procedure
4. Directions to straighten the legs slowly during the procedure

5 The ambulatory clinic nurse assesses a client who reports the presence of a pounding headache. The client is known to have a T4 level spinal cord injury that occurred some time ago. The nurse should first assess for additional signs of which problem?

1. Sinus infection
2. Spinal shock
3. Upper motor neuron deficit
4. Autonomic hyperreflexia

6 The nurse plans to prevent corneal abrasion in the client with myasthenia gravis by taking which action?

1. Applying saline soaks every shift
2. Instilling artificial tears in the eyes every 1–2 hours
3. Ensuring the client's contact lenses are on while awake
4. Providing sunglasses when sunlight is entering the room

7 To reduce the risk of contracting meningitis, the nurse's best instruction to an older adult client is to do which of the following?

1. Avoid being in any situations in which there are large crowds.
2. Get *pneumococcal pneumonia, influenza,* and *meningococcal* vaccinations.
3. Drink at least 2,000 mL fluids per day.
4. Exercise 15 to 30 minutes most days of the week.

8 The nurse working on a neurological nursing unit overhears that a client will be scheduled for plasmapheresis. The nurse concludes that this discussion is most likely applying to clients with which health problems? Select all that apply.

1. Meningitis
2. Parkinson's disease
3. Myasthenia gravis
4. Amyotrophic lateral sclerosis
5. Guillain-Barré syndrome

9 The client with newly diagnosed Parkinson's disease states, "I just don't think I can handle having Parkinson's disease." What is the best first response by the nurse?

1. "It sounds as though you are feeling overwhelmed."
2. "I am sure you can. A lot of other people do."
3. "What do you think will be the hardest thing to handle?"
4. "The entire health care team will help you manage the disease."

10 A client is admitted to the emergency department with acute onset of loss of sensation and weakness in the left side. What other symptoms would alert the nurse to the presence of a stroke (cerebrovascular accident or CVA) or transient ischemic attack (TIA)? Select all that apply.

1. Difficulty speaking
2. Hyperglycemia and history of type 2 diabetes
3. Loss of coordination and trouble walking
4. Sudden difficulty with vision
5. Facial weakness and an asymmetrical smile

➤ *See pages 129–131 for Answers and Rationales.*

ANSWERS & RATIONALES

Pretest

1 **Answer: 3** **Rationale:** Although a ventilator is not absolutely required for spinal cord injury below the level of C3, the innervation of intercostal muscles is affected. Hemorrhage and cord swelling extends the level of injury and deficit, making it likely that this client could need a ventilator temporarily. The client will also require cervical traction but may not yet be ready for a halo brace. A kinetic bed is not the priority at this time. A catheterization tray will be needed but has lesser priority than a ventilator to maintain an airway when planning care. **Cognitive Level:** Analyzing **Client Need:** Physiological Adaptation **Integrated Process:** Nursing Process: Planning **Content Area:** Adult Health **Strategy:** Focus on the level of spinal cord injury and recall that cervical injury increases the risk of airway impairment. Anticipate this type of complication as life threatening to choose the option that protects the airway over the others. **Reference:** LeMone, P., Burke, K., & Bauldoff, G. (2011). *Medical-surgical nursing: Critical thinking in patient care* (5th ed.). Upper Saddle River, NJ: Pearson Education, pp. 1483–1484.

2 **Answer: 2** **Rationale:** Keeping the head of the bed elevated to 30 degrees promotes venous drainage from the brain, which is important in decreasing intracranial pressure (ICP). Alignment of the head prevents obstruction of the jugular veins. Obstruction would impede venous drainage and raise the ICP. Although the airway is also maintained, it is not the reason for the positioning. This position does not prevent pulmonary embolism. The client would not be positioned on the side to obtain ICP readings. **Cognitive Level:** Applying **Client Need:** Physiological Adaptation **Integrated Process:** Teaching and Learning **Content Area:** Adult Health **Strategy:** Recall that proper positioning of a client often involves principles of gravity, particularly when it affects blood flow. With this in mind, select the option that reflects this theme. **Reference:** LeMone, P., Burke, K., & Bauldoff, G. (2011). *Medical-surgical nursing: Critical thinking in patient care* (5th ed.). Upper Saddle River, NJ: Pearson Education, pp. 1441–1443.

3 **Answer: 1** **Rationale:** Momentary loss of consciousness followed by a lucid period and rapid deterioration is a classic picture resulting from a torn cerebral artery, producing an epidural bleed. This pattern of symptoms is not displayed with conditions such as reticular activating system concussion, diffuse axonal injury or expanding pericardial hematoma. **Cognitive Level:** Applying **Client Need:** Physiological Adaptation **Integrated Process:** Nursing Process: Implementation **Content Area:** Adult Health **Strategy:** Use the history of head trauma as a clue. Eliminate wrong options using pathophysiology and the pattern of symptoms presented. **Reference:** Huether, S. E., & McCance, K. L. (2012). *Understanding pathophysiology* (5th ed.). St. Louis, MO: Mosby, Inc., an imprint of Elsevier Inc., p. 380.

4 **Answer: 4** **Rationale:** The period after the clonic phase of a seizure is the post-ictal period. Typically, the client slowly regains consciousness, moving from a relaxed, quiet state to confusion or disorientation on awakening. The nurse does not change a medication dose without an order. Although it is appropriate to notify the health care provider of seizure activity, it is unnecessary to do so regarding a post-ictal state. It is unnecessary to call the rapid response team, since the client's condition is not quickly deteriorating. **Cognitive Level:** Applying **Client Need:** Management of Care **Integrated Process:** Nursing Process: Implementation **Content Area:** Adult Health **Strategy:** Recall the usual findings in a client following a tonic-clonic (grand mal) seizure to make the appropriate selection. **Reference:** LeMone, P., Burke, K., & Bauldoff, G. (2011). *Medical-surgical nursing: Critical thinking in patient care* (5th ed.). Upper Saddle River, NJ: Pearson Education, pp. 1442–1444.

5 **Answers: 1, 2, 5** **Rationale:** Protective pads/undergarments should be used only after all other treatment modes have been tried. Early dependency on incontinence products may decrease motivation to seek evaluation and treatment. The client, with the same risks as for the first stroke, may have another. Teaching is needed to control the modifiable risk factors, such as cigarette smoking. Walking and safety measures are desirable. **Cognitive Level:** Applying **Client Need:** Health Promotion and Maintenance **Integrated Process:** Nursing Process: Evaluation **Content Area:** Adult Health **Strategy:** The wording of the question indicates the correct options will be incorrect statements. Note the presence of critical words such as *a year's supply* and *never* and select these options. Then note that cigarette smoking adds to the risk of recurrence of stroke to select this option also. **Reference:** LeMone, P., Burke, K., & Bauldoff, G. (2011). *Medical-surgical nursing: Critical thinking in patient care* (5th ed.). Upper Saddle River, NJ: Pearson Education, pp. 1448–1449.

6 Answer: 3 Rationale: Clients with meningitis will be less able to protect themselves from both internal and external injury. Providing cognitive stimulation and increasing cardiac output are contraindicated with meningitis. Enhancing coping skills may be a focus if the client has residual effects from meningitis but is not a major focus during the acute phase. **Cognitive Level:** Applying **Client Need:** Safety and Infection Control **Integrated Process:** Nursing Process: Planning **Content Area:** Adult Health **Strategy:** Use Maslow's hierarchy of needs to address physiological needs before psychosocial needs to eliminate one option. Use knowledge of factors that increase intracranial pressure to eliminate 2 options. **Reference:** LeMone, P., Burke, K., & Bauldoff, G. (2011). *Medical-surgical nursing: Critical thinking in patient care* (5th ed.). Upper Saddle River, NJ: Pearson Education, pp. 1498–1499.

7 Answers: 1, 3, 5 Rationale: The cause of Guillain-Barré syndrome (GBS) is unknown, but precipitating events include a respiratory or gastrointestinal viral or bacterial infection. Lower extremity weakness or paralysis that progresses upward is classic in GBS. Preventing problems from immobility and altered respiratory function is important. Autonomic nervous system involvement may be manifested by bradycardia and hypotension. Fatigue and low blood glucose are not usually seen, nor are seizures. **Cognitive Level:** Analyzing **Client Need:** Physiological Adaptation **Integrated Process:** Nursing Process: Assessment **Content Area:** Adult Health **Strategy:** Begin the nursing process with assessment. Note that the paralysis is ascending upward, which involves the brain. **Reference:** LeMone, P., Burke, K., & Bauldoff, G. (2011). *Medical-surgical nursing: Critical thinking in patient care* (5th ed.). Upper Saddle River, NJ: Pearson Education, pp. 1543–1545.

8 Answer: 3 Rationale: The client should know the signs of crisis and should report them immediately. There is often more fatigue and weakness later in the day than in the morning, so the client should plan important activities for early in the day. Exercise should be done carefully to avoid fatigue, which can precipitate symptoms. It may be easier to eat 3 small meals with added snacks because chewing may cause fatigue. **Cognitive Level:** Applying **Client Need:** Physiological Adaptation **Integrated Process:** Nursing Process: Implementation **Content Area:** Adult Health **Strategy:** The critical word in the stem of

the question is *priority*. Use nursing knowledge and the process of elimination noting the corresponding critical word *crisis* in the correct option. **Reference:** LeMone, P., Burke, K., & Bauldoff, G. (2011). *Medical-surgical nursing: Critical thinking in patient care* (5th ed.). Upper Saddle River, NJ: Pearson Education, pp. 1539–1540.

9 Answer: 3 Rationale: The resting or nonintentional tremor may be controlled with purposeful movement, such as holding an object. Deep breathing, a warm bath, and diazepam will promote relaxation but are not specific interventions for the tremor. **Cognitive Level:** Applying **Client Need:** Physiological Adaptation **Integrated Process:** Teaching and Learning **Content Area:** Adult Health **Strategy:** Note that 3 options are focused on relaxation. The correct option is different. **Reference:** LeMone, P., Burke, K., & Bauldoff, G. (2011). *Medical-surgical nursing: Critical thinking in patient care* (5th ed.). Upper Saddle River, NJ: Pearson Education, pp. 1526–1528.

10 Answers: 2, 4 Rationale: It is important to always believe the client's report and rating of pain. The client tolerated the last full dose of medication so he should be given a dose now without delay. The nurse would reassess the client's pain level within 30 minutes of administering pain medication depending on peak action time of the drug. The pain level would be recorded at 9, not 5. It is unnecessary to initiate patient-controlled analgesia because the analgesic last used was effective. **Cognitive Level:** Analyzing **Client Need:** Management of Care **Integrated Process:** Nursing Process: Implementation **Content Area:** Adult Health **Strategy:** The level of pain is subjective data. Follow the order for the drug if it is safe for the client and appropriate. Identify the opposite options as incorrect and eliminate the patient-controlled analgesia as unnecessary with the information in the question. **Reference:** LeMone, P., Burke, K., & Bauldoff, G. (2011). *Medical-surgical nursing: Critical thinking in patient care* (5th ed.). Upper Saddle River, NJ: Pearson Education, pp. 65–66.

Posttest

1 Answer: 4 Rationale: Fatigue affects almost all clients with multiple sclerosis (MS). Stressors such as pregnancy can increase fatigue and risk of exacerbation. Signs of an exacerbation include spasticity, weakness, visual changes and fatigue. Guillain-Barré syndrome is manifested by weakness that progresses upward in the extremities. A change in level of consciousness, severe headache or slow pulse indicates increased intracranial pressure or hematoma. A sore or stiff neck and pain when the neck is flexed indicate meningitis. **Cognitive Level:** Analyzing **Client Need:** Physiological Adaptation **Integrated Process:** Teaching and Learning **Content Area:** Adult Health **Strategy:** Eliminate the options that are appropriate for neurological problems other than multiple sclerosis (MS). **Reference:** LeMone, P., Burke, K., & Bauldoff, G. (2011). *Medical-surgical nursing: Critical thinking in* *patient care* (5th ed.). Upper Saddle River, NJ: Pearson Education, pp. 1518–1526.

2 **Answer: 2** **Rationale:** Status epilepticus can develop during seizure activity. The seizure activity becomes continuous with only very short periods of calm between intense and persistent seizures. This progression to a state of epilepticus is life threatening. Nursing interventions focus on prevention of hypoxia, acidosis, hypoglycemia, hyperthermia, and exhaustion. The progression of symptoms is not entitled anticonvulsant syndrome. Brain herniation is of concern when a client has increased intracranial pressure. There is no evidence the client has syphilis. **Cognitive Level:** Applying **Client Need:** Physiological Adaptation **Integrated Process:** Nursing Process: Diagnosis **Content Area:** Adult Health **Strategy:** Make an association between the term *seizure* in the stem of the question and *epilepticus* in the correct option. **Reference:** LeMone, P., Burke, K., & Bauldoff, G. (2011). *Medical-surgical nursing: Critical thinking in patient care* (5th ed.). Upper Saddle River, NJ: Pearson Education, p. 1444.

3 **Answers: 1, 2, 5** **Rationale:** A positive Kernig sign, positive Babinski reflex, and headache, drowsiness, and confusion are all indicative of an intracranial hematoma. Cogwheel and lead pip rigidity describe Parkinson's disease. Muscle aches and cramps are vague and can be symptoms of a variety of health problems. **Cognitive Level:** Analyzing **Client Need:** Physiological Adaptation **Integrated Process:** Nursing Process: Assessment **Content Area:** Adult Health **Strategy:** Choose options that reflect an acute central nervous system problem. Cogwheel and lead pipe rigidity are classis for Parkinson's disease. **Reference:** LeMone, P., Burke, K., & Bauldoff, G. (2011). *Medical-surgical nursing: Critical thinking in patient care* (5th ed.). Upper Saddle River, NJ: Pearson Education, pp. 1465–1466.

4 **Answer: 3** **Rationale:** The client has to maintain bed rest for a prescribed time after the lumbar puncture. This will help prevent spinal headache and allow some time for production and replacement of the CSF. The spinal needle is inserted into the area below the spinal cord eliminating the likelihood of paralysis. There is no need to maintain a full bladder. The client must maintain the knees to chest position until completion of the lumbar puncture. **Cognitive Level:** Applying **Client Need:** Reduction of Risk Potential **Integrated Process:** Nursing Process: Implementation **Content Area:** Adult Health **Strategy:** Note that the wording of the question indicates that the correct answer is also a true statement. Recall that bed rest with the head positioned according to the type of dye used (oil or water based) will help minimize meningeal irritation and subsequent headache. **Reference:** LeMone, P., Burke, K., & Bauldoff, G. (2011). *Medical-surgical nursing: Critical thinking in patient care* (5th ed.). Upper Saddle River, NJ: Pearson Education, p. 1417.

5 **Answer: 4** **Rationale:** Spinal cord injury at or above the level of T6 can experience an exaggerated sympathetic

response, seen only after recovery from spinal shock. Autonomic hyperreflexia is a clinical emergency. Without prompt treatment severe hypertension progresses and coma or death can occur. There is no indication the client has a sinus infection or upper motor neuron deficit. Spinal shock happens after complete transaction of the spinal cord. **Cognitive Level:** Analyzing **Client Need:** Physiological Adaptation **Integrated Process:** Nursing Process: Assessment **Content Area:** Adult Health **Strategy:** Assessment for life-threatening complications such as autonomic hyperreflexia is always a priority. Note the critical words *some time ago* to discriminate between the correct option and spinal shock. **Reference:** LeMone, P., Burke, K., & Bauldoff, G. (2011). *Medical-surgical nursing: Critical thinking in patient care* (5th ed.). Upper Saddle River, NJ: Pearson Education, pp. 1481–1483.

6 **Answer: 2** **Rationale:** Corneal abrasion in the client with myasthenia gravis is caused by dryness of the cornea from inability to close the eyelids and blink. It can be prevented by application of artificial tears every 1–2 hours. Saline soaks and use of contact lenses or sunglasses are not helpful for dry eyes. **Cognitive Level:** Applying **Client Need:** Physiological Adaptation **Integrated Process:** Nursing Process: Planning **Content Area:** Adult Health **Strategy:** Apply the pathophysiology of muscle weakness to the face and eyelids. Determine which action best prevents corneal trauma. **Reference:** LeMone, P., Burke, K., & Bauldoff, G. (2011). *Medical-surgical nursing: Critical thinking in patient care* (5th ed.). Upper Saddle River, NJ: Pearson Education, pp. 1538–1539.

7 **Answer: 2** **Rationale:** Meningitis bacteria or viruses often gain entry into the cerebrospinal fluid secondary to an upper respiratory tract infection. Avoidance of large crowds, drinking at least 2,000 mL of fluids per day and exercising 15–30 minutes most days of the week are generally healthy practices for the older adult client but not specific health promotion for prevention of meningitis. Immunizations are recommended. **Cognitive Level:** Applying **Client Need:** Health Promotion and Maintenance **Integrated Process:** Teaching and Learning **Content Area:** Adult Health **Strategy:** Note which action specifically prevents the infection. Keep in mind the age of the client and the presence of the word *any*. **Reference:** LeMone, P., Burke, K., & Bauldoff, G. (2011). *Medical-surgical nursing: Critical thinking in patient care* (5th ed.). Upper Saddle River, NJ: Pearson Education, pp. 1498–1499.

8 **Answers: 3, 5** **Rationale:** Plasmapheresis is performed to remove autoantibodies that attack the myelin sheaths of motor and sensory nerves in Guillain-Barré syndrome and acetylcholine receptors at the neuromuscular junction in myasthenia gravis. Meningitis, Parkinson's disease, and amyotrophic lateral sclerosis have not been identified as being autoimmune disorders. **Cognitive Level:** Analyzing **Client Need:** Physiological Adaptation **Integrated Process:** Nursing Process: Implementation **Content Area:** Adult Health **Strategy:** The core issue of the question is knowledge of plasmapheresis as a treatment option and the underlying pathophysiology of the health problems listed. Use this information and the process of elimination to make a selection. **Reference:** LeMone, P., Burke, K., & Bauldoff, G. (2011). *Medical-surgical nursing: Critical thinking in patient care* (5th ed.). Upper Saddle River, NJ: Pearson Education, pp. 314, 675, 1107.

9 **Answer: 1** **Rationale:** The nurse should first encourage the client experiencing a loss to express his feelings. Providing a broad opening that reflects what the client has said acknowledges the client's feelings and promotes further discussion. The incorrect options provide false reassurance or do not respond to the client's feelings. **Cognitive Level:** Analyzing **Client Need:** Psychosocial Integrity **Integrated Process:** Communication and Documentation **Content Area:** Adult Health **Strategy:** First recall information about the course of Parkinson's disease. Then apply therapeutic communication techniques and note the clue word *first* in the stem of the question.

Reference: LeMone, P., Burke, K., & Bauldoff, G. (2011). *Medical-surgical nursing: Critical thinking in patient care* (5th ed.). Upper Saddle River, NJ: Pearson Education, pp. 1526–1530.

10 **Answers: 1, 3, 4, 5** **Rationale:** Weakness, numbness, confusion, difficulty speaking, trouble with coordination and ambulation, and visual difficulties are warning signs of a cerebrovascular accident (CVA) or transient ischemic attack (TIA). Although uncontrolled type 2 diabetes increases the risk of stroke, its presence does not indicate a stroke. **Cognitive Level:** Applying **Client Need:** Physiological Adaptation **Integrated Process:** Nursing Process: Assessment **Content Area:** Adult Health **Strategy:** Identify the neurological manifestations of a cerebral problem and use the process of elimination to make your selection(s). **Reference:** LeMone, P., Burke, K., & Bauldoff, G. (2011). *Medical-surgical nursing: Critical thinking in patient care* (5th ed.). Upper Saddle River, NJ: Pearson Education, pp. 1450–1451.

References

Adams, M., Holland, L., & Bostwick, P. (2011). *Pharmacology for nurses: A pathophysiologic approach* (3rd ed.). Upper Saddle River, NJ: Pearson Education.

Ball, J., & Binder, R. (2012). *Pediatric nursing: Caring for children* (5th ed.). Upper Saddle River, NJ: Pearson Education.

Corbett, J. V. (2013). *Laboratory tests and diagnostic procedures with nursing diagnoses* (8th ed.). Upper Saddle River, NJ: Pearson Education.

Ignatavicius, D., & Workman, L. (2012). *Medical surgical nursing: Patient-centered collaborative care* (7th ed.). Philadelphia, PA: W. B. Saunders.

LeMone, P., Burke, K. M., & Bauldoff, G (2011). *Medical-surgical nursing: Critical thinking in patient care* (5th ed.). Upper Saddle River, NJ: Pearson Education.

Lewis, S., Dirksen, S., Heitkemper, M., Bucher, L., & Camera, I. (2011). *Medical-surgical nursing: Assessment and management of clinical problems* (8th ed.). St. Louis, MO: Elsevier.

McCaffery, M. (1999). *Pain: Clinical manual* (2nd ed.). St. Louis, MO: Mosby, pp. 15–34, 36–102, 121–122.

McCance, K., & Huether, K. (2010). *Understanding pathophysiology: The biologic basis for disease in adults and children* (6th ed.) St. Louis, MO: Elsevier.

Porth, C., & Matfin, G. (2010). *Pathophysiology: Concepts of altered health states* (8th ed.). Philadelphia, PA: Lippincott Williams & Wilkins.

Venes, D., Thomas, C. L., & Taber, C. (2009). *Taber's cyclopedic medical dictionary* (21st ed.). Philadelphia: F. A. Davis.

ANSWERS & RATIONALES

5 Musculoskeletal Health Problems

Chapter Outline

Risk Factors Associated with Musculoskeletal Health Problems
Osteoarthritis (OA)
Rheumatoid Arthritis (RA)
Gouty Arthritis
Osteomyelitis

Paget's Disease (Osteitis Deformans)
Muscular Dystrophy (MD)
Fibromyalgia
Bone Tumors
Systemic Lupus Erythematosus (SLE)

Scleroderma (Systemic Sclerosis)
Fractures
Compartment Syndrome
Osteoporosis

NCLEX-RN® Test Prep

Use the accompanying online resource, NursingReviewsandRationales, to test yourself with hundreds of NCLEX®-style practice questions.

Objectives

➤ Define key terms associated with musculoskeletal health problems.
➤ Identify risk factors associated with the development of musculoskeletal health problems.
➤ Explain the common etiologies of musculoskeletal health problems.
➤ Describe the pathophysiologic processes associated with specific musculoskeletal health problems.
➤ Distinguish between normal and abnormal musculoskeletal findings obtained from nursing assessment.
➤ Prioritize nursing interventions associated with specific musculoskeletal health problems.

Review at a Glance

ankylosis joint immobility or fixation secondary to an underlying disease process
articular cartilage connective tissue covering an epiphysis where joint surfaces meet; acts as a cushion between joint surfaces
bone remodeling formation of new bone by osteoblasts and removal of old bone by osteoclasts; regulated by actions of parathyroid hormone, calcitonin, and vitamin D
Bouchard's node formation of hard nodules in proximal interphalangeal (PIP) joints resulting in joint deformity characteristic of osteoporosis
boutonnière deformity joint deformity associated with rheumatoid arthritis, characterized by flexion of PIP joint and hyperextension of distal interphalangeal (DIP) joint

calcinosis abnormal deposits of calcium salts on skin
diaphysis long portion or shaft of long bones; inner portion of diaphysis contains medullary cavity, which is comprised of bone marrow; surrounded by cortical bone
epiphysis proximal and distal end of long bones, comprised of cancellous bone surrounded by cortical bone
fascia fibrous connective tissue responsible for supporting and connecting structures of musculoskeletal system
Heberden's node formation of a hard nodule in distal interphalangeal (DIP) joints resulting in joint deformity characteristic of osteoarthritis (OA)
metaphysis located in area of flaring between epiphysis and diaphysis of long bones; contains growth plates

responsible for longitudinal growth of bones during growth years
osteolysis softening and breakdown of bone
osteophytes outgrowth of bony tissue often referred to as spurs
pannus vascular granulation tissue that forms in synovial membrane of clients with rheumatoid arthritis (RA); is responsible for destruction of bones and surrounding tissue in affected joints
periosteum membrane covering bone, except in areas where articular cartilage is present; it contains nerve, lymph, and blood vessels
rheumatoid nodules subcutaneous masses found in some clients with rheumatoid arthritis; characterized as firm, nontender masses usually found on olecranon bursae or along extensor surface of forearm

scleradactyly scleroderma that is localized within fingers

swan neck deformity joint deformity associated with rheumatoid arthritis, characterized by hyperextension of PIP joint with flexion of DIP joints

telangiectasis small, dilated blood vessels with a bright-red center point and spider-like branches that may occur in clients with scleroderma

ulnar drift joint deformity characteristic of rheumatoid arthritis, characterized by displacement of fingers laterally toward little finger of same hand

PRETEST

1 The nurse concludes that a client with osteoarthritis understood instructions on health maintenance if the client states that participation in which sport would be beneficial?

1. Tennis
2. Jogging
3. Swimming
4. Volleyball

2 The nurse would document which expected health history and physical assessment data findings on an adult client with rheumatoid arthritis (RA)? Select all that apply.

1. Heberden's nodes
2. Morning stiffness lasting longer than 30 minutes
3. Asymmetric joint swelling
4. Swan neck deformities
5. Weight loss, anorexia, fatigue, and weakness

3 A client diagnosed with gouty arthritis is receiving medications to treat an acute attack. What action by the nurse will facilitate the excretion of urates and help prevent uric acid renal calculi?

1. Encourage client to eat acid-forming foods to acidify the urine.
2. Give liberal fluids as tolerated to maintain a daily urine output of 2,000 mL or more.
3. Ensure an intake of fluids that equals approximately 1,000 mL in 24 hours.
4. Keep client on bed rest with the affected joint elevated as much as possible.

4 Which interventions should the nurse expect to include in a plan of care for a client with acute osteomyelitis? Select all that apply.

1. Apply heat compresses to affected area.
2. Immobilize affected area in functional position.
3. Administer opioid analgesics as ordered for severe pain.
4. Administer acetaminophen (Tylenol) as prescribed for mild pain.
5. Maintain strict hand hygiene practices.

5 The nurse interprets that which laboratory or diagnostic test data would be most significant in the client with Paget's disease?

1. Elevated white blood count (WBC)
2. Elevated erythrocyte sedimentation rate (ESR)
3. Positive tissue biopsy for *Staphylococcus*
4. Elevated serum alkaline phosphatase

6 The nurse considers that which clients seen in the ambulatory clinic are at high risk for developing an osteosarcoma? Select all that apply.

1. Male, age 34
2. Female, age 15
3. Male, age 52, history of Paget's disease
4. Male, age 58
5. Female, age 34, and pregnant

PRETEST

7 The nurse who is taking a medication history in a client with systemic lupus erythematosus (SLE) makes special note of the client's use of which drug?

1. Procainamide (Procan SR)
2. Acetylsalicylic acid (aspirin, ASA)
3. Diazepam (Valium)
4. Azathioprine (Imuran)

8 To prevent occurrences of Raynaud's phenomenon, what instruction should the nurse give to a client diagnosed with systemic sclerosis (scleroderma)?

1. Wear gloves if the temperature is cold.
2. Perform range-of-motion (ROM) exercises weekly.
3. Limit sodium intake.
4. Avoid warm temperatures.

9 A client viewing x-rays of a healing bone fracture asks the nurse if the bone will ever be normal again. The nurse's response will be based on knowledge of which events in the remodeling phase of bone healing?

1. Callus formation occurs.
2. Callus is replaced with mature bone.
3. Osteoclasts resorb excess callus to return the bone to its original shape.
4. Proliferation of osteoblast and fibroblasts occurs within the hematoma at the fracture site.

10 The nurse is caring for a client who had a cast applied to immobilize a tibia fracture that occurred 6 hours ago. The client reports severe leg pain that is unrelieved by the opioid analgesic. The nurse suspects that what cycle of events may be causing compartment syndrome and jeopardizing the limb?

1. Increased pressure within tissues results from excessive edema at fracture site, compressing the vascular network.
2. Nerves are damaged by trauma, and narcotics will not relieve pain.
3. Peripheral pulses will become accelerated to compensate for inadequate oxygen supply to injured tissue.
4. Injured fascia is elastic and expands with fluid so the cast becomes too tight, causing pain and compromising circulation.

➤ *See pages 154–156 for Answers and Rationales.*

I. RISK FACTORS ASSOCIATED WITH MUSCULOSKELETAL HEALTH PROBLEMS

A. **Osteoarthritis (OA)**: obesity, age, gender (affects genders equally up to age 55, incidence increases in women after this time), heredity

B. **Rheumatoid arthritis (RA)**: gender (occurs 2–3 times more often in females); middle age years (although can occur at any time); possible genetic link

 C. **Gouty arthritis**: gender (increased frequency in men, may occur postmenopausal or in women with a genetic link), obesity, heavy alcohol intake, familial trait, disease states (malignancies, diabetes mellitus [DM], kidney disease, hypertension [HTN], acidosis); drug-induced gout from thiazide diuretics, cytotoxic drugs, low-dose acetylsalicylic acid (aspirin), and ethambutol (Myambutol)

D. **Osteomyelitis**
  1. Hematogenous: children under age 10 with recent history of throat, ear, or skin infections; debilitated clients with recurrent upper respiratory infections (URIs), urinary tract infections (UTIs), and skin infections; and intravenous (IV) drug abusers
  2. Direct entry: recent history of puncture wound, gunshot wound, fracture, or surgery

E. **Paget's disease**: adults over 40 years of age, more common in males

F. **Muscular dystrophy (MD)**: male children with family history

G. **Fibromyalgia**: more common in women; stress

H. Bone tumors: genetic link, exposure to chemotherapy or radiation (osteosarcomas), Paget's disease

I. Systemic lupus erythematosus (SLE): women of childbearing years, family history, ethnicity (African Americans, Asians, and Hispanics)

J. Scleroderma: women of childbearing years; African American women; coal miners; occupational exposure to polyvinyl chloride, epoxy resins, and aromatic hydrocarbons; genetic link probable

K. Fractures: trauma, active participation in sports, older adult clients at risk for falls, clients with bone disease

L. Compartment syndrome: more frequent in crushing injuries and fractures of forearm or lower leg

M. Osteoporosis: postmenopausal women; ethnicity (Caucasian and Asian descent); both genders over 80 years of age; endocrine disorders such as hyperparathyroidism, hyperthyroidism, Cushing's disease, and diabetes mellitus; use of glucocorticoids, caffeine, nicotine, tetracycline, and aluminum-containing antacids; sedentary lifestyle

II. OSTEOARTHRITIS (OA)

A. Overview

1. Defined as a form of arthritis with progressive destruction of cartilage in both synovial joints and vertebrae
2. Characteristics
   a. Most common form of arthritis, also referred to as *degenerative arthritis*; is a chronic, progressive, nonsystemic disease
   b. Characterized by degeneration of **articular cartilage** (connective tissue covering **epiphysis** [proximal and distal end of long bones] where joint surfaces meet) in hands: proximal interphalangeal (PIP) and distal interphalangeal (DIP) joints, feet (metatarsophalangeal [MTP] joints), shoulder, lumbar and cervical spine, hips, and knees
3. Classifications and causes
   a. *Primary idiopathic*: unknown etiology but risk factors usually present
   b. *Secondary disorder*: results from conditions that predispose to degenerative changes in joints, such as RA, DM, congenital deformities, joint trauma, or repetitive joint movement during sports or work activities

B. Pathophysiology

1. Primary idiopathic OA: articular cartilage decreases friction during joint movement and displaces force of workload onto subchondral bone, thereby decreasing stress within joint itself
   a. Type II collagen (normally present in healthy articular cartilage) contains proteoglycans (macromolecules that provide elasticity and stiffness to articular cartilage, allowing it to resist compression)
   b. Clients with primary idiopathic OA may have some type of malfunction in production of proteoglycans; body attempts to compensate by producing more proteoglycans and collagen; however, these substances are destroyed faster than they can be synthesized
   c. Type II collagen is eventually replaced with Type I collagen (normally present in skin and tendons); with disease progression, composition of articular cartilage is altered and unable to perform its original function
   d. In response to changes in articular cartilage, synovitis (inflammation of a synovial joint) often occurs within joint; subchondral bone responds to cartilage damage by producing **osteophytes** (outgrowths of bony tissue often referred to as spurs)

    2. Secondary OA

      a. Repetitive movements that apply excessive workload to joints result in breakdown of cartilage and changes in subchondral bone

      b. Ability of cartilage to lubricate joint becomes depleted and friction increases between joint surfaces during joint motion

      c. Joint narrowing occurs with cartilage breakdown, and synovitis and formation of osteophytes occurs with disease progression

    3. Signs and symptoms

      a. Dull, aching pain in affected joint with movement and weight bearing and relieved with rest

      b. Numbness or tingling at night, associated with disease progression secondary to nerve damage

      c. Crepitus with joint movement

      d. Edema and stiffness in affected joint

      e. Decreased range of motion (ROM) and ability to participate in activities of daily living (ADLs)

      f. Joint deformities: **Heberden's nodes** (formation of hard nodules in DIP joints, resulting in joint deformity) and **Bouchard's nodes** (formation of hard nodules in PIP joints, resulting in joint deformity)

      g. Symptoms vary in severity and may range from mild intermittent discomfort to complete disability

C. Nursing assessment

    1. Assessment includes baseline ROM, performance of ADLs and work/leisure activities, pain assessment, safety with ambulation, baseline weight and dietary habits, presence of Heberden's and Bouchard's nodes

    2. Diagnostic tests

      a. X-ray: loss of joint cartilage, narrowing of space between adjacent bones, and formation of osteophytes in progressive disease states

      b. Eosinophil sedimentation rate (ESR): normal, slight increase with synovitis, used to differentiate other forms of arthritis

D. Nursing management

    1. Medications include acetaminophen (Tylenol), which is preferred, or acetylsalicylic acid (aspirin), corticosteroids (intra-articular injection or other forms), nonsteroidal anti-inflammatory drugs (NSAIDs)

    2. Instruct on weight reduction

    3. Collaborate with physical therapy (PT) regarding an aerobic exercise program to reduce and eliminate strain on joints: swimming, biking, walking, water aerobics

    4. Collaborate with occupational therapy (OT) for assistive devices for ADLs

    5. Implement and assess effectiveness of pain relief measures

      a. Teach action and side effects of medications used for pain control

      b. Application of heat before exercising and cold after exercising

      c. Splints designed to immobilize joint

      d. Cotton gloves at night

      e. Paraffin wax treatments

      f. Warm water soaks

      g. Neck collar and lumbar corsets for OA of vertebrae

      h. Firm mattress for sleeping

    6. Preoperative teaching as required for surgery:

      a. Arthroscopy (use of an arthroscope to examine interior of a joint)

      b. Total or partial joint replacements for OA of hip and knee

      c. Joint fusions for OA of cervical spine

    7. Instruct on safety in home (see Box 5-1)

Box 5-1	• Eliminate throw rugs in home.
Home Safety Tips for Clients with Musculoskeletal Health Problems	• Use proper body mechanics when performing ADLs and work/leisure activities. • Use a shower chair and hand rails when bathing. • Use cane and walker as directed to decrease workload on hips and knees. • Use well-fitting, supportive shoes when ambulating.

III. RHEUMATOID ARTHRITIS (RA)

A. Overview

1. Defined as a chronic, progressive, systemic, autoimmune disease with inflammation of joints and deformity
2. Characteristics
   a. Onset is insidious and characterized by periods of remissions and exacerbations
   b. Characterized by chronic inflammation of bilateral joints and surrounding structures; multiple joints are usually involved
3. Unknown etiology, but seems to be related to autoimmune processes in middle age
4. Systemic complications: vasculitis, anemia, and extrasynovial rheumatoid nodules on heart, lungs, eyes, or spleen

B. Pathophysiology

1. Exposure to a virus may initiate inflammatory response; immunoglobulin G (IgG) is formed in response to antigen, but for an unknown reason, body produces autoantibodies (called rheumatoid factors) against IgG
   a. Rheumatoid factors combine with IgG to form immune complexes
   b. Continued presence of immune complexes within joint cavity results in chronic inflammation and destruction of articular cartilage and surrounding joint structures
2. Synovial membrane (located within joint capsule and responsible for producing synovial fluid to lubricate joint structures) hypertrophies and thickens secondary to chronic inflammation
   a. Blood supply to area is occluded and cellular necrosis occurs
   b. These events lead to formation of **pannus** (vascular granulation tissue that forms in synovial membrane of clients with RA)
   c. Pannus gradually extends from synovial membrane and surface of articular cartilage into joint capsule and subchondral bone causing bone destruction
3. Fibrous adhesions and bony **ankylosis** (joint immobility or fixation secondary to an underlying disease process) occurs as involved bone is destroyed; inflammatory process extends to support structures of bone, tendons and ligaments, and joint instability and deformities occur
4. Signs and symptoms
   a. Initially may present with vague systemic symptoms such as anorexia, weight loss, fever, and loss of energy
   b. Early in disease there is inflammation, swelling, and decreased movement of joints in hand (PIP and MCP), feet (MTP), wrists, and elbows; as RA progresses, joints of knees, hips, and cervical spine may be involved
   c. The American Rheumatism Association has developed diagnostic criteria for RA; evidence of 4 out of 7 criteria must be present to confirm diagnosis (see Box 5-2)

Box 5-2	• Morning stiffness lasting for at least 1 hour and persisting over at least 6 weeks

Diagnostic Criteria for Rheumatoid Arthritis

- Morning stiffness lasting for at least 1 hour and persisting over at least 6 weeks
- Arthritis with swelling or effusion of 3 or more joints persisting for at least 6 weeks
- Arthritis of wrist, MCP, or PIP joints persisting for at least 6 weeks
- Symmetric arthritis with simultaneous involvement of corresponding joints on both sides of the body
- Rheumatoid nodules
- Positive serum rheumatoid factor
- Characteristic radiologic changes (erosions or decalcifications) of rheumatoid arthritis noted in hands and wrists

Source: LeMone, R. E., Burke, K., & Bauldoff, G. *Medical-surgical Nursing: Critical Thinking in Patient Care,* 5th ed., © 2011. Reprinted and Electronically reproduced by permission Pearson Education Inc., Upper Saddle River, NJ.

C. Nursing assessment

1. Assessment includes low-grade temperature; decreased ROM; signs and symptoms of inflammation (tenderness, swelling, redness) involving multiple joints bilaterally; morning stiffness lasting longer than 1 hour; reduced energy level and ability to participate in ADLs and work or leisure activities; pain assessment; neurological assessment (headache, numbness, or tingling with involvement of cervical vertebrae); baseline weight and history of recent weight loss; presence of:
   a. Joint deformities
      1) **Swan neck deformity** (hyperextension of PIP joints with flexion of DIP joints)
      2) **Ulnar drift** (joint deformity characteristic of RA; characterized by displacement of fingers laterally toward little finger of same hand)
      3) **Boutonnière deformity** (flexion of PIP joint and hyperextension of DIP joint)
   b. **Rheumatoid nodules** (firm, nontender subcutaneous masses found on olecranon bursae or extension surface of forearm) over pressure areas
2. Diagnostic tests
   a. X-ray: minimal changes early in disease, but narrowing of joint space, bone erosion, and bone deformities are evident bilaterally as disease progresses
   b. Serum rheumatoid factor: not exclusive for RA but positive in majority of clients
   c. Evidence of anemia with complete blood count (CBC)
   d. Elevated ESR
   e. Synovial fluid analysis: increased white blood cells (WBCs), increased turbidity, decreased viscosity

D. Nursing management

1. Medications
   a. NSAIDs, used early in disease
   b. Systemic corticosteroids: long-term use is associated with severe side effects; they are usually utilized when NSAIDs are no longer effective
   c. Disease-modifying drugs (DMARDs): being used earlier in treatment because newer evidence suggests they may help stop disease progression; most DMARDs are contraindicated in clients with kidney and liver disease
2. Instruct on disease process and treatment regimen
3. Refer to support groups including Arthritis Foundation
4. Emphasize rest to decrease joint stress: pace activities and perform activities while sitting when able; use splints for hands and wrists; use relaxation techniques and guided imagery

Practice to Pass

When providing health maintenance teaching to the client with rheumatoid arthritis (RA), what information should the nurse include regarding the best methods to increase joint mobility and maintain joint function?

5. Collaborate with physical therapist (PT) regarding therapeutic exercise program, isotonic exercises, passive and active ROM exercise to maintain muscle strength and joint ROM
6. Collaborate with occupational therapist (OT) regarding assistive devices for ADLs, tips for joint protection and work simplification
7. Teach action and side effects of medications used for pain control
8. Implement and assess effectiveness of pain relief measures (medication, heat or cold applications, paraffin dips, and firm mattress with proper positioning)
9. Preoperative teaching as needed for surgery: synovectomy (removal of synovial membrane), total joint replacements of hip or knee, and joint fusions for RA of cervical spine
10. Instruct on home safety (refer back to Box 5-1)
11. Instruct on hazards of immobility if bedridden and teach prevention

IV. GOUTY ARTHRITIS

A. Overview

1. Defined as a metabolic disease marked by increased serum uric acid levels (hyperuricemia) and joint inflammation
2. Characteristics

   a. Not all clients with hyperuricemia will develop gouty arthritis
   b. Acute, painful episodes of monoarticular joint inflammation lasting about 10–14 days
   c. Acute episodes vary in frequency and are often precipitated by some stress: surgery, joint trauma, and emotional stress; it is self-limiting with treatment
3. Classifications and causes
   a. *Primary*: genetic alteration in purine metabolism resulting in increased production of uric acid or decreased excretion of uric acid
   b. *Secondary*: hyperuricemia secondary to disease state or medications

B. Pathophysiology

1. Increased levels of serum uric acid precipitate within joint and initiate inflammatory response; sodium urates are deposited around or within joints
2. Phagocytosis of urate crystals occurs, leading to cell death and release of lysosomal enzymes
3. If untreated, chronic inflammation will lead to involvement of multiple joints, destruction of cartilage, bone, and formation of tophi
4. Signs and symptoms
   a. Sudden onset of severe pain in a single joint (most often great toe but may occur in instep, wrist, tarsal joints, knees, elbows, and ankles)
   b. Joint appears red or dusky, swollen, edematous, and is very tender to touch
   c. Tophi: hard, movable, nodules with irregular surfaces occur most often in synovium, helix of ear, olecranon bursa, and Achilles' tendon; associated with chronic untreated gout; can resolve with treatment

C. Nursing assessment

1. Assessment includes: complete health history, risk factors, pain assessment, inspection of affected joint for signs of inflammation, and mobility and safety with ADLs
2. Diagnostic tests
   a. Serum uric acid level greater than 7.5 mg/dL (normal: male 2.1–8.5 mg/dL; female 2–6.6 mg/dL)
   b. Increased WBC and ESR during acute episodes
   c. 24-hour urine to evaluate uric acid excretion
      1) Levels will correlate with increased serum uric acid levels if there is an overproduction of uric acid

2) In cases where excretion of uric acid is a problem, serum uric acid will be increased; however, 24-hour urine levels will be decreased

   d. Synovial fluid analysis (positive for urate crystals)

D. Nursing management

1. Medication

   a. Uric acid inhibiting drugs: allopurinol (Zyloprim), probenecid (Benemid), colchicine (also used for acute attacks), and sulfinpyrazone (Anturane)

   b. Narcotic analgesics and NSAIDs relieve pain from acute attacks; acetylsalicylic acid (aspirin) is contraindicated because it decreases excretion of uric acid and interferes with action of uricosuric drugs

2. Instruct client on disease process and treatment plan; emphasize that disease prognosis is good with adherence to treatment

3. Administer medications as prescribed and instruct on medication regimen; instruct to increase fluid intake to 3 L/day to decrease risk of kidney stones associated with use of uricosuric agents, unless contraindicated by other conditions

4. Instruct on strict bedrest for first 24 hours of acute attack (activity may aggravate and prolong acute symptoms); provide a bed cradle to relieve pressure from linens on affected area

5. Assist with weight reduction

6. Instruct on limiting intake of alcohol

Practice to Pass

Explain how the results of a 24-hour urine for uric acid assists the health care provider in determining the etiology of gout.

V. OSTEOMYELITIS

A. Overview

1. Defined as an acute or chronic infection of bone

2. Characteristics: most common causative agent is *Staphylococcus aureus*; early diagnosis is critical to prevent disease progression

3. Classifications and causes: osteomyelitis is classified by mode of entry as well as course of disease

   a. Entry

     1) Hematogenous: bloodborne infection localized in bone

     2) Direct entry: contamination through an open wound; most common form in adults

   b. Course: acute (less than 6 weeks) or chronic (more than 6–8 weeks, can last years)

B. Pathophysiology

1. Entry of pathogen occurs; organism lodges in bone, multiplies, and initiates inflammatory response

2. As pus accumulates, pressure within bone cavity increases and blood supply to area diminishes

3. If infection enters chronic stage, infection spreads through bone

4. Bone cells become necrotic and break off into segments called sequestra

5. Sequestra remain surrounded by pus and become a great medium for spread of bacteria to surrounding bone tissue

6. New bone formation, called involucrum, develops around necrotic bone cells and sinus tract formation often occurs

7. Signs and symptoms

   a. Hematogenous

     1) Acute onset of fever, chills, pain, and limited ROM at site

     2) Involvement of **metaphysis** (growth plates located in area of flaring between epiphysis [proximal and distal end of long bones] and **diaphysis** [shaft or long portion of long bones]) of tibia, humerus, or femur in children

     3) Involvement of vertebrae in adults

   b. Direct entry: afebrile or low-grade temperature, erythema, pain, tenderness at site of infection

C. Nursing assessment
1. Health history: recent episode of *Staphylococcus* infection in children under 10 years old; illicit IV drug use; or recent trauma, surgery, or puncture wound in adults
2. Assessment includes drug allergies; pain assessment (abrupt onset of pain, guarding of affected site); vital signs (VS); discomfort; decreased ROM at affected site; wound drainage; and decreased activity level
3. Diagnostic tests
   a. X-ray: no changes in early stages, elevation of **periosteum** (membrane covering bone that contains nerve, lymph, and blood vessels) and increased osteoclastic activity (bone breakdown) with disease progression
   b. Bone scan (positive for active infection)
   c. Computed tomography (CT) scan or magnetic resonance imaging (MRI) (positive for sinus tracts, abscesses, and may assist in determining boundaries of infection)
   d. ESR and WBC (elevated)
   e. Blood and tissue cultures (positive)

D. Nursing management
1. Medications include: antibiotics as prescribed, over-the-counter (OTC) or opioid analgesics for pain relief; assess degree of therapeutic effects
2. Immobilize affected area
3. Prevent spread of infection
   a. Implement aseptic technique
   b. Instruct on importance of proper hand hygiene

   c. Instruct on strict bedrest, mobility may mobilize bacteria
   d. Application of heat during acute infection is contraindicated; bacteria may spread as a result of vasodilation
4. Splint foot to prevent foot drop
5. Preoperative teaching as required for incision and drainage (I&D) of wound
6. Instruct on nutritious diet (increased protein, calcium, and vitamin C) for optimal wound healing
7. Instruct on safety measures with use of assistive devices (crutches, walkers, wheelchair)

VI. PAGET'S DISEASE (OSTEITIS DEFORMANS)

A. Overview

1. Defined as a chronic bone disease with inflammation of bone, hypertrophy of long bones, and deformity of flat bones; cause is unknown but may be viral in origin
2. Characteristics
   a. Early diagnosis is important to arrest disease progression
   b. Occurs most commonly in spine, cranium, hips, pelvis, thighs, and lower extremities
3. Long-term complications
   a. Heart failure secondary to increased demand for blood to achieve **bone remodeling** (formation of new bone by osteoblasts and removal of old bone by osteoclasts)
   b. Lung disease if ribs are involved
   c. Neurological deficits due to pressure on brain from enlarged cranium
   d. Increased incidence of sarcoma
   e. Arthritis and renal calculi secondary to hypercalcemia

B. Pathophysiology
1. Osteolytic phase: characterized by rapid growth of abnormal osteoclasts; formation of new bone cannot occur as fast as bone resorption (destruction of bone) and healthy bone is replaced with vascular, fibrous connective tissue
2. Osteoblastic sclerotic phase: deformities occur as bone eventually becomes enlarged, rough, thicker, and weaker; bone assumes a mosaic pattern called cement lines

3. Signs and symptoms: bone pain (most common), fatigue, increased head size, bowing of legs, and headache and hearing loss if cranium is involved; may remain asymptomatic for years

C. Nursing assessment

   1. Assessment

   a. Pain assessment: increasing pain with weight bearing may indicate long bone involvement; headaches may indicate cranial bone involvement

   b. Waddling gait, bone deformities (kyphosis, enlarged skull, and bowing of legs), and pathological fractures

   c. Decrease in height

   d. Cardiac assessment: hypertension and arteriosclerosis

   e. Hearing or vision loss secondary to pressure on cranial nerves

   f. Complaints of fatigue

   2. Diagnostic tests

   a. Serum alkaline phosphatase (elevated)

   b. Urine for hydroxyproline (elevated), an amino acid present in urine of clients with Paget's disease

   c. X-rays (reveal bone deformities, bone enlargement, widening of bone cortex)

   d. Bone scans (reveal active bone remodeling)

D. Nursing management

   1. Medications include NSAIDs; bone metabolism regulators such as calcitonin (Calcimar), and bisphosphonates such as alendronate (Fosamax), pamidronate (Aredia) and tiludronate (Skelid)

   2. Implement and assess effectiveness of pain relief measures: medications and heat and massage therapy

   3. Encourage client to remain active

   4. Assess for hypercalcemia caused by increased osteoclast activity (fatigue, depression, mental confusion, nausea, vomiting, increased urination, and electrocardiogram [ECG] changes)

   5. Instruct on safety to prevent pathological fractures

   6. Instruct client to increase fluid intake 2–3 liters/day to prevent renal calculi unless contraindicated because of other conditions

   7. Collaborate with PT or OT regarding proper fitting for a brace or corset; assist with adaptation to hearing or vision loss

VII. MUSCULAR DYSTROPHY (MD)

A. Overview

   1. Defined as a genetically transmitted disease that is progressive and involves specific muscles

   2. Characteristics

   a. Condition includes several disease states characterized by progressive muscle wasting

   b. Has an insidious onset associated with progressive muscle weakness

   3. Genetically transmitted by recessive gene on X chromosome (mother to son) or spontaneous mutation form may occur in females

   4. Classifications: there are several forms, which characterized by age of onset, clinical manifestations, and disease progression

   a. Rapidly progressing: Duchenne's muscular dystrophy (DMD)

   1) X-linked recessive, onset usually by age 5

   2) Most common form

   b. Slower-progressing forms

   1) Becker's: onset 5–15 years of age; X-linked recessive

Practice to Pass

A client diagnosed with Paget's disease wants to know why physical therapy is needed. Relate the bone deformities common in clients with Paget's disease to the disease's pathophysiology.

  2) Facioscapulohumeral: onset 10–30 years; autosomal dominant

  3) Limb-girdle: onset 10–30 years; cause varies

B. Pathophysiology

1. Defect in gene that produces dystrophin (a protein), which affects muscle contraction and is normally found next to sarcolemma membrane
2. Muscle cells die, are phagocytized, and eventually replaced with fatty tissue
3. Muscle size increases causing pseudohypertrophy (false appearance of being enlarged), muscles become progressively weakened because of fatty deposits and connective tissue that enters muscle fibers
4. Signs and symptoms
   a. Duchenne's MD
   1) Symptoms present around 2–3 years of age with frequent falls
   2) Waddling gait and toe walking
   3) Pseudohypertrophy of muscles in lower extremities
   4) Kyphosis
   5) Progressive immobility, confined to wheelchair by teen years
   6) Death in early adulthood secondary to respiratory or cardiac failure
   7) Cardiac involvement in later stage of illness
   b. Becker's MD: generalized muscle involvement; normal life span
   c. Facioscapulohumeral MD: face, neck, and shoulder muscles involved with muscle inflammation
   d. Limb-girdle MD: shoulder and pelvic muscle involvement; upper- and lower-extremity weakness in proximal muscles

C. Nursing assessment

1. Assessment includes: family history; gait and walking in toddlers; kyphosis in preteen years; muscle strength; history of recurrent URIs with aging
2. Diagnostic tests
   a. Elevated serum creatinine phosphokinase (CPK), lactic dehydrogenase (LDH), glutamic transaminase, and glucose phosphate
   b. Electromyograms (reveals decreased electrical signals within muscles)
   c. Muscle biopsy (muscle cell necrosis and scar tissue present)
   d. Prenatal testing for dystrophin gene for prevention

D. Nursing management

1. No medications are recommended
2. Access available resources and refer client and family to support groups
3. Prevent upper respiratory infections
4. Goal is to maintain mobility and prevent contractures: collaborate with PT for therapeutic exercise program and OT for splints to prevent contractures
5. Instruct on safe use of wheelchair
6. Incorporate growth and developmental activities appropriate for age

VIII. FIBROMYALGIA

A. Overview

1. Defined as a condition of muscles and joints resulting in chronic pain without evidence of arthritis
2. Characteristics: may be precipitated or aggravated by stress or exertion; onset is usually gradual, but it can occur suddenly
3. Cause: unknown etiology, may be associated with endocrine disorders, affective disorders, and disturbances in sleep; may be acute or chronic

B. **Pathophysiology**
1. Unclear; inappropriate levels of neurotransmitters have been investigated
2. Lacks characteristics of arthritis such as inflammation or structural changes in muscles or joints

 3. Signs and symptoms
    a. Muscle pain: local or generalized over entire body; most commonly occurs in neck, shoulders, lower back, and hips
    b. Fatigue and sleep disturbances, especially lack of stage 4 non-REM sleep
    c. Headache
    d. Irritable bowel syndrome
    e. Muscle spasms

C. **Nursing assessment**
1. Assessment includes: pain, mobility, sleep patterns, sources of stress, bowel patterns, and psychosocial assessment
2. Diagnostic tests: physical exam and the presence of 11 consistent tender points; tests to rule out other disorders such as OA or RA possible

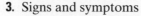 D. **Nursing management**
1. Medications include: NSAIDs for pain; antidepressants for sleep, pregabalin (Lyrica) benzodiazepine derivatives such as clonazepam (Klonopin), or mild analgesics
2. Encourage activity and assist with exercise program
3. Refer to support groups as indicated
4. Teach importance of basic health measures such as adequate rest, nutritious diet, and stress management

IX. BONE TUMORS

A. **Overview**
1. Defined as a tumor or neoplasm involving skeletal tissue
2. Characteristics
    a. *Primary bone tumors*: account for 1% of cancer in adults and 15% in children; commonly called sarcomas; may be malignant or benign
    b. *Metastatic bone tumors*: originate from a tumor elsewhere in body
        1) Occur more commonly than primary bone tumors
        2) Associated with primary cancer of breast, lung, prostate, and kidney
        3) Usually located in spine, pelvis, femur, humerus, or ribs
3. See Table 5-1 for comparison of osteosarcoma, chondrosarcoma, and Ewing's sarcoma

B. **Pathophysiology**
1. Growth of neoplastic cells in tissue of origin causes **osteolysis** (softening and breakdown of bone)

Table 5-1	Comparison of Malignant Bone Tumors			
Type of Tumor	**Description**	**Incidence**	**Tissue of Origin**	**Common Sites**
Osteosarcoma	Rapidly growing primary malignant bone tumor; etiology unknown; often discovered after injury	Higher in males age 10–25 years (highest in teen years)	Metaphysis of long bones	Distal femur, proximal tibia, and proximal humerus
Chondrosarcoma	Slow growing malignant bone tumor; etiology unknown	Higher in adult males	Cartilage	Pelvis, femur, and humerus
Ewing's sarcoma	Primary malignant bone tumor with rapid metastasis to lungs; etiology unknown	Higher at ages 10–25 years (highest in teen years)	Nerve tissue within bone marrow	Pelvis, humerus, femur, and ribs

2. Alteration in bone remodeling process results in destruction of normal bone tissue
3. Enlargement of bony surfaces occurs with tumor growth; bones become weak, leaving client at risk for pathological fractures
4. Structures surrounding bone tissue are invaded as neoplastic cells continue to multiply

5. Signs and symptoms vary based on size and location of tumor and include:
   a. Pain or tenderness and swelling at site of tumor; neuralgia secondary to nerve compression
   b. Decreased ROM and function
   c. Palpable mass and pathological fractures
   d. Temperature elevation

C. **Nursing assessment**
1. Assessment includes symptom analysis of pain or swelling at affected site, activity level, weakness, risk factors, vital signs; palpate for masses
2. Diagnostic tests: x-rays, CT scan, MRI, bone scans, bone biopsy and labs (elevated serum calcium, alkaline phosphatase, and red blood cell [RBC] count)

Practice to Pass

Identify the characteristics that differentiate osteosarcomas, chondrosarcomas, and Ewing's sarcomas.

D. **Nursing management**
1. Medications include nonopioid and opioid analgesics and chemotherapy prior to surgery
2. Monitor clients receiving opioids for constipation and use preventive measures such as increased fiber and fluids

3. Ensure proper positioning and use of assistive devices for ambulation
4. Instruct on safety in home
5. Provide rest periods between activities
6. Instruct on chemotherapy and radiation therapies as treatment options
7. Preoperative teaching as required for surgery: limb-salvage surgery (surgical removal of a bone tumor that prevents limb amputation) and limb amputation
8. Incorporate growth and developmental stage in nursing interventions
9. Collaborate with PT and/or OT for therapeutic exercise regime after surgery
10. Assist client and family in developing strategies to cope with diagnosis and treatment plans; refer to cancer support groups

X. SYSTEMIC LUPUS ERYTHEMATOSUS (SLE)

A. **Overview**
1. Defined as a chronic inflammatory, rheumatic, autoimmune disease, characterized by remissions and exacerbations
2. Characteristics
   a. Prognosis improves with early diagnosis and treatment
   b. May affect connective tissue of any body organ, disease progression varies from mild to severe depending on organ involvement
3. Classifications
   a. *Drug-induced lupus*: associated with use of procainamide (Procan SR), hydralazine (Apresoline), isoniazid (INH), and some antiepileptic drugs; symptoms usually subside after drugs are discontinued
   b. *Discoid lupus*: limited to involvement of skin
   c. *Systemic lupus*: involvement of 1 or more of these systems: musculoskeletal, lungs, kidneys, CNS, cardiovascular, hematological
4. Causes
   a. Etiology is unknown but may be attributed to exposure to ultraviolet rays, genetic defect, or hormonal imbalance (which may explain increased incidence during pregnancy)
   b. Infections from leukemia and renal failure are major causes of mortality

B. Pathophysiology

1. Body produces autoantibodies, specifically against DNA, secondary to hyperactivity of B-cells
2. Autoantibodies combine with antigens to form immune complexes and accumulate within connective tissue to trigger an inflammatory response
3. Chronic inflammation destroys connective tissue; tissue damage varies with organ involvement
4. Signs and symptoms
   a. May be unpredictable and vary with organs involved
   b. General presenting symptoms include; fever, malaise, fatigue, weakness, and weight loss
   c. Musculoskeletal: polyarthralgia, symmetrical arthritis
   d. Integumentary: alopecia, butterfly rash, sclerosis of skin on fingers, discoid lesions
   e. Painless lesions in oral mucosa
   f. Cardiac: pericarditis
   g. Lungs: pleural effusions, pleuritis
   h. Kidney: glomerulonephritis, renal failure
   i. CNS: seizures, psychosis, cerebrovascular accident (CVA), senile dementias
   j. Hematological: anemia, leukopenia, and thrombocytopenia
   k. Infections

C. Nursing assessment

1. Assessment includes identifying risk factors; complete drug history; nutrition (baseline weight and history of recent weight loss) and fluid balance (intake and output or I & O); skin (rashes, hair loss, photosensitivity; ecchymosis and petechiae may indicate hematologic involvement); respiratory (pleural effusion and pleuritis); renal status; neurological (seizure activity, changes in affect and/or cognitive abilities); cardiovascular (VS, signs and symptoms of pericarditis); musculoskeletal (symmetrical joint pain, ability to participate in ADLs, history of weakness)
2. Diagnostic tests
   a. X-ray of affected joints (will not show degenerative changes or bone deformities characteristic of arthritis)
   b. Serum syphilis (false positive)
   c. Serum antinuclear antibody (ANA) (positive), but not exclusive to SLE
   d. Anti-DNA antibody (positive), which is definitive for SLE
   e. Serum complement levels (decreased)
   f. CBC (positive for anemia, leukopenia, and/or thrombocytopenia)
   g. Urinalysis (UA): positive for proteinuria and/or hematuria
   h. Blood urea nitrogen (BUN) and creatinine (Cr): elevated
   i. ESR (elevated)

D. Nursing management

1. Medications
   a. NSAIDs: used to treat joint pain
   b. Antimalarials: used to treat joint pain and skin disorders
   c. Corticosteroids: used during acute exacerbations, may also use a low-maintenance dose during remissions
   d. Immunosuppressive drugs: toxic drugs used during acute life-threatening exacerbations only
2. Instruct on disease process and treatment regimen
3. Instruct on factors that may trigger exacerbations
   a. Pregnancy: provide counseling regarding family planning and alternatives to birth control pills

      b. Exposure to UV rays: use sunscreen with sun protection factor (SPF) of 15, wear sun hats, avoid sunbathing, and use a beach umbrella

      c. Medication: avoid use of birth control pills, sulfonamides, penicillin

  4. Refer to support groups

  5. Implement and assess effectiveness of joint pain relief measures, including medications, application of heat, and therapeutic exercise program

  6. Administer medications as directed and assess therapeutic and nontherapeutic responses

      a. Educate about side effects of corticosteroids (cushingoid effects, hypertension, weight gain) and immunosuppressive drugs

      b. Blindness can occur with antimalarials; routine eye exams should be done

  7. Explain importance of nutrition and oral care as general health measures

  8. Instruct on hand hygiene and infection control at home to prevent infection

  9. If alopecia occurs from SLE, make referral for hair wig if appropriate to maintain positive body image

  10. Assist family and client in developing safety interventions as well as coping strategies to deal with cognitive changes

XI. SCLERODERMA (SYSTEMIC SCLEROSIS)

A. Overview

  1. Defined as an uncommon, chronic, autoimmune connective tissue disorder involving skin and other organs, characterized by remissions and exacerbations

  2. Classifications are systemic sclerosis, CREST syndrome, and localized

  3. Unknown etiology; may include genetic, immune, or environmental factors

B. Pathophysiology

  1. Unknown etiology

  2. Overproduction of collagen leads to fibrosis and inflammation resulting in damage to affected area

  3. Types of scleroderma

      a. *Systemic sclerosis* (SS): involves visceral organs (most commonly esophagus, intestines, lungs, heart, and kidney) and skin of fingers, hands, face, and trunk; may progress quickly; may be life threatening depending on extent of organ involvement

      b. *CREST syndrome*: acronym representing:

         1) Calcinosis (abnormal deposits of calcium salts on skin)

         2) Raynaud's disease

         3) Esophageal dysfunctions

         4) Sclerodactyly (scleroderma localized within fingers)

         5) Telangiectasis (small, dilated blood vessels with a bright-red center point and spider-like branches)

         6) Prognosis is good and disability is limited

      c. Localized or limited: involvement of skin on fingers, hands, and face; self-limiting with good prognosis

  4. Signs and symptoms

      a. Skin: shiny, thick skin on fingers, hands progressing to arms, trunk, and face, nonpitting edema of affected areas, calcium deposits on skin, telangiectasis, hyperpigmentation, and pursed lips

      b. Vascular: Raynaud's disease

      c. Musculoskeletal: polyarthralgia and joint stiffness

      d. Esophageal: heartburn and dysphagia

      e. Intestinal: constipation, diarrhea, malabsorption, abdominal distention

      f. Heart: ECG changes, signs and symptoms of pericarditis

        g. Lungs: shortness of breath (SOB) on exertion

        h. Kidneys: renal failure

C. Nursing assessment

   1. Assessment

        a. Skin assessment: for changes previously listed

        b. Baseline height and weight; recent weight loss

        c. Gastrointestinal (GI): dietary intake, bowel patterns, abdominal assessment, complaints of heartburn and dysphagia

        d. Musculoskeletal: decreased ROM in affected areas, reports of polyarthralgia and joint stiffness, clawlike appearance of hands

        e. Respiratory assessment for exertional dyspnea

        f. Cardiac: heart rate and rhythm, hypertension

        g. Renal: I & O for fluid retention

   2. Diagnostic tests: ESR (elevated), urinalysis (proteinuria), BUN and creatinine (elevated with renal failure), ANA (elevated), skin biopsy (results indicate dermal collagen thickening, confirms diagnosis) and pulmonary function tests (abnormal if decreased lung function)

D. Nursing management

   1. Medications

        a. NSAIDs or analgesics for joint pain

        b. H_2-antagonists and proton pump inhibitors for GI symptoms

        c. Antibiotics if needed; may be used prophylactically as indicated

        d. Corticosteroids and immunosuppressive drugs are used in advanced life-threatening disease states

        e. Stool softeners to decrease constipation from analgesics, if appropriate

        f. Anticoagulants to prevent deep vein thrombosis

   2. Instruct on disease process and treatment regimen

   3. Refer to support groups

   4. Musculoskeletal symptoms: collaborate with PT for therapeutic exercises to maintain joint mobility and OT for assistive devices and ADL training

   5. GI symptoms: consult dietitian for nutritional support; maintain high-Fowler's position during and following meals; give small frequent meals

   6. Raynaud's disease: instruct to avoid cold temperatures, wear gloves and socks to warm hands and improve circulation, and avoid smoking

   7. Skin care: inspect skin daily for breakdown, and utilize skin moisturizers

XII. FRACTURES

A. Overview

   1. Defined as a break in a bone, which occurs secondary to trauma or bone disease

   2. Classifications: according to location of break, angle of break, and/or relationship with external environment; see Box 5-3

   3. A client may be able to move affected area even though a fracture exists

   4. Causes include accidents, trauma, motor vehicle accidents, abuse, neglect, and disease processes such as osteoporosis or metastatic disease

B. Pathophysiology

   1. Hematoma formation: bleeding occurs immediately following fracture because of ruptured blood vessels within bone and trauma to surrounding tissue; presence of clotting factors within hematoma leads to formation of a fibrin mesh around fracture site

   2. Granulation tissue: during first 48–72 hours, new capillary beds form and proliferation of osteoblasts (bone cell responsible for formation of new bone) and fibroblasts occurs within hematoma

        a. Granulation tissue replaces hematoma

        b. Phagocytosis also occurs and removes necrotic bone tissue

Box 5-3	Fractures can be classified or described in the following ways:
Terminology Related to Fractures	*Relationship to external environment* • Open or compound: penetration of skin, bone protrudes through • Closed: no penetration of bone through skin *Type of break* • Complete: bone broken all the way through • Incomplete: partially broken or splintered *Name of fracture* • Comminuted: bone shatters into pieces • Compression: bone is crushed • Impacted: ends of broken pieces are jammed together • Spiral: bone twists and causes jagged break • Greenstick: incomplete break • Transverse: complete break at right angle to long axis of bone

Practice to Pass

A 10-year-old client diagnosed with a fractured humerus is discharged from the emergency department after application of a cast. Develop a teaching plan for the child and caregivers regarding cast care.

3. Callus formation: within a week, granulation tissue changes and becomes callus (composed of new cartilage, calcium, phosphorus, and osteoblasts)
   a. Callus becomes interlaced among bony fragments and delicately links distal ends of fracture
   b. Eventually callus formation extends beyond fracture and serves as a temporary splint
   c. The process continues leading to increased strengthening of bone
   d. X-rays confirm this stage of bone healing and help to determine treatment regimen
4. Ossification: formation of mature bone replaces callus; the delicate link between distal ends of fracture solidifies and a strong connection is restored
5. Remodeling: osteoclasts resorb excess callus and bone returns to preinjury strength and shape
6. Signs and symptoms
   a. Pain and muscle spasms
   b. Asymmetrical appearance of limb secondary to bone displacement
   c. Numbness and or tingling at affected site secondary to nerve compression
   d. Loss of function
   e. Edema ecchymosis, and tenderness at site secondary to tissue trauma
   f. Crepitus with movement

C. Nursing assessment
1. Assessment includes signs and symptoms noted in section above, subjective data describing event, pain assessment including guarding of affected site, and presence of pulses
2. Diagnostic test: X-ray will confirm fracture

D. Nursing management
1. Medications include analgesics to control pain, antibiotics for open fracture

2. Emergency nursing care: immobilize fracture, control bleeding, and clean wound (unless an open fracture exists, which will be cleaned in surgery)

3. Assess 5 Ps (see Figure 5-1)
4. Client teaching as required for closed reduction or for surgery (open reduction)
5. Teach action and side effects of medications

6. Elevate extremity and apply an ice pack to relieve edema
7. Assess and provide client teaching on prevention of hazards of immobility

8. Recognize and treat early complications: hypovolemic shock, fat emboli (petechial rash, tachycardia, tachypnea), deep vein thrombosis, and compartment syndrome (see next section)

9. Instruct on cast care if applicable (see Box 5-4)

10. Provide traction care if applicable (see Box 5-5)
11. Maintain nutritional status
12. Instruct on safety and use of assistive devices

Figure 5-1

5 Ps in assessing circulation

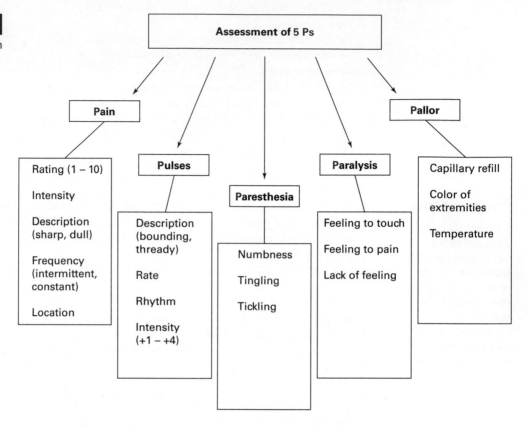

Box 5-4

Teaching Tips for Clients with Casts

- During the first 24 hours after application of the cast, apply ice directly over the fracture, elevate the extremity, and promote drying of the cast by leaving it exposed to air and supporting it on pillows.
- Report any of the following symptoms to your health care provider: increased pain, change in color, coolness of extremity, lack of movement, or numbness and tingling.
- Do not place any item in the cast; use a blow dryer on the cool setting to relieve itching.
- Keep plaster casts dry at all times; cover with plastic during bathing.
- Fiberglass casts may get wet; be sure to dry them completely with a blow dryer on cool setting.
- Report drainage or cast odor to your health care provider.

Box 5-5

Nursing Implications for Clients Receiving Traction

- Maintain correct alignment at all times.
- All weights should clear the floor at all times.
- Inspect the skin at pressure points for skin breakdown.
- Implement skin care measures that prevent skin breakdown.
- Implement nursing interventions that prevent hazards of immobility.
- Inspect pin sites for signs and symptoms of infection.
- Provide pin care according to agency policy.

XIII. COMPARTMENT SYNDROME

A. Overview

1. Defined as muscle and nerve damage related to excessive swelling in area of a fracture
2. Classifications
   a. *Acute*: occurs after a crush injury or cast application for bone fracture
   b. *Chronic*: occurs most often in adults who engage in activities requiring repetitive motion, causing excessive strain on extremities; for example, long-distance running or typing on keyboard (repetitive motion injury)

B. Pathophysiology

1. Two factors leading to compartment syndrome
   a. Hemorrhage and edema occur following a fracture, causing a reduction in ability of **fascia** (fibrous connective tissue responsible for supporting and connecting structures of musculoskeletal system) to accommodate excessive edema
   b. A closed compartment may be created by applying a tight-fitting external dressing, splint, or cast, causing increased pressure on limb
2. As pressure within compartment increases, both venous and arterial circulation become obstructed and tissue perfusion is diminished
3. Consequently, tissue ischemia, loss of function, and nerve damage occur; pressures of 30 mmHg or more can result in permanent muscle and nerve damage
4. Signs and symptoms
   a. Severe pain unrelieved by analgesics and aggravated by elevation
   b. Paresthesias
   c. Loss of function and decreased reflexes
   d. Pallor with extremity cool to touch
   e. Pulse that is decreased in volume or absent

C. Nursing assessment

1. Assessment
   a. Symptom analysis of pain
   b. Neurovascular checks following fractures; pulses may be present during early stages of compartment syndrome
   c. Assess external dressings, splint, or cast for tightness
   d. Excessive edema at fracture site
2. Diagnostic tests: no tests are recommended

D. Nursing management

1. Medications include analgesics for pain
2. Notify health care provider
3. Elevate extremity and apply ice immediately to increase venous return and decrease edema as a means of *preventing* compartment syndrome
4. Remove or loosen constrictive dressings and or splint, assist with bivalving cast if directed once it has occurred
5. Conduct preoperative teaching as indicated for a fasciotomy (surgical procedure to cut and divide a fascia)

XIV. OSTEOPOROSIS

A. Overview

1. Defined as a musculoskeletal disorder characterized by loss of bone mass
2. Disease process predisposes clients to fractures

3. Classifications
   a. *Type I*: associated with early postmenopausal estrogen deficiency
   b. *Type II*: senile osteoporosis associated with calcium deficiency
4. Cause related to endocrine disorder, malignancy, or aging process

B. **Pathophysiology**
   1. An increase in osteoclast activity and a decrease in osteoblast activity lead to rate of bone resorption that exceeds rate of bone formation
   2. Outer cortex (outer surface of bone composed of hard, cortical bone) of diaphysis and metaphysis become thinner secondary to enlargement of bone
   3. Advanced disease process leads to loss of trabeculae (spongy bone containing red bone marrow located in metaphysis of long bones) from cancellous bone (spongy bone located towards interior of bone containing red or yellow bone marrow) and thinning of cortex; these changes increase risk for bone fracture
   4. Signs and symptoms: loss of height, kyphosis, low back pain, fractures of forearm, spine, and hip

C. **Nursing assessment**
   1. Assessment includes analysis of possible risk factors; height (pattern of decrease); pain assessment; and any recent fractures
   2. Diagnostic test: bone density studies; x-rays (will not show changes in bone mass until a loss greater than 30% exists)

D. **Nursing management**
   1. Medications include calcium supplements; calcitonin and fluoride; selective estrogen receptor modulators (SERMs) such as raloxifene hydrochloride (Evista); bisphosphonates such as alendronate (Fosamax), etidronate (Didronel), and pamidronate (Aredia)
   2. Instruct clients at risk and those diagnosed on the following:
      a. Implement an exercise regimen that incorporates weight-bearing exercises, jogging, walking, rowing, and weight lifting
      b. Instruct on adequate calcium intake through diet or supplements (premenopausal women 1,000 mg/day and postmenopausal women 1,500 mg/day)
      c. Instruct older adult clients at risk about safety with ambulation in home (see Box 5-1 again)

Case Study

A 45-year-old client sustains fractures of the right leg and arm because of a motor vehicle crash. The client is treated in the emergency department and then admitted to an orthopedic unit for observation.

1. What are the priorities of care at the scene of the accident?

2. Outline the nursing care of the client after casts are placed on the right arm and leg.

3. What discharge instructions should the nurse give to the client?

4. Forty-eight hours after the accident, the client complains of excruciating pain in his right arm unrelieved by analgesics. What complication should the nurse suspect?

5. What are the priorities of care in question 4?

For suggested responses, see page 463.

POSTTEST

1 A client has had a fracture reduced and immobilized. Which of the following is a priority area for assessment by the nurse to detect a classic hallmark manifestation of compartment syndrome as a complication?

1. Assessing for edema at the fracture site
2. Palpation of a pulse distal to the fracture site
3. Performing a pain assessment
4. Assessing for the presence of drainage on the cast

2 In reviewing the medication order sheet for a client with systemic sclerosis (scleroderma), the nurse concludes that the ordered calcium channel blocker and alpha-adrenergic blocker are being given to treat which of the following problems accompanying this disease?

1. Renal failure
2. Pericarditis
3. Bradycardia
4. Raynaud's phenomenon

3 Which of the following laboratory values is most significant to the nurse when assessing a client for complications associated with Paget's disease?

1. Calcium level of 15 mg/dL
2. Positive rheumatoid factor (RF)
3. Blood urea nitrogen (BUN) of 90 mg/dL
4. Eosinophil sedimentation rate (ESR) of 30 mm/h

4 A female client has breast cancer that has metastasized to the bones. The nurse would develop which goals of nursing care for this client? Select all that apply.

1. Treat primary cancer and prevent further metastasis.
2. Control pain associated with the disease.
3. Promote maximal function and mobility.
4. Prevent pathological fractures.
5. Prevent complications from hypercalcemia.

5 An adult male limps into the ambulatory clinic reporting a red, hot, swollen joint in his great toe. The problem developed after a night of heavy alcohol use. He asks the nurse what caused his gout pain to return. The nurse formulates a response based on what underlying pathophysiology?

1. Increased immune complexes are deposited within the joint cavity.
2. Alteration in purine metabolism results in hyperuricemia; alcohol consumption may trigger it.
3. Excessive bone remodeling is secondary to increased levels of phosphorus, related to overeating.
4. Presence of fibrous adhesions within bony cartilage causes pain and a limping gait.

6 A client is diagnosed with osteomyelitis involving the foot. The wound is draining, and dressing changes are being done daily or more often as needed. What is the nurse's highest priority at this time?

1. Maintaining adequate pain control
2. Implementing aseptic technique
3. Promoting adequate nutrition
4. Splinting the foot to prevent foot drop

7 The nurse is counseling the parents of a child diagnosed with muscular dystrophy (MD). Which statement by the nurse most accurately describes the disease progression?

1. "Prognosis is favorable with early detection."
2. "With aggressive physical therapy and the use of a walker, your child will remain ambulatory through adulthood."
3. "The muscles and the lungs may also become involved, and this can shorten your child's life span."
4. "Muscle weakness is progressive and rapid, and your child will most likely be confined to a wheelchair by the age of 5."

POSTTEST

8 The nurse is explaining osteoarthritis (OA, or degenerative joint disease) to a client. The nurse incorporates which information about the underlying pathology in the discussion?

1. Changes in composition of the articular cartilage contribute to increased friction during joint movement
2. Joint inflammation occurs secondary to the presence of immune complexes within the joint cavity
3. Excessive bone necrosis within the joint occurs secondary to increased osteoclastic activity
4. Bone damage occurs secondary to osteolysis and excessive bone remodeling

9 An adult client is being treated in the early stages of rheumatoid arthritis (RA). Which of the following drugs would the nurse expect to be included in the client's drug regime? Select all that apply.

1. Nonsteroidal anti-inflammatory drugs (NSAIDs) such as ibuprofen (Motrin) or aspirin
2. Systemic corticosteroids such as prednisone (Deltasone)
3. Disease-modifying anti-rheumatoid drugs (DMARDs) such as methotrexate (Trexall)
4. Oral opioid analgesics such as oxycodone (Oxycontin)
5. Routine injections of an opioid such as morphine sulfate

10 The nurse is explaining the pathophysiology of osteoporosis to a female client. Which statement should the nurse include in the discussion to best describe the disease process?

1. "Increased amounts of estrogen in postmenopausal women contribute to bone loss."
2. "There is an imbalance between formation of new bone and the absorption of existing bone."
3. "A decrease in blood supply to the bone results in bony necrosis or the death of bone cells."
4. "An invasion by a pathogen leads to infection and destruction of bone."

➤ *See pages 156–157 for Answers and Rationales.*

ANSWERS & RATIONALES

Pretest

1 **Answer: 3** **Rationale:** Activities should be chosen that allow range of motion (ROM) but do not further injure a joint. Swimming is an aerobic exercise that does not stress the joints but allows full ROM. Weight-bearing exercises such as tennis, jogging, and volleyball place excessive strain on diseased joints and should not be activities of choice. **Cognitive Level:** Applying **Client Need:** Health Promotion and Maintenance **Integrated Process:** Nursing Process: Evaluation **Content Area:** Adult Health **Strategy:** Consider what activity is aerobic and puts less stress on damaged joints. The correct option stands out from the others. **Reference:** LeMone, P., Burke, K., & Bauldoff, G. (2011). *Medical-surgical nursing: Critical thinking in patient care* (5th ed). Upper Saddle River, NJ: Pearson Education, p. 1360.

2 **Answer: 2, 4, 5** **Rationale:** Swan neck deformities of the hand are classic deformities associated with rheumatoid arthritis (RA) secondary to the presence of fibrous connective tissue within the joint space. Clients with RA experience morning stiffness lasting from 30 minutes up

to several hours. Systemic manifestations include weakness, fatigue, and weight loss. RA is characterized by symmetrical joint involvement. Heberden's nodes and morning stiffness lasting less than 30 minutes are characteristic of osteoarthritis. **Cognitive Level:** Analyzing **Client Need:** Physiological Adaptation **Integrated Process:** Communication and Documentation **Content Area:** Adult Health **Strategy:** The core issue of the question is the ability to distinguish between rheumatoid arthritis (RA) and osteoarthritis (OA). Use nursing knowledge and the process of elimination to make a selection. **Reference:** LeMone, P., Burke, K., & Bauldoff, G. (2011). *Medical-surgical nursing: Critical thinking in patient care* (5th ed). Upper Saddle River, NJ: Pearson Education, pp. 1353–1370.

3 **Answer: 2** **Rationale:** A liberal fluid intake (to maintain a urine output of 2,000 mL or more daily) is recommended to reduce calculi formation and increase urate excretion. Alkalizing agents such as bicarbonate or citrate may also minimize uric acid stone formation; acidifying urine may be of some use in preventing urinary tract infection. Bed rest is indicated during an acute attack to rest the joint, but rest does not prevent renal problems. **Cognitive Level:** Applying **Client Need:** Physiological Adaptation **Integrated Process:** Nursing Process: Implementation **Content Area:** Adult Health **Strategy:** Utilize principles of fluid balance and renal excretion to answer the question. Critical words include *facilitate* and *excretion*. Identify options that are opposite in nature if the correct answer is unknown because one of these would have to be incorrect. **Reference:** LeMone, P., Burke, K., & Bauldoff, G. (2011). *Medical-surgical nursing: Critical thinking in patient care* (5th ed). Upper Saddle River, NJ: Pearson Education, pp. 1347–1351.

4 **Answer: 2, 3, 4, 5** **Rationale:** Immobilizing the joint, providing analgesia for mild or severe pain, and maintaining strict hand hygiene practices are appropriate nursing interventions to manage pain and prevent the spread of infection for a client diagnosed with osteomyelitis. The application of heat is contraindicated because it can increase edema and pain in the affected area and spread bacteria through vasodilatation. **Cognitive Level:** Applying **Client Need:** Physiological Adaptation **Integrated Process:** Nursing Process: Implementation **Content Area:** Adult Health **Strategy:** Identify the actions that provide comfort and maintain function. These will be the correct options in the question. **Reference:** LeMone, P., Burke, K., & Bauldoff, G. (2011). *Medical-surgical nursing: Critical thinking in patient care* (5th ed). Upper Saddle River, NJ: Pearson Education, pp. 1383–1384.

5 **Answer: 4** **Rationale:** Serum alkaline phosphatase is elevated because of increased activity of bone cells. Inflammation is in the bone and usually does not reveal an elevated serum white blood cell count, erythrocyte sedimentation rate, or the presence of *Staphylococcus*. **Cognitive Level:** Applying **Client Need:** Reduction of Risk Potential **Integrated Process:** Nursing Process: Diagnosis **Content Area:** Adult Health **Strategy:** Choose the option that reflects loss of bone tissue. Eliminate the options related to infection. **Reference:** Huether, S. E., & McCance, K. L. (2012). *Understanding pathophysiology* (5th ed). St. Louis, MO: Elsevier Inc., p. 994.

6 **Answer: 2, 3, 4** **Rationale:** The incidence of osteosarcoma, the most commonly diagnosed primary bone tumor, peaks around puberty in both boys and girls with a slight preference for males. A secondary peak incidence occurs in the 50–60 year age group, primarily in individuals with a history of radiation therapy, malignancies, or Paget's disease of bone. Adult males and females of child-bearing age are less likely to develop osteosarcoma. **Cognitive Level:** Applying **Client Need:** Health Promotion and Maintenance **Integrated Process:** Nursing Process: Assessment **Content Area:** Adult Health **Strategy:** If this question is difficult and you need to make an educated guess, note that one option stands out as different from the others. **Reference:** Huether, S. E., & McCance, K. L. (2012). *Understanding pathophysiology* (5th ed). St. Louis, MO: Elsevier Inc., pp. 1015–1016.

7 **Answer: 1** **Rationale:** Although the etiology of systemic lupus erythematosus (SLE) is unknown, certain environmental factors have been associated with the onset of symptoms. The administration of procainamide (Procan SR), an antidysrhythmic, and hydralazine (Apresoline), an antihypertensive, have been associated with SLE symptoms, which usually subside after the drug is discontinued. **Cognitive Level:** Applying **Client Need:** Pharmacological and Parenteral Therapies **Integrated Process:** Nursing Process: Assessment **Content Area:** Adult Health **Strategy:** The core issue of the question is knowledge of which drugs have adverse effects resembling systemic lupus erythematosus (SLE). Use this knowledge and the process of elimination to make a selection. **Reference:** Huether, S. E., & McCance, K. L. (2012). Understanding pathophysiology (5th ed). St. Louis, MO: Elsevier Inc., p. 198. LeMone, P., Burke, K., & Bauldoff, G. (2011). *Medical-surgical nursing: Critical thinking in patient care* (5th ed). Upper Saddle River, NJ: Pearson Education, p. 1377.

8 **Answer: 1** **Rationale:** Systemic sclerosis is characterized by functional and structural abnormalities of small arteries that lead to progressive vessel obstruction. Initial manifestations are usually noted in the skin, which thickens. Arthralgias and Raynaud's phenomenon are common early manifestations of systemic sclerosis. Attacks are usually triggered by cold temperatures. Clients with scleroderma should perform range of movement exercises daily, and avoid cold temperatures. Limiting sodium intake is not directly related to scleroderma. **Cognitive Level:** Applying **Client Need:** Physiological Adaptation **Integrated Process:** Teaching and Learning **Content Area:** Adult Health **Strategy:** Recall that treatment is supportive to prevent vascular spasms due to cold temperatures. Identify options that are opposite and consider whether one of them may be the correct option. **Reference:** Huether, S. E., & McCance, K. L. (2012). *Understanding pathophysiology* (5th ed). St. Louis, MO: Elsevier Inc., p. 1056. LeMone, P., Burke, K., & Bauldoff, G. (2012). *Medical-surgical nursing: Critical thinking in patient care* (5th ed). Upper Saddle River, NJ: Pearson Education, Inc., pp. 1388–1389.

9 **Answer: 3** **Rationale:** During earlier stages of bone healing, overproduction of callus enlarges the bone and acts as a splint. Callus is eventually replaced with mature bone during the ossification phase of bone healing, and then the excess callus is resorbed during the remodeling phase to return the bone to its original shape. **Cognitive Level:** Applying **Client Need:** Physiological Adaptation **Integrated Process:** Nursing Process: Diagnosis **Content Area:** Adult Health **Strategy:** Apply principles of healing. Recall that remodeling is the last stage. **Reference:** Huether, S. E., & McCance, K. L. (2012). *Understanding pathophysiology* (5th ed). St. Louis, MO: Elsevier Inc., p. 980. LeMone, P., Burke, K., & Bauldoff, G. (2012). *Medical-surgical nursing: Critical thinking in patient care* (5th ed). Upper Saddle River, NJ: Pearson Education, Inc., pp. 1312–1313.

10 Answer: 1 Rationale: Edema is expected immediately following a fracture, but because the fascia is nonelastic, excessive swelling will lead to increased capillary pressure within the area, resulting in nerve and muscle damage if left untreated. Damage is irreversible if the capillary pressure reaches 30 mmHg. A pulse may still be present during early stages of compartment syndrome. One factor that can differentiate pain associated with trauma from the fracture and that from compartment syndrome is the ineffectiveness of analgesics when compartment syndrome occurs. **Cognitive Level:** Applying **Client Need:** Physiological Adaptation **Integrated Process:** Nursing Process: Diagnosis **Content Area:** Adult Health **Strategy:** Consider the hemorrhage and edema that occur at a fracture site and use the process of elimination to make a selection. **Reference:** LeMone, P., Burke, K., & Bauldoff, G. (2012). *Medical-surgical nursing: Critical thinking in patient care* (5th ed). Upper Saddle River, NJ: Pearson Education, Inc., pp. 1310–1311.

Posttest

1 Answer: 3 Rationale: Compartment syndrome usually develops within the first 48 hours of injury, when edema is at its peak. Early manifestations include pain and normal or decreased peripheral pulse. The nurse should assess for edema, pulses, and presence of drainage as routine assessments; however, pain unrelieved by analgesics is a symptom most indicative of compartment syndrome. **Cognitive Level:** Analyzing **Client Need:** Physiological Adaptation **Integrated Process:** Nursing Process: Assessment **Content Area:** Adult Health **Strategy:** Identify the critical word *priority* in the stem of the question. With this in mind, expect all options to be plausible. Select the best one after reading all the options. **Reference:** LeMone, P., Burke, K., & Bauldoff, G. (2011). *Medical-surgical nursing: Critical thinking in patient care* (5th ed). Upper Saddle River, NJ: Pearson Education, pp. 1310–1312.

2 Answer: 4 Rationale: When clients with scleroderma develop Raynaud's phenomenon, which is characterized by vasospasms of the arteries and veins of the hands, calcium channel blockers (such as nifedipine) or alpha-adrenergic blockers (such as prazosin) are the treatment of choice. Angiotensin-converting enzyme (ACE) inhibitors would be used for renal involvement. Bradycardia is not specific to scleroderma. Clients may experience pericarditis, but this is not treated with calcium channel or alpha adrenergic blockers. **Cognitive Level:** Applying **Client Need:** Pharmacological and Parenteral Therapies **Integrated Process:** Nursing Process: Diagnosis **Content Area:** Adult Health **Strategy:** Recognize that all the options are possible concerns for a client with scleroderma. Consider which complication may be treated with the drugs in the stem of the question. **Reference:** Huether, S. E., & McCance, K. L. (2012). *Understanding pathophysiology* (5th ed). St. Louis, MO: Elsevier Inc., pp. 594–595. LeMone, P., Burke, K., & Bauldoff, G. (2011). *Medical-surgical nursing: Critical*

thinking in patient care (5th ed). Upper Saddle River, NJ: Pearson Education, pp. 1374–1377.

3 Answer: 1 Rationale: Hypercalcemia can occur as a complication of Paget's disease secondary to increased osteoclast activity. The other tests are not specific to Paget's disease although they are all abnormal values. **Cognitive Level:** Analyzing **Client Need:** Reduction of Risk Potential **Integrated Process:** Nursing Process: Diagnosis **Content Area:** Adult Health **Strategy:** Find the laboratory test result that reflects the abnormal bone reabsorption and formation seen in Paget's disease. **Reference:** LeMone, P., Burke, K., & Bauldoff, G. (2011). *Medical-surgical nursing: Critical thinking in patient care* (5th ed). Upper Saddle River, NJ: Pearson Education, pp. 1345–1347.

4 Answer: 2, 3, 4, 5 Rationale: Metastatic bone disease weakens the bones, predisposing the client to pathological fractures. The major symptom is pain. The goals are to prevent pathological fractures, maximize function, maintain mobility, and control pain as much as possible. Hypercalcemia occurs in 10% to 20% of clients with metastatic bone disease because of demineralization, so this may also need to be controlled. A nursing goal would not be to prevent further metastasis. **Cognitive Level:** Applying **Client Need:** Physiological Adaptation **Integrated Process:** Nursing Process: Planning **Content Area:** Adult Health **Strategy:** Do not choose goals that are unrealistic. **Reference:** Huether, S. E., & McCance, K. L. (2012). *Understanding pathophysiology* (5th ed). St. Louis, MO: Elsevier Inc., pp. 1014–1015.

5 Answer: 2 Rationale: The pathophysiology of gouty arthritis is related to overproduction or decreased excretion of uric acid in the primary form. Alteration in purine metabolism results in hyperuricemia; alcohol consumption may trigger it. The pathophysiology does not involve deposits of immune complexes, increased phosphorus, or fibrous adhesions. **Cognitive Level:** Applying **Client Need:** Physiological Adaptation **Integrated Process:** Nursing Process: Diagnosis **Content Area:** Adult Health **Strategy:** The critical words in the question are *gout* and *alcohol*. Use nursing knowledge and the process of elimination to make a selection. **Reference:** LeMone, P., Burke, K., & Bauldoff, G. (2011). *Medical-surgical nursing: Critical thinking in patient care* (5th ed). Upper Saddle River, NJ: Pearson Education, p. 1349.

6 Answer: 2 Rationale: Although all the items listed are important in the plan of care for the client diagnosed with osteomyelitis, maintaining aseptic technique and preventing the spread of infection is crucial to resolving the disease process. Maslow's hierarchy may identify adequate pain control as the highest priority, but infection is the cause of the pain, making infection the primary focus. Implementation of aseptic technique the highest priority. **Cognitive Level:** Analyzing **Client Need:** Physiological Adaptation **Integrated Process:** Nursing Process: Planning **Content Area:** Adult Health **Strategy:** Think of what causes the problem and deal with that first in a question such as this. **Reference:** Huether, S. E., & McCance, K. L. (2012). *Understanding pathophysiology* (5th ed). St. Louis, MO: Elsevier Inc., pp. 1026–1027.

7 Answer: 3 Rationale: Symptoms of muscular dystrophy (MD) usually manifest in early childhood. The child has a waddling gait and experiences frequent falls. There is no cure for the disease and muscles become progressively weaker. Most children are wheelchair confined by the teen years. As the disease progresses, heart and lung muscle are affected, resulting in cardiac and pulmonary failure. The child lives, on average, 15 years after onset. **Cognitive Level:** Applying **Client Need:** Physiological Adaptation **Integrated Process:** Communication and Documentation **Content Area:** Adult Health **Strategy:** Recall that this is a progressive disease and the options are linear. Use this information and the process of elimination to make a selection. **Reference:** LeMone, P., Burke, K., & Bauldoff, G. (2011). *Medical-surgical nursing: Critical thinking in patient care* (5th ed). Upper Saddle River, NJ: Pearson Education, pp. 1362–1363.

8 Answer: 1 Rationale: Articular cartilage is responsible for decreasing friction during joint movement and displacing the force of the workload onto the subchondral bone. In osteoarthritis (OA), the composition of the articular cartilage is changed because of a malfunction in the release of cytokines and proteases. Consequently, the articular cartilage can no longer perform its original function. The pathology does not involve immune complexes, excessive bone necrosis or osteolysis, and extensive bone remodeling. **Cognitive Level:** Applying **Client Need:** Physiological Adaptation **Integrated Process:** Nursing Process: Diagnosis **Content Area:** Adult Health **Strategy:** Eliminate the options that describe other diseases. Another clue lies in the other name for the disease. **Reference:** LeMone, P., Burke, K., & Bauldoff, G. (2011).

Medical-surgical nursing: Critical thinking in patient care (5th ed). Upper Saddle River, NJ: Pearson Education, p. 1354.

9 Answer: 1, 3 Rationale: Disease-modifying anti-rheumatoid drugs (DMARDs) are now being used earlier in the treatment regime for rheumatoid arthritis (RA) because evidence suggests that they may play a role in arresting the disease process. Nonsteroidal anti-inflammatory drugs (NSAIDs) are used in combination with this drug classification for pain management. Systemic corticosteroids are not used until NSAIDs are no longer effective because of the severe side effects associated with their use. Opioid analgesics are not indicated early in the disease process. **Cognitive Level:** Applying **Client Need:** Pharmacological and Parenteral Therapies **Integrated Process:** Nursing Process: Implementation **Content Area:** Adult Health **Strategy:** Note the clue words *early stages* in the stem. With this in mind, select agents that are useful to the disease process and analgesics that are milder in nature. **Reference:** LeMone, P., Burke, K., & Bauldoff, G. (2011). *Medical-surgical nursing: Critical thinking in patient care* (5th ed). Upper Saddle River, NJ: Pearson Education, pp. 1363–1370.

10 Answer: 2 Rationale: Osteoporosis is characterized by a decrease in the number and activity of osteoblasts that form new bone and an increase in number of osteoclasts that absorb bone. It is more prevalent in postmenopausal women with low levels of estrogen. Bony necrosis and pathogens are not involved. **Cognitive Level:** Applying **Client Need:** Physiological Adaptation **Integrated Process:** Teaching and Learning **Content Area:** Adult Health **Strategy:** Eliminate the options that relate to other diseases. **Reference:** LeMone, P., Burke, K., & Bauldoff, G. (2011). *Medical-surgical nursing: Critical thinking in patient care* (5th ed). Upper Saddle River, NJ: Pearson Education, pp. 1338–1341.

References

Adams, M., Holland, L., & Bostwick, P. (2011). *Pharmacology for nurses: A pathophysiologic approach* (3rd ed). Upper Saddle River, NJ: Pearson Education.

D'Amico, D., & Barbarito, C. (2012). *Health & physical assessment in nursing* (2nd ed). Upper Saddle River, NJ: Pearson Education.

Ignatavicius, D. D., & Workman, M. L. (2010). *Medical-surgical nursing: Patient-centered collaborative care* (6th ed). St. Louis, MO: Elsevier.

Huether, S.E., & McCance, K. L. (2012). *Understanding pathophysiology* (5th ed). St. Louis, MO: Mosby, Inc.

Kee, J. (2009). *Laboratory and diagnostic tests with nursing implications* (8th ed). Upper Saddle River, NJ: Pearson Education.

LeMone, P., Burke, K.M., & Bauldoff, G. (2011). *Medical-surgical nursing: Critical thinking in client care* (5th ed). Upper Saddle River, NJ: Pearson Education.

Porth, C. M. (2010). *Pathophysiology: Concepts of altered health states* (8th ed). Philadelphia, PA: Lippincott Williams & Wilkins.

Roberts, D. (2011). *Nursing management: Arthritis and connective tissue diseases*. In S. Lewis, M. Heitkemper, & S. Dirkson (Eds), *Medical-surgical nursing: Assessment and*

management of clinical problems (8th ed). St. Louis, MO: Mosby.

Venes, C. & Thomas, C. L. (2009). *Taber's cyclopedic medical dictionary* (21st Ed). Philadelphia, PA: F. A. Davis.

Wilson, B. A., Shannon, M. T., & Shields, K. M. (2012). *Pearson nurse's drug guide 2012*. Upper Saddle River, NJ: Pearson Education.

ANSWERS & RATIONALES

6 Eye, Ear, Nose, and Throat Health Problems

Chapter Outline

Risk Factors Associated with
Eye, Ear, Nose, and Throat
Problems
Glaucoma
Cataracts
Eye Injury
Macular Degeneration

Retinal Detachment
Sensorineural Hearing
Impairment
Conductive Hearing Impairment
Otitis Media
External Otitis
Ménière's Disease

Epistaxis
Sinusitis
Epiglottitis
Peritonsillar Abscess
Laryngeal Cancer

NCLEX-RN® Test Prep

Use the accompanying online resource,
NursingReviewsandRationales, to test
yourself with hundreds of NCLEX®-style
practice questions.

Objectives

➤ Define key terms associated with eye, ear, nose, and throat health
problems.
➤ Identify risk factors associated with the development of eye, ear,
nose, and throat health problems.
➤ Explain the common etiologies of eye, ear, nose, and throat health
problems.
➤ Describe the pathophysiologic processes associated with specific
eye, ear, nose, and throat health problems.
➤ Distinguish between normal and abnormal eye, ear, nose, and
throat findings obtained from nursing assessment.
➤ Prioritize nursing interventions associated with specific eye, ear,
nose, and throat health problems.

Review at a Glance

audiometry test used to evaluate ability to hear pure tones of varying intensity
cholesteatoma an inflamed cyst or mass filled with epithelial cells and debris that remains infected, enlarges, and may destroy ossicles, causing permanent hearing loss; results from chronic otitis media
endolymph pale, transparent fluid within membranous labyrinth of ear
gonioscopy test used to measure depth of anterior chamber of eye; used to differentiate open-angle from narrow (angle-closure) glaucoma
intraocular pressure (IOP) pressure of aqueous humor within eye; normally ranges from 12–21 mmHg

labyrinth term used to describe inner ear; composed of 2 parts: bony labyrinth, a system of open channels that houses second part (membranous labyrinth); bony labyrinth contains vestibule, semicircular canals, and cochlea
laryngectomy removal of all or part of larynx; partial is done when tumor is confined to a specific portion of larynx; total involves removal of entire larynx and surrounding structures when tumor extends beyond vocal cords; requires creation of permanent tracheostomy
miotics pharmacological agents that cause pupil constriction
mydriatics pharmacological agents that cause pupil dilation

myringotomy incision into tympanic membrane to relieve pressure
nystagmus involuntary, rapid movements of eye
otosclerosis familial condition of stapes (ossicles of middle ear) characterized by resorption of bone followed by overgrowth of new, hard sclerotic bone; sclerotic changes impact stapes and oval window and impair sound transmission into inner ear
presbycusis age-related loss of ability to hear high-frequency sounds; may impair ability to hear normal speech
Rinne test test done by alternately placing a tuning fork on mastoid bone and in front of ear canal to compare air

and bone conduction; with conductive hearing loss, bone conduction is greater than air conduction; with sensorineural loss, the opposite results are noted

stapedectomy surgical removal and replacement of diseased stapes to restore hearing

tonometry indirect measure of intra-ocular pressure using contact or noncontact methods

tympanocentesis aspiration of fluid/pus from middle ear using a needle

tympanometry an indirect measurement of compliance of middle ear to sound transmission; an audiometer with a sealed probe tip is used to deliver a continuous tone to tympanic membrane; an instrument records energy reflected from surface of membrane; also known as impedance audiometry

tympanoplasty surgical reconstruction of ossicles and tympanic membrane of middle ear to help restore hearing

Weber test diagnostic test using a tuning fork held against midline of top of head to differentiate conductive hearing loss from sensorineural hearing loss

PRETEST

1 A client has just been diagnosed with angle closure (narrow-angle or closed-angle) glaucoma. The nurse assesses the client for which common presenting symptoms of this disorder? Select all that apply.

1. Halo vision
2. Dull eye pain
3. Severe eye and face pain
4. Impaired night vision
5. Sudden loss of vision

2 The nurse notes a cloudy appearance to the lens of an 80-year-old client's eye. Which additional assessment finding would help confirm the diagnosis of cataracts?

1. Sense of a curtain falling over the visual field
2. Persistent, dull eye pain
3. Loss of red reflex
4. Double vision

3 The nurse would take which priority action for the client with a penetrating eye injury from a visible foreign body?

1. Patch both eyes.
2. Immobilize the foreign body and cover the eye.
3. Irrigate the eye with copious amounts of water.
4. Administer carbonic anhydrase inhibitors as prescribed.

4 A client is diagnosed with conductive hearing loss and asks how this occurred. The nurse's response should include which statement about conductive hearing loss?

1. Has an unknown etiology
2. Occurs as a result of damage to the hair cells of the inner ear
3. Usually results from chronic exposure to loud noise
4. Occurs as a result of damage to the middle ear structures

5 The nurse should anticipate that a client with suspected sensorineural hearing loss will be evaluated using which of the following methods? Select all that apply.

1. Tympanocentesis
2. Transillumination of the sinuses
3. Electronystagmography
4. Weber and Rinne tests
5. Audiometry

6 The nurse should include which items of information in a teaching plan for the parents of an infant with acute otitis media? Select all that apply.

1. Antibiotics can be discontinued when infant is afebrile.
2. When bottle-feeding, infant should be maintained in an upright position.
3. Orange juice and other fruit juices should be eliminated from the diet.
4. Cigarette smoke in the home is a significant risk factor in acute otitis media.
5. Infants should be fed in a horizontal position, not upright.

7 The nurse developing a teaching plan for a client with atrophic macular degeneration should include information about which of the following?

1. Surgical treatment options
2. Availability of aids to enhance vision and promote safety
3. Risks associated with the loss of peripheral vision
4. Antibiotic therapy

8 The nurse notes uvular deviation when examining the oropharynx of a client reporting dysphasia and throat pain. The nurse concludes that this is consistent with which health problem?

1. Pharyngitis
2. Peritonsillar abscess
3. Esophagitis
4. Epiglottitis

9 A 60-year-old man presents to the clinic reporting having a cough and hoarseness for at least 2 months. His spouse states his voice has changed in the last few months. The nurse interprets that the client's symptoms are consistent with which health problem?

1. Gastroesophageal reflux disease (GERD)
2. Coronary heart disease (CAD)
3. Laryngeal cancer
4. Chronic sinusitis

10 The nurse is caring for a client immediately after surgery. The client has nasal packing. What is the most important action that the nurse should take to provide safe care to this client?

1. Provide frequent oral care.
2. Ensure adequate intake of oral fluids.
3. Monitor respiratory function and oxygen saturation.
4. Administer analgesics as prescribed.

See pages 180–182 for Answers and Rationales.

I. RISK FACTORS ASSOCIATED WITH EYE, EAR, NOSE, AND THROAT PROBLEMS

A. **Glaucoma**: advancing age, ethnicity, diabetes, and family history
B. **Cataracts**: advancing age, tobacco smoking associated with alcohol consumption, exposure to ultraviolet light, ocular trauma, and family history
C. **Eye injury**: environmental and workplace hazards, motor vehicle crashes, sports injuries, and physical assault
D. **Macular degeneration**: advancing age, family history, and nutritional factors have been implicated
E. **Retinal detachment**: advancing age, myopia, and trauma (i.e., sudden blows to head)
F. **Sensorineural hearing impairment**: advancing age, ototoxic medications, and persistent exposure to loud noise
G. **Conductive hearing impairment**: otosclerosis, infections of external or middle ear, trauma to tympanic membrane and middle ear
H. **Otitis media**: age (i.e., common in infants and children), upper respiratory infection (URI), and allergies
I. **Ménière's disease**: age (i.e., increased incidence in middle age) and family history
J. **Epistaxis**: nasal trauma (i.e., blunt trauma or mild irritation from manipulation), nasal allergies, substance abuse (i.e., cocaine) sinusitis, upper respiratory infections (URIs), tobacco smoking, use of oxygen, certain climates or altitudes, prescription drugs, and anatomic variations (i.e., deviated nasal septum, nasal polyps)
K. **Laryngeal cancer**: tobacco smoking, alcohol consumption associated with tobacco smoking, occupational exposure to chemicals and toxins, and family history

II. GLAUCOMA

A. Overview

1. Defined as a group of conditions characterized by increased **intraocular pressure (IOP)**; normal IOP is 12–21 mmHg; if untreated, it results in ischemia and degeneration of retina and optic nerve, loss of vision, and complete blindness
2. Caused by alterations in circulation and resorption of aqueous humor
3. Classified as *open-angle* (wide-angle) or *closed-angle* (narrow-angle or acute-angle closure)
4. Manifests as a *primary* or *secondary* disorder and may be congenital or acquired
   a. Primary glaucoma occurs without preexisting eye or systemic disease
   b. Secondary glaucoma results from inflammatory processes, tumors, long-term steroid use, or ocular trauma

B. Pathophysiology

1. Aqueous humor serves to maintain IOP and support metabolism of lens and posterior cornea
2. Formation/secretion of aqueous humor is an active process that begins at ciliary body (ciliary epithelium) in posterior chamber; aqueous humor flows through pupil into anterior chamber; resorption into venous system occurs through trabecular meshwork of anterior chamber into Canal of Schlemm (Figure 6-1)
3. Open-angle (wide-angle) glaucoma
   a. Etiology is unclear; there is no obstruction between trabecular meshwork and anterior chamber
   b. May occur because of an abnormality of trabecular meshwork (network) that impairs flow of aqueous humor into Canal of Schlemm; the resulting increased IOP in anterior chamber causes increased IOP in posterior chamber
   c. Usually affects both eyes, has a genetic component, and is frequently seen in adults over 60 years of age

Figure 6-1

Internal structures of the eye

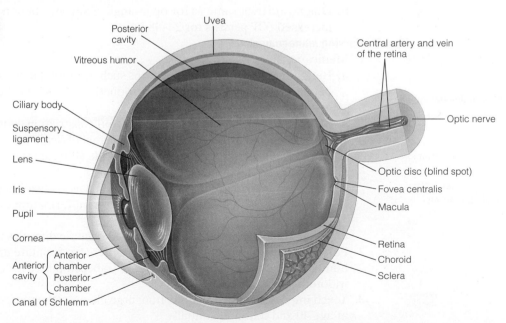

Uvea

Posterior cavity

Vitreous humor

Central artery and vein of the retina

Ciliary body

Suspensory ligament

Lens

Iris

Pupil

Cornea

Anterior cavity

Anterior chamber

Posterior chamber

Canal of Schlemm

Optic nerve

Optic disc (blind spot)

Fovea centralis

Macula

Retina

Choroid

Sclera

        d. Onset is insidious with no symptoms in early stages

        e. Signs and symptoms: tunnel vision (an initial symptom) from loss of peripheral vision, pain (persistent, dull eye pain, lasting over 20 minutes), halo and/or blurred vision, inability to detect colors, and mild headaches

    4. Closed-angle (narrow-angle or acute-angle closure) glaucoma

        a. An *acute medical emergency* resulting in narrowing of angle between pupil and lateral cornea resulting in impaired outflow of aqueous humor

        b. Symptoms relate to sudden, intermittent increases in IOP and may occur following prolonged sitting in a darkened room, during emotional upset or stress, or any condition causing prolonged pupil dilation

        c. Often unilateral; other eye may be affected at a later time; accounts for 5–10% of cases

        d. Signs and symptoms: sudden, severe eye and face pain, severe headache accompanied by nausea and vomiting (N/V) (may be confused with migraine), blurred vision and/or seeing halos around lights, redness of eye, haziness (steaminess) of cornea, and fixed dilated pupil at midpoint that is nonreactive to light

C. Nursing assessment

    1. Open-angle (wide-angle) glaucoma

        a. Eye examination for loss of peripheral vision, tunnel vision, or complaints of seeing halos around lights; ability to focus on near objects or differentiate colors, symptom analysis of headaches and eye or face pain, and family history of glaucoma

        b. Diagnostic tests: intraocular pressure measurement (**tonometry**), examination of optic disk, visual field testing, and **gonioscopy** (visualization and measurement of angle of anterior chamber) to differentiate open-angle from closed-angle glaucoma

    2. Closed-angle (narrow-angle or acute-angle closure) glaucoma

        a. Assessment includes symptom analysis of acute onset of severe eye pain, headaches associated with N/V, assessment of eye for color, clarity and pupil response, and recent history of prolonged exposure to darkened room, high stress, or emotional distress

        b. Diagnostic tests: same as for open-angle glaucoma; blindness can occur if increased IOP persists for 24–48 hours

D. Nursing management

    1. Medications

        a. Beta-adrenergic blocking eye drops such as timolol maleate (Timoptic) or betaxolol (Betoptic) to decrease production of aqueous humor; watch for systemic effects

        b. **Miotics** (drugs that constrict pupil); pupil constriction causes ciliary muscle to pull on trabecular meshwork surrounding Canal of Schlemm, which facilitates flow of aqueous humor; pilocarpine hydrochloride (Pilocar) is a typical drug in anticholinergic drug class

        c. Carbonic anhydrase inhibitors (CAIs) such as acetazolamide (Diamox) are used in closed-angle glaucoma to reduce secretion/formation of aqueous humor by ciliary body

        d. Sympathomimetics, prostaglandins, and osmotic diuretics may be used

    2. For closed-angle glaucoma, surgical procedures to facilitate drainage of aqueous humor can include trabeculectomy, laser trabeculoplasty, iridectomy, or laser iridotomy

    3. Teach importance of early detection; urge clients to begin regular eye examinations at age 40 and continue annually

Practice to Pass

A client who has just been diagnosed with open-angle glaucoma states that her mother "went blind" from glaucoma and that she fears the same will happen to her. How should the nurse respond?

4. Avoid **mydriatics** (drugs that dilate pupils) such as atropine sulfate (Isopto Atropine); memory trick: "d" is in both mydriatic and dilate
5. Obtain MedicAlert card or bracelet
6. Use safety precautions (i.e., lights, handrails) to compensate for reduced vision
7. Client teaching
   a. Importance of daily adherence to drug therapy; noncompliance may lead to permanent loss of vision
   b. Actions and side effects of specific medications (i.e., systemic effects of ophthalmic beta blockers)
   c. Procedures for correct and safe self-administration of eye drops
   d. Postoperative home care
   e. Importance of reading over-the-counter (OTC) labels since many of these drugs can increase IOP

III. CATARACTS

A. Overview
1. A progressive clouding or opacity of lens of eye that interferes with transmission of light to retina, leading to painless loss of vision
2. Cataracts due to aging (senile cataracts) are most common; other causes are foreign body ocular trauma causing lens swelling and rupture, congenital factors (i.e., Down syndrome, intrauterine rubella infection, and fetal exposure to radiation), metabolic disorders (i.e., diabetes mellitus, hypoparathyroidism), exposure to ultraviolet light (UV-B), drugs such as systemic corticosteroids, chlorpromazine (Thorazine) and busulfan (Myleran)

B. Pathophysiology
1. As a result of aging or injury, cells in lens degenerate beginning at periphery and moving to center; with progression, entire lens becomes involved
2. Cellular debris from deteriorating lens escapes through lens capsule into aqueous humor and may contribute to obstruction of outflow of aqueous humor resulting in increased IOP
3. Partial opacity is termed "immature cataract"; opacity of entire lens is termed "mature cataract"
4. Age-related (senile) cataracts are usually bilateral but may be asymmetrical in development
5. Signs and symptoms: blurred vision, visual distortion, decreased night vision, glare and/or abnormal presence of light in visual field, decline in near and distant vision, white or gray opacity filling pupil opening (aperture); as cataract matures, retina becomes impossible to visualize; loss of red reflex

C. Nursing assessment
1. Assessment includes an eye exam, determining client's knowledge of cause, symptoms, and treatment options for cataracts, and client's fears of blindness and/or permanent disability from cataracts and proposed cataract surgery
2. Diagnostic tests: eye examination using an ophthalmoscope or slit-lamp (lens opacity and absence of red reflex) and Snellen vision testing to assess loss of visual acuity

D. Nursing management
1. Medications include postoperative analgesics, anti-inflammatories, and antibiotics to decrease discomfort and prevent infection; no effective medicine is available to remove a cataract

Practice to Pass

Following cataract surgery with lens implantation, the client asks the nurse to explain at-home activity restrictions. What specific instructions should be given to the client?

2. Surgical interventions: lens extraction and intraocular lens implantation or use of convex corrective lens (rare); methods utilized include:
    a. Extracapsular extraction: removal of lens nucleus and cortex; posterior lens capsule remains intact to help support lens implant; currently is most popular method
    b. Phacoemulsification: use of sound waves to break up lens; has enhanced success of extracapsular extraction
    c. Cryoextraction: use of forceps or supercooled probe to extract lens through small incision in cornea
    d. Intracapsular extraction: removal of entire lens and surrounding capsule
    e. Newer technology involves laser removal of lens opacities
3. Surgical procedures are done on outpatient basis using local anesthesia; performed on one eye at a time with second procedure completed within several weeks or months
4. Identify safety concerns in environment related to loss of visual acuity and propose adaptive measures; if a lens implant is not performed, reinforce safety measures because of loss of accommodation
5. Caution clients to avoid night driving prior to surgical correction
6. Client teaching related to surgery (see Box 6-1)

IV. EYE INJURY
A. Overview
1. Any injury to a part of eye; even minor injuries can threaten vision, so all should be considered emergencies requiring immediate evaluation and care
2. Major causes: corneal abrasion, blunt or penetrating trauma, and burns
B. Pathophysiology
1. Corneal abrasion
    a. Characterized by a disruption of superficial epithelium of cornea
    b. Common causes: contact lenses, foreign bodies (i.e., dust, dirt, fingernails, eyelashes), and chemical irritants
    c. Drying of surface of eye contributes to corneal abrasion
    d. Superficial abrasions are extremely painful but generally heal without scarring; deeper abrasions may lead to infection and scar formation
    e. Signs and symptoms: pain, tearing, photophobia, and visual impairment (usually temporary)

Box 6-1	The following should be included when teaching clients undergoing cataract surgery:
Teaching Clients Undergoing Cataract Surgery	• Anticipated pre- and postoperative procedures • Importance of leaving eye patch in place until changed or removed by surgeon at postoperative visit, usually within 24 to 48 hours • Importance and procedure for administering eye drops and/or ointments during the postoperative period • Need for eye protection such as sunglasses during the day and eye shields at night; photophobia is common after eye surgery • Need to avoid sleeping on operative side and bending over • Insertion and care of postoperative contact lenses if prescribed • If convex corrective lens are prescribed, explain the loss of peripheral visual fields and need for *turning* the head from side to side to prevent accidents; measures to compensate for loss of depth perception should be emphasized • Teach symptoms to report to health care provider: eye pain or pressure, redness, cloudiness, drainage, decreased vision, floaters, halos around objects

2. Blunt trauma
   a. Common causes: sports injuries from baseballs, tennis rackets, handballs, and contact sports such as basketball, football, boxing, and wrestling; motor vehicle crashes, physical assault, and falls
   b. Signs and symptoms: lid ecchymosis (black eye), subconjunctival hemorrhage, hyphema, and orbital blowout fracture
      1. Subconjunctival hemorrhage is caused by blood vessel rupture under conjunctiva (membrane lining inner surface of eye); is a well-defined, red, painless area; usually requires no treatment; blood reabsorbs in 2–3 weeks
      2. Hyphema is characterized by bleeding into anterior chamber of eye; symptoms include pain, decreased visual acuity and reddish tint in visual field; blood is visible to examiner when visualized at an angle
      3. Orbital blowout fracture is caused by fracture of any part of orbit; ethmoid bone on orbital floor is most common site; with fracture, orbital contents including fat, muscles, and eye can herniate into maxillary sinus; symptoms include diplopia, pain with upward movement, decreased sensation on affected cheek, limited eye movement with upward movement, and enophthalmos (sunken appearance to eye)
3. Penetrating trauma
   a. Common causes: shards of glass, pieces of metal produced from high-speed drilling, gunshot wounds (including BBs), arrows, and knives
   b. In penetrating injuries, layers of eye reapproximate immediately after injury, and injury may not be readily apparent
   c. In perforating injuries, layers of eye do not reapproximate and rupture of globe and loss of ocular contents may occur
   d. Symptoms: pain, loss of vision, bleeding, and possible loss of eye contents
4. Burns
   a. Causes: chemicals (most common), heat, radiation, and explosions
   b. Sources of chemical burns include both acids (i.e., acid from car batteries) and alkaline substances (i.e., ammonia, lye from oven cleaners)
   c. Alkaline burns are generally more serious because of progressive damage from particles of offending agent that remain in contact with conjunctival sac; acid burns are generally less serious
   d. Symptoms: eye pain, decreased vision, swollen eyelids, conjunctival reddening, and edema and cloudiness of cornea; corneal ulcerations and sloughing of conjunctival tissue may occur with chemical burns

C. **Nursing assessment**
   1. Presence of other injuries (i.e., nasal fractures, skin abrasions, facial and scalp lacerations/burns), eye movement, and visual acuity
   2. Diagnostic tests: eye exam under magnification using topical anesthetics, fluorescein staining to identify abrasions, and facial x-rays or computed tomography (CT) scan to identify/evaluate orbital fractures or foreign bodies

D. **Nursing management**
   1. Corneal abrasions
      a. Medications: ophthalmic antibiotics with application of eye pad to reduce pain and photophobia
      b. If foreign body present, remove with sterile applicator and/or irrigate with sterile solution
      c. Client education to prevent reinjury
   2. Blunt trauma
      a. Medications: CAIs to reduce IOP as prescribed
      b. Place client on bedrest in semi-Fowler's position

!
> c. Patch affected eye; unaffected eye may also be patched to decrease eye movement
> d. Client education about use of protective eyewear during sports activities

3. Penetrating trauma

!
> a. Medications: opioid analgesics, sedatives and/or antiemetics for vomiting, topical and/or intravenous antibiotics to prevent infection
> b. Do not attempt to remove embedded foreign body

!
> c. Immobilize foreign body and cover eye with metal eye shield to protect from further injury; paper cup may be substituted for metal shield if foreign body is too large
> d. Patching unaffected eye decreases movement of affected eye

!
> e. Institute bed rest to prevent further injury
> f. Client education to avoid future injuries

4. Burns
> a. Medication: topical anesthetics to decrease pain during irrigation; after irrigation, apply topical antibiotics as prescribed

!
> b. Immediately flush chemical burns with copious amounts of saline or water; evert eyelid to ensure thorough irrigation of conjunctival sac
> c. After irrigation, evaluate vision with and without any corrective eyeglasses
> d. Client education on importance of protective eyewear

V. MACULAR DEGENERATION

A. Overview
1. Degeneration of macular area of retina in eye; most common cause of blindness; most common type is age-related macular degeneration (ARMD)
2. Macula (located in center of retina) receives light from center of visual field and has greatest visual acuity
3. Causes of ARMD are unknown; injury, inflammation, nutritional and hereditary factors are implicated; males and females are affected equally

B. Pathophysiology
1. In ARMD, gradual failure of outer layer of retina (pigmented epithelium, which attaches to choroid layer and functions to remove cellular wastes) occurs; as outer layer fails, photoreceptor cells are lost, waste products and toxins accumulate in subretinal space, and cell death occurs
2. Types
> a. Atrophic ("dry") form: gradual, progressive bilateral loss of vision caused by atrophy and degeneration of outer pigmented layer of retina
> b. Exudative ("wet") form: more rapid, severe loss of vision from accumulation of serous or hemorrhagic fluid in subretinal space; accumulated fluid leads to separation of retina from choroid; scar formation leads to death of retinal cells and loss of vision

3. Signs and symptoms: loss of central vision (peripheral vision intact), pale yellow spots called "drusen" on macula, visual distortion of images (i.e., straight lines may appear wavy), and difficulty with activities requiring close central vision (i.e., reading and sewing)

C. Nursing assessment
1. Assessment includes eye exam and symptom analysis of appearance of wavy lines and changes in ability to perform close-up work
2. Diagnostic tests: ophthalmologic exam, visual acuity, visual field and color vision tests, and electroretinography (ERG) to measure retinal responses to light

D. Nursing management
1. No medications are required; treatment modalities include:
> a. Laser photocoagulation for exudative macular degeneration
> b. No current therapy for atrophic macular degeneration

Practice to Pass

The client asks the nurse to explain the term "macular degeneration." How should the nurse respond?

2. Early referral for ophthalmologic exam and early intervention may preserve vision and slow progression of disease

 3. Assessment of home environment to prevent injuries related to loss of vision
4. Client education

   a. Aids to enhance vision and promote safety (i.e., magnification devices, enhanced lighting)
   b. Availability of large-print books and newspapers as well as audio books
   c. Importance of home safety evaluation to minimize risk of injury and falls
   d. Loss of central vision does not progress to loss of peripheral vision

VI. RETINAL DETACHMENT

A. Overview
1. Defined as separation of sensory layer of retina from choroid
2. Often occurs spontaneously (most frequent after age 50) but may result from trauma such as sudden blows to head

Practice to Pass

A client is admitted to the outpatient surgery unit for scleral buckling of a detached retina. How should the nurse explain retinal detachment and respond to the client's fears about permanent loss of vision?

3. Causes include eye tumors, inflammatory disorders, myopia, and cataract extraction

B. Pathophysiology
1. Retina may tear and fold back onto itself or remain intact and be pulled away from choroid as vitreous humor shrinks because of aging
2. Breaks in retina allow fluid from vitreous cavity to seep into defect; additionally, fluids from choroid vessels, pull of gravity, and traction imposed by vitreous enhance separation
3. Separation of retina from choroid causes ischemia, death of retinal neurons, and permanent loss of vision
4. Retinal damage can progress slowly or can enlarge quickly resulting in complete detachment
5. It is considered a medical emergency requiring immediate intervention
6. Signs and symptoms: is usually painless; sudden appearance of floaters, irregular lines and/or flashes of light in visual field, sensation of a curtain drawn across field of vision, progressive deterioration of vision, blurred vision, weeping of eye (if trauma), loss of central vision (if macula is involved), and hemorrhage into vitreous; ophthalmic exam may reveal gray opaque appearance of retina and/or evidence of tears, holes, or folds in retina

C. Nursing assessment
1. Symptom analysis of visual changes such as floating spots and/or flashing lights, loss of visual acuity, blurred vision, and/or sense of curtain or veil coming down into visual field, any history of trauma to eye, and physical exam for weeping and visual redness
2. Diagnosis based on ophthalmoscopic exam

D. Nursing management
1. Medications: antibiotics, anti-inflammatories, and analgesics as prescribed
2. Treatment modalities include various surgical interventions:
   a. Scleral buckling utilizes laser photocoagulation or cryothermy to produce adhesions that seal retinal layers; silicone is used to indent or "buckle" sclera to enhance contact between layers
   b. Pneumatic retinopexy involves injecting air/gas into vitreous to force detached retina to come into contact with choroid
   c. Laser photocoagulation or cryothermy can also be used without scleral buckling to create areas of inflammation and adhesions, which fuse separated layers together
   d. Surgical instrumentation is used to manipulate detached retina into place

3. Provide for emergency care with an ophthalmologist
4. Ensure that client's head is positioned with detached area in a dependent (downward) position to assist gravity to pull retina back closer to choroid
5. Instruct client to avoid bending forward or making sudden head movements
6. Cover both eyes with patches to limit ocular movement
7. Protect client from injury (i.e., bed in low position, side rails up, call bell within reach)
8. Provide pre- and postoperative instructions
9. Offer psychological support to alleviate anxiety related to sudden loss of vision and fear of permanent blindness
10. Provide diversional activities for distraction such as books on tape or mirror to view television while lying in head-dependent position

VII. SENSORINEURAL HEARING IMPAIRMENT

A. Overview

1. Abnormality of cochlear apparatus or auditory nerve decreasing and/or distorting transfer of sounds to brain, resulting in loss of hearing; sound transmission to inner ear is normal
2. Occurs with disorders affecting inner ear, auditory nerve, or auditory pathways to brain
3. Characterized by loss of perception of high-frequency tones, making speech recognition difficult in noisy environments
4. Causes: persistent exposure to loud noise, trauma to head or inner ear, vascular lesions, drug ototoxicity (i.e., aminoglycosides, salicylates, diuretics, vancomycin, antineoplastic agents); infections (i.e., bacterial meningitis), Ménière's disease, **presbycusis** (degenerative changes resulting from aging), endocrine disorders (i.e., diabetes mellitus, hypothyroidism), intrauterine infections (i.e., maternal rubella), developmental malformations, and tumors (i.e., acoustic neuroma, meningioma, metastatic brain tumors)
5. In presbycusis, degenerative changes may begin in early adulthood but not be clinically significant until later in life; men are affected earlier and experience greater hearing loss than women
6. Hearing loss is usually permanent
7. May occur along with conductive hearing loss; termed mixed hearing loss

B. Pathophysiology

1. Inner ear (**labyrinth**) contains vestibule, semicircular canals, and cochlea; cochlea contains organ of Corti (see Figure 6-2)
2. Exposure to constant or intermittent high level of noise damages hair cells of organ of Corti
3. With presbycusis, hair cells of organ of Corti degenerate; gradual, progressive hearing loss results in difficulty hearing high-pitched tones and conversational speech; eventually, ability to hear middle and lower tones is lost
4. Signs and symptoms: deafness (usually bilateral), inability to hear low, middle and/or high-pitched sounds, tinnitus (ringing in ear), dizziness, and pain

C. Nursing assessment

1. Signs of hearing loss (i.e., increased voice volume, requests for information to be repeated, inappropriate responses to questions, lack of response, and turning head to direction of a speaker)
2. Diagnostic tests: **audiometry** to assess hearing, **Weber** and **Rinne tests** (tuning fork tests) to differentiate sensorineural from conductive hearing loss, brainstem auditory evoked response (BAER), and brain imaging studies to rule out intracranial lesions

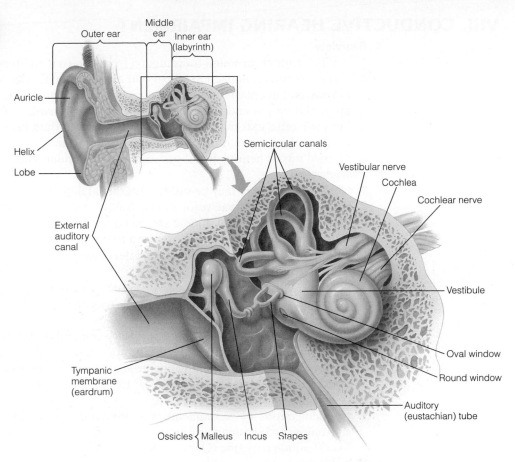

Figure 6-2

Structures of the external ear, middle ear, and inner ear

Outer ear
Middle ear
Inner ear (labyrinth)

Auricle

Helix

Lobe

External auditory canal

Semicircular canals

Vestibular nerve

Cochlea

Cochlear nerve

Vestibule

Oval window

Round window

Auditory (eustachian) tube

Tympanic membrane (eardrum)

Ossicles { Malleus Incus Stapes

D. Nursing management
   1. Medications are not indicated; treatment modalities are limited but include:
      a. Cochlear implants: provide clients with perception of sound but not normal hearing; allow clients to recognize warning sounds of telephones, sirens, and automobiles; alert clients to incoming communication; and provide some help for clients even if no auditory nerve function exists
      b. Hearing aids not generally helpful; serve only to intensify distorted sounds
      c. Use of devices that provide "white noise" to mask unpleasant or distressing sounds associated with tinnitus (such as tinnitus marker)
   2. Avoid shouting; address clients in normal, low-pitched voice
   3. Provide adequate visual contact and lighting when communicating with clients to foster speech lip-reading; face client directly
   4. Provide alternate means of communication (sign language, pad and paper, computer)
   5. Reduce background noises when communicating with clients
   6. Use short sentences and gestures (i.e., pointing) when appropriate
   7. Educate family about social isolation associated with sensorineural hearing loss, including apparent inattention, withdrawal, and/or disinterest
   8. Evaluate safety of home environment (i.e., ability to hear smoke detectors, telephones)

VIII. CONDUCTIVE HEARING IMPAIRMENT

A. Overview
1. An interruption in sound transmission from external auditory canal to inner ear
2. Causes: cerumen impaction of external auditory canal; edema of canal lining, foreign objects, and neoplasms; rupture or scarring of tympanic membrane; disruption or fixation of bones in middle ear from trauma or **otosclerosis** (a familial disorder of hearing loss); otitis externa or otitis media, presence of fluid in middle ear; and congenital malformations of external or middle ear
3. Termed mixed hearing loss if occurs with sensorineural hearing loss

B. Pathophysiology
1. Changes in hearing may be sudden or gradual depending upon cause
2. With otosclerosis, bone resorption is followed by overgrowth of new, hard sclerotic bone; stapes (ossicle in middle ear) becomes immobilized against oval window thus decreasing transmission of sound to inner ear; pressure of otosclerotic bone on inner ear structures or 8th cranial nerve may also result in sensorineural hearing loss
3. Often unilateral; may be bilateral if caused by otosclerosis
4. Signs and symptoms: loss of sound at all frequencies and tinnitus with otosclerosis

C. Nursing assessment
1. Assess for presence of foreign bodies, infection and/or cerumen in external auditory canal, integrity of tympanic membrane and presence of otitis media
2. Diagnostic tests: Weber and Rinne tests, audiometry, **tympanometry** (indirect measurement of compliance of middle ear to sound transmission), and otoscopic exam

D. Nursing management
1. No medications are recommended; treatment modalities include:
    a. Removal of cerumen or foreign body by health care provider; medications such as carbamide peroxide (Debrox) help with dry cerumen
    b. Hearing aids to amplify sound
    c. Assistive listening devices ("pocket talker")
    d. Reconstructive procedures to restore hearing: **stapedectomy** (making an incision in stapes to improve hearing) for otosclerosis and **tympanoplasty** (surgical procedure to restore function of middle ear to transmit sound more efficiently)
2. Client teaching related to conductive hearing loss (see Box 6-2)
3. Utilize techniques appropriate for hearing impaired as noted in section on nursing management of sensorineural hearing loss
4. Provide appropriate pre- and postoperative care

Box 6-2	The following points should be included in a teaching plan for clients with conductive hearing loss:
Teaching Clients with Conductive Hearing Loss	• Technique for proper insertion and cleaning of hearing aids • Proper insertion of hearing aid batteries; need for extra batteries • Availability of assistive listening devices (i.e., "pocket talkers") • Postoperative and home care following stapedectomy or tympanoplasty • Methods to protect ears from injury; use of ear plugs while swimming and diving • Care of ears and ear canal, including cleaning and removal of cerumen • Signs of middle ear infection and the importance of early and complete treatment

IX. OTITIS MEDIA

A. Overview

1. Inflammation and/or infection of middle ear that primarily affects infants and young children; may occur in adults; is a major cause of conductive hearing loss

2. Two common forms: *serous otitis media* and *acute otitis media*

3. Causes

   a. Serous otitis media: URIs, allergies, and narrow or edematous Eustachian tubes

   b. Acute otitis media: *Streptococcus pneumoniae*, *Haemophilus influenzae*, and *Streptococcus pyogenes*

B. Pathophysiology

1. Tympanic membrane protects middle ear from external auditory canal; Eustachian tube (auditory tube) connects middle ear with nasopharynx and equalizes pressure in middle ear with atmospheric pressure

2. *Serous otitis media*

   a. Occurs when Eustachian tube is obstructed for a prolonged period of time, causing impaired equalization of air pressure within middle ear

   b. Air in middle ear is absorbed; continued obstruction of Eustachian tube prevents more air from entering, and negative pressure in middle ear results; serous fluid moves into middle ear forming a sterile effusion

   c. Signs and symptoms: decreased hearing and possible reports of "snapping" or "popping" in affected ear, decreased mobility of tympanic membrane, tympanic membrane bulging (from fluid or air) or retraction, pain, bleeding and/or rupture of tympanic membrane, rupture of round window with sensory hearing loss, and vertigo

3. *Acute otitis media*

   a. Results from entry of pathogens from oronasopharynx via Eustachian tube into normally sterile middle ear; typically follows URI

   b. Common in infants and children because of short, straight Eustachian tubes; higher incidence noted in bottle-fed infants/toddlers who maintain a more horizontal position during feeding and in those living with smokers

   c. Bacterial colonization and white blood cell invasion lead to pus formation, which increases middle ear pressure and may lead to rupture of tympanic membrane

   d. Signs and symptoms: pain, often severe, in affected ear; infants and young children may pull at affected ear; fever; impaired hearing; dizziness and vertigo; red, inflamed or dull, bulging tympanic membrane; decreased movement of membrane; tenderness over mastoid area indicating development of mastoiditis

4. Chronic, recurring otitis media may result in permanent perforation of tympanic membrane, permanent hearing loss, and/or formation of a benign epithelial-cell tumor, called **cholesteatoma**

5. Complications of untreated acute otitis media include meningitis, osteomyelitis of skull, and facial paralysis

C. Nursing assessment

1. Visualization of tympanic membrane using otoscope, pain (intensity, description, and location); note that pain associated with otitis media, unlike external otitis, is not aggravated by ear movement; check for history of recurrent otitis media

2. Diagnostic tests: visualization of tympanic membrane with pneumatic otoscope, tympanometry, elevated white blood cell count, and culture of middle ear effusion if membrane has ruptured or **myringotomy** (incision into tympanic membrane) has been done

D. Nursing management

1. Serous otitis media

Practice to Pass

A young mother brings her 12-month-old child in with recurrent acute otitis media. What should the nurse suggest to help prevent recurrence of these middle ear infections?

a. Medications: systemic or intranasal decongestants to reduce edema and maintain patency of Eustachian tube, analgesics, and antipyretics

b. Treatment: autoinflation of middle ear by forcefully exhaling against closed nostrils; avoiding air travel and underwater diving

2. Acute otitis media

a. Medications: antibiotic therapy (often for 10–12 days) with or without decongestants; analgesics, and antipyretics

b. **Tympanocentesis**: aspiration of fluid from middle ear

c. Myringotomy with or without insertion of tympanostomy tubes (ventilation tubes)

3. Stress importance of completing full course of antibiotic therapy, increasing fluid intake, and good nutrition to enhance immune system and hasten resolution of symptoms

4. Alert clients or parents of possibility of superinfections due to antibiotic therapy, such as diarrhea or thrush

5. If tympanostomy tubes are present, caution clients to avoid swimming, diving, or allowing water to enter ear

6. Provide appropriate pre- and postoperative care for myringotomy and/or insertion of tympanostomy tubes

X. EXTERNAL OTITIS

A. Overview

1. An inflammation of outer ear canal; known as swimmer's ear

2. Caused by excess moisture in ear canal, fungi or bacteria, trauma, or local hypersensitivity; common organisms include *Pseudomonas aeruginosa*

B. Pathophysiology

1. Removal of cerumen, which has water-repellant and antimicrobial properties, leaves ear canal susceptible to infection; excess moisture, vigorous cleaning, or excess drying of ear canal tends to remove cerumen

2. Signs and symptoms: severe pain, fullness in ear, and decreased hearing; pain with application of pressure on tragus is a hallmark sign; visual exam shows clusters of white particles on side of canals and edema; tympanic membrane may be difficult to see but will appear normal and pearly gray

C. Nursing assessment

1. Symptom analysis of when pain began (frequency, description), occupation or frequency in swimming, physical palpation of tragus

2. Diagnostic tests: ear examination with otoscope

D. Nursing management

1. Medications: topical antibiotics, topical corticosteroids such as polymixin B-neomycin hydrocortisone (Cortisporin otic), benzocaine and antipyrine (Auralgan), analgesic as needed, and aluminum sulfate and calcium acetate (Dome Burrow) solution to irrigate ear

2. Instruct client to use topical antibiotic for prescribed time in order to completely eliminate organism and avoid swimming for 7–10 days

3. Educate client to use drying agents before and after swimming (such as Swimmer's Ear™ or a 2% acetic acid solution with alcohol), earplugs should be used for clients with ear tubes

XI. MÉNIÈRE'S DISEASE

A. Overview

1. A chronic inner ear disorder characterized by a triad of symptoms (vertigo, tinnitus, and sensorineural hearing loss), also called *endolymphatic hydrops*

2. Usually unilateral, affecting men and women equally; high-risk group includes adults between ages of 35 and 60

3. Causes include trauma, infection, allergies, adrenal-pituitary insufficiency, hypothyroidism, immune system dysfunction, increased sodium intake, stress, and premenstrual fluid retention; a genetic predisposition may exist

B. **Pathophysiology**

1. Most common form is idiopathic
2. An overaccumulation of fluid (**endolymph**) in membranous labyrinth of inner ear results in dilation of lymphatic channels and labyrinth dysfunction; autonomic nervous system control of labyrinthine circulation may be impaired, also contributing to labyrinth dysfunction
3. Excess fluid may be caused by an impaired absorption of endolymph
4. Onset of symptoms may be gradual or sudden
5. Signs and symptoms: severe rotary vertigo (lasting minutes to hours, may be associated with N/V and may cause immobility), tinnitus, sensorineural hearing loss, sense of fullness in ears, hypotension, diaphoresis, and **nystagmus** (irregular eye movements) during acute attacks

C. **Nursing assessment**

1. Subjective reports of dizziness, N/V, sweating, tinnitus, incapacitating vertigo, blurred vision, photosensitivity, and roaring sensation in ears; history often includes past otitis media, allergies, and arteriosclerosis; objective assessment for heart rate (HR) (bradycardia), diarrhea, and disequilibrium
2. Diagnostic tests
   a. Electronystagmography (ENG): a series of tests used to evaluate vestibular-ocular reflexes by identifying nystagmus as a response to specific stimuli; cold caloric test is one part of ENG
   b. Cold caloric testing involves instillation of cold water into external auditory canal; in clients with impaired inner ear function, normal nystagmus response is blunted or absent; this test is not recommended if tympanic membrane is perforated
   c. X-rays and CT scans evaluate anatomic changes of central portion of inner ear known as the vestibule
   d. Rinne and Weber tests utilize a tuning fork to test hearing
   e. Auditory dehydration test involves administering a fast-acting diuretic or hyperosmolar substance (i.e., glycerin) orally to decrease fluid pressure in inner ear; temporary improvement is considered diagnostic
   f. Audiometry testing

D. **Nursing management**

1. Medications for *acute attacks*
   a. Anticholinergics: atropine sulfate (Isopto Atropine) and scopolamine (Isopto Hyoscine) to decrease response peripheral nervous system
   b. Central nervous system (CNS) depressants: diazepam (Valium), lorazepam (Ativan) as an alternative to anticholinergics
   c. Antiemetics: prochlorperazine (Compazine), meclizine (Antivert)
   d. Sedatives/antiemetics: droperidol (Inapsine)
   e. Antihistamines: diphenhydramine (Benadryl)
   f. Antibiotics in large doses for bacterial labyrinthitis
2. Medications *between attacks* include oral diuretics such as furosemide (Lasix) or hydrochlorothiazide with triamterene (Dyazide) to decrease pressure in labyrinth, as well as vasodilators; monitor electrolyte balance
3. Ensure client safety *during attacks* (assist with ambulation, side rails up, bed in low position, call bell within reach), limit movement, and replace fluid and electrolytes
4. Medical treatment options *between* acute attacks focus on prevention; interventions include a sodium-restricted diet and avoiding substances causing vasoconstriction (i.e., tobacco, alcohol, and caffeine)

5. Surgical interventions
   a. Endolymphatic sac decompression and shunting (releases pressure in labyrinth by shunting endolymph from membranous labyrinth to subarachnoid space)
   b. Vestibular nerve resection: removal of part of 8th cranial nerve
   c. Labyrinthectomy: complete removal of labyrinth

6. Ensure adequate hydration and nutrition if attacks are frequent
7. Client teaching
   a. Signs of impending attack (i.e., feeling of ear fullness, increasing tinnitus, vertigo, N/V)
   b. Avoidance of attack triggers (i.e., stress, fatigue, blinking lights, loud noises, quick or jerky body movements)
   c. Safety measures if attack occurs while driving (i.e., pull off to side of road, need for cell phone and "HELP POLICE" sign)
   d. Need for adequate rest and sleep; avoid tobacco
   e. Relaxation techniques
   f. Availability of organizations offering information and support (i.e., Vestibular Disorders Association and Ménière's Network)
   g. Need for MedicAlert bracelet, card, or necklace
   h. Salt-restricted diet

XII. EPISTAXIS

A. Overview
1. Defined as bleeding from nose, which is highly vascular (receives arterial blood flow from vessels originating at internal and external carotid arteries)
2. Men are affected by nosebleeds more often than women
3. Bleeding may originate in anterior or posterior nose
4. Identified by area where bleeding originates: *anterior epistaxis* or *posterior epistaxis*
5. Causes include medications such as antiplatelets or anticoagulants and the following:
   a. Anterior epistaxis: drying of nasal passages, infection, blunt trauma or trauma from manipulation, cocaine use, and local infection
   b. Posterior epistaxis: blood dyscrasias, hypertension, diabetes, and trauma

B. Pathophysiology
1. Most nosebleeds (90%) arise from Kiesselbach's area, a rich vascular plexus in anterior nasal spectum or from rupture of vessels caused by trauma
2. Posterior epistaxis tends to be more severe; occurs more often in older adults

C. Nursing assessment

1. Client's health history, medication history including herbal products, and vital signs; identify amount of blood lost and source of bleeding by examining both nares and back of throat to rule out posterior bleeding
2. There are no diagnostic tests; a CBC may be obtained if severe blood loss

D. Nursing management
1. Medications: topical vasoconstrictors such as phenylephrine (Neo-Synephrine), oxymetazoline hydrochloride (Afrin), or adrenaline; chemical cauterization using silver nitrate or Gelfoam, topical antibacterial ointment to inner nares, and analgesics (particularly if packing has been placed)
2. Treatment options
   a. First aid measures
      1) Assess for respiratory distress; administer supplemental oxygen as indicated
      2) Instruct client to sit upright with head tilted forward
      3) Apply pressure, by pinching nose toward septum, for 5–10 minutes
      4) Apply ice packs to nose and/or forehead to promote vasoconstriction
      5) Encourage client to expectorate blood to prevent N/V from swallowed blood

      6) Estimate blood loss when possible

      7) Maintain an attitude of calm reassurance

    b. Nasal packing

    c. Surgery including cauterization and ligation of vessels (i.e., *Caldwell-Luc procedure*, which involves entering maxillary sinus through an incision under upper lip; involves ligating artery responsible for bleeding in epistaxis; involves creating a window to increase aeration of sinus and promote drainage if used for sinusitis)

  3. Following nasal packing

    a. Monitor respiratory function and oxygen saturation

    b. Assess packing for odor, color, and amount of drainage

    c. Administer analgesics as needed

    d. Monitor vital signs to assess for cardiovascular complications and infection

    e. Monitor position of catheter (i.e., rubber or inflatable type) if used to provide hemostasis

    f. Provide frequent oral care; use bedside humidifier or high humidity face mask to reduce drying of oral mucous membranes

  4. Provide pre- and postoperative teaching and care as indicated

XIII. SINUSITIS

A. Overview

  1. Inflammation with resulting infection of mucous membranes of 1 or more paranasal sinuses; often follows URIs or viral rhinitis

  2. Classified as *acute*, *subacute*, or *chronic*

    a. Acute: lasts from 1 day to 3 weeks

    b. Subacute: persists from 3 weeks to 3 months

    c. Chronic: lasts longer than 3 months

  3. Immunocompromised clients may be at greater risk for sinusitis and may be more difficult to treat

  4. Causes: URIs, viral rhinitis, nasal polyps, deviated nasal septum, tooth abscess, prolonged nasotracheal or nasogastric intubation, abuse of nasal decongestants, swimming and diving, frequent changes in barometric pressure (i.e., pilots, flight attendants), smoking, nasal packing (epistaxis), and allergies

B. Pathophysiology

  1. Paranasal sinuses are air cells that connect with nasal cavity; are named for bone in which they are located (i.e., frontal, sphenoid, ethmoid, maxillary)

  2. Sinuses are lined with cilia, which facilitate movement of fluids and microorganisms into nasal cavity for exit from body

  3. Viral illness produces inflammation of sinus mucosa causing obstruction of normal ciliary action, creating an ideal environment for bacterial growth

  4. After bacterial invasion of sinuses, inflammatory response increases swelling and congestion, further compromising normal ciliary action; bacterial growth continues

  5. Common causative organisms: *Streptococcus pyogenes*, *Staphylococcus aureus*, *Streptococcus pneumoniae*, and *Haemophilus influenzae*; gram-negative species and fungi may also be causative

  6. Signs and symptoms

    a. Acute sinusitis: constant, often severe pain and tenderness over infected sinuses, pain in teeth may indicate maxillary sinusitis, headache, fever, malaise, and fatigue, nasal congestion, purulent nasal discharge, halitosis, sore and inflamed throat because of swallowed secretions (postnasal drip)

    b. Subacute or chronic sinusitis: dull, intermittent or constant pain, purulent nasal discharge, chronic cough, and loss of sense of smell

7. Local and intracranial complications: periorbital abscesses and/or cellulitis, osteomyelitis of facial bones, cavernous sinus thrombosis, meningitis, brain abscess, and sepsis

C. Nursing assessment
1. Frequency of sinusitis, precipitating factors, pain, and need for analgesics
2. Diagnostic tests: inspection of nose and throat, cultures of nasal discharge, transillumination of sinuses, x-rays and CT scans to detect opacity of sinuses, and nasal endoscopy to visualize anterior nasal cavity and sinus openings

D. Nursing management

1. Medications: antibiotics, oral or intranasal decongestants, intranasal corticosteroids, expectorants such as guaifenesin (Robitussin) to liquefy secretions, saline nasal sprays and/or steam inhalation, saline irrigation of maxillary sinus (i.e., antral irrigation) using needle access to sinus, and analgesics; clients with allergies may use nonsedating antihistamines to decrease allergic response, such as desloratidine (Clarinex) and others
2. Surgical interventions
   a. Include endoscopic sinus surgery, Caldwell-Luc procedure, and external sphenoethmoidectomy (removal of diseased tissue from sphenoid or ethmoid sinuses via a surgical incision alongside of nose)
   b. Administer analgesics prn and comfort measures (i.e., ice packs, head elevation)
   c. Provide teaching
      1) Importance of completing full course of antibiotic therapy
      2) Uses and hazards of nasal decongestants, such as rebound effect
      3) Signs and symptoms of recurrent infection
      4) Importance of adequate hydration
      5) Postoperative management including avoidance of strenuous activity and blowing the nose

XIV. EPIGLOTTITIS

A. Overview
1. A severe, life-threatening, rapidly progressive infection of epiglottis and surrounding area
2. Often caused by *H. influenzae* type B; with advent of *H. influenzae* type B vaccine, incidence has dropped to 10–20% of former levels
3. Formerly a disease of children, now affects both children and adults

B. Pathophysiology
1. Epiglottis is an inflammation of supraglottic structures in upper airway
2. In children, smaller diameter of airway and large size of upper airway structures pose a significant threat to airway patency, even when there is less swelling
3. Bacterial illness produces edema in epiglottis
4. Common organisms associated with epiglottitis include *Haemophilus influenzae and* Group A *streptococcus*
5. Signs and symptoms

   a. Severe sore throat, high fever, toxic appearance, muffled voice, inability to handle oral secretions, assumes position of comfort (erect and quiet), stridor, dysphagia, respiratory distress
   b. Symptoms may be of rapid or gradual onset
6. Complications of epiglottitis: airway obstruction, death, pneumonia, meningitis, brain abscess, and sepsis

C. Nursing assessment

1. Assessment includes frequent monitoring of airway patency; use caution in visualization of throat, which may cause further obstruction
2. Soft-tissue radiography of neck reveals "thumb sign"

   D. Nursing management
      1. Medications: antibiotics, analgesics; dexamethasone (Decadron) to decrease swelling
      2. Anticipate intubation if there are signs of impending airway compromise
      3. Explain importance of completing full course of antibiotic therapy and signs and symptoms of recurrent infection

XV. PERITONSILLAR ABCESS

   A. Overview
      1. Infection of tonsils causes unilateral swelling and can occlude airway; is a complication of acute tonsillitis
      2. Often caused by group A beta-hemolytic streptococcus or *Staphylococcus aureus*
   B. Pathophysiology
      1. Tonsils are structures of upper airway
      2. In children, smaller diameter of airway and large size of upper airway structures pose a significant threat to airway patency, even when there is less swelling
      3. Common organisms associated with peritonsillar abscess include *Staphylococcus aureus* and Group A beta-hemolytic *streptococcus*
      4. Signs and symptoms
         a. Sore throat, high fever, trismus, muffled voice, inability to handle oral secretions, assumes position of comfort (erect and quiet), dysphagia, respiratory distress, unilateral peritonsillar bulging, uvular deviation
         b. Symptoms may be of rapid or gradual onset
      5. Complications of peritonsillar abscess: airway obstruction, death, aspiration pneumonia, and sepsis
   C. Nursing assessment
      1. Frequent monitoring of airway patency
      2. Uvular deviation away from affected side; use caution in visualization of throat, which may cause further obstruction
   D. Nursing management
      1. Medications: antibiotics, analgesics; dexamethasone (Decadron) to decrease swelling
      2. Incision and drainage (I&D) of abscess
      3. Explain importance of completing full course of antibiotic therapy and signs and symptoms of recurrent infection

XVI. LARYNGEAL CANCER

   A. Overview
      1. Defined as cancer of glottis (true vocal cords), supraglottis, or subglottis
      2. Causes are prolonged use of tobacco and alcohol, chronic laryngitis, occupational exposure to chemicals and toxins, exposure to selected types of human papilloma virus, and genetic predisposition
      3. Squamous cell carcinoma is most common type of laryngeal malignancy
      4. With early diagnosis and treatment, 80–90% of small lesions can be cured
   B. Pathophysiology
      1. Exposure to irritants (i.e., tobacco smoke, chemicals, toxins) result in changes to laryngeal mucosa
      2. Precancerous leukoplakia (white, patchy lesions) and erythroplakia (red, velvet-like patches) appear on laryngeal mucosa
      3. Lesions may occur in any of 3 areas of larynx (i.e., glottis, supraglottis, or subglottis); lesions along edges of glottis (true vocal cords) are most common (see Figure 6-3)
      4. Lesions of glottis are usually well differentiated and slow growing

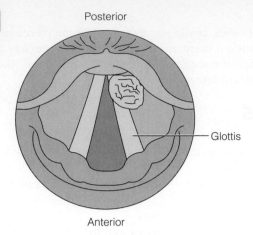

Figure 6-3

Visualization of lesion along edge of glottis

Posterior

Glottis

Anterior

5. Structures in supraglottis include epiglottis, arytenoid muscles and cartilage, and false vocal cords; subglottis is located below vocal cords and terminates at tracheal ring; tumors of supraglottis are often large before symptoms are noted and very rare
6. Laryngeal tumors initially metastasize to regional lymph nodes; metastasis to lungs may follow
7. Signs and symptoms: hoarseness, change in voice, dyspnea, pain and burning in throat when drinking hot liquids or citrus juices, dysphagia, foul-smelling breath, pain radiating to ear, persistent cough, and palpable lump in neck

C. **Nursing assessment**
1. Early recognition of signs and symptoms (early diagnosis is critical to survival), signs of respiratory distress, nutritional status, and psychosocial needs; prompt assessment and early referral of clients presenting with symptoms of laryngeal cancer
2. Diagnostic tests
   a. Laryngoscopy with biopsy of leukoplakia (precancerous lesions) and erythroplakia (precancerous patches)
   b. X-ray studies of head, neck, and chest; CT or MRI scans
   c. Barium swallow to evaluate swallowing and/or presence of tumor in esophagus

D. **Nursing management**
1. Medications include adjunctive chemotherapy
2. Treatment options
   a. Surgical interventions: partial, supraglottic, or total **laryngectomy** (removal of part or all of larynx) depending upon tumor location; radical neck dissection with cervical lymph node involvement
   b. External beam radiation or implants for early tumors
3. Monitor respiratory status
4. Provide supplemental nutrition
5. Assess emotional status and possible grieving, encourage client to ventilate feelings and concerns
6. Provide postoperative care as indicated and client teaching as follows:
   a. Postoperative and home care following partial or total laryngectomy (i.e., tracheotomy care, enteral nutrition)
   b. Need for radiation treatments and/or chemotherapy
   c. Options available for restoration of speech (i.e., esophageal speech, battery-operated speech generator)
   d. Availability of support services (i.e., American Cancer Society, support groups, pastoral care)

Practice to Pass

The client asks the nurse about the methods available to restore speech following total laryngectomy. How should the nurse respond?

Case Study

R. M., a 48-year-old female client, has been admitted to the Emergency Department with severe vertigo accompanied by nausea and vomiting. She also reports tinnitus and a sense of fullness in the left ear. She is diagnosed with acute Ménière's disease.

1. What other assessment findings can be expected?

2. What medical interventions can be anticipated during the acute phase of this illness?

3. What diagnostic tests can be anticipated for this client?

4. How should the nurse explain Ménière's disease to the client?

5. What discharge instructions should be given to the client?

For suggested responses, see pages 463–464.

POSTTEST

1 A client reports sudden onset of continuous eye pain and impaired vision. Pupil dilation is noted. The nurse concludes that this assessment data is consistent with which disorder?

1. Closed-angle (narrow-angle) glaucoma
2. Open-angle glaucoma
3. Cataracts
4. Retinal detachment

2 The nurse is assessing a client with Ménière's disease. What subjective assessment data does the nurse expect to obtain?

1. Bilateral hearing impairment
2. Vertigo and nausea
3. Pain when the tragus is touched
4. Tenderness over the mastoid area

3 A male client has just had a cataract operation with a lens implant. In discharge teaching, the nurse will instruct the client's wife to do which of the following?

1. Prepare only soft foods for several days to prevent facial movement.
2. Encourage sleeping on the affected side for greater comfort.
3. Have her husband resume all normal activities starting the next day.
4. Instill eye drops correctly.

4 An adult client presents to the emergency department a few hours after a sizeable rock hit his eye while weeding along a ditch near a busy highway. The nurse assesses the eye and finds redness and weeping, but the client denies any pain. Which early symptoms would help confirm retinal detachment? Select all that apply.

1. Pain
2. Floaters
3. Subconjunctival hemorrhage
4. Sensation of curtain drawn across the vision
5. Dark lines or spots in the field of vision

5 A young child has had a recent upper respiratory infection. The child now reports severe pain in the right ear and says, "I can't hear." The nurse concludes that the pathology that led to this problem is most likely which of the following?

1. Tympanic membrane has ruptured causing hearing loss
2. Child has been exposed to secondhand smoke, which caused an acute allergic response
3. Narrowed auditory tube impaired equalization of pressure in the middle ear, stopping air from entering
4. Edema of the auditory tube followed the respiratory infection, impairing drainage of the middle ear

6 The community health nurse interprets that which client is at highest risk for macular degeneration?

1. Biochemist exposed to various toxins
2. Older adult client
3. Youth hit in the eye with a baseball
4. Young adult with multiple allergies

7 A client presents to the clinic with reports of pain in the cheekbones that is worse when bending forward. What other symptoms should the nurse expect if the diagnosis is acute sinusitis? Select all that apply.

1. Nausea and food intolerances
2. Nasal congestion and purulent discharge
3. Bad breath
4. Nuchal rigidity
5. Pain in the upper teeth

8 Which of the following is a priority nursing diagnosis that the nurse should address for a client with epistaxis?

1. Risk for Aspiration
2. Risk for Infection
3. Acute Pain
4. Impaired Verbal Communication

9 The community health nurse interprets that which client is at highest risk for laryngeal cancer?

1. A client who has an injury to the larynx.
2. An older adult who is 85 years old.
3. A man who has chewed tobacco and smoked for 20 years.
4. A woman who has chronic sinusitis and seasonal allergies.

10 The nurse would include which interventions in the plan of care for a client with sensorineural hearing loss?

1. Provide information about availability of hearing aids to amplify sound.
2. Educate family members about social isolation and depression.
3. Administer antibiotics as prescribed.
4. Prepare client for tympanoplasty.

➤ *See pages 182–183 for Answers and Rationales.*

ANSWERS & RATIONALES

Pretest

1 **Answer: 3, 5** **Rationale:** Angle closure or narrow-angle glaucoma develops abruptly and manifests with sudden loss of vision and acute face and eye pain. It is a medical emergency. Halo vision, dull eye pain, and impaired night vision are symptoms commonly associated with open-angle glaucoma. **Cognitive Level:** Applying **Client Need:** Physiological Adaptation **Integrated Process:** Nursing Process: Assessment **Content Area:** Adult Health **Strategy:** Use nursing knowledge to answer the question. If none of the options are recognizable, keep in mind that when options are opposite, one of them is more likely to be correct. **Reference:** LeMone, P., Burke, K., and Bauldoff, G.

(2011). *Medical-surgical nursing: Critical thinking in patient care* (5th ed.). Upper Saddle River, NJ: Pearson Education, p. 1592.

2 **Answer: 3** **Rationale:** A cloudy-appearing lens is symptomatic of cataract development. As the cataract matures, the red reflex is lost. A sense of a curtain falling over the visual field is associated with detached retina. Eye pain and double vision are not associated with cataracts. **Cognitive Level:** Applying **Client Need:** Physiological Adaptation **Integrated Process:** Nursing Process: Assessment **Content Area:** Adult Health **Strategy:** Recall normal assessment findings related to the eye. Consider what other assessment changes would occur if the lens is clouding. **Reference:** LeMone, P., Burke, K., and Bauldoff, G. (2011). *Medical-surgical thinking in patient care* (5th ed.). Upper Saddle River, NJ: Pearson Education, p. 1589.

3 **Answer: 2** **Rationale:** The foreign body should not be removed or manipulated. It should be immobilized if possible and the eye covered to protect from further injury. A paper cup can be used in place of an eye patch. Patching both eyes is an appropriate intervention to prevent ocular movement but follows immobilization of the foreign body. Irrigation with water is an intervention for chemical burns to the eyes. Carbonic anhydrase inhibitors are used to decrease intraocular pressure following blunt trauma. **Cognitive Level:** Analyzing **Client Need:** Physiological Adaptation **Integrated Process:** Nursing Process: Implementation **Content Area:** Adult Health **Strategy:** For emergency actions, choose the option that stabilizes the client and prevents further injury. **Reference:** LeMone, P., Burke, K., and Bauldoff, G. (2011). *Medical-surgical nursing: Critical thinking in patient care* (5th ed.). Upper Saddle River, NJ: Pearson Education, p. 1586.

4 **Answer: 4** **Rationale:** Conductive hearing loss results from changes that occur in the external or middle ear. Hearing aids, assistive listening devices (i.e., "pocket talkers"), and reconstructive surgeries can improve or correct hearing loss. Exposure to high levels of noise on an intermittent or constant basis damages the hair cells of the organ of Corti, resulting in sensorineural hearing loss. **Cognitive Level:** Applying **Client Need:** Physiological Adaptation **Integrated Process:** Teaching and Learning **Content Area:** Adult Health **Strategy:** Note the clarifying word *conductive* in the stem of the question that identifies the type of hearing loss. Read the question carefully and choose the option that is consistent with this form of hearing loss. **Reference:** LeMone, P., Burke, K., and Bauldoff, G. (2011). *Medical-surgical nursing: Critical thinking in patient care* (5th ed.). Upper Saddle River, NJ: Pearson Education, p. 1614.

5 **Answer: 4, 5** **Rationale:** Weber and Rinne tests are used to differentiate conductive hearing loss from sensorineural. Audiometry is used to evaluate and diagnose sensorineural and conductive hearing loss. Tympanocentesis is the aspiration of fluid or pus from the middle ear

to identify the causative organism of acute otitis media. Transillumination of the sinuses is a diagnostic tool used to assess for sinusitis. The diagnosis of Ménière's disease is confirmed by electronystagmography, a series of tests to evaluate vestibular-ocular reflexes. **Cognitive Level:** Applying **Client Need:** Reduction of Risk Potential **Integrated Process:** Nursing Process: Assessment **Content Area:** Adult Health **Strategy:** Decode unfamiliar terms by finding the root word and prefixes or suffixes. Note the wording of the question indicates that more than one option is correct. **Reference:** LeMone, P., Burke, K., and Bauldoff, G. (2011). *Medical-surgical nursing: Critical thinking in patient care* (5th ed.). Upper Saddle River, NJ: Pearson Education, pp. 1573–1574.

6 **Answer: 2, 4** **Rationale:** A higher incidence of acute otitis media is noted in infants who are bottle-fed in a horizontal position and who live in homes with smokers. The full 10- to 12-day course of antibiotic therapy must be administered. There is no relationship between the ingestion of fruit juices and acute otitis media. **Cognitive Level:** Applying **Client Need:** Physiological Adaptation **Integrated Process:** Teaching and Learning **Content Area:** Adult Health **Strategy:** The wording of the question indicates the correct options contain true information. Use nursing knowledge and the process of elimination to make selections. **Reference:** LeMone, P., Burke, K., and Bauldoff, G. (2011). *Medical-surgical nursing: Critical thinking in patient care* (5th ed.). Upper Saddle River, NJ: Pearson Education, p. 1606.

7 **Answer: 2** **Rationale:** Atrophic macular degeneration causes loss of central vision. Magnification devices and enhanced lighting help to promote safety. Peripheral vision remains intact. Although laser photocoagulation is effective for exudative macular degeneration, there is no treatment for the atrophic form. Since macular degeneration is not an infectious process, antibiotic therapy is not indicated. **Cognitive Level:** Applying **Client Need:** Physiological Adaptation **Integrated Process:** Teaching and Learning **Content Area:** Adult Health **Strategy:** Apply knowledge of anatomy and physiology and determine what the macula does. Choose the option that can assist with the lost function. **Reference:** LeMone, P., Burke, K., and Bauldoff, G. (2011). *Medical-surgical nursing: Critical thinking in patient care* (5th ed.). Upper Saddle River, NJ: Pearson Education, p. 1599.

8 **Answer: 2** **Rationale:** Peritonsillar abscess is a complication of tonsillitis and can cause unilateral swelling, which can in turn cause uvular deviation away from the affected side. Pharyngitis, epiglottitis, and esophagitis can all cause swelling and throat pain, but it is bilateral. Additionally, the nurse would not attempt to visualize the oropharynx of a client with suspected epiglottitis. **Cognitive Level:** Applying **Client Need:** Physiological Adaptation **Integrated Process:** Nursing Process: Assessment **Content Area:** Adult Health **Strategy:** The question asks for a particular presentation. Unilateral swelling, causing uvular deviation, is found only in peritonsillar abscess. Epiglottitis and pharyngitis both cause throat pain, and all 4 conditions could cause dysphagia. **Reference:** LeMone, P., Burke, K., and Bauldoff, G. (2011). *Medical-surgical nursing: Critical thinking in patient care* (5th ed.). Upper Saddle River, NJ: Pearson Education, p. 1151.

9 **Answer: 3** **Rationale:** These symptoms, along with dysphagia, foul-smelling breath, and pain when drinking hot or acidic fluids, are common signs of laryngeal cancer. Chronic sinusitis can produce foul breath and pain or burning in the throat. Gastroesophageal reflux disease and coronary heart disease may produce epigastric and/or chest pain, but hoarseness and change of voice do not occur. **Cognitive Level:** Applying **Client Need:** Physiological Adaptation **Integrated Process:** Nursing Process: Diagnosis **Content Area:** Adult Health **Strategy:** Recall that these are classic warning signs of cancer. **Reference:** LeMone, P., Burke, K., and Bauldoff, G. (2011). *Medical-surgical nursing: Critical thinking in patient care* (5th ed.). Upper Saddle River, NJ: Pearson Education, p. 1164.

10 **Answer: 3** **Rationale:** All of the nursing actions listed are appropriate for the client following nasal packing for epistaxis or surgery; however, the risk of respiratory and cardiovascular complications is high, and monitoring respiratory function is essential, and therefore of highest priority. **Cognitive Level:** Analyzing **Client Need:** Physiological Adaptation **Integrated Process:** Nursing Process: Implementation **Content Area:** Adult Health **Strategy:** Notice the question asks for the priority intervention. Use the process of elimination and physiological priorities in making a selection. **Reference:** LeMone, P., Burke, K., and Bauldoff, G. (2011). *Medical-surgical nursing: Critical thinking in patient care* (5th ed.). Upper Saddle River, NJ: Pearson Education, p. 1156.

Posttest

1 **Answer: 1** **Rationale:** Closed- or narrow-angle glaucoma has an abrupt onset and is characterized by severe pain of sudden onset that usually lasts longer than 20 minutes. Open-angle glaucoma occurs gradually with no initial manifestations but subsequent loss of peripheral visual fields. Pain is not associated with cataracts or retinal detachment. **Cognitive Level:** Applying **Client Need:** Physiological Adaptation **Integrated Process:** Nursing Process: Diagnosis **Content Area:** Adult Health **Strategy:** Eliminate the diseases that do not cause pain. **Reference:** LeMone, P., Burke, K., and Bauldoff, G. (2011). *Medical-surgical nursing: Critical thinking in patient care* (5th ed.). Upper Saddle River, NJ: Pearson Education, p. 1592.

2 **Answer: 2** **Rationale:** Ménière's disease is associated with vertigo that may last for hours, as well as fluctuating hearing loss, nausea, and vomiting. The disorder is unilateral, but because hearing is bilateral, the client often does not realize the extent of the hearing loss. Pain when the tragus is touched is indicative of otitis externa

or swimmer's ear, and tenderness over the mastoid area is indicative of acute otitis media. **Cognitive Level:** Applying **Client Need:** Physiological Adaptation **Integrated Process:** Nursing Process: Assessment **Content Area:** Adult Health **Strategy:** Note that the incorrect options are found with other ear disorders. **Reference:** LeMone, P., Burke, K., and Bauldoff, G. (2011). *Medical-surgical nursing: Critical thinking in patient care* (5th ed.). Upper Saddle River, NJ: Pearson Education, p. 1611.

3 **Answer: 4** **Rationale:** Postoperative information includes limitations on reading, lifting, strenuous activity, and sleeping on the affected side. A family member needs to be taught to instill eye drops. There are no dietary restrictions. **Cognitive Level:** Applying **Client Need:** Physiological Adaptation **Integrated Process:** Teaching and Learning **Content Area:** Adult Health **Strategy:** Consider which activities are necessary and which restrictions are needed for safety and home care after eye surgery. **Reference:** LeMone, P., Burke, K., and Bauldoff, G. (2011). *Medical-surgical nursing: Critical thinking in patient care* (5th ed.). Upper Saddle River, NJ: Pearson Education, p. 1591.

4 **Answer: 2, 4, 5** **Rationale:** Retinal detachment is painless, but eventually floaters, lines or spots, and visual loss will be manifested, especially if hemorrhage has occurred. Dark lines, spots, or sensation of a curtain drawn across the field of vision is a common manifestation. Subconjunctival hemorrhage is a manifestation of blunt trauma to the eye and not of retinal detachment. **Cognitive Level:** Analyzing **Client Need:** Physiological Adaptation **Integrated Process:** Nursing Process: Assessment **Content Area:** Adult Health **Strategy:** Consider the consequences of damage to the retina, which receives visual stimuli. **Reference:** LeMone, P., Burke, K., and Bauldoff, G. (2011). *Medical-surgical nursing: Critical thinking in patient care* (5th ed.). Upper Saddle River, NJ: Pearson Education, pp. 1600–1601.

5 **Answer: 4** **Rationale:** In acute otitis media, the auditory tube provides entry of pathogens. This infection typically follows an upper respiratory infection. Edema of the tube causes mucus and fluid to accumulate and the pathogens to grow. There is no evidence in the question to indicate rupture of the tympanic membrane or exposure to secondhand smoke. Impaired pressure equalization is not suggested by these symptoms. **Cognitive Level:** Analyzing **Client Need:** Physiological Adaptation **Integrated Process:** Nursing Process: Diagnosis **Content Area:** Adult Health **Strategy:** Consider the history of upper respiratory infection (URI) and apply knowledge of complications. Also remember that the client is a child. **Reference:** LeMone, P., Burke, K., and Bauldoff, G. (2011). *Medical-surgical nursing: Critical thinking in patient care* (5th ed.). Upper Saddle River, NJ: Pearson Education, pp. 1606–1607.

6 **Answer: 2** **Rationale:** Age-related macular degeneration is the leading cause of loss of vision in clients over 50 years of age. Blunt trauma, exposure to toxins, and allergies are not known causes of macular degeneration. **Cognitive Level:** Applying **Client Need:** Health Promotion and Maintenance **Integrated Process:** Nursing Process: Diagnosis **Content Area:** Adult Health **Strategy:** Consider the factors associated with macular degeneration. Note that 3 of the options include the age of the client. **Reference:** LeMone, P., Burke, K., and Bauldoff, G. (2011). *Medical-surgical nursing: Critical thinking in patient care* (5th ed.). Upper Saddle River, NJ: Pearson Education, pp. 1598–1599.

7 **Answer: 2, 3, 5** **Rationale:** Manifestations of acute sinusitis include nasal congestion with postnasal drip and purulent discharge. Bad breath is a frequent finding. With involvement of the maxillary sinuses, pain and pressure may be felt in the upper teeth. Food intolerances are not related. Nuchal rigidity would indicate a more serious problem, such as meningitis. **Cognitive Level:** Applying **Client Need:** Physiological Adaptation **Integrated Process:** Nursing Process: Assessment **Content Area:** Adult Health **Strategy:** Consider upper respiratory symptoms of infection. **Reference:** LeMone, P., Burke, K., and Bauldoff, G. (2011). *Medical-surgical nursing: Critical thinking in patient care* (5th ed.). Upper Saddle River, NJ: Pearson Education, p. 1148.

8 **Answer: 1** **Rationale:** Blood draining into the nasopharynx poses a Risk for Aspiration. Risk for Infection and Acute Pain are appropriate nursing diagnoses related to nasal packing but are not the priorities because they do not address airway and breathing. Impaired Verbal Communication is unlikely in the client with epistaxis. **Cognitive Level:** Analyzing **Client Need:** Physiological Adaptation **Integrated Process:** Nursing Process: Diagnosis **Content Area:** Adult Health **Strategy:** Consider which diagnosis poses the most immediate threat. **Reference:** LeMone, P., Burke, K., and Bauldoff, G.

(2011). *Medical-surgical nursing: Critical thinking in patient care* (5th ed.). Upper Saddle River, NJ: Pearson Education, p. 1157.

9 **Answer: 3** **Rationale:** The 2 major risk factors for laryngeal cancer are prolonged smoking along with concomitant use of alcohol. Although the majority of cases occur in men ages 50 to 75, advancing age does not significantly increase risk. Injury to the larynx, seasonal allergies, and chronic sinusitis are not risk factors. **Cognitive Level:** Applying **Client Need:** Health Promotion and Maintenance **Integrated Process:** Nursing Process: Diagnosis **Content Area:** Adult Health **Strategy:** Consider unhealthy lifestyle as etiology for many disorders. **Reference:** LeMone, P., Burke, K., and Bauldoff, G. (2011). *Medical-surgical nursing: Critical thinking in patient care* (5th ed.). Upper Saddle River, NJ: Pearson Education, p. 1165.

10 **Answer: 2** **Rationale:** The client with sensorineural hearing loss experiences social isolation and depression and may appear withdrawn. Amplification devices such as hearing aids are helpful for clients with conductive hearing loss but only amplify noxious sounds for the client with sensorineural hearing loss. Antibiotics would not be helpful for sensorineural hearing loss, and tympanoplasty is used to correct damage to structures in the middle ear. **Cognitive Level:** Applying **Client Need:** Psychosocial Integrity **Integrated Process:** Nursing Process: Implementation **Content Area:** Adult Health **Strategy:** The critical word *sensorineural* in the stem of the question tells what type of hearing loss is being tested. Consider the psychological as well as physical problems and then determine the nursing actions needed. **Reference:** LeMone, P., Burke, K., and Bauldoff, G. (2011). *Medical-surgical nursing: Critical thinking in patient care* (5th ed.). Upper Saddle River, NJ: Pearson Education, pp. 1618–1619.

References

Adams, M., Holland, L., & Bostwick, P. (2011). *Pharmacology for nurses: A pathophysiologic approach* (3rd ed.). Upper Saddle River, NJ: Pearson Education.

Davidson, M., London, M., & Ladewig, P. (2012). *Olds' maternal-newborn nursing & women's health across the lifespan* (9th ed.). Upper Saddle River, NJ: Pearson Education.

Guyton, A., & Hall, J. E. (2011). *Textbook of medical physiology* (12th ed.). Philadelphia, PA: W. B. Saunders.

Huether, S. E., & McCance, K. L. (2012). *Understanding pathophysiology* (5th ed.). St. Louis, MO: Elsevier.

Ignatavicius, D., & Workman, L. (2012). *Medical surgical nursing: Patient-centered collaborative care* (7th ed.). Philadelphia, PA: W. B. Saunders.

LeMone, P., Burke, K., & Bauldoff, G. (2011). *Medical-surgical nursing: Critical thinking in patient care* (5th ed.). Upper Saddle River, NJ: Pearson Education.

McCance, K., & Huether, K (2010). *Understanding pathophysiology: The biologic basis for disease in adults and children* (6th ed.) St. Louis, MO: Elsevier.

Porth, C., & Matfin, G. (2010). *Pathophysiology: Concepts of altered health states* (8th ed.). Philadelphia, PA: Lippincott Williams & Wilkins.

Wilson, B., Shannon, M., & Shields, K. (2012). *Pearson's nurse's drug guide 2012.* Upper Saddle River, NJ: Pearson Education.

ANSWERS & RATIONALES

7 Gastrointestinal Health Problems

Chapter Outline

Risk Factors Associated with Gastrointestinal Health Problems

Gastroesophageal Reflux Disease (GERD)

Peptic Ulcer Disease (PUD)

Hiatal Hernia

Crohn's Disease (Regional Enteritis)

Ulcerative Colitis

Diverticular Disease

Intestinal Obstruction

Appendicitis

Peritonitis

Neoplasms of Gastrointestinal Tract

Celiac Disease

NCLEX-RN® Test Prep

Use the accompanying online resource, NursingReviewsandRationales, to test yourself with hundreds of NCLEX®-style practice questions.

Objectives

➤ Define key terms associated with gastrointestinal health problems.

➤ Identify risk factors associated with the development of gastrointestinal health problems.

➤ Explain the common etiologies of gastrointestinal health problems.

➤ Describe the pathophysiologic processes associated with specific gastrointestinal health problems.

➤ Distinguish between normal and abnormal gastrointestinal findings obtained from the nursing assessment.

➤ Prioritize nursing interventions associated with specific gastrointestinal health problems.

Review at a Glance

borborygmus rumbling sounds in gastrointestinal (GI) tract

Crohn's disease an inflammatory bowel condition in which there are patchy areas of inflammation anywhere along entire GI tract; also known as regional enteritis

dumping syndrome rapid emptying of stomach contents into small intestine, causing sweating and weakness after a meal; may occur after gastric resection

dyspepsia burning, epigastric pain

erythroplakia red patches in mouth

fecalith a hard piece of stool that is stonelike and may cause bleeding

gastroparesis delayed gastric emptying time

hematemesis vomiting up blood

Helicobacter pylori Gram-negative bacteria that play a role in development of peptic ulcers

intussusception intrusion of one part of intestine into another part that is distal to it

leukoplakia white patches on mouth

McBurney's point point halfway between umbilicus and right iliac crest

melena black, tarry feces caused by presence of blood

peptic ulcer disease (PUD) an ulcer that may be located in lower end of esophagus, stomach, or duodenum

peritonitis infection of membrane that lines peritoneum or abdominal cavity

pyrosis severe epigastric pain or heartburn

rebound tenderness severe pain over an area of tenderness when pressure is applied to that area by examiner and quickly released

volvulus obstruction a twisting of bowel resulting in a large bowel obstruction

Zollinger-Ellison syndrome a condition in which a pancreatic tumor causes secretion of excess amounts of gastrin, which stimulates secretion of hydrochloric acid and pepsin; these events can lead to formation of a peptic ulcer

PRETEST

1 A client being admitted to the hospital with reports of severe lower abdominal pain is lying on the bed with the knees flexed. Temperature on admission is 101.2°F orally. The nurse should conclude that which additional finding is consistent with a diagnosis of appendicitis?

1. Pain is localized halfway between umbilicus and right iliac crest
2. Client describes pain as occurring 2 hours after eating
3. Pain radiates from the mid-abdomen to the back
4. Pain is in left lower quadrant

2 An older adult client presents with fever, leukocytosis, left lower quadrant pain, and diarrhea alternating with constipation. The nurse concludes that these are frequently seen in clients with which health problem?

1. Appendicitis
2. Diverticulitis
3. Peptic ulcer disease
4. Irritable bowel syndrome

3 A client says to the nurse, "My health care provider told me my ulcer may have been caused by bacteria. I thought ulcers were caused by diet and too much stress." Which response by the nurse is best?

1. "If it was caused by bacteria, you would have a fever as a result of the inflammatory process."
2. "We know that ulcers are communicable. They can be spread easily. Be careful you don't spread them to your children."
3. "Diet and stress usually do not play a role in ulcer development."
4. "The bacteria *Helicobacter pylori* causes inflammation, which can then lead to ulcer formation."

4 The nurse is caring for a client with a hiatal hernia. The client asks what could have prevented the problem. The nurse provides a response that considers which possible etiologies of the disorder? Select all that apply.

1. Heavy lifting over a period of time
2. A diet high in saturated fats
3. Young adult age
4. History of upper abdominal surgery
5. Frequent use of nonsteroidal inflammatory drugs (NSAIDs)

5 An older adult male client is worried about bright red blood in his stool, along with feeling "tired and worn out." The nurse considers that these symptoms are consistent with which health problems? Select all that apply.

1. Ascending (right-sided) colon cancer
2. Descending (left-sided) colon cancer
3. Sigmoid colon cancer
4. Gastric ulcers
5. Hemorrhoids

6 A client states, "My doctor told me to stop taking aspirin since I've developed this ulcer. I usually take aspirin to keep my arthritis from hurting. I'm not sure what to do." Which response by the clinic nurse is best?

1. "At this time the treatment of your ulcer is the highest priority and you should focus on it."
2. "Aspirin can make an ulcer worse. Let's ask your health care provider about which drug would be best for you."
3. "Go ahead and take the aspirin if it helps, but watch closely for bleeding."
4. "The doctor knows what is best for you, and you should follow those instructions."

7 A female client recently diagnosed with a duodenal ulcer suddenly experiences severe abdominal pain, increased heart rate, increased respiratory rate, and diaphoresis. On palpation, the abdomen is rigid; bowel sounds are faint and diminished. Which nursing action is most appropriate?

1. Immediately place her in high Fowler's position to facilitate breathing.
2. Help her walk to the bathroom to get rid of any flatus.
3. Check to see if she has food allergies and see if she ate anything to which she might be allergic.
4. Establish IV access and call the provider to report the assessment data.

8 A female client reports a burning, cramping pain in the upper abdomen that worsens in midafternoon and sometimes awakens her at night. She reports that eating something usually relieves the pain but that it is now becoming more intense. What is the best conclusion for the nurse to draw?

1. Symptoms are consistent with peptic ulcer disease.
2. Client is probably developing cholelithiasis.
3. Client probably has indigestion and needs to watch what she eats.
4. Symptoms are indicative of a gastrointestinal bleeding episode.

9 The nurse considers that which of the following clients would be most at risk for an intestinal obstruction?

1. Jewish client who smokes and consumes large amounts of caffeine
2. Older adult client on postoperative bed rest after abdominal surgery
3. A client whose diet includes eating low-fiber, high-fat foods
4. Adult client diagnosed with cirrhosis of the liver

10 The nurse suspects which condition when a client reports dyspepsia, frequent belching, and increased salivation?

1. Peptic ulcer disease (PUD)
2. Ulcerative colitis
3. Paraesophageal hiatal hernia
4. Gastroesophageal reflux disease (GERD)

➤ *See pages 201–202 for Answers and Rationales.*

I. RISK FACTORS ASSOCIATED WITH GASTROINTESTINAL HEALTH PROBLEMS

    A. **Gastroesophageal reflux disease (GERD)**: prolonged gastric intubation, infections, systemic diseases, systemic lupus erythematosus (SLE), ingestion of corrosive substances, acidic foods, obesity, smoking, and alcohol intake

    B. *Peptic ulcer disease (PUD)*: chronic diseases such as COPD, rheumatoid arthritis (RA), or cirrhosis; stress; smoking; continued or excessive use of nonsteroidal anti-inflammatory drugs (NSAIDs) or aspirin products; *Helicobacter pylori* infection; duodenal ulcers are more prominent with type O blood and may be genetically transmitted

    C. **Hiatal hernia**: aging, trauma, surgery, hereditary, obesity

    D. *Crohn's disease*: genetic and familial predisposition, race (Jewish highest), stress

    E. **Ulcerative colitis**: race, genetic predisposition, stress, autoimmune disease

    F. **Diverticular disease**: diseases such as ulcerative colitis and Crohn's disease; obesity; poor dietary habits (high intake of refined foods), especially in elderly

    G. **Intestinal obstruction**: clients having abdominal surgeries; older adults; trauma

    H. **Appendicitis**: fecal impactions, kinking of bowel, parasites, infections

    I. *Peritonitis*: diseases such as Laënnec's cirrhosis, tuberculosis, PUD, inflammatory conditions, trauma or perforation of abdominal viscus, surgery

J. Neoplasms of gastrointestinal (GI) tract: tobacco use (oral cancer); excessive alcohol and tobacco consumption; diet lacking fruits and vegetables; esophageal disorders (esophageal cancer); genetic predisposition; diet high in gastric irritants; conditions such as chronic gastritis or achlorhydria (stomach cancer); low-fiber, high-fat diet and diseases such as Crohn's disease, polyps, ulcerative colitis (intestinal cancer)

K. Celiac disease: people with genetic predisposition (first and second degree relatives of persons with celiac disease), type 1 diabetes mellitus, other autoimmune endocrine disorders, and/or Turner syndrome

II. GASTROESOPHAGEAL REFLUX DISEASE (GERD)

A. Overview

1. Defined as a backflow of gastric contents into esophagus; also known as heartburn or esophagitis
2. Etiologies include high-fat diet; hiatal hernia; pregnancy, obesity; conditions that reduce lower esophageal sphincter (LES) tone (such as excess caffeine intake); congenital defects; **gastroparesis** (delayed gastric emptying time); activities such as vomiting, coughing, lifting, or bending

B. Pathophysiology

1. Gastric contents that are regurgitated into esophagus are acidic and irritate esophageal lining; LES should close completely when food is consumed into stomach; when LES is weakened or incompetent, higher pressure within stomach forces contents into esophagus where pressure is lower; this same concept of a higher pressure area emptying into a lower pressure area accounts for incidence of GERD in conditions such as pregnancy, obesity, and overindulgence of food
2. Esophagus has mucus-producing cells to protect its lining, but in less quantity than in stomach, where a high acid environment is normal
3. Severe GERD can cause epithelial cell damage and erosion of muscularis
4. Complications include strictures, bleeding, reflux-induced asthma, laryngitis
5. Signs and symptoms include **dyspepsia** (burning, epigastric pain); frequent belching with a sour taste; pain after eating, when lying down, and after straining or lifting; increased salivation; flatulence; history of high stress level
6. Drugs that relax LES: calcium channel blockers, nicotine, and peppermint

C. Nursing assessment

1. Assessment includes symptom analysis of pain (1–2 hours after eating) and other symptoms, nutritional assessment, and evidence of complications
2. Diagnostic tests: pH probe test is used to determine number and length of declines in pH of stomach contents (less than 4.0); barium swallow; otherwise history determines diagnosis

D. Nursing management

1. Medications include antacids, H_2-receptor blockers, proton pump inhibitors, antihistamines; separate all antacids from meals by 1 hour and from other medications by 1–2 hours
2. Teach client about possible surgery (fundoplication)
3. Offer several small meals rather than 3 large ones; suggest weight loss if necessary; limit or eliminate caffeine, heavy spices, and smoking
4. Elevate head of bed while sleeping
5. Instruct client to avoid eating in a supine position and to drink extra fluids unless contraindicated
6. Instruct client to keep a diary of foods that seem to increase symptoms and avoid these when determined
7. Discuss stress reduction methods and resources, as well as weight reduction

Practice to Pass

A 42-year-old male client is diagnosed with GERD after being admitted with severe pains in his chest, frequent indigestion, and pain after meals. Since he thought he was having a heart attack, how should the nurse explain the difference in the symptoms between the 2 diagnoses?

III. PEPTIC ULCER DISEASE (PUD)

A. Overview

1. Defined as an ulcer, which may be located in lower end of esophagus, stomach, or duodenum
2. Occurs equally between males and females; mortality increases with age over 75
3. Causes include: excessive stress, *H. pylori* infection (a gram-negative bacteria), excessive use of NSAIDs and aspirin products; any situation where there is damage to mucosa; and **Zollinger-Ellison syndrome** (a pancreatic tumor that causes excess amounts of gastrin to be excreted)
4. Three main types are gastric, duodenal, and stress; may be acute or chronic
   a. Gastric ulcers: etiologies include ingestion of medications, tobacco, caffeine, alcohol; *H. pylori* infection; chronic bile reflux and increased serum gastrin
   b. Duodenal ulcers: etiologies include hypersecretion of pepsinogen, autosomal dominant trait, *H. pylori* infection (95–100% of cases)

B. Pathophysiology

1. Three main factors contribute to ulcer development
   a. *Excess acid* can lead to a break or ulceration in mucosa of stomach or duodenum; this break allows mucosa to be subjected to an acid environment and thus autodigestion occurs
   b. *Decreased mucus production* can leave mucosal cells unprotected from acid environment; hypoxia, shock, severe burns, etc., can lead to injury of mucus-producing cells
   c. *Increased delivery of acid* can cause protective mucus layer to be irritated because of rapid movement of stomach contents, such as in **dumping syndrome** (rapid emptying of stomach contents into small intestine causing sweating, weakness, etc., after a meal)
2. Ulcers can be superficial or deep
   a. Superficial ulcers are also called erosions
   b. Deep lesions extend through musculature and penetrate blood vessels causing hemorrhage; can also cause perforation of wall of stomach or intestines
3. Infection with bacteria *H. pylori* is a major factor in gastric and duodenal ulcers, causing death of mucosal epithelial cells; it also releases toxins and enzymes that produce inflammation and ulcer development; increased levels of gastrin and/or pepsinogen have been attributed to presence of bacteria
4. Rapid gastric emptying (such as in dumping syndrome) may cause increased acid in duodenum and aid ulcer development (Figure 7-1)
5. Stress, caffeine, cigarette smoking, and alcohol consumption increase acid production; aspirin and NSAID medications inhibit prostaglandin, which helps protect lining of stomach
6. Gastric ulcers are usually small and singular, located at lesser curvature of stomach; duodenal ulcers are usually deep and occur at beginning area of duodenum near to pyloric sphincter
7. A Curling's ulcer is an acute stress ulcer that usually follows a severe illness (especially burns, trauma, surgery, shock, renal failure); tends to be multiple, superficial, and tends to erode several areas of gastric mucosa
8. Signs and symptoms
   a. Gastric ulcers: severe **pyrosis** (epigastric pain or heartburn); may radiate to back or flank; usually occurs during or immediately after a meal; food usually does not relieve pain
   b. Duodenal ulcers: right epigastric pain; radiates to back or thorax; often occurs when stomach is empty; food and antacids relieve pain

Practice to Pass

A client asks the nurse, "How can I prevent development of an ulcer? My father had lots of trouble with them." How should the nurse answer the client?

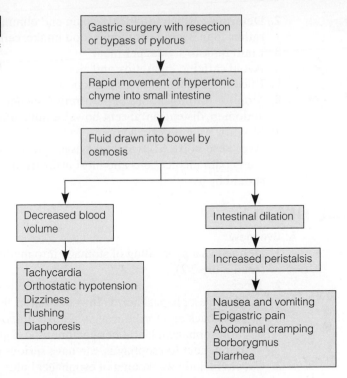

Figure 7-1

The pathophysiology of dumping syndrome

Gastric surgery with resection or bypass of pylorus

↓

Rapid movement of hypertonic chyme into small intestine

↓

Fluid drawn into bowel by osmosis

↓

Decreased blood volume

↓

Tachycardia
Orthostatic hypotension
Dizziness
Flushing
Diaphoresis

Intestinal dilation

↓

Increased peristalsis

↓

Nausea and vomiting
Epigastric pain
Abdominal cramping
Borborygmus
Diarrhea

c. Other: fullness after eating, nausea, vomiting, bloating, anorexia, gnawing type of pain; weight loss or weight gain (with duodenal ulcers because eating relieves pain); pain may come and go; **hematemesis** (vomiting up blood), **melena** (black, tarry feces because of presence of blood) or hematochezia (blood in stool)

C. Nursing assessment

  1. Assessment includes symptom analysis of pain; relationship of pain to food intake; any hematemesis or melena; use of NSAIDs, all medications taken at home; intake of alcohol or use of cigarettes; history of stress level

  2. Diagnostic tests: bloodwork for electrolytes, CBC (decreased RBC, hemoglobin, hematocrit), and presence of *H. pylori* antibodies; endoscopy; barium studies and upper GI (ulcer craters present); stool specimen (positive for occult blood)

D. Nursing management

  1. Medications

  a. H₂-blockers such as cimetidine (Tagamet), ranitidine (Zantac), famotidine (Pepcid) or nizatidine (Axid); may be administered without regard to meals

  b. Proton pump inhibitor such as omeprazole (Prilosec), lansoprazole (Prevacid), esomeprazole (Nexium), pantoprazole (Protonix), or rabeprazole (Aciphex); give 30 minutes before meals

  c. Mucosal barrier such as sucralfate (Carafate); give 30 minutes before meals

  d. Antacids to neutralize gastric acid (with exception of bicarbonate of soda)

  e. Cytoprotective agent such as synthetic *E. prostaglandin* (Cytotec) to promote mucus production for healing

  f. Antibiotics to destroy *H. pylori*

   1) Frequently this disorder can be treated by giving two antibiotics such as tetracycline hydrochloride (Achromycin) or clarithromycin (Biaxin) and metronidazole (Flagyl)

   2) Often recommended to give bismuth compound (Pepto-Bismol) with the antibiotics (but may make stools appear as melena)

2. Determine which foods cause pain and eliminate them; suggest 6 small meals daily rather than 3 large ones; limit food intake, caffeine, and alcohol late at night

3. Limit milk to 1 glass per meal

4. Avoid caffeine, cigarettes, and alcohol

5. Encourage rest and stress reduction

 6. Monitor for indications of perforation such as severe abdominal pain, rigidity in abdomen, distention, absent bowel sounds, and signs of shock

7. Monitor weight periodically

 8. Avoid use of NSAIDs and acetylsalicylic acid (aspirin) products; instruct client that many pain medications and most arthritis medications contain these agents and should be avoided

IV. HIATAL HERNIA

A. Overview

1. Defined as a protruding of stomach into mediastinal cavity by way of diaphragm (see Figure 7-2)

2. Types

   a. Sliding esophageal hernia (most common, 90%): herniated section of stomach slides back and forth through hiatus with position changes and increased peristalsis

   b. Paraesophageal hiatal hernia: fundus and greater curvature of stomach roll into thorax next to esophagus; can have serious complications

3. Causes include weakening of esophageal muscles due to aging, trauma, surgery or an anatomic defect; heavy straining or lifting

Figure 7-2

Two types of hernias.
A. Sliding esophageal hernia.
B. Rolling esophageal hernia.

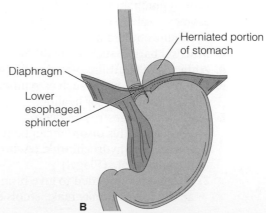

B. Pathophysiology

1. In a sliding esophageal hernia, there is gastroesophageal reflux caused by weakened esophageal hiatus muscles; this accounts for symptoms experienced
2. In a paraesophageal hernia, increased intrathoracic pressure occurs because of protrusion of thoracic contents by hernia

3. It may be asymptomatic, or signs and symptoms may vary according to type of hernia
   a. Sliding: dysphagia, pyrosis, regurgitation, bloating, and heartburn
   b. Rolling: shortness of breath, chest pain (similar to anginal pain), and tachycardia

C. Nursing assessment

1. Assessment includes symptom analysis of pain, vital signs (VS), complaints of shortness of breath, analysis of symptoms that would suggest angina versus GI pain (description of pain)
2. Diagnostic tests: upper GI, arterial blood gases (ABGs) if shortness of breath is experienced, CXR shows stomach in thorax

D. Nursing management

1. Medications include antacids, H_2-receptor blockers, analgesics
2. Monitor and educate about proper diet and taking 6 small meals rather than 3 large ones; advise weight reduction program if necessary

3. Educate client about head elevation for sleep and eating
4. Explain surgery if indicated

5. Discourage intake of alcohol, high amounts of caffeine, and cigarettes

V. CROHN'S DISEASE (REGIONAL ENTERITIS)

A. Overview

1. Defined as a chronic inflammatory condition of bowel; patchy areas of inflammation occur most commonly in ileum or colon, but may occur along entire GI tract; referred to as a chronic inflammatory bowel disease (IBD) and grouped with ulcerative colitis because symptoms are similar
2. Incidence is higher among young adults and adolescents; occurs equally in both genders; more often seen in clients of Jewish and Caucasian backgrounds

3. Develops slowly, with remissions and exacerbations; emotional factors related to family matters or work aggravate the illness
4. Cause is uncertain but may be multifactoral, probably involving an infectious process (bacteria, viruses, mycobacteria), allergy or immune disorder, psychosomatic, dietary, hormonal, and environmental factors

B. Pathophysiology

1. Inflammatory lesions may occur anywhere from mouth to anus; more often lesions occur in ascending colon and terminal ileum
2. Lesions are local and involve all layers of intestinal wall; wall contains shallow long ulcers with long or short areas of stricture
3. Lesions involve some areas of bowel but not all areas (called skip lesions)
4. Because of involvement of submucosal layers, mucosa has a granuloma (tumor-like growth) that gives tissue a cobblestone appearance
5. Bowel wall becomes congested, thickened, and may develop abscesses; fistulas may develop between infected area and bladder or other areas of intestine, resulting in malabsorption of nutrients (see Figure 7-3)
6. Scar tissue may interfere with movement of chyme and perforation or obstruction may occur

7. Complications caused by excessive diarrhea include fluid and electrolyte imbalance as well as dehydration; deficiency in absorption of folic acid, calcium, and vitamin D; anal fissures, perianal abscesses, fistula, and obstruction

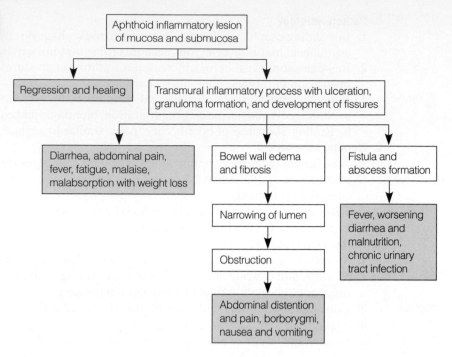

Figure 7-3

Pathophysiology leading
to the symptoms of
Crohn's disease

8. Signs and symptoms include nausea, vomiting, flatulence, malaise, weight loss cause by anorexia, 3–5 semisolid foul-smelling stools/day; intermittent, localized pain in right lower quadrant (worsening as disease progresses); mucus in stools with possible pus (blood may also be present); urgency at night to defecate; fluid and electrolyte imbalance, dehydration, fever, elevated WBC, iron-deficiency anemia, perianal abscesses and fistulas, and hypoalbuminemia

C. **Nursing assessment**

1. Assessment includes nutritional and fluid status, symptom analysis of pain and other symptoms, bowel pattern assessment, daily weight, activity tolerance, visual examination of stool, history of risk factors/stress level and emotional factors, VS, skin/nail color changes secondary to anemia

2. Diagnostic tests: CBC (elevated WBC, low RBC, Hgb, and Hct), barium enema (reveals characteristic "string sign," or skip lesions) colonoscopy, low albumin level, high erythrocyte sedimentation rate (ESR), electrolytes (hypocalcemia), folic acid level, possibly serum levels of vitamins

D. **Nursing management**

1. Medications include GI anti-inflammatory drugs such as sulfasalazine (Azulfidine), mesalamine (Asacol, Rowasa), or olsalazine (Dipentum); corticosteroids to decrease inflammation; analgesics to control abdominal pain; anticholinergics to control diarrhea; vitamin, mineral, and electrolyte replacements as needed; antipyretics if fever occurs; immunosuppressants

2. Attempt to control diarrhea since distended intestinal wall may lead to perforation; monitor temperature

3. Fluid replacement may be given to correct dehydration; monitor for symptoms of dehydration; TPN may be added if necessary to provide for nutritional needs while allowing GI tract to rest

4. Give low-residue, low-fat, high-protein, high-calorie diet

5. Instruct about lifestyle management to reduce stress

Practice to Pass

How should the nurse determine whether a client with Crohn's disease is becoming dehydrated?

VI. ULCERATIVE COLITIS

A. Overview

1. Defined as an inflammatory disease affecting mucous membranes of colon; affects part of or all of colon and rectum
2. Often occurs at ages 10–40; more common in those of Caucasian and Jewish backgrounds
3. Considered under general heading of chronic inflammatory bowel disease (IBD) along with Crohn's disease; disease has stages of exacerbations and remissions
4. Disease is labeled as mild, moderate, or fulminating
5. Disease is of uncertain etiology; suggested causes include a genetic basis, viruses, bacteria, autoimmunity, and stress

B. Pathophysiology

1. Ulcerated lesions form small erosions in mucosal layer; there are no skip lesions as in Crohn's disease; affects large bowel in a continuous pattern progressing from distal to proximal
2. These cavities may feature small hemorrhages and abscesses
3. Wall of bowel thickens and ulcerations are fibrotic in later stages of illness
4. Complications can include intestinal obstruction, dehydration, fluid and electrolyte imbalances, malabsorption and iron-deficiency anemia
5. Signs and symptoms include chronic, bloody diarrhea mixed with mucus (worsens as disease increases in severity); fever; weight loss; abdominal cramping and pain; nausea and vomiting; urge to defecate
6. Acute complications include hemorrhage, toxic megacolon, and colon perforation

C. Nursing assessment

1. Assessment includes bowel habits, visual inspection of stool, VS, recent or progressive weight loss, symptom analysis of pain, activity tolerance, bowel sounds, and nutritional status
2. Diagnostic tests: CBC (low RBC, Hgb, Hct), electrolytes (low potassium), colonoscopy, stool for occult blood

D. Nursing management

1. Medications include antipyretics; GI anti-inflammatory drugs such as sulfasalazine (Azulfidine); corticosteroids; antibiotics such as metronidazole (Flagyl); antidiarrheals; antispasmodics
2. Offer bulk-free diet and nutritional supplements as necessary; weigh client weekly, individualizing plan of care as needed
3. Offer psychological support and counseling
4. Monitor bowel sounds and bowel movements
5. Assess for signs of dehydration; monitor intake and output; administer IV fluids as ordered

VII. DIVERTICULAR DISEASE

A. Overview

1. Defined as *diverticula* or *diverticulum*: an outpouching of walls of colon; *diverticulitis*: inflammation of a diverticulum within intestinal tract; *diverticulosis*: condition of having diverticula within colon without any inflammation or symptoms
2. More common in clients over age 60 who eat a low-residue diet
3. May be *acute* (similar to appendicitis) or *chronic* (characterized by severe constipation and pain, distention, and flatulence)
4. Causes include severe constipation, obesity, inadequate dietary fiber or roughage

B. Pathophysiology
1. An increase in intraluminal pressure causes outpouching of colon wall; there is usually a weakness in intestinal wall from effects of diet
2. Bacteria from food that becomes trapped in pouches then causes diverticulitis
3. A lack of adequate blood supply or nutrients from diet may also contribute to development of this disease
4. Chronic diverticulitis may cause thickening of intestinal walls and possibly obstruction
5. Complications include rupture of intestinal wall leading to peritonitis; obstruction, and abscesses (rare)
6. Signs and symptoms include constipation, lower left-sided abdominal pain, signs of peritonitis (fever, guarding, abdominal rigidity); occasional rectal bleeding; diarrhea (not as common as constipation); elevated WBC; may be asymptomatic

C. Nursing assessment
1. Assessment includes: symptom analysis of pain and any other symptoms, VS, palpation of abdomen, auscultation of bowel sounds, bowel habits, any posturing
2. Diagnostic tests: ultrasound, colonoscopy, guaiac stool, barium enema, CT scan, flexible sigmoidoscopy

D. Nursing management
1. Medications include antidiarrheals and antispasmodics (occasionally), stool softeners, analgesics, antipyretics if fever occurs, broad-spectrum antibiotics for acute stage: metronidazole (Flagyl), ciprofloxacin (Cipro), or trimethoprim/sulfamethoxazole (Septra, Bactrim)
2. Monitor vital signs and treat fever as necessary

3. Encourage 2–3 liters of fluid per day unless contraindicated by another condition

4. Assess stools for color, consistency, frequency, presence of blood
5. Encourage rest periods and discourage lifting, straining, or bending
6. Offer high dietary roughage (fruit, vegetables, fiber)
7. Educate client about symptoms of disease and a lifestyle that can decrease these symptoms
8. Encourage cessation of smoking and alcohol use for general GI health

VIII. INTESTINAL OBSTRUCTION

A. Overview
1. Defined as inability of intestinal contents to progress through bowel in a normal manner; sites of blockage may be located in small intestine (high blockage) or colon (low blockage)
2. Classified as mechanical or paralytic obstructions
   a. *Mechanical* is caused by any condition that hinders patency of bowel lumen (tumors, adhesions); most common type overall
      1) A **volvulus obstruction** refers to a twisting of bowel and results in a large bowel obstruction; most common in elderly clients
      2) Intussusception is intrusion of a part of intestine into another part that lies distal to it; most common in infants 10–15 months
   b. *Functional* or *paralytic* (adynamic) is caused by neurogenic or muscular impairment that hinders peristalsis (postsurgery, prolonged bed rest)
3. Children most commonly have mechanical obstructions (especially younger than 2 years) rather than paralytic obstructions
4. Causes include intestinal adhesions, hernias, tumors, severe constipation, surgery, debilitated state with prolonged bed rest

B. Pathophysiology
1. Blockage of intestine (regardless of cause) leads to intestinal distention by gas and air, pooling of gastric and biliary secretions, and loss of fluids, electrolytes, and proteins

2. Distention caused by pooling of secretions leads to decreased absorption of water and electrolytes through bowel wall; vomiting and pooling lead to hypovolemia, dehydration, and ultimately hypovolemic shock
3. Impaired blood supply leads to increased peristalsis initially, ischemia and acidosis, bacterial invasion, and possibly subsequent necrosis and peritonitis
4. Cellular disruption and tissue hypoxia, along with stasis of secretions, provide an excellent medium for bacteria growth
5. Complications include fluid and electrolyte imbalances, gangrene of bowel, strangulation of a bowel segment, and perforation
6. Signs and symptoms include colicky pain, distention of bowel; bowel sounds may be **borborygmus** (rumbling sounds) initially, then change to hypoactive or absent; nausea and vomiting (bilious, feculent); anorexia; diarrhea or lack of bowel movement; abdominal tenderness, rigidity, fever; restlessness; electrolyte abnormalities; hypovolemic or septic shock may occur

C. Nursing assessment

1. Assessment includes bowel habits and patterns, symptom analysis of pain, bowel sounds, palpation of abdomen, visual inspection of stool, intake and output (I & O), nutritional status, VS and oxygen (O_2) saturation, abdominal girth
2. Diagnostic tests: CBC, electrolytes, abdominal x-ray, amylase level, barium enema, CT scan (use gastrografin if obstruction suspected; check for allergies), ultrasound of abdomen, ABGs

D. Nursing management

1. Medications include laxatives (oral or suppository), enemas, and electrolyte replacements as needed
2. Monitor bowel sounds and bowel movements; check for a fecal impaction and remove if possible
3. Measure I & O; weight, and amount of food consumed each meal
4. Provide privacy to have a bowel movement; offer air freshener
5. Decompression of bowel through a nasogastric or nasoenteric tube or surgical intervention may be needed
6. Postsurgery, encourage early ambulation and increased fluid intake
7. Monitor VS; provide IV fluids as ordered
8. Educate client about need to prevent constipation (use of natural laxatives, stool softeners, increased fluid intake, and increased activity)
9. Monitor use and frequency of opioid analgesics that decrease motility

> **Practice to Pass**
>
> An elderly female client presents with a distended abdomen, hypoactive bowel sounds, tenderness and pain upon palpation, and states her last bowel movement was 7 days ago. What changes could occur within the next few hours that would warrant immediate attention if the obstruction is not treated?

IX. APPENDICITIS

A. Overview

1. Defined as an inflammation of vermiform appendix
2. Occurs often in children and young adults ages 10–30 years; males are affected more often than females
3. May be acute (sudden, severe), chronic (follows an acute attack), or gangrenous (extreme inflammation); an appendix may rupture
4. Symptoms in females must be differentiated from ovarian cysts, ectopic pregnancy, and pelvic inflammatory disease
5. Causes include unknown etiology, obstruction of appendix from stool, or necrosis of organ

B. Pathophysiology

1. Appendix is attached to cecum just below ileocecal valve and normally is small, serving no known purpose
2. Obstruction of lumen can occur due to stool (**fecalith**—a hard piece of stool that is stonelike), tumors, parasites, or foreign bodies

3. Obstruction can lead to inflammation and bacterial invasion can occur
4. Occlusion of capillaries and venules leads to increased intraluminal pressure, decreased blood flow to mucosa, and hypoxic tissue
5. Gangrene can develop from thrombosis of luminal blood vessels, which may lead to perforation and possibly resultant peritonitis (infection of membrane that lines peritoneum or abdominal cavity)

6. Signs and symptoms include pain in right lower quadrant of abdomen that may localize at **McBurney's point** (halfway between umbilicus and right iliac crest); GI disturbances (anorexia, nausea, vomiting, diarrhea, or sometimes constipation); **rebound tenderness** (severe pain over area of tenderness when pressure is applied to appendix area and quickly released); posturing by lying on side or back with knees flexed; fever, elevated BP and/or heart rate caused by pain and fever; malaise
7. If a confirmed diagnosis of appendicitis is made and pain suddenly stops without any intervention, appendix may have ruptured; pain is lessened because appendix is no longer distended; surgery is still needed and is an emergency to reduce risk of peritonitis

C. Nursing assessment
1. Assessment includes VS, symptom analysis of pain, palpation of abdomen (rebound tenderness) until diagnosis is made, history of bowel movements, history of menses in women, and activity tolerance
2. Diagnostic tests: CBC (elevated WBC [note differential] with rupture), ultrasound, CT scan

D. Nursing management
1. Medications include IV antibiotics, analgesics for pain, and antipyretics for fever
2. Comfort measures until a diagnosis is confirmed; surgery is recommended treatment
3. Administer IV fluids in preparation for surgery if diagnosis is confirmed; in absence of rebound tenderness, IV fluids are given to confirm a possible GI virus (pain improves after fluids are given if etiology is viral)

4. Avoid enemas, cathartics, heating pads, or abdominal palpation with a confirmed diagnosis to prevent a rupture
5. Monitor vital signs, especially temperature

6. Administer standard postoperative care: turn, cough, deep breathing; early ambulation, assess bowel sounds, monitor urinary output, and provide wound care

X. PERITONITIS

A. Overview
1. Defined as local or generalized inflammation of peritoneum (lining that covers abdominal viscera)
2. May be primary (bacterial infection), secondary (trauma, surgical injury, chemical irritation), or as a complication of GI accessory organ disease
3. Caused by a ruptured appendix or peptic ulcer, diverticulitis, bowel obstruction, ruptured urinary bladder, infection from reproductive tract, or as a postoperative complication resulting in leakage from an intestinal anastomosis

B. Pathophysiology
1. Peritoneum is a semipermeable membrane; as an attempt to maintain homeostasis, fluid shifts may occur with third-spacing into peritoneal cavity; dehydration, decreased urinary output, hypovolemia, electrolyte imbalance, and even shock may occur
2. If secretions or chemical irritants leaking into peritoneum are sterile, irritation is primarily chemical; if they are infected, an intense inflammatory response is generated
3. Generalized peritonitis progresses to septicemia, which leads to septic shock and multiple organ failure; symptoms may be overlooked in an older adult client until condition is severe

Practice to Pass

A 15-year-old is brought to the emergency department reporting right lower quadrant pain and diarrhea. There are no other signs and symptoms present. What assessment and nursing intervention would help to rule out appendicitis?

4. Signs and symptoms include abdominal pain that is intense, often localized at site of involvement; chills and fever; anorexia, nausea, and vomiting; guarding and rigidity of abdomen; abdominal distention; diminished or absent bowel sounds; sweating, tachycardia, tachypnea; oliguria; restlessness, disorientation; elevated WBC; pallor; reduced urine output from dehydration

C. Nursing assessment
   1. Assessment includes symptom analysis of pain and other symptoms, VS, auscultation of bowel sounds, palpation of abdomen, urinary output, mental status, skin color, and nutritional assessment
   2. Diagnostic tests: CBC, electrolytes, abdominal ultrasound, BUN, creatinine, peritoneal aspiration with cultures, blood cultures, flat plate x-ray (supine and standing)

D. Nursing management
   1. Medications: antibiotics (after cultures are obtained); analgesics for pain control; potassium replacement if kidney function is adequate
   2. Replacement of fluid and electrolytes
   3. Monitor urine output and venous pressure
   4. Mechanical ventilation or monitoring of pulmonary artery pressure by a Swan-Ganz catheter may be necessary for severely ill clients
   5. Total parenteral nutrition (TPN) may be used for nutritional needs
   6. NG tube is often necessary for abdominal distention and reduced peristalsis; postoperative feeding may be done by jejunostomy tube if client is unable to take an oral diet
   7. Emotional support for both client and family is important
   8. Routine postoperative care, discharge planning, and referrals are essential

XI. NEOPLASMS OF GASTROINTESTINAL TRACT

A. Overview
   1. Defined as oral cancer (lips, pharynx, tongue, soft palate, and uvula); esophageal, stomach, or colon and rectum (colorectal) cancer
   2. **Leukoplakia** (white patches on mouth) and **erythroplakia** (red patches in mouth) are precancerous lesions that should be reported; ulcers on lips or in mouth that don't heal, as well as enlarged lymph nodes, should be investigated as possible harmful lesions
   3. Early diagnosis is essential in both oral and colorectal cancer for higher survival rates to be achieved
   4. Causes include tobacco and alcohol use; diet low in fiber, high in fat, and low in fruits and vegetables; genetic disposition

B. Pathophysiology
   1. Squamous cells in mouth are susceptible to developing squamous cell carcinoma; oral cancer spreads very rapidly because of rich vascular supply in mouth
   2. Esophageal tumors encircle esophagus and invade lymphatic system
   3. Stomach cancer includes adenocarcinoma occurring within pyloric region of stomach; spreads through lymphatic system and into other organs
   4. Most colorectal cancers are moderately differentiated adenocarcinomas; colorectal cancers tend to grow slowly; start in mucosa and most extend over a considerable amount of tissue before reaching lymph channel and metastasizing
   5. Signs and symptoms
      a. Oral: difficulty or pain in chewing, swallowing, or speaking; presence of a precancerous lesion or an ulcer in the tissue
      b. Esophageal: dysphagia, pulmonary complications, regurgitation, aspiration, or fistula formation

c. Stomach: loss of appetite, weight loss, gastric discomfort, weakness, and pain
d. Colorectal
  1) Right-sided (ascending): mild bleeding; weakness, fatigue, lack of energy; anorexia and weight loss
  2) Left-sided (descending): change in bowel habits such as going from diarrhea to constipation; small or pencil-shaped stools, gas or bloating, dark blood in stool or rectal bleeding; another complaint is a feeling of incomplete emptying on defecation
e. Anorexia, weakness, and weight loss are indications of any tumor growth; in advanced stages, tumor mass would be palpable

C. Nursing assessment
  1. Assessment includes changes in bowel habits, nutritional status, weight loss or gain, activity tolerance, palpation of abdomen, symptom analysis of any pain, inspection of any oral lesions (frequently can be palpated with a gloved finger before they are visible; any firm, asymmetric enlargement should be reported); visual inspection of stool specimen
  2. Diagnostic tests: guaiac test for occult blood, biopsy, colonoscopy or sigmoidoscopy, barium enema, CBC, liver function tests, CT scan/MRI, bronchoscopy, endoscopy, carcinoembryonic antigen (CEA), upper and lower GI series, coagulation panel

D. Nursing management
  1. Medications and other treatment
    a. Radiation and/or surgery is often the treatment recommended
    b. Chemotherapy may be given alone or in combination with radiation therapy and surgery
    c. Other: analgesics, antiemetics, stool softeners, antibiotics if indicated
  2. Client teaching: detection measures for any GI cancer, use of sunscreens, need for annual physical exam and to avoid potential risk factors such as smoking, tobacco, or snuff
  3. At age 40, a colonoscopy is recommended and then every 10 years, especially if a family history exists or a client has rectal polyps or diverticulosis; an annual guaiac test is recommended for clients over age of 50
  4. If surgery is performed, provide standard postoperative care
  5. Provide pain management
  6. Maintain patent airway after oral surgery
  7. Monitor nutritional status; provide good oral care; hydrate well after an endoscopy or GI series
  8. Provide emotional support and referral as needed for client and family
  9. After surgery for colorectal cancer, monitor bowel patterns closely (frequency, volume, and consistency) or provide ostomy care if created

XII. CELIAC DISEASE
A. Overview
  1. Defined as a chronic immune mediated disorder of small intestine triggered by ingestion of gluten containing grains, including barley, rye, and wheat
  2. Also known as *celiac sprue*, *tropical sprue*, and *gluten sensitive enteropathy*
  3. Manifestations often develop in childhood, but may develop at any age
B. Pathophysiology
  1. There is an inappropriate T cell-mediated immune response against the gliadin fraction of gluten, a cereal protein in foods ingested
  2. Immune response produces an intense inflammatory reaction, leading to loss of absorptive villi in small intestine, thus villi shorten and atrophy; if lesions become extensive, impaired absorption of macro- and micronutrients may occur

3. Small bowel involvement is most prominent in proximal small intestine, where exposure to gluten is greatest
4. Gastrointestinal malignancies and intestinal lymphoma are potential complications

C. **Nursing assessment**

1. Infants and young children commonly present with diarrhea, abdominal distention, failure to thrive, and possibly malnutrition; assess children for impaired growth, dental enamel defects, anemia, muscle wasting, vitamin deficiencies, and rickets
2. Adults classically present with diarrhea, abdominal pain, bloating and cramps or discomfort, and may manifest iron deficiency anemia, vitamin deficiencies, osteoporosis
3. Diagnosis is based on clinical manifestations, serological tests, and intestinal biopsy; manifestations often resolve when gluten is removed from diet
4. Fecal fat may be measured; it is increased in malabsorptive disorders
5. Immunoglobulin A antihuman tissue transglutaminase (TTG) and IgA endomysial antibody immunofluorescence (EMA) test show a high sensitivity; IgG and IgA antigliadin antibodies will be present; proximal small biopsy is indicated when antibody tests are positive

D. **Nursing management**

1. Removal of gluten and related proteins from the diet; severe nutritional deficits are treated with vitamin, mineral, iron, and folic acid replacement
2. Teach client about foods containing gluten (wheat, barley, and rye), and products which may become contaminated with wheat when processed, such as oats
3. Teach client to check food labels for gluten containing foods and hidden sources of gluten; dietary consult and teaching may be indicated
4. Lactose may need to be restricted to compensate for loss of lactase-containing microvilli

Case Study

A 34-year-old female is admitted who reports abdominal pain and diarrhea. She is very pale and emaciated. Her admitting diagnosis is rule out Crohn's disease.

1. What specific questions should the nurse ask her as part of the admission history?
2. What objective data should the nurse collect?
3. What information will be helpful regarding the client's social history? Why?
4. What nursing measures are important to prevent the complication of dehydration?
5. What other nursing interventions should the nurse anticipate providing?

For suggested responses, see page 464.

POSTTEST

1 A client presents to the clinic with "bad pain" in midabdomen, vomiting, and "not knowing what is wrong." Palpation reveals rebound tenderness with increased pain halfway between the umbilicus and the top of the pelvis. The client reports less pain when lying on the left side and flexing the knees. What is the best conclusion for the nurse to draw?

1. The client needs an enema to make sure client does not have an impaction.
2. Since client is vomiting, the problem is probably gastroenteritis.
3. Client should be checked for possible appendicitis.
4. Since client has been vomiting, nourishment may help.

2 A client with Zollinger-Ellison syndrome thinks she has a rare form of cancer. The nurse explains that this syndrome is characterized by which of the following?

1. Destruction of mucus-protecting cells of the stomach that could lead to an ulcer
2. Condition that causes increased secretion of pepsin and hydrochloric acid
3. Twisting of bowel that leads to intestinal obstruction
4. Crohn's disease, which is an inflammatory bowel disorder

3 A client who is exhibiting borborygmi, cramping pain, and diarrhea recently underwent gastric resection for severe peptic ulcer disease (PUD) that included the pyloric area. The nurse considers that the client is probably experiencing which of the following?

1. Dumping syndrome
2. Complications of the peptic ulcer disease (PUD)
3. Perforation of the stomach
4. Peritonitis

4 A client diagnosed with peptic ulcer disease (PUD) wants to know why antibiotics are being given. What is the best reply by the nurse?

1. "Antibiotics help to reduce the acidity of the stomach."
2. "Antibiotics decrease dumping syndrome, which can lead to peptic ulcer disease (PUD)."
3. "*H. pylori* is a bacterial cause for peptic ulcer disease (PUD), and antibiotics will treat the cause."
4. "The excess acid can be decreased when the stomach is sterile."

5 A client is being treated for peptic ulcer disease (PUD). The nurse anticipates prescriptions for which medications that might be used to decrease gastric acid content or protect the stomach? Select all that apply.

1. Proton pump inhibitors such as omeprazole (Prilosec) or lansoprazole (Prevacid)
2. Bismuth compounds (Pepto-Bismol) to stimulate mucosal bicarbonate
3. Nonsteroidal anti-inflammatory drugs (NSAIDs) such as ibuprofen (Motrin) to reduce the inflammation
4. Laxatives such as bisacodyl (Dulcolax) to prevent constipation
5. Sucralfate (Carafate) to form a barrier against acid and pepsin in the ulcer base

6 The nurse plans to monitor a client with celiac disease for which complication?

1. Anemia
2. Peptic ulcer disease (PUD)
3. Polyps
4. Renal failure

7 The nurse explains to the family of a 76-year-old client that older adults are more prone to developing diverticulitis for which reason?

1. Poor, deficient diet and constipation
2. Chronic diarrhea with resulting infection
3. Frequent use of stimulating laxatives
4. Sedentary lifestyle

8 The nurse should caution a client who has Crohn's disease and does not adhere to the treatment plan about the risk for which of the following health problems?

1. Perforation of the bowel
2. Cancer of the small intestine or colon
3. Peptic ulcer disease (PUD)
4. Ulcerative colitis

9 Prior to giving an analgesic for pain to a postoperative client who has a history of peptic ulcer disease (PUD), the nurse should check to see that the medication does not contain which of the following?

1. Codeine
2. Acetaminophen (Tylenol)
3. Acetylsalicylic acid (aspirin)
4. Hydrocodone

10 A client is admitted to the unit with a large, distended bowel, acute tenderness with abdominal palpation, fever, rigidity, and absent bowel sounds. Soon after admission, the client's level of consciousness decreases, and he begins to have feculent vomit. The nurse anticipates the need for what therapeutic interventions? Select all that apply.

1. Reduce fever through oral antipyretics.
2. Insert NG tube to suction and monitor the output.
3. Administer opioid pain medication for comfort.
4. Begin to prepare client for surgery.
5. Insert IV line to begin fluid administration.

➤ *See pages 203–204 for Answers and Rationales.*

ANSWERS & RATIONALES

Pretest

1 **Answer: 1** **Rationale:** Pain over McBurney's point, the point halfway between the umbilicus and the iliac crest, is diagnostic for appendicitis. Assessment for rebound tenderness would also assist in the diagnosis. Pain after eating may be associated with a gastric ulcer. Pain radiating to the back could reflect peptic ulcer, perforation of an ulcer, or pancreatitis. Pain in the left lower quadrant may be associated with diverticulitis. **Cognitive Level:** Applying **Client Need:** Physiological Adaptation **Integrated Process:** Nursing Process: Assessment **Content Area:** Adult Health **Strategy:** Consider the anatomical location of the appendix and determine where the pain should be felt. **Reference:** LeMone, P., Burke, K., & Bauldoff, G. (2011). *Medical-surgical nursing: Critical thinking in patient care* (5th ed.). Upper Saddle River, NJ: Pearson Education, pp. 664–666.

2 **Answer: 2** **Rationale:** Fever and diarrhea accompany diverticulitis. Fever indicates an infection, which would rule out peptic ulcer disease and irritable bowel syndrome. Appendicitis typically causes pain in the umbilical area or right lower quadrant and is not usually accompanied by diarrhea. **Cognitive Level:** Applying **Client Need:** Physiological Adaptation **Integrated Process:** Nursing Process: Diagnosis **Content Area:** Adult Health **Strategy:** Eliminate the incorrect options considering the fever, elevated white blood cells, and pain. **Reference:** LeMone, P., Burke, K., & Bauldoff, G. (2011). *Medical-surgical nursing: Critical thinking in patient care* (5th ed.). Upper Saddle River, NJ: Pearson Education, pp. 633–641, 664–666, 692–695.

3 **Answer: 4** **Rationale:** *Helicobacter pylori* causes release of toxins and enzymes that promote inflammation and ulceration. Gastric ulcers are not accompanied by fever. Ulcers are not spread from one person to another. Diet and stress can contribute to ulcer development, although they are not the primary causes. **Cognitive Level:** Applying **Client Need:** Physiological Adaptation **Integrated Process:** Communication and Documentation **Content Area:** Adult Health **Strategy:** Apply current knowledge of the pathophysiology of peptic ulcers. Look for the broadest answer. **Reference:** LeMone, P., Burke, K., & Bauldoff, G. (2011). *Medical-surgical nursing: Critical thinking in patient care* (5th ed.). Upper Saddle River, NJ: Pearson Education, pp. 633–641.

4 **Answer: 1, 4** **Rationale:** Factors contributing to hiatal hernia include weakening of the diaphragm muscle, either due to trauma, aging, or prior surgeries, as well as anything that places an increased intra-abdominal pressure, such as straining and heavy lifting. Dietary fat, young adult age, and use of nonsteroidal anti-inflammatory drugs (NSAIDs) do not predispose to hiatal hernia. **Cognitive Level:** Applying **Client Need:** Physiological Adaptation **Integrated Process:** Teaching and Learning **Content Area:** Adult Health **Strategy:** Recall specific information about hiatal hernias and factors contributing to their formation to choose the correct options. Note the wording of the question indicates that more than one option is correct. **Reference:** LeMone, P., Burke, K., & Bauldoff, G. (2011). *Medical-surgical nursing: Critical thinking in patient care* (5th ed.). Upper Saddle River, NJ: Pearson Education, pp. 627–630.

5 **Answer: 2, 3, 5** **Rationale:** Red blood in the stool is more characteristic of left-sided colon cancer, including the sigmoid colon. If blood occurs in the stool in right-sided colon cancer or gastric ulcers, it will be black and tarry. Bright red blood can also occur with hemorrhoids. **Cognitive Level:** Applying **Client Need:** Physiological Adaptation **Integrated Process:** Nursing Process: Diagnosis **Content Area:** Adult Health **Strategy:** Consider the appearance of digested heme or older blood. Where must bleeding be in order to be seen as red in the stool? **Reference:** Porth, C. M. (2011). *Essentials of pathophysiology.* Philadelphia, PA: Lippincott, Williams & Wilkins, pp. 700–726.

6 **Answer: 2** **Rationale:** Aspirin is one of the nonsteroidal anti-inflammatory drugs (NSAIDs). These drugs are predisposing or contributing factors in the development of a peptic ulcer, because of the effect on prostaglandins. Many medications used for arthritis may also irritate an ulcer; therefore, the health care provider should be consulted. Telling the client to take the aspirin places the client at risk and the alternative responses fail to address the client's concern. **Cognitive Level:** Applying **Client Need:** Pharmacological and Parenteral Therapies **Integrated Process:** Communication and Documentation **Content Area:** Adult Health **Strategy:** The treatment for one health problem may aggravate another condition. Comorbidities must be managed. **Reference:** LeMone, P., Burke, K., & Bauldoff, G. (2011). *Medical-surgical nursing: Critical thinking in patient care* (5th ed.). Upper Saddle River, NJ: Pearson Education, pp. 633–641.

7 **Answer: 4** **Rationale:** The client is exhibiting signs of peritonitis, which constitutes an emergent event. A history of a duodenal ulcer indicates a possible perforation, and IV access should be established and the primary care provider notified. If a client has a possible perforation, she should be in low Fowler's position to contain the secretions in the abdomen. Walking is not recommended, and food allergies are not likely to be the problem. **Cognitive Level:** Analyzing **Client Need:** Physiological Adaptation **Integrated Process:** Nursing Process:

Implementation **Content Area:** Adult Health **Strategy:** This is an emergency situation. What is needed most to support the anticipated emergency care? **Reference:** LeMone, P., Burke, K., & Bauldoff, G. (2011). *Medical-surgical nursing: Critical thinking in patient care* (5th ed.). Upper Saddle River, NJ: Pearson Education, pp. 667–670.

8 **Answer: 1** **Rationale:** This description of pain is consistent with ulcer pain. The pain is epigastric and is worse when the stomach is empty and is relieved by food. These symptoms are not common with cholelithiasis or gastrointestinal bleeding. Ordinary indigestion does not present with this clinical scenario. **Cognitive Level:** Applying **Client Need:** Physiological Adaptation **Integrated Process:** Nursing Process: Diagnosis **Content Area:** Adult Health **Strategy:** Consider the factors related to the timing of the pain, such as an empty stomach. **Reference:** LeMone, P., Burke, K., & Bauldoff, G. (2011). *Medical-surgical nursing: Critical thinking in patient care* (5th ed.). Upper Saddle River, NJ: Pearson Education, pp. 633–641.

9 **Answer: 2** **Rationale:** One form of intestinal obstruction is paralysis, caused by decreased movement of the intestinal contents by normal peristalsis. The client who smokes and consumes large amounts of caffeine is at high risk for Crohn's disease and ulcerative colitis. Eating a low-fiber, high-fat diet enhances the risk of cancer of the colon and diverticular disease. A client with cirrhosis is at risk for ascites and spontaneous bacterial peritonitis. **Cognitive Level:** Applying **Client Need:** Physiological Adaptation **Integrated Process:** Nursing Process: Assessment **Content Area:** Adult Health **Strategy:** Intestinal obstruction may be mechanical or functional—that is, from problems outside the intestine or from failure of peristalsis. What clients are at risk for either of these? **Reference:** LeMone, P., Burke, K., & Bauldoff, G. (2011). *Medical-surgical nursing: Critical thinking in patient care* (5th ed.). Upper Saddle River, NJ: Pearson Education, pp. 680–681, 667–670, 692–695, 711–715.

10 **Answer: 4** **Rationale:** Gastroesophageal reflux disease (GERD) causes epigastric pain usually described as burning; it is accompanied by belching with a sour taste, pain after eating, increased salivation, and flatulence. The symptoms of a sliding hiatal hernia are similar to GERD, but not those of a paraesophageal hiatal hernia. Symptoms of peptic ulcer disease are more pronounced and reflective of a full or empty stomach. Ulcerative colitis symptoms are related to pain and bowel movements. **Cognitive Level:** Applying **Client Need:** Physiological Adaptation **Integrated Process:** Nursing Process: Diagnosis **Content Area:** Adult Health **Strategy:** Eliminate options that present with different symptoms. **Reference:** LeMone, P., Burke, K., & Bauldoff, G. (2011). *Medical-surgical nursing: Critical thinking in patient care* (5th ed.). Upper Saddle River, NJ: Pearson Education, pp. 680–681, 622–626, 633–641.

Posttest

1 **Answer: 3** **Rationale:** Lying on the side with legs flexed, pain over McBurney's point, and rebound tenderness are characteristic symptoms of appendicitis. Vomiting frequently accompanies the pain. Administering an enema could be dangerous and stimulate rupture of the appendix. The client has more serious symptoms than those indicative of gastroenteritis, including rebound tenderness at a point between the umbilicus and pelvis. If surgery is needed for appendicitis, the client needs to be NPO. **Cognitive Level:** Analyzing **Client Need:** Physiological Adaptation **Integrated Process:** Nursing Process: Diagnosis **Content Area:** Adult Health **Strategy:** The findings described in the question are common characteristics of a problem. What organ is in the anatomic area where the pain is located? **Reference:** LeMone, P., Burke, K., & Bauldoff, G. (2011). *Medical-surgical nursing: Critical thinking in patient care* (5th ed.). Upper Saddle River, NJ: Pearson Education, pp. 664–666.

2 **Answer: 2** **Rationale:** Zollinger-Ellison syndrome is a condition usually caused by a gastrin-secreting tumor of the pancreas, stomach, or intestines that leads to the increased secretion of pepsin and hydrochloric acid. Peptic ulcer disease is often caused by destruction of mucus-protecting cells in the stomach. A volvulus is produced when the bowel twists upon itself, causing an intestinal obstruction. Crohn's disease is characterized by inflammation, not secretion of gastrin. **Cognitive Level:** Applying **Client Need:** Physiological Adaptation **Integrated Process:** Nursing Process: Diagnosis **Content Area:** Adult Health **Strategy:** The nurse must identify the description of Zollinger-Ellison syndrome. If the disease is unfamiliar, eliminate the options that describe diseases that are known. **Reference:** LeMone, P., Burke, K., & Bauldoff, G. (2011). *Medical-surgical nursing: Critical thinking in patient care* (5th ed.). Upper Saddle River, NJ: Pearson Education, pp. 633–641.

3 **Answer: 1** **Rationale:** Dumping syndrome is the rapid influx of stomach contents into the duodenum or jejunum after gastric resection, causing increased peristalsis and dilation of the intestines. The client has just had surgery to treat the peptic ulcer disease (PUD), so complications of PUD are not as likely to occur. The client would be experiencing profound pain and shock with perforation of the stomach. The abdomen becomes painful and rigid with peritonitis; bowel sounds are often diminished or absent. **Cognitive Level:** Applying **Client Need:** Physiological Adaptation **Integrated Process:** Nursing Process: Diagnosis **Content Area:** Adult Health **Strategy:** The clue event is the recent surgery. Review complications following gastric surgery. **Reference:** LeMone, P., Burke, K., & Bauldoff, G. (2011). *Medical-surgical nursing: Critical thinking in patient care* (5th ed.). Upper Saddle River, NJ: Pearson Education, pp. 633–641, 667–670.

4 **Answer: 3** **Rationale:** The bacteria *H. pylori* has been discovered to be the leading cause of many ulcers and can be treated with success by antibiotics. Antibiotics will not reduce stomach acidity. Dumping syndrome does not result in peptic ulcer disease (PUD). Creating a "sterile" environment in the stomach is not realistic and would not reduce acid production or secretion. **Cognitive Level:** Applying **Client Need:** Physiological Adaptation **Integrated Process:** Communication and Documentation **Content Area:** Adult Health **Strategy:** Review the actions of antibiotics if this question was difficult. **Reference:** LeMone, P., Burke, K., & Bauldoff, G. (2011). *Medical-surgical nursing: Critical thinking in patient care* (5th ed.). Upper Saddle River, NJ: Pearson Education, pp. 633–641.

5 **Answer: 1, 2, 5** **Rationale:** Proton pump inhibitors, histamine receptor blockers, sucralfate (Carafate), and bismuth compounds are all used to treat peptic ulcer disease (PUD). Nonsteroidal anti-inflammatory drugs (NSAIDs) are contraindicated because they block production of prostaglandins, which has a cytoprotective effect on gastric mucosa. Some drugs cause constipation, but laxatives are not routinely given to treat PUD. **Cognitive Level:** Applying **Client Need:** Pharmacological and Parenteral Therapies **Integrated Process:** Nursing Process: Planning **Content Area:** Adult Health **Strategy:** Choose the drugs that reduce gastric acid content or protect the gastric mucosa. **Reference:** LeMone, P., Burke, K., & Bauldoff, G. (2011). *Medical-surgical nursing: Critical thinking in patient care* (5th ed.). Upper Saddle River, NJ: Pearson Education, pp. 633–641.

6 **Answer: 1** **Rationale:** Celiac disease is characterized by an inability to metabolize gluten-containing foods, leading to inflammatory changes in the bowel and flattening of the intestinal villi. The client with celiac disease experiences malabsorption of nutrients, which can lead to fluid and electrolyte imbalances, anemia, nutrient deficiencies, and osteoporosis. **Cognitive Level:** Applying **Client Need:** Physiological Adaptation **Integrated Process:** Nursing Process: Planning **Content Area:** Adult Health **Strategy:** Recall the pathophysiology of celiac disease to determine possible consequences of the malabsorption that occurs. **Reference:** LeMone, P., Burke, K., & Bauldoff, G. (2011). *Medical-surgical nursing: Critical thinking in patient care* (5th ed.). Upper Saddle River, NJ: Pearson Education, pp. 696–698.

7 **Answer: 1** **Rationale:** A high-fiber diet reduces the risk of complications with diverticulosis such as development of diverticulitis. Older adults often eat less food with less roughage and fiber and therefore do not obtain the proper nutrients from their diet, which can aid in the development of the disease. Most often chronic constipation, not diarrhea, is a cause. Sedentary lifestyle may contribute to the constipation but is not a direct etiology. **Cognitive Level:** Applying **Client Need:** Physiological Adaptation **Integrated Process:** Teaching and Learning **Content Area:** Adult Health **Strategy:** Consider the relationship of diet and disease. Identify the opposite options. **Reference:** LeMone, P., Burke, K., & Bauldoff, G. (2011).

Medical-surgical nursing: Critical thinking in patient care (5th ed.). Upper Saddle River, NJ: Pearson Education, pp. 692–695.

8 **Answer: 2** **Rationale:** Clients with long-standing Crohn's disease have 4–5 times the risk of developing cancer of the small intestine or colon. Reducing complications and exacerbations of the disease can reduce this risk. Fistulas are common but perforation of the bowel is not. Although Crohn's disease produces an added stress, the risk for peptic ulcer disease (PUD) is not as great as cancer. Ulcerative colitis is a different type of inflammatory bowel disorder. **Cognitive Level:** Applying **Client Need:** Health Promotion and Maintenance **Integrated Process:** Nursing Process: Diagnosis **Content Area:** Adult Health **Strategy:** Consider the cell changes that result from chronic inflammation such as Crohn's disease. **Reference:** LeMone, P., Burke, K., & Bauldoff, G. (2011). *Medical-surgical nursing: Critical thinking in patient care* (5th ed.). Upper Saddle River, NJ: Pearson Education, pp. 681–684.

9 **Answer: 3** **Rationale:** A client with any GI disorder, especially a peptic ulcer, should not receive an analgesic that contains aspirin or a nonsteroidal anti-inflammatory drug (NSAID). Many pain medications contain aspirin or ibuprofen and are combined with an opioid analgesic. The nurse administering the pain medication should know what ingredients are in it. Hydrocodone and codeine are opioid analgesics and are acceptable if used singly or if combined with acetaminophen for a client with peptic ulcer disease (PUD). **Cognitive Level:** Analyzing **Client Need:** Pharmacological and Parenteral Therapies **Integrated Process:** Nursing Process: Implementation **Content Area:** Adult Health **Strategy:** What classification of analgesic is contraindicated in peptic ulcer disease (PUD)? That is the correct answer. **Reference:** LeMone, P., Burke, K., & Bauldoff, G. (2011). *Medical-surgical nursing: Critical thinking in patient care* (5th ed.). Upper Saddle River, NJ: Pearson Education, pp. 633–641.

10 **Answer: 2, 4, 5** **Rationale:** This is an urgent situation; the client probably has an obstructed or ruptured bowel. NPO status must be maintained because of the nonfunctioning GI tract and need to prepare for surgery. Opioid analgesics may mask worsening level of consciousness and are not indicated at this time. Inserting an NG tube will decompress the bowel, which may help relieve the vomiting and pain. Vomiting fecal matter can be dangerous (as well as unpleasant) because of the possibility of aspiration, especially with a decreasing level of consciousness. An IV line is needed if not already present. **Cognitive Level:** Analyzing **Client Need:** Physiological Adaptation **Integrated Process:** Nursing Process: Implementation **Content Area:** Adult Health **Strategy:** What actions are needed to manage this emergency situation? What is contraindicated? **Reference:** LeMone, P., Burke, K., & Bauldoff, G. (2011). *Medical-surgical nursing: Critical thinking in patient care* (5th ed.). Upper Saddle River, NJ: Pearson Education, pp. 667–670, 711–715.

References

Adams, M., Holland, L., & Bostwick, P. (2011). *Pharmacology for nurses: A pathophysiologic approach* (3rd ed.). Upper Saddle River, NJ: Pearson Education.

Ignatavicius, D., & Workman, M. (2010). *Medical surgical nursing: Critical thinking for collaborative care* (6th ed.). Philadelphia, PA: W. B. Saunders, pp. 1159–1297.

LeMone, P., Burke, K. M., & Bauldoff, G. (2011). *Medical-surgical nursing: Critical thinking in patient care* (5th ed.). Upper Saddle River, NJ: Pearson Education.

Lewis, S., Dirksen, S. Heitkemper, M., Bucher, L., & Camera, I. (2011). *Medical surgical nursing: Assessment and management of clinical problems* (8th ed.). St. Louis, MO: Elsevier.

McCance, K. L., & Huether, S. E. (2010). *Pathophysiology: The biologic basis for disease in adults and children* (6th ed.). St. Louis, MO: Mosby, Inc.

Osborn, K. S., Wraa, C. E., & Watson, A. (2010). *Medical surgical nursing: Preparation for practice*. Upper Saddle River, NJ: Pearson Education.

Porth, C., & Matfin, G. (2010) *Pathophysiology: Concepts of altered health states* (8th ed.). Philadelphia, PA: Lippincott Williams & Wilkins, pp. 700–726.

Wilson, B.A., Shannon, M.T., & Shields, K.M. (2012). *Pearson nurse's drug guide 2012*. Upper Saddle River, NJ: Pearson Education.

Hepatobiliary Health Problems

8

Chapter Outline

Objectives

➤ Define key terms associated with hepatobiliary health problems.
➤ Identify risk factors associated with the development of hepatobiliary health problems.
➤ Explain the common etiologies of hepatobiliary health problems.
➤ Describe the pathophysiologic processes associated with specific hepatobiliary health problems.
➤ Distinguish between normal and abnormal hepatobiliary findings obtained from nursing assessment.
➤ Prioritize nursing interventions associated with specific hepatobiliary health problems.

NCLEX-RN® Test Prep

Use the accompanying online resource, NursingReviewsandRationales, to test yourself with hundreds of NCLEX®-style practice questions.

Review at a Glance

ascites increased amount of fluid in abdominal cavity

bile a thick, yellow-green fluid secreted from biliary tract and duodenum; responsible for digestion of food, absorption of fats and fat-soluble vitamins, and stimulation of peristalsis

biliary cirrhosis cirrhosis characterized by a prolonged state of jaundice because of retention of bile and bile duct inflammation

cholecystitis inflammation of gallbladder

cholelithiasis condition in which there are stones present in gallbladder

cirrhosis scarring of liver tissue, which interferes with normal liver function and results in structural changes within liver

fulminant hepatitis necrosis and shrinking of liver, possibly resulting in liver failure; a complication of viral hepatitis

hemochromatosis a genetically transmitted disease where iron is excessively absorbed and accumulated

hepatic encephalopathy damage to brain tissue, which occurs as a complication of cirrhosis of liver caused by ammonia in brain tissue

hepatitis an inflammation of liver

jaundice yellow-tinged color of skin, body organs, or body fluids caused by abnormally high accumulation of bile pigment (bilirubin) in blood

nonalcoholic fatty liver disease fatty infiltration of liver that can lead to cirrhosis and end stage liver disease; not caused by alcohol ingestion

pancreatitis inflammation of pancreas

portal hypertension increase in pressure in portal vein caused by obstruction or congestion; a complication of cirrhosis of liver

splenomegaly an enlarged spleen

steatorrhea excessive elimination of fat; fatty stools

varices dilation of a vein that is usually tortuous

Wilson's disease an autosomal recessive disorder where ceruloplasmin is decreased, which leads to increased copper in several organs (liver, brain, kidney, and cornea)

PRETEST

1 The nurse is reviewing a client's liver biopsy report, which confirmed a fatty liver and the diagnosis of nonalcoholic fatty liver disease (NAFLD). The nurse checks laboratory data expecting to find elevation of which value?

1. Bilirubin
2. Triglycerides
3. Amylase
4. White blood cell count (WBC)

2 A concerned mother does not understand how her child acquired hepatitis A, when the child was perfectly healthy up to a week ago. The nurse identifies which characteristic of hepatitis A that may help her to understand the infection?

1. An incubation period of 60–180 days
2. A fecal–oral mode of transmission
3. A positive carrier state
4. A sexual mode of transmission

3 The nurse is analyzing the physical assessment findings of spider angiomas, palmar erythema, peripheral edema, ascites, and change in mental status of an assigned client. These findings are consistent with which disorder?

1. Cholelithiasis
2. Cholecystitis
3. Cirrhosis
4. Pancreatitis

4 A 45-year-old female hospitalized with acute pancreatitis has a prescription for morphine sulfate 8 mg IM every 3 hours prn for pain. The nurse explains that morphine has been prescribed for which reason?

1. It has a slower onset of action than oxycodone (Percocet).
2. It is less addictive than meperidine (Demerol).
3. The pain of acute pancreatitis is severe.
4. It has fewer cognitive side effects.

5 A 65-year-old female with a history of hepatic encephalopathy is hospitalized for pneumonia and dehydration. When she says that the portions of meat ordered by the dietitian are too small, what is the nurse's best response?

1. "Ask your health care provider about it in the morning."
2. "I will call and order larger portions for you."
3. "The amount of meat on your tray is dictated by certain blood test results."
4. "Your protein is being limited, but you can have more food that is not meat or protein."

6 A 55-year-old female with end-stage cirrhosis has a protuberant abdomen with bulging flanks and dullness to percussion on the dependent side while lying laterally. What terminology should the nurse use to document this assessment?

1. Fluid overload
2. Malnutrition
3. Ascites
4. Distention

7 The nurse is teaching a client who has been diagnosed with advanced pancreatic cancer. When the client asks the nurse why it was not diagnosed earlier, which responses by the nurse would be correct? Select all that apply.

1. "The onset of pancreatic cancer is usually insidious."
2. "Pancreatic cancer causes black tarry stools as a later sign."
3. "Pancreatic cancer presents with slow weight loss that might not be noticed immediately and jaundice."
4. "Pancreatic cancer often is diagnosed early and rarely metastasizes."
5. "The pain of pancreatic cancer is a dull epigastric pain that may not be reported right away."

8 When providing discharge teaching to a client with chronic cirrhosis, the spouse asks the nurse to explain why there is so much emphasis on bleeding precautions. Which response by the nurse is most appropriate?

1. "The liver affected by cirrhosis is unable to produce clotting factors."
2. "The low-protein diet will result in reduced clotting factors."
3. "The increased production of bile decreases clotting factors."
4. "The required medications reduce clotting factors."

9 A nurse sustained a needle stick injury with a client's used intramuscular needle. The nurse has previously had the 3 doses of hepatitis B vaccine but requests postexposure prophylaxis for hepatitis B. What advice should the occupational health nurse give to this nurse?

1. The nurse needs a booster vaccination to provide protection for this new exposure.
2. If the nurse's hepatitis B titer is positive, the nurse does not need prophylactic treatment.
3. The real risk is hepatitis A, which requires an immune globulin injection for prophylaxis.
4. An antiviral drug is needed for 6 months to prevent development of any type of hepatitis.

10 A male client with a history of alcoholism and long-time intravenous drug use has been diagnosed with primary liver cancer. He asks the nurse to explain the cause of his cancer. Which risk factors might fit this client's history? Select all that apply.

1. Chronic hepatitis C infection
2. Chronic hepatitis B infection
3. Drinking from the city's treated water supply
4. Alcoholic cirrhosis of the liver
5. Taking folic acid and vitamins as a dietary supplement

➤ *See pages 221–223 for Answers and Rationales.*

I. RISK FACTORS ASSOCIATED WITH HEPATOBILIARY HEALTH PROBLEMS

A. ***Cirrhosis***: alcoholism (primary); viral hepatitis, toxic reactions to drugs and chemicals, biliary obstruction, cardiac disease; **hemochromatosis** (a genetically transmitted disease where iron is excessively absorbed and accumulated); **Wilson's disease** (an autosomal recessive disorder where ceruloplasmin is decreased, leading to increased copper in several organs [liver, brain, kidney, and cornea])

B. ***Hepatitis***

1. Hepatitis A: drinking contaminated milk or water and consumption of shellfish from contaminated waters; children in day care centers and institutionalized adults are at increased risk

2. Hepatitis B: contact with blood or serum and oral or sexual contact
3. Hepatitis C: intravenous (IV) drug abusers, persons receiving blood transfusions, health care workers, persons on hemodialysis, those with high-risk sexual behavior, and organ transplant recipients
4. Hepatitis D: IV drug users and those receiving clotting factor concentrates
5. Hepatitis E: pregnant women in developing countries

C. **Cancer of liver**: persons with chronic hepatitis B infection, hepatitis C, or cirrhosis, and consumption of hepatocarcinogens in food such as aflatoxin in moldy peanuts

D. ***Cholecystitis***: diet high in fat content, cholelithiasis

E. ***Cholelithiasis***: aging process, family history, cirrhosis, Crohn's disease, sickle-cell anemia, hyperlipidemia, congenital malformation of biliary ducts, obesity and rapid weight loss, diabetes mellitus, drugs that reduce cholesterol, and total parenteral nutrition (TPN); other risk factors include Native American, Caucasian, or Mexican American ethnicity, and female gender (pregnancy or use of oral contraceptives)

    F. *Pancreatitis*: alcohol in men, gallstones in women, hyperlipidemia, hyperparathyroidism, viral infections, and abdominal trauma

    G. Cancer of pancreas: smoking (major risk); industrial chemicals, environmental toxin exposure, high-fat diet, pancreatitis, age, and diabetes mellitus

    H. *Nonalcoholic fatty liver disease (NAFLD)*: metabolic syndrome, high-fat diet, and elevated triglyceride levels

II. CIRRHOSIS

A. Overview

1. Cirrhosis is defined as scarring of liver tissue, which interferes with normal liver function and results in structural changes within lobes of liver
2. Characterized by structural and functional disorganization as a result of diffuse fibrosis and nodules of regenerated tissue
3. Four types of cirrhosis: alcoholic (formerly called Laënnec's cirrhosis), biliary, posthepatic, and cardiac
4. Causes of cirrhosis
   a. Alcoholic: consumption of a pint or more of alcohol per day
   b. Biliary: hepatotoxins, any obstruction of common bile duct, severe congestive heart failure (CHF)
   c. Posthepatic: results from chronic hepatitis B or C
   d. Cardiac: secondary to end stage heart failure

B. Pathophysiology

1. Alcoholic: associated with chronic alcoholism
   a. Alcohol is transformed to acetaldehyde, which begins to alter hepatocyte function
   b. Acetaldehyde inhibits removal of proteins from liver and alters metabolism of vitamins and minerals
   c. As large amounts of alcohol are consumed, fat accumulates in liver, known as "fatty liver"
2. **Biliary cirrhosis** is characterized by a prolonged state of bile duct inflammation and jaundice (late manifestation) because of retention of **bile** (a thick, yellow-green fluid secreted from biliary tract to duodenum; responsible for digestion of food, absorption of fat and fat-soluble vitamins, and stimulation of peristalsis)
   a. *Primary*: inflammation, destruction, fibrosis, and obstruction of intrahepatic bile ducts results in nodular regeneration and cirrhosis; women are more often affected than men; does not usually begin before age 30
   b. *Secondary*: inflammation and scarring of bile ducts occurs proximal to an obstruction caused by neoplasms, strictures, or gallstones
3. Posthepatic cirrhosis: fibrous, nodular scar tissue replaces necrotic tissue because of viral hepatitis B or C, drugs, toxins, or autoimmune disease
4. Metabolic and cardiac cirrhosis: inflammation and scarring, which is a result of defects or storage diseases; examples are antitrypsin deficiency, glycogen storage disease, Wilson's disease, and galactosemia; cardiac cirrhosis develops secondary to advanced heart failure; fluid backup from vena cava produces increased pressure and infiltration of hepatic tissue
5. Progression of disease
   a. Fatty infiltration results in inflammation, which in turn results in necrosis and fibrosis of liver, followed by regeneration and scarring
   b. Damage is increased if client has a poor nutritional state

   c. Normal structure of liver is lost and replaced by disorganized arrangement of scars and nodules
   d. Widespread scarring puts pressure on and obstructs blood vessels and biliary ducts

e. Increased capillary pressure causes increased fluid in abdomen and development of **portal hypertension** (increased pressure in portal vein caused by obstruction or congestion; a complication of cirrhosis of liver)

f. Decreased production of albumin results in decreased colloidal osmotic pressure; fluid leaves blood vessels and enters abdomen (third spacing)

g. Decreased metabolism of aldosterone results in sodium retention and increased fluid retention

h. Portal hypertension causes collateral blood vessels to develop in stomach, rectum, and esophagus; they become distended and cause **varices** (tortuous dilation of a vein); esophagus varices are irritated by alcohol and food causing rupture and excessive bleeding and hematemesis and melena (black, tarry-colored feces); bleeding is also aggravated by coughing, vomiting, lifting, or straining

i. Portal hypertension causes stasis of blood in splenic vein, which results in **splenomegaly** (enlarged spleen), and increased breakdown of white blood cells (WBCs) (leukopenia), red blood cells (RBCs) (anemia), and platelets (thrombocytopenia), and thus decreased defenses against infection

j. Decreased liver function results in inability to inactivate adrenocortical hormones, estrogen, testosterone, and aldosterone

k. Normally, ammonia is produced by bacteria and enzymes, which break down amino acids
   1) Ammonia goes to liver to be converted to urea and eliminated
   2) If liver is not functioning, ammonia is not broken down; it accumulates in bloodstream, crosses blood–brain barrier and goes into brain tissue, leading to **hepatic encephalopathy** (damage to brain tissue caused by ammonia in brain tissue); precipitated by any major hemodynamic insult to body such as bleeding, shock, toxins to body, hypovolemia, or anything that can increase metabolic needs on liver

6. Signs and symptoms of cirrhosis include weakness, fatigue, fever, anorexia, weight loss, nausea and vomiting (N/V), indigestion, flatulence, change in memory or level of consciousness (LOC), sexual dysfunction (loss of libido, change in menstrual pattern), gynecomastia, edema, ascites, bruising or hematoma, spider angiomas (a telangiectasis with a red, elevated center and small radiating blood vessels), palmar erythema (redness of palm), jaundice, dark urine, light-colored feces, enlarged liver and spleen, muscle wasting, decreased strength, insomnia

7. Signs and symptoms of hepatic encephalopathy include restlessness, change in LOC, inability to concentrate, altered sleep, forgetfulness, confusion, asterixis (flapping tremor of hands when extending arms), muscle twitching, and coma

C. **Nursing assessment**
1. Assessment includes vital signs (VS), bowel sounds, abdominal girth, dilation of abdominal wall veins, pulse quality, **ascites** (increased amount of fluid in abdominal cavity), sodium and water retention, peripheral edema, color, mental status, reproductive history, urine and stool color, weight, and gastrointestinal (GI) complaints
2. Diagnostic tests
   a. Labs: electrolytes, blood urea nitrogen (BUN), creatinine (CR), complete blood count (CBC), clotting studies including prothrombin time (PT), partial thromboplastin time (PTT), international normalized ratio (INR), arterial blood gases (ABGs), liver function tests (alanine aminotransferase [ALT], aspartate aminotransferase [AST], alkaline phosphatase, gamma-glutamyl transpeptidase [GGT]), bilirubin levels, protein, albumin, ammonia levels, glucose, cholesterol, and urine specific gravity
   b. Diagnostic studies: electrocardiogram (ECG), ultrasound (US) of abdomen, stool for occult blood, liver biopsy (to verify cirrhosis and only if necessary), esophagoscopy

D. Nursing management
  1. Medications
    a. Diuretics for ascites: spironolactone (Aldactone) is drug of choice and furosemide (Lasix)
    b. Lactulose (Chronulac) and neomycin (Mycifradin) to reduce high ammonia levels by metabolism of lactulose to organic acids by intestinal bacteria and decreasing pH of colon; a more acid pH converts ammonia to a nonabsorbable food so it is expelled in feces
    c. Ferrous sulfate and folic acid
    d. Vitamin K (Aquamephyton) to enhance clotting
    e. Antacids if gastritis is present
    f. Beta blocker such as nadolol (Corgard) with isosorbide mononitrate (Imdur)
  2. Avoid medications highly metabolized by liver such as barbiturates, sedatives, acetaminophen (Tylenol), and alcohol-containing products
  3. Monitor weight, abdominal girth, and peripheral edema daily
  4. Administer low-sodium, low-protein diet of 500–2,000 mg of sodium with restricted fluids; control protein to reduce ammonia and sodium to limit fluid accumulation
  5. Inspect skin integrity every 8 hours
  6. Be cautious about amount and frequency of medications administered (especially acetaminophen, barbiturates, sedatives, and hypnotics)
  7. Monitor neurologic functioning for early signs of encephalopathy
  8. Check VS every 8 hours
  9. Institute bleeding precautions
    a. Avoid manipulation of rectum, including prevention of constipation
    b. Avoid injections and coordinate timing of lab work to prevent excess venipunctures
    c. Assess and report ecchymosis and purpura
    d. Apply extra pressure for areas that begin to bleed
    e. Use a soft toothbrush and assess gums for bleeding
    f. Avoid harsh blowing of nose
  10. Position in high Fowler's with feet elevated, avoid supine position
  11. Monitor respiratory status and administer O_2 as indicated
  12. Use warm—not hot—water for bathing to reduce pruritus
  13. Institute skin protocols to prevent breakdown
  14. Be cautious in administering antihistamines for itching because of liver disease and impaired metabolism
  15. Priority nursing diagnoses are Excess Fluid Volume, Impaired Tissue Perfusion, Risk for Injury: Bleeding, Risk for Impaired Gas Exchange, Impaired Skin Integrity

E. Complications
  1. Portal hypertension
    a. Overview
      1) Defined as an abnormally high blood pressure in portal venous system
      2) Occurs when blood flow through portal system is obstructed or impeded due to thrombosis, inflammation, or fibrous changes in hepatic sinuses with cirrhosis or hepatitis; other causes are parasitic diseases and right-sided heart failure
    b. Pathophysiology
      1) Portal veins carry blood from GI tract, pancreas, and spleen to liver
      2) Blood then flows through liver, empties into inferior vena cava, and is delivered to right atrium
      3) Normal pressure in this system is 3 mmHg; with portal hypertension, pressure reaches 10 mmHg

Practice to Pass

How should the nurse determine if a client is developing ascites? What lab data are important?

4) Obstruction causes blood to back up into portal circulation and increase pressure; high pressure in portal veins causes collateral circulation to develop between portal veins and systemic veins

5) Decreased protein synthesis results in a decrease in albumin, which leads to edema and ascites

6) Long-term portal hypertension causes distended, twisted collateral veins; gradually these become transformed to varicosities

7) Major complication is hemorrhage

c. Nursing assessment

1) Assess abdomen for distention of collateral veins radiating over abdomen; hematemesis, melena; signs of shock (cool, pale skin, drop in blood pressure [BP], increase in heart rate [HR] and respirations) review history for jaundice, hepatitis, or alcoholism

2) Diagnostic tests: CBC, clotting factors

d. Nursing management

1) There is no effective medical treatment for portal hypertension, and nursing care is same as treatment of cirrhosis

2) Nursing diagnoses are Risk for Injury: Bleeding, Risk for Impaired Gas Exchange, Risk for Impaired Skin Integrity, and Imbalanced Nutrition: Less than Body Requirements

2. Esophageal varices

a. Overview: distended, tortuous collateral veins that occur from prolonged elevation of pressure; most commonly located in stomach and lower esophagus but may also be found in rectum: mortality from ruptured varices ranges from 30–60%, and many die within 1 year

b. Pathophysiology

1) Increased pressure in portal veins causes development of collateral vessels to occur between portal and systemic veins, where blood pressure is lower

2) Blood then bypasses obstructed portal vessels and is carried via collateral veins in esophagus, anterior abdominal wall, and rectum

3) First sign of esophageal varices is usually vomiting of copious amounts of dark-colored blood; ruptured varices do not cause pain and are usually precipitated by increased venous pressure and gastric acid

c. Nursing assessment

1) Assessment includes: hematemesis and melena

2) Diagnostic tests: CBC, clotting studies, type and cross-match

d. Nursing management

1) Medications include: vasopressin (Pitressin) to stop bleeding; beta blockers to lower portal BP; antacids; lactulose (Chronulac) or neomycin (Mycifradin) to decrease production of ammonia if caused by cirrhosis; vitamin K (AquaMephyton) for clotting

2) Ruptured esophageal varices are a medical emergency, and management includes compression with insertion of a Sengstaken-Blakemore tube; varices may be managed by injecting a sclerosing agent (sclerotherapy), banding of varices, or surgical construction of a portacaval shunt

3) Replace blood loss with administration of blood and IV fluids

4) Maintain patent airway

5) Monitor VS every 30 minutes

6) Use gastric lavage with cool saline to control bleeding

7) Monitor for signs of shock

Practice to Pass

A known client with alcoholism is admitted with a BP of 210/110, strong ammonia odor, tenderness in the abdomen, anorexic look, and reports eating only one meal per day containing less than nutritional foods. The client develops a GI hemorrhage and is treated for a GI bleed. Relate the signs and symptoms to alcoholic cirrhosis.

III. HEPATITIS

A. Overview

1. Hepatitis is defined as an inflammation of liver, usually viral in nature

 2. Known hepatitis viruses cause hepatitis A (HAV), B (HBV; causes large amount of liver damage), B-associated delta virus (HDV), C (also cause large amount of liver damage), E (HEV), F, and G (see Table 8-1 for overview of more common forms of hepatitis)

3. Each virus differs in mode of transmission, incubation period, degree of liver damage, and ability to create a carrier state

a. HAV and HEV are both spread by fecal–oral contamination; major sources of infection are inadequate hand hygiene, infected food handlers, contaminated food or water, and improper cleaning of utensils

b. HBV, HCV, and HDV are all spread by bloodborne organisms; control of contaminated needles, standard precautions for health care workers, and control of blood administration are primary means to control infection

c. Hepatitis F and G: less is known about transmission and mechanism of hepatic injury; hepatitis F is an enteric virus isolated from human stool, and hepatitis G is associated with acute and chronic non-ABCDE hepatitis; hepatitis G is transmitted parenterally

d. Depending upon cause, hepatitis can exist in either an acute or chronic form; chronic form results in cirrhosis

e. Causes other than viruses include hepatobiliary obstruction from gallstones or from toxic effects of alcohol, drugs, toxins, or infectious agents

B. Pathophysiology

1. Viral infections of liver create same pathologic lesions as in other parts of body; hepatic cell necrosis, scarring, Kupffer cell hyperplasia, and infiltration by mononuclear phagocytes occur in varying amounts and severity

2. Cytotoxic T-cells and natural killer cells become activated by immune response and promote cellular injury; hepatic cells begin to regenerate within 48 hours of injury

3. Distortion of normal structure of liver interferes with flow of blood and bile

Table 8-1	**Classification and Characteristics of Viral Hepatitis**				
	Hepatitis A HAV	**Hepatitis B HBV**	**Hepatitis C HCV**	**Hepatitis D HDV**	**Hepatitis E HEV**
Onset	Abrupt	Insidious	Insidious	Abrupt	Abrupt
Transmission	Fecal–oral	Blood and body fluids	Blood and body fluids	Blood and body fluids; perinatal	Fecal-oral
Incubation Period	2–6 weeks	6 weeks to 4 months	2–12 weeks	1–6 months	3 weeks to 2 months
Antibody-Antigens	Anti-HAV*	Anti-HBs, HBsAg⁺	Anti-HCV (indicates infection, no confirmation of immunity), +HCV RNA	Anti-HDV*, HDVAg⁺	Anti-HEV*
Carrier State	No	Yes	Yes	Yes	No
Post-Exposure Treatment	Gamma globulin	Hepatitis B immune globulin	None available	Immune globulin	Gamma globulin does not offer protection
Vaccination	Immune globulin HAV vaccine	HBV vaccine	None	HBV vaccine	None

*Demonstrates immunity⁺
Presence of this antigen signifies acute infection or carrier state

4. Obstruction of portal and hepatic blood flow increases portal pressure causing engorgement, hepatomegaly, and splenomegaly

5. Cholestasis and obstructive **jaundice** (yellow-tinged color of skin, body organs, or body fluids caused by abnormally high accumulation of bile [bilirubin] in blood) are a result of inflammatory effect on bile canaliculi

6. Signs and symptoms are specific to stages
   a. Preicteric stage (before jaundice occurs): malaise, fatigue, N/V, diarrhea, anorexia (and aversion to food, especially protein and fat), enlarged liver and lymph nodes, electrolyte imbalances; conjunctivitis; skin rash; pain (headache, muscle aches, painful joints, fever, and sore throat)
   b. Icteric stage (onset of jaundice): jaundice, pruritus, light-colored stools, brown urine, malaise, preicteric symptoms improve or subside
   c. Posticteric stage (convalescent phase): decrease in fatigue, appetite returns to normal, laboratory work improves, and pain subsides

7. A complication of hepatitis is **fulminant hepatitis** (necrosis and shrinking of liver, possibly resulting in liver failure): develops 6–8 weeks after initial symptoms, anorexia, vomiting, abdominal pain, progressive jaundice followed by ascites, GI bleeding, lethargy, disorientation, and coma develop; mortality rate is high

C. Nursing assessment

1. Assessment
   a. Preicteric: assess for energy level; nutritional status; GI complaints; genitourinary (GU) patterns; presence of any pain; palpate liver and lymph nodes; VS
   b. Icteric phase: assess skin for color and integrity; stools and urine characteristics; VS; GI symptoms; nutritional status
   c. Posticteric: assess for improvement in all laboratory results and symptoms

2. Diagnostic tests
   a. Preicteric stage: abnormal electrolytes, elevated liver function tests (AST, ALT, alkaline phosphatase [ALP]); virus and antibodies present in serum
   b. Icteric stage: elevated total, conjugated, and unconjugated serum bilirubin; bilirubinuria in urinalysis
   c. Posticteric stage: normalizing serum bilirubin and enzymes; elevated serum antibodies
   d. Other diagnostic tests
      1) Hepatitis A: anti-HAV (antibody to HAV demonstrates immunity); IgM anti-HAV (antibody to HAV in recent infections to 6 months)
      2) Hepatitis B: HBsAG (hepatitis B surface-antigen indicating active disease); HBeAg (antigen in chronic carriers of hepatitis B); anti-HBs (immunity following hepatitis B vaccine); anti-HBc-IgM (indicates core infection in hepatitis B)
      3) Hepatitis C: anti-HCV (antibody found in hepatitis C clients that indicates an infection but not necessarily immunity)
      4) Hepatitis D: HDAg (antigen in acute infection); anti-HDV (antibody found in hepatitis D)

D. Nursing management

1. Medications for symptom control: antiemetics for nausea; antihistamines such as diphenhydramine (Benadryl), dimenhydrinate (Dramamine) or trimethobenzamide (Tigan) for itching; and emollient skin creams and lotions

2. Avoid acetaminophen (Tylenol), prochlorperazine (Compazine), or other drugs detoxified in liver

3. Eliminate risk for infection (transmission): standard precautions and meticulous hand hygiene are essential to prevent transmission of hepatitis A and E

Practice to Pass

A client asks, "How can I keep from developing hepatitis B?" What should the nurse tell him?

!▸ 4. Diet should consist of 16 carbohydrate kcal/kg of ideal body weight; calories should be consumed in morning hours since most clients are nauseated by afternoon and evening; decrease fat content as fat is generally not appetizing

5. Monitor fluid and electrolytes
6. Prevent skin breakdown and avoid use of hot water for bathing
7. In fulminant hepatitis, protein is restricted
8. Supportive care with rest and gradual return to normal activities

!▸ 9. Prevention for health care workers includes use of standard precautions, meticulous hand hygiene, and hepatitis A and B vaccines

IV. NONALCOHOLIC FATTY LIVER DISEASE

A. Overview

1. A fatty liver disease that can progress to cirrhosis and end-stage liver disease
2. Ranges from a simple steatosis (fatty infiltration of liver) to steatohepatitis (fatty infiltration with inflammation and hepatocyte necrosis); the latter is often referred to as NASH, or nonalcoholic steatohepatitis

B. Pathophysiology

1. Obesity increases synthesis and reduces oxidation of free fatty acids
2. Type 2 diabetes or insulin resistance increases adipose tissue lipolysis and production of free fatty acids
3. When liver's capacity to export triglyceride is exceeded, excess fatty acids contribute to development of steatosis and fatty liver disease
4. Alcohol must be excluded as a cause to determine diagnosis

C. Nursing assessment

1. May be asymptomatic
2. Fatigue, right upper quadrant discomfort
3. Elevated triglyceride levels noted on lipid panel
4. Mild to moderately elevations in AST, and/or ALT levels is common; hypoalbumininemia, prolonged PT, and hyperbilirubinemia may be present
5. Liver biopsy may be done to confirm diagnosis

!▸ D. Nursing management

1. Stress to client changes needed to slow progression of liver disease
2. Encourage weight loss and exercise to alleviate insulin resistance; reduce intake of calorie dense foods, including simple sugars and processed foods
3. Teach client to avoid alcohol (although not a cause, alcohol will exacerbate condition)

V. CANCER OF LIVER

A. Overview

1. Defined as metastatic carcinoma or primary neoplasm of liver
2. Liver cancer as a primary site is not common in United States, but frequently metastasis occurs from pulmonary, breast, and GI primary sites
3. Primary cancers arise from bile duct in 10% of cases; alcohol-induced cirrhosis and hepatitis A or B account for most primary liver cancers in United States
4. Causes include chronic cirrhosis, vinyl chloride exposure, inorganic arsenic, aflatoxins, nitrosamines, pesticides, prolonged androgen therapy, and contraceptive steroids

B. Pathophysiology

1. Major types
   a. Hepatocellular carcinoma, arising from liver cells
   b. Cholangiocarcinoma, primary cancer of cells of bile duct

2. Hepatocellular carcinoma is classified as nodular, massive, or diffuse
3. Metastasis to heart, lung, brain, kidney, and spleen is rapid because of invasion of hepatic and portal veins
4. Benign tumors of liver are adenomas often affecting women and related to oral contraceptives
5. Manifestations are usually related to effects of tumor or functional changes in liver
   a. Bile products are secreted because of secretion of substances by tumors
   b. Tumor secretes hormones that lead to polycythemia, hypoglycemia, and hypercalcemia
   c. Obstruction of biliary system leads to jaundice, portal hypertension, ascites
   d. Impairment of hepatocytes results in metabolic disturbances
   e. Invasion of tumor into liver, which is often inoperable, causes hepatomegaly, hemorrhage, and liver failure
   f. Other signs and symptoms
      1) GI: N/V, fullness, pressure, and dull ache in right upper abdomen, anorexia, malaise, fever of unknown origin (FUO)
      2) Pain from enlarging tumor
      3) Debilitation, weight loss, cachexia
      4) Symptoms of cirrhosis

C. **Nursing assessment**
1. Assessment includes presence of GI symptoms, pain, weight, nutritional status, fluid status (I & O), abdominal girth, and presence of bleeding
2. Diagnostic tests: magnetic resonance imaging (MRI), computed tomography (CT) scans, US, and alpha-fetoprotein serum markers (specific to detecting hepatocellular carcinoma)

D. **Nursing management**
1. Medications include narcotics and analgesics for pain; chemotherapeutic agents [5-fluorouracil (5-FU), methotrexate (MTX), doxorubicin (Adriamycin)]
2. There is no cure; palliative care is the goal
3. Monitor for and prevent infection
4. Inspect skin and prevent breakdown
5. Manage pain and instruct client to ask for pain medication prior to onset of severe pain
6. Offer support for client and family for grief and coping

VI. CHOLELITHIASIS

A. **Overview**
1. Cholelithiasis is defined as a formation of stones in biliary duct system or gallbladder
2. Approximately 10–20% of men and 20–40% of women are affected
3. Causes include obesity, oral contraceptives and estrogen therapy, family history, diseases (cirrhosis, Crohn's disease, hyperlipidemia, diabetes mellitus), or TPN

B. **Pathophysiology**
1. Gallstones form when cholesterol and calcium precipitate as solid crystals within mucous lining of gallbladder; process is enhanced by delayed gallbladder emptying
2. If gallstone obstructs cystic duct, acute cholecystitis occurs
3. Manifestations result from presence and location of stones (see Figure 8-1)
   a. Stones lodged in cystic duct cause distention of gallbladder and colicky pain (severe, cramplike)
   b. Pain may radiate to subscapular area

Practice to Pass

A client with cholelithiasis is admitted to the medical-surgical unit. What nursing diagnoses are appropriate for the plan of care and what specific interventions would be necessary to institute?

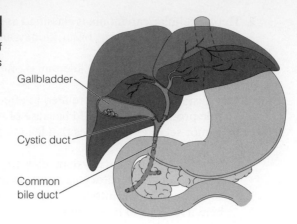

Figure 8-1

Common location of gallstones

Gallbladder

Cystic duct

Common bile duct

    c. Obstruction of common bile duct causes reflux of bile into liver and jaundice

    d. Other symptoms include N/V, epigastric pain, heartburn, and intolerance to fat-containing foods

C. Nursing assessment

    1. Assessment includes pain, color, stool characteristics, nutritional status, GI symptoms (epigastric pain, heartburn, N/V, right upper abdominal pain)

    2. Diagnostic tests: serum bilirubin (direct bilirubin elevated if biliary ducts involved, indirect bilirubin elevated if liver damage occurs), alkaline phosphatase (elevated), cholangiography or radioactive gallbladder scan, US of gallbladder

D. Nursing management

    1. Medications include: oral bile acids or dissolvers: ursodiol (Actigall) and chenodiol (Chenix); analgesics such as morphine sulfate; cholestyramine (Questran) for pruritis

    2. Clients should be taught to avoid high-fat foods because these stimulate gallbladder contractions: avoid whole-milk products, fried foods, nuts, gravies, cooking oils, hot dogs, chocolate, and cheese

    3. Obese or overweight clients should be instructed in weight loss

    4. Goal is to reduce inflammation and blockage

VII. CHOLECYSTITIS

A. Overview

    1. Cholecystitis is defined as an inflammation of cystic duct caused by lodging of a gallstone in duct

    2. May be acute or chronic

    3. Causes: cholelithiasis; or trauma, fasting, TPN, or surgery in absence of cholelithiasis

B. Pathophysiology

    1. A lodged gallstone in cystic duct exerts pressure against wall of gallbladder, decreasing blood flow

    2. Ischemia follows with possibility of necrosis and perforation of gallbladder

    3. Chemical irritation from obstruction or presence of a bacterial infection prevents outflow of bile from gallbladder

    4. Signs and symptoms include pain that suddenly or gradually develops (classically in back or right shoulder), fever, N/V, jaundice, clay-colored stools, intolerance to fat-containing foods, epigastric pain, heartburn

C. Nursing assessment

    1. Assessment includes rebound tenderness, VS, abdominal muscle guarding, GI distress (epigastric pain, heartburn, N/V, right upper quadrant abdominal pain), skin color, stool characteristics, and nutritional status

2. Diagnostics tests: serum bilirubin (direct bilirubin elevated if biliary ducts involved, indirect bilirubin elevated if liver damage), alkaline phosphatase (elevated), serum amylase (normal unless pancreas involved), CBC (elevated WBC), electrolytes, cholangiography or radioactive scan, gallbladder US

D. Nursing management
1. Medications such as oral bile acids or dissolvers (ursodiol [Actigall] and chenodiol [Chenix]); antibiotics, antipyretics; analgesics such as morphine sulfate; cholestyramine (Questran) for pruritis
2. Assist clients to avoid whole-milk products, fried foods, nuts, gravies, cooking oils, hot dogs, chocolate, and cheese
3. Explain need for weight loss for obese or overweight clients
4. For clients undergoing surgery, focus on Deficient Knowledge, both pre-and postoperatively; other nursing diagnoses include Pain, Risk for Impaired Gas Exchange, and Risk for Infection
5. Teaching for home care
   a. Nonsurgical intervention focuses on diet management and instructions for stone-dissolving medications; include information about function of gallbladder and purpose of bile

   b. Teaching for postoperative client is focused upon pain control, monitoring for infection, eating low-fat foods, and managing a T-tube by:
      1) Ensuring patency of tube
      2) Monitoring amount of drainage: as much as 500 mL within first 24 hours, 200 mL the next 2 to 3 days, and minimal after that
      3) Maintaining a Fowler's position to promote drainage
      4) Assessing skin around tube for integrity
      5) Assisting and teaching client to ambulate with tube
      6) Monitoring for signs of infection

VIII. PANCREATITIS

A. Overview
1. Pancreatitis is defined as an inflammation of pancreas
2. Classification
   a. Acute: necrosis, suppuration (abscesses), gangrene, and hemorrhage occurs
   b. Chronic: scar tissue forms that interferes with organ function
3. Causes
   a. Alcoholism (excessive intake of liquor or wine for 6 years or more)
   b. Biliary (obstruction of pancreatic duct by a gallstone)
   c. Other: high triglyceride levels, hypercalcemia, or infections

B. Pathophysiology
1. Acute

   a. When pancreas is injured and/or function is disrupted, pancreatic enzymes (phosopholipase A, lipase, and elastase) leak into pancreatic tissue and initiate autodigestion
   b. Trypsin and elastase are activated proteolases and along with lipases, break down tissue and cell membranes, resulting in edema, vascular damage, hemorrhage and necrosis
   c. Fibrous changes to pancreatic tissue causes exocrine and endocrine changes with loss of function of islets of Langerhans (which secrete insulin), resulting in diabetes mellitus
   d. Multiple-organ failure and mortality occurs when toxic enzymes are released into bloodstream and distributed by vessels into major organs
      1) Activation of kinin occurs, resulting in vasodilation
      2) Increased stickiness of leukocytes occurs, causing emboli

        3) Coagulopathy occurs, which causes disseminated intravascular coagulopathy (DIC)

        4) Increased permeability causes movement of fluid and circulatory insufficiency

        5) Myocardial depressant factor (MDF) is released, which decreases cardiac function

        6) Activation of renin-angiotensin system decreases kidney function as a result of decreased renal perfusion

    e. Types

        1) Acute interstitial: pancreas and surrounding tissue are engorged with interstitial fluid; this form may progress to hemorrhagic

        2) Acute hemorrhagic: bleeding into gland and other structures occurs

2. *Chronic*: a structural or functional impairment of pancreas, most commonly associated with chronic alcohol abuse

    a. Chronic form is irreversible with connective tissue replacing pancreatic tissue

    b. Pancreatic cysts are common lesions found in chronic pancreatitis, which are walled-off pockets of pancreatic juice, necrotic debris, or blood

    c. Types

        1) Chronic calcifying pancreatitis is associated with alcoholism; alcohol causes spasm of sphincter of Oddi, which blocks passage of secretions out of pancreas; enzymes then pass into pancreas, leading to autodigestion of pancreatic tissue

        2) Chronic obstructive pancreatitis is associated with gallstones in women

3. Signs and symptoms

    a. Acute pancreatitis

        1) Sudden onset of severe epigastric and abdominal tenderness and pain that radiates to back; may be relieved by sitting up and leaning forward, flexing left leg or by walking; may be initiated by fatty meal or excessive alcohol intake

        2) GI: N/V and distention

        3) Cardiac: tachycardia, hypotension

        4) Other: anxiety, weakness, pallor, fever, decreased bowel sounds, and cold, clammy skin; mild jaundice may occur within 24 hours of acute symptoms, retroperitoneal bleeding after 3–6 days

    b. Chronic pancreatitis

        1) Left upper abdominal pain radiating to back

        2) GI: N/V, weight loss, flatulence, constipation, **steatorrhea** (excessive elimination of fat, fatty stools), malabsorption

C. Nursing assessment

1. Assessment includes symptom analysis of pain, GI complaints, nutritional status, energy level, stool characteristics, VS, skin color, bleeding—positive Turner's sign (flank bruising) or Cullen's sign (umbilical bruising)

2. Diagnostic tests

    a. Acute: elevated serum amylase, serum lipase: decreased serum calcium

    b. Chronic: elevated serum bilirubin and serum and urinary amylase levels

D. Nursing management

1. Medications: pancreatic enzyme replacement such as pancrelipase (Lipancreatin), opioid analgesics such as morphine sulfate, antibiotics, antacids, H$_2$-blockers such as ranitidine (Zantac) or famotidine (Pepcid), proton pump inhibitors such as omeprazole (Prilosec), carbonic anhydrase inhibitor such as acetazolamide (Diamox), antispasmodics such as dicyclomine (Bentyl), antiemetics, and antipyretics

2. Assess and reassess pain at regular intervals for location, radiation, duration, character, and intensity

3. Maintain nothing by mouth (NPO) status (3–7 days) in order to reduce gastric secretions and aggravation of pancreatic pain; gastric suction may be ordered to minimize secretions

4. Decrease physical movement and mental stimulation to minimize gastric secretions and pain
5. Provide moisture to dry mucous membranes, which result from NPO status
6. Prevent visualization of food since gastric secretions are stimulated by sight of food
7. Encourage a position of comfort, which is elevation of head at 45 degrees, side lying with knees flexed
8. Daily weight
9. Assess bowel sounds
10. Assess cardiovascular status at regular intervals, monitor VS
11. Assess respiratory function at regular intervals because abdominal pain causes shallow respirations; pleural effusion is also a complication of pancreatitis
12. IV fluid replacement with electrolytes and possibly TPN
13. IV albumin may be needed to combat third-spacing
14. Monitor O_2 saturation

IX. CANCER OF PANCREAS

A. Overview
1. Defined as tumors of pancreas that are ductal adenocarcinomas; nearly all cases are fatal; 70% of tumors are located in pancreatic head, 20% in body of pancreas, and 10% in tail
2. Causes include longstanding diabetes mellitus, chronic pancreatitis, and smoking; it is not associated with coffee, alcoholism, and cholelithiasis

B. Pathophysiology
1. Pancreatic cancer has a slow onset and is usually not detected until tumor has spread
2. Cancer of head of pancreas obstructs bile flow while tumors in body of pancreas press on celiac ganglion
3. Cancer cells often invade stomach, duodenum, bile duct, colon, spleen, kidney, and major blood vessels
4. Signs and symptoms

   a. Common symptoms: weight loss, anorexia, N/V, flatulence, epigastric pain, malaise, diarrhea and constipation, palpable abdominal mass, hematemesis, and melena
   b. Cancer of head of pancreas specifically causes jaundice (from biliary obstruction), clay-colored stools, dark urine, and pruritus
   c. Cancer in tail of pancreas may cause no symptoms until metastasis has occurred
   d. Tumors in body of pancreas may cause pain and nausea during eating or when lying supine

C. Nursing assessment
1. Assessment includes weight, GI symptoms, pain, stool and urine characteristics, skin color, fluid and electrolyte status, nutritional status, energy level
2. Diagnostic tests: carcinoembryonic antigen (elevated), bilirubin levels (increased), urine urobilinogen (decreased), alkaline phosphatase (elevated), ultrasonography

D. Nursing management
1. Medications: opioid analgesics and antiemetics
2. Client may be a candidate for Whipple procedure (surgical removal of head of pancreas, entire duodenum, one-third of stomach, part of jejunum, and lower-half of common bile duct with restructuring of pancreas, stomach, and common bile duct); postoperative care is similar to any abdominal surgery and demands special attention to
   a. Pain management
   b. Respiratory expansion
   c. Monitoring of complications related to oxygenation

    d. Renal function
    e. Level of consciousness
    f. Blood chemistries
  3. Have dietitian evaluate client's needs, especially during NPO status
  4. Palliative care if appropriate (terminally ill client)

Case Study

M. S. is a 55-year-old female presenting as a hospital admission for surgery in the morning. She is a divorced mother of 3 adult children and has smoked 1 pack of cigarettes daily for 30 years. In the past month, she has lost 20 pounds, cannot sleep lying on her back, and is unable to tolerate solid foods. The client became jaundiced in the past 48 hours and computed tomography (CT) scan confirmed a mass in the pancreas.

1. What are the primary risk factors present for pancreatic cancer?

2. Where is the likely location of the tumor based upon the client's symptoms?

3. What are the primary preoperative nursing interventions?

4. What are the primary postoperative nursing interventions?

5. What is the likely prognosis for this client?

For suggested responses, see page 464.

POSTTEST

1 When considering risk factors for pancreatitis, the nurse determines that which assigned client is most likely to develop chronic pancreatitis?

  1. 59-year-old male with a history of excessive alcohol use
  2. Client with renal problems and hypocalcemia
  3. Client recovering from a myocardial infarction with hypercholesterolemia
  4. Client with a stone lodged in the pancreatic duct

2 The nurse concludes a diagnosis of nonalcoholic fatty liver disease (NAFLD) is supported when the client's laboratory values reflect which values?

  1. White blood cell count (WBC) 12,5000/mm^3
  2. Triglycerides 250mg/dL
  3. Albumin 2.8 mg/dL
  4. Amylase 100 units/dL

3 The following laboratory results were returned on a client who is suspected of having pancreatitis. The nurse concludes that which result gives positive evidence of pancreatitis?

  1. Lipase 230 IU/liter
  2. Calcium 9.3 mg/dL
  3. Blood glucose 75 mg/dL
  4. White blood cell count 5,000/mm^3

4 An adult female is diagnosed with cholecystitis and is being treated conservatively. What diet should the nurse recommend when teaching the client about dietary measures for healthy weight loss and reducing episodes of pain?

  1. Very low-calorie diet to promote faster weight loss
  2. Higher-fat diet to stimulate the gallbladder to empty
  3. Low-carbohydrate, low-fat, higher-protein diet
  4. Low-protein diet with adequate carbohydrate and no fat at all

5 Which of the following assessment findings would strongly indicate to the nurse the possibility of cirrhosis in a client?

1. Dry skin
2. Hepatomegaly
3. Peripheral edema
4. Pruritus

6 The nurse is reviewing the laboratory reports for a female client with cirrhosis of the liver. What abnormal results does the nurse note that are consistent with severe cirrhosis? Select all that apply.

1. Albumin 3.7
2. Arterial pH of 7.48
3. Prothrombin time (PT) 20 seconds; international normalized ratio (INR) 1.8
4. White blood cells (WBCs) 3,000 mm^3
5. Red blood cells (RBCs) 3.23 million/mm^3; hemoglobin 10.4 grams/dL

7 The nurse elicits asterixis in a client with advanced cirrhosis by asking client to perform which action?

1. Instruct client to extend arms and dorsiflex the wrists.
2. Observe hands for a carpopedal spasm when the blood pressure is taken.
3. Have the client hold arms above the head for 15 seconds.
4. Ask client to open and close hands rapidly.

8 In reviewing the possible causes of hepatitis A in a 24-year-old male, the nurse concludes that which of the following would be the most likely factor?

1. Contact with blood during work as a police officer
2. Receiving a blood transfusion during surgery
3. Eating shrimp at the local pub
4. Admitting to being sexually active

9 A client is admitted to the unit with reports of malaise, nausea, vomiting, anorexia, and headaches. The laboratory results show abnormal electrolytes and elevated aspartate aminotransferase (AST), alanine aminotransferase (ALT), and alkaline phosphatase (ALP). Hepatitis B surface antigen (HbsAG) is also present. The nurse would conclude that the client has which condition?

1. Hepatitis A
2. Hepatitis B
3. Cirrhosis
4. Pancreatitis

10 A client is admitted with possible liver cancer. The nurse interprets that which test would be the most confirming of this diagnosis and tumor type?

1. Abdominal ultrasound (US)
2. Liver biopsy
3. Alpha-fetoprotein markers
4. Computed tomography (CT) scan

➤ *See pages 223–224 for Answers and Rationales.*

ANSWERS & RATIONALES

Pretest

1 **Answer: 2** **Rationale:** Fatty liver infiltration occurs with nonalcoholic fatty liver disease (NAFLD). Typical laboratory findings include an elevation in triglycerides and liver enzymes. Bilirubin levels and white blood cell count are not elevated in NAFLD. Amylase is elevated with pancreatitis. **Cognitive Level:** Applying **Client Need:** Physiological Adaptation **Integrated Process:** Nursing Process: Assessment **Content Area:** Adult Health **Strategy:** Recall what nonalcoholic fatty liver disease (NAFLD) is and correlate the causes of the condition to choose

the correct answer. **Reference:** Porth, C. M. (2011). *Essentials of pathophysiology* (3rd ed.). Philadelphia, PA: Lippincott Williams & Wilkins, pp. 744–745.

2 **Answer: 2** **Rationale:** Hepatitis A has an acute onset and accounts for about 25% of hepatitis cases in the United States. The usual incubation period is 15–40 days. The disease is spread where there is fecal contamination of water supplies and from oral contamination (such as from day care or in contaminated food). Hepatitis B, C, and D can be transmitted sexually. A positive carrier state is associated with hepatitis B, not A. **Cognitive Level:** Applying **Client Need:** Physiological Adaptation **Integrated Process:** Teaching and Learning **Content Area:** Adult Health **Strategy:** Relate the answer to hepatitis type A and eliminate the options that refer to other types of hepatitis. **Reference:** LeMone, P., Burke, K., & Bauldoff, G. (2011). *Medical-surgical nursing: Critical thinking in patient care* (5th ed.). Upper Saddle River, NJ: Pearson Education, p. 730.

3 **Answer: 3** **Rationale:** Portal hypertension and liver cell failure contribute to the late manifestations of cirrhosis. Cholelithiasis and cholecystitis will be accompanied by pain, food intolerances, and/or vomiting. Pancreatitis presents with pain radiating to the back, mild cardiovascular changes, and hypocalcemia. **Cognitive Level:** Applying **Client Need:** Physiological Adaptation **Integrated Process:** Nursing Process: Diagnosis **Content Area:** Adult Health **Strategy:** Recognize that 2 options relate to gallbladder disease, which is not manifested with the findings in the question. Eliminate those options. **Reference:** LeMone, P., Burke, K., & Bauldoff, G. (2011). *Medical-surgical nursing: Critical thinking in patient care* (5th ed.). Upper Saddle River, NJ: Pearson Education, pp. 722–724, 736–742.

4 **Answer: 3** **Rationale:** The pain of acute pancreatitis is severe and requires early intervention with opioid (narcotic) analgesics. Both morphine and meperidine have the potential for addiction. Oxycodone (Percocet) is an oral preparation with a slower onset of action. All opioid analgesics have side effects. **Cognitive Level:** Applying **Client Need:** Pharmacological and Parenteral Therapies **Integrated Process:** Nursing Process: Planning **Content Area:** Adult Health **Strategy:** One option stands out as different from the others. This option answers what is asked. **Reference:** LeMone, P., Burke, K., & Bauldoff, G. (2011). *Medical-surgical nursing: Critical thinking in patient care* (5th ed.). Upper Saddle River, NJ: Pearson Education, pp. 751–756.

5 **Answer: 4** **Rationale:** Ammonia is a by-product of protein metabolism and is not converted to urea by a damaged liver. The client is at increased risk for a return of the encephalopathy because of the diagnosis of pneumonia and dehydration. Dietary protein intake must be controlled to minimize the ammonia levels in the bloodstream. The nurse should not order additional protein. Referring to blood test results provides a vague response that is not helpful. The nurse should not defer

questions to other health care providers that the nurse can answer. **Cognitive Level:** Analyzing **Client Need:** Physiological Adaptation **Integrated Process:** Communication and Documentation **Content Area:** Adult Health **Strategy:** Usually options that defer to the health care provider are incorrect if the nurse can implement the care. Look for the option that is client centered. **Reference:** LeMone, P., Burke, K., & Bauldoff, G. (2011). *Medical-surgical nursing: Critical thinking in patient care* (5th ed.). Upper Saddle River, NJ: Pearson Education, pp. 740–748.

6 **Answer: 3** **Rationale:** Decreased serum proteins and increased aldosterone, along with portal hypertension, causes ascites, an accumulation of fluid in the abdominal cavity. Gravity causes the fluid to sink, creating the shifting dullness during assessment. This is different than distention and not related to nutrition or fluid overload. **Cognitive Level:** Analyzing **Client Need:** Physiological Adaptation **Integrated Process:** Communication and Documentation **Content Area:** Adult Health **Strategy:** Only one option fits the percussion findings. Associate dullness that shifts with position changes to indicate ascites. **Reference:** LeMone, P., Burke, K., & Bauldoff, G. (2011). *Medical-surgical nursing: Critical thinking in patient care* (5th ed.). Upper Saddle River, NJ: Pearson Education, p. 736.

7 **Answer: 1, 3, 5** **Rationale:** Most cancers of the pancreas have already metastasized by the time of diagnosis. The onset is insidious with dull epigastric pain and slow onset of jaundice and weight loss as the classic symptoms. Black tarry stools are caused by GI bleeding such as from gastric or intestinal cancers. **Cognitive Level:** Applying **Client Need:** Physiological Adaptation **Integrated Process:** Teaching and Learning **Content Area:** Adult Health **Strategy:** Select options that are general and fit for any area of the pancreas. **Reference:** Porth, C. M. (2011). *Essentials of pathophysiology* (3rd ed.). Philadelphia, PA: Lippincott Williams & Wilkins, pp. 756–757.

8 **Answer: 1** **Rationale:** Clotting is altered by vitamin K deficiency and impaired liver production of clotting factors II, VII, IX, and X. Increased platelet destruction secondary to splenomegaly is also a factor. Everyone with cirrhosis does not have to follow a low-protein diet; this is sometimes restricted in the presence of hepatic encephalopathy. Bile production is not increased with cirrhosis. Medications associated with cirrhosis therapy, such as aldosterone antagonists, are not a cause of reduced clotting factors. **Cognitive Level:** Applying **Client Need:** Physiological Adaptation **Integrated Process:** Communication and Documentation **Content Area:** Adult Health **Strategy:** Consider the role of the liver in the coagulation process. In chronic cirrhosis the liver function is impaired. **Reference:** LeMone, P., Burke, K., & Bauldoff, G. (2011). *Medical-surgical nursing: Critical thinking in patient care* (5th ed.). Upper Saddle River, NJ: Pearson Education, pp. 736–738.

9 **Answer: 2** **Rationale:** Hepatitis B prophylaxis is not needed if the exposed person has been vaccinated and is known to be immune because of a positive hepatitis B titer. Hepatitis immune globulin is given for short-term immunity to persons who are not already immune. Hepatitis A is transmitted by the fecal–oral route. **Cognitive Level:** Applying **Client Need:** Safety and Infection Control **Integrated Process:** Nursing Process: Planning **Content Area:** Adult Health **Strategy:** How can the immune status be determined? Consider the epidemiology of hepatitis A and B. **Reference:** LeMone, P., Burke, K., & Bauldoff, G. (2011). *Medical-surgical nursing: Critical thinking in patient care* (5th ed.). Upper Saddle River, NJ: Pearson Education, pp. 729–735.

10 Answer: 1, 2, 4 Rationale: With the history of IV drug use, it is likely that he has either chronic hepatitis B or C, which are risk factors for liver cancer. His alcoholism predisposes him to cirrhosis, which is another risk factor for liver cancer. Although arsenic-containing water and carcinogens in food are risk factors, food supplements and municipal water are considered safe. **Cognitive Level:** Analyzing **Client Need:** Physiological Adaptation **Integrated Process:** Nursing Process: Implementation **Content Area:** Adult Health **Strategy:** Look at the client's lifestyle and determine what liver disorders he may have as a consequence. Which of these are risk factors for liver cancer? **Reference:** LeMone, P., Burke, K., & Bauldoff, G. (2011). *Medical-surgical nursing: Critical thinking in patient care* (5th ed.). Upper Saddle River, NJ: Pearson Education, pp. 749–751.

Posttest

1 Answer: 1 Rationale: Causes of pancreatitis include alcohol abuse with excessive intake of liquor or wine for 6 years or more; high triglyceride levels, and hypercalcemia. Myocardial infarction and hypercholesterolemia are not contributing factors to chronic pancreatitis, although high triglyceride levels are a contributing factor. Stones lodged in the pancreatic duct can cause obstruction and lead to inflammation of the pancreas; these are a common cause of acute pancreatitis. **Cognitive Level:** Analyzing **Client Need:** Physiological Adaptation **Integrated Process:** Nursing Process: Diagnosis **Content Area:** Adult Health **Strategy:** Note the question asks about *chronic* pancreatitis. Eliminate options that do not represent a primary risk factor. **Reference:** LeMone, P., Burke, K., & Bauldoff, G. (2011). *Medical-surgical nursing: Critical thinking in patient care* (5th ed.). Upper Saddle River, NJ: Pearson Education, pp. 751–753.

2 Answer: 2 Rationale: Risk factors for the development of nonalcoholic fatty liver disease (NAFLD) include elevated triglyceride levels, obesity, and the metabolic syndrome. Laboratory values reflect elevated liver enzymes and triglycerides. Changes in white blood cell count (WBC) count, albumin level, and amylase are not associated with NAFLD. **Cognitive Level:** Analyzing **Client Need:** Reduction of Risk Potential **Integrated Process:** Nursing Process: Assessment **Content Area:** Adult Health **Strategy:** Recall the factors contributing to nonalcoholic

fatty liver disease (NAFLD). **Reference:** Porth, C. M. (2011). *Essentials of pathophysiology* (3rd ed.). Philadelphia, PA: Lippincott, Williams & Wilkins, pp. 744–745.

3 Answer: 1 Rationale: In pancreatitis, the lipase, amylase, glucose, and white blood cell count (WBC) are all elevated. The calcium is low for 7 to 10 days and is a sign of severe pancreatitis. The calcium, blood glucose, and WBC values in the incorrect options are within normal limits. **Cognitive Level:** Analyzing **Client Need:** Reduction of Risk Potential **Integrated Process:** Nursing Process: Assessment **Content Area:** Adult Health **Strategy:** This question draws on knowledge of laboratory results and what is normal and abnormal. If this question was problematic, review normal lab values for each of these tests. **Reference:** LeMone, P., Burke, K., & Bauldoff, G. (2011). *Medical-surgical nursing: Critical thinking in patient care* (5th ed.). Upper Saddle River, NJ: Pearson Education, pp. 751–753.

4 Answer: 3 Rationale: A low-carbohydrate, low-fat, higher-protein diet will reduce symptoms of cholecystitis. The goal is a healthy rate of weight loss and reduced pain episodes. Fasting and very low-carbohydrate diets are contraindicated. Fat is an essential nutrient and is needed in a balanced diet. **Cognitive Level:** Applying **Client Need:** Health Promotion and Maintenance **Integrated Process:** Teaching and Learning **Content Area:** Adult Health **Strategy:** Consider a moderate, healthy diet for gradual weight loss while controlling the fat. **Reference:** LeMone, P., Burke, K., & Bauldoff, G. (2011). *Medical-surgical nursing: Critical thinking in patient care* (5th ed.). Upper Saddle River, NJ: Pearson Education, pp. 722–726.

5 Answer: 2 Rationale: Hepatomegaly is an enlarged liver and would be the most suggestive of cirrhosis. Pruritus and dry skin can occur for many reasons. Although the client with cirrhosis may develop peripheral edema, edema is also associated with many cardiovascular conditions, such as heart failure, and so would not be specific to cirrhosis. **Cognitive Level:** Applying **Client Need:** Physiological Adaptation **Integrated Process:** Nursing Process: Diagnosis **Content Area:** Adult Health **Strategy:** Read carefully. One word may change the meaning and make an option wrong. **Reference:** LeMone, P., Burke, K., & Bauldoff, G. (2011). *Medical-surgical nursing: Critical thinking in patient care* (5th ed.). Upper Saddle River, NJ: Pearson Education, pp. 736–740.

6 Answer: 3, 4, 5 Rationale: Clients with cirrhosis have impaired production of clotting factors. A prothrombin time (PT) is an indication of the time needed for blood to clot; the high PT and international normalized ratio (INR) indicate slow clotting. Low white blood cell (WBC) count, red blood cell (RBC) count, and a low albumin level also are seen with cirrhosis. Arterial blood gas levels are not related to liver function. **Cognitive Level:** Analyzing **Client Need:** Reduction of Risk Potential **Integrated Process:** Nursing Process: Diagnosis **Content Area:** Adult Health **Strategy:** Although most of these results are abnormal, only some are the result of impaired liver function. Continue to review normal and abnormal labs if this question was difficult. **Reference:** LeMone, P., Burke, K., & Bauldoff, G. (2011). *Medical-surgical nursing: Critical thinking in patient care* (5th ed.). Upper Saddle River, NJ: Pearson Education, pp. 736–738.

7 Answer: 1 Rationale: Asterixis, or liver flap, occurs in hepatic encephalopathy and is associated with cirrhosis. To elicit the sign, the client is asked to extend the arms and dorsiflex the wrists, which elicits the flapping tremor. Carpopedal spasm during blood pressure measurement is called Trousseau sign and accompanies hypocalcemia. Holding the arms above the head and opening and closing the hands rapidly may give a general idea of client motor strength and neurological status, respectively. **Cognitive Level:** Understanding **Client Need:** Physiological Adaptation **Integrated Process:** Nursing Process: Implementation **Content Area:** Adult Health **Strategy:** Specific information is needed to answer the question. Recall how to test for asterixis to choose correctly. **Reference:** LeMone, P., Burke, K., & Bauldoff, G. (2011). *Medical-surgical nursing: Critical thinking in patient care* (5th ed.). Upper Saddle River, NJ: Pearson Education, p. 741.

8 Answer: 3 Rationale: Hepatitis A is transmitted by fecal–oral route. The virus is excreted in oropharyngeal secretions (nose and throat) and transmitted by direct contact person to person, or by fecal contamination of food or water. A worker could have hepatitis A and transfer it to food. Hepatitis B, C, and D are transmitted by contact with blood or body fluids. **Cognitive Level:** Applying **Client Need:** Physiological Adaptation **Integrated Process:** Nursing Process: Diagnosis **Content Area:** Adult Health **Strategy:** Consider the type of hepatitis and the modes of

transmission. Remember the correct option is one that is different from the others. **Reference:** LeMone, P., Burke, K., & Bauldoff, G. (2011). *Medical-surgical nursing: Critical thinking in patient care* (5th ed.). Upper Saddle River, NJ: Pearson Education, pp. 729–731.

9 Answer: 2 Rationale: The symptoms in preicteric hepatitis are vague and more flulike as described above. The health care provider usually needs laboratory tests to verify a diagnosis. In this case, the presence of the antigen HBsAG concludes that the client has an active form of the disease since the hepatitis B surface antigen is present. **Cognitive Level:** Analyzing **Client Need:** Reduction of Risk Potential **Integrated Process:** Nursing Process: Assessment **Content Area:** Adult Health **Strategy:** Evaluate the laboratory findings in the question along with vague symptoms. The options are all hepatobiliary problems—which one fits the description? A clue is the surface antigen result. **Reference:** LeMone, P., Burke, K., & Bauldoff, G. (2011). *Medical-surgical nursing: Critical thinking in patient care* (5th ed.). Upper Saddle River, NJ: Pearson Education, pp. 730–733.

10 Answer: 2 Rationale: Abdominal ultrasound (US), x-ray, and computed tomography (CT) scans are useful in the diagnosis of cancer of the liver. The alpha-fetoprotein serum markers are specific to detecting primary hepatocellular carcinoma. To confirm the diagnosis and identify the tumor type or origin, a biopsy is done. **Cognitive Level:** Applying **Client Need:** Reduction of Risk Potential **Integrated Process:** Nursing Process: Assessment **Content Area:** Adult Health **Strategy:** Consider what would be the best diagnostic test to confirm almost any type of cancer. **Reference:** LeMone, P., Burke, K., & Bauldoff, G. (2011). *Medical-surgical nursing: Critical thinking in patient care* (5th ed.). Upper Saddle River, NJ: Pearson Education, pp. 749–751.

References

Adams, M., Holland, L., & Bostwick, P. (2011). *Pharmacology for nurses: A pathophysiologic approach* (3rd ed.). Upper Saddle River, NJ: Pearson Education.

D'Amico, D., & Barbarito, C. (2012). *Health & physical assessment in nursing* (2nd ed.). Upper Saddle River, NJ: Pearson Education, Inc.

Ignatavicius, D., & Workman, M. (2013). *Medical-surgical nursing: Critical thinking for collaborative care* (7th ed.) Philadelphia: W. B. Saunders Company.

Kee, J. L. (2009). *Laboratory and diagnostic tests* (8th ed.). Upper Saddle River, NJ: Pearson Education.

LeMone, P., Burke, K., & Bauldoff, G. (2011). *Medical-surgical nursing: Critical thinking in patient care* (5th ed.). Upper Saddle River, NJ: Pearson Education.

McCance, K., & Huether, K. (2010) *Understanding pathophysiology: The biologic basis for disease in adults and children* (6th ed.) St. Louis, MO: Elsevier.

Osborn, K. S., Wraa, C. E., & Watson, A. (2010). *Medical surgical nursing: Preparation for practice.* Upper Saddle River, NJ: Pearson Education.

Porth, C. (Ed.). (2011). *Essentials of pathophysiology* (3rd ed.). Philadelphia, PA: Lippincott Williams & Wilkins.

Porth, C., & Matfin, G. (2010) *Pathophysiology: Concepts of altered health states* (8th ed.). Philadelphia, PA: Lippincott Williams & Wilkins.

Ralph, S., & Taylor, C. (2010). *Sparks and Taylor's nursing diagnosis reference manual* (8th ed.). Philadelphia, PA: Lippincott William & Wilkins.

Wilson, B. A., Shannon, M. T., & Shields, K. M. (2012). *Pearson nurse's drug guide 2012.* Upper Saddle River, NJ: Pearson Education.

ANSWERS & RATIONALES

Endocrine and Metabolic Health Problems

9

Chapter Outline

Risk Factors Associated with
  Endocrine and Metabolic
  Health Problems
Thyroid Hyperfunction
  Disorders
Thyroid Hypofunction Disorders

Parathyroid Disorders
Adrenal Cortex Hyperfunction
  Disorders
Adrenal Cortex Hypofunction
  Disorder: Addison's Disease

Adrenal Medulla
  Hyperfunction Disorder:
  Pheochromocytoma
Anterior Pituitary Disorders
Posterior Pituitary Disorders
Diabetes Mellitus

Objectives

➤ Define key terms associated with endocrine and metabolic
  health problems.
➤ Identify risk factors associated with the development of endocrine
  and metabolic health problems.
➤ Explain the common etiologies of endocrine and metabolic
  health problems.
➤ Describe the pathophysiologic processes associated with specific
  endocrine and metabolic health problems.
➤ Distinguish between normal and abnormal endocrine and metabolic
  findings obtained from nursing assessment.
➤ Prioritize nursing interventions associated with specific endocrine
  and metabolic health problems.

NCLEX-RN® Test Prep

Use the accompanying online resource,
NursingReviewsandRationales, to test
yourself with hundreds of NCLEX®-style
practice questions.

Review at a Glance

Addison's disease chronic
adrenocortical insufficiency from
destruction of adrenal glands
Addisonian crisis acute
adrenocortical insufficiency precipitated
by stress or abrupt withdrawal of
glucocorticoids; signs and symptoms
include hypotension and shock
antidiuretic hormone (ADH)
hormone secreted by posterior pituitary
gland to control water balance and
serum osmolality
**Conn syndrome
(hyperaldosteronism)** primary
hyperaldosteronism; hypersecretion of

aldosterone in which hypertension is a
major complication
Cushing's disease symptoms
produced by excess cortisol from
adrenal cortex; classic signs and
symptoms are moon face, truncal obesity,
and "buffalo hump"
diabetes insipidus (DI) disorder
caused by antidiuretic hormone
(ADH) insufficiency, results in excess
fluid excretion
diabetes mellitus (DM)
a pancreatic disorder caused by lack of
secretion or inadequate secretion of
insulin, or insulin resistance, resulting in
hyperglycemia and multisystem effects

diabetic ketoacidosis (DKA)
life-threatening state of hyperglycemia
and metabolic acidosis
exophthalmos abnormal protrusion
of eyeballs in hyperthyroidism; may affect
one or both eyes
goiter enlargement of thyroid gland,
most often seen in hyperthyroidism, but
also may occur in hypothyroidism
or euthyroidism
Graves' disease hyperthyroidism
leading to a hypermetabolic state
hyperparathyroidism increase in
secretion of parathyroid hormone (PTH)

hyperthyroidism increase in secretion of thyroid hormone (TH)

hypoparathyroidism decrease in secretion of parathyroid hormone (PTH)

hypothyroidism decrease in secretion of thyroid hormone (TH)

insulin hormone produced by pancreas, responsible for controlling serum glucose level

myxedema form of hypothyroidism characterized by non-pitting edema that is generally found in periorbital and pretibial areas

myxedema coma life-threatening state of hypothyroidism

pheochromocytoma tumor (usually benign) of adrenal medulla resulting in excessive secretion of catecholamines, which leads to severe hypertension

syndrome of inappropriate antidiuretic hormone (SIADH) excessive secretion of antidiuretic hormone (ADH) from pituitary gland; results in excessive water retention

thyroid storm life-threatening form of hyperthyroidism, characterized by extreme state of hypermetabolism

PRETEST

1 The nurse is obtaining a health history on a 36-year-old female who reports an increase in appetite, weight loss, intolerance to heat, and nervousness. On physical assessment, the client is noted to have thin hair and moist skin. Based on this information, the nurse would suspect which disorder?

1. Hypothyroidism
2. Hyperthyroidism
3. Hypoparathyroidism
4. Hyperparathyroidism

2 A client is returning from a subtotal thyroidectomy for the treatment of hyperthyroidism. The immediate priority of the nurse who is assigned to this client is to assess for which of the following?

1. Respiratory distress
2. Fluid volume status
3. Neurological status
4. Incisional pain

3 The nurse has given medication instructions to a client newly diagnosed with hypothyroidism who will be taking levothyroxine sodium (Synthroid). Which statement made by the client would indicate additional teaching is required?

1. "I know I will be on this medication for the rest of my life."
2. "I won't eat excessive amounts of cabbage or spinach."
3. "I'll take my Synthroid with food."
4. "I'll take my Synthroid in the morning."

4 In providing care for a client being admitted for severe hyperparathyroidism, the nurse anticipates implementing which of the following actions?

1. Administering intravenous (IV) calcium gluconate
2. Administering large amounts of IV saline
3. Maintaining strict fluid restriction
4. Monitoring for tetany

5 A client is receiving supplemental calcium as treatment for hypoparathyroidism. The nurse concludes that the client has achieved therapeutic results of drug therapy when the serum calcium level has reached at least how many mg/dL? Provide a numeric answer with no decimal places.

_____ mg/dL

6 A client with Cushing's disease is admitted with the symptoms of hypertension, fatigue, and edema. The priority nursing diagnosis for this client would be which of the following?

1. Imbalanced Nutrition: More than Body Requirements
2. Excess Fluid Volume
3. Anxiety
4. Deficient Knowledge

7 A client with Conn syndrome (hyperaldosteronism) who will not be treated surgically is receiving spironolactone (Aldactone). The nurse explains to the client that the purpose of this drug is to do which of the following?

1. Reverse the hyperaldosteronism.
2. Decrease the serum potassium level.
3. Promote fluid retention.
4. Treat hypertension and hypokalemia.

8 A client with Addison's disease is being discharged home and will be taking hydrocortisone (Cortisol). Which statements by the client indicate that client teaching about the disease and its management was successful? Select all that apply.

1. "I will monitor closely for any signs of infection."
2. "I will wear a MedicAlert bracelet indicating disease and treatment."
3. "I will report any rapid weight gain or fluid in my legs if it persists for over two weeks."
4. "I will take safety measures at home to prevent injuries."
5. "I will have to take this medicine for the rest of my life."

9 The nurse is establishing a plan of care for a client newly admitted with syndrome of inappropriate antidiuretic hormone secretion (SIADH). The priority nursing diagnosis for this client would be which of the following?

1. Deficient Fluid Volume
2. Anxiety
3. Excess Fluid Volume
4. Risk for Injury

10 The nurse is discussing the treatment regimen for a client newly diagnosed with type 1 diabetes mellitus. While discussing insulin administration, the client asks, "Why can't I just take a pill like my friend does?" Which followup client statement indicates the client understands the nurse's explanation?

1. "Because my body does not produce insulin, I must receive the injections."
2. "I will be on insulin for a short while, then I can take the pills."
3. "The pills are not as effective as the insulin injections."
4. "When my body starts making insulin again, I can stop taking the injections."

➤ *See pages 250–252 for Answers and Rationales.*

I. RISK FACTORS ASSOCIATED WITH ENDOCRINE AND METABOLIC HEALTH PROBLEMS

A. **Thyroid hyperfunction disorders**
   1. Graves' disease: immunological factors, genetic predisposition, infection, stress, excessive intake of thyroid medications; occurs 8 times more frequently in females
   2. Goiter: inadequate intake of iodine, increase in thyroid hormone demand
   3. Thyroid storm: stress, injury, infection, surgery

B. **Thyroid hypofunction disorders**
   1. Hypothyroidism: congenital defect, immunological factors, older adults, infection, iodine deficiency, antithyroid drugs
   2. Myxedema: undiagnosed or untreated hypothyroidism

C. **Parathyroid disorders**
   1. Hyperparathyroidism: older adults, female, thyroid adenoma
   2. Hypoparathyroidism: accidental removal or damage to parathyroid during thyroidectomy

D. **Adrenal cortex hyperfunction disorders**
   1. Cushing's disease: tumor of pituitary gland, excess administration of corticosteroids or adrenocorticotropic hormone (ACTH), although exogenous hormone may also suppress endogenous function
   2. Conn syndrome: tumors of adrenal gland

E. **Adrenal cortex hypofunction disorder (Addison's disease)**: immunological factors; surgical removal, infection or tumor of adrenal gland(s); head trauma (affects pituitary gland); withdrawal of exogenous glucocorticoids or ACTH

F. **Adrenal medulla hyperfunction disorder (pheochromocytoma)**: genetic predisposition, middle age

G. **Anterior pituitary disorders**
1. Gigantism: pituitary adenoma (hyperfunction)
2. Acromegaly: pituitary adenoma (hyperfunction)
3. Dwarfism: pituitary adenoma, congenital inheritance, trauma, and radiation (hypofunction)

H. **Posterior pituitary disorders**
1. Diabetes insipidus (hypofunction of ADH secretion): head trauma, brain tumor, removal or irradiation of pituitary gland, genetic predisposition, renal disease
2. Syndrome of inappropriate antidiuretic hormone (SIADH; hyperfunction of ADH): head trauma, brain tumor, infection, brain surgery, some pharmacologic agents

I. **Diabetes mellitus (DM)**
1. Type 1 diabetes mellitus: genetic predisposition, immunological factors, environmental factors, age under 30 years, increased in African Americans and Native Americans; hypertension and elevated cholesterol are common associated conditions
2. Type 2 diabetes mellitus: age older than 30 years, obesity, and genetic predisposition
3. Diabetic ketoacidosis: increased insulin requirements, insufficient exogenous insulin
4. Hyperosmolar hyperglycemic non-ketotic syndrome (HHNS): stressors such as infection, trauma, surgery coupled with underlying (and perhaps unknown) hyperglycemia, and type 2 DM; also called hyperosmolar coma (HOC)

II. THYROID HYPERFUNCTION DISORDERS

A. **Overview**
1. Thyroid gland is located in lower neck anterior to trachea; its primary function is to produce, store, and secrete hormones:
   a. Thyroxine (T_4)—responsible for cellular metabolism
   b. Triiodothyronine (T_3)—responsible for regulating cellular metabolism
   c. Thyrocalcitonin (calcitonin)—role is calcium regulation
   d. T_3 and T_4 are known collectively as thyroid hormone
2. Iodine is necessary for thyroid gland to synthesize and secrete hormones
3. Thyroid hormone (T_3 and T_4) stimulates body growth, increases metabolic rate, heart rate, and glucose; overall role is to maintain metabolism and regulate growth and development
4. Calcitonin acts on kidneys and bones to decrease serum calcium levels
5. Causes of thyroid hyperfunction disorders include autoimmune responses, neoplasms, excessive intake of thyroid medications, and excess secretion of thyroid-stimulating hormone (TSH) from anterior pituitary gland

B. **Pathophysiology**
1. Thyroid hormone (TH) production depends on adequate secretion of TSH from anterior pituitary; hypothalamus regulates TSH secretion by negative feedback
2. **Hyperthyroidism** (hyperfunction of thyroid gland) leads to an excess of TH
   a. Excess TH leads to a hypermetabolic state, which causes an increase in metabolic function, O_2 consumption by tissues, and heat production
   b. Thyroid hyperfunction disorders include Graves' disease, toxic goiter, and thyroid storm, which lead to increased protein, lipid, carbohydrate, and vitamin metabolism

3. Graves' disease (most common cause of hyperthyroidism) is seen most often in women under age 40
  a. Exact cause is unknown, but is considered an autoimmune disorder in response to stimulation of thyroid gland from a long-acting thyroid stimulator (LATS)
  b. An excess production of TH results, which leads to a *hypermetabolic state*
4. Goiter describes an enlargement of thyroid gland in an attempt to compensate for inadequate TH, and may be present in hyperthyroidism or hypothyroidism
  a. Goiter may result from response to excess TSH stimulation, excess growth-stimulating immunoglobulins, or presence of substances that inhibit TH synthesis
  b. A goiter may become so large that respiratory complications arise as a result of compression to neck and chest
  c. *Toxic multinodular goiter* exists when small, independently functioning nodules (either benign or malignant) in thyroid gland are present and secrete TH; signs develop more slowly than in Grave's disease; is most often seen in women age 60 or older who have had goiter for several years
5 Thyroid storm (also known as thyroid crisis or thyrotoxicosis) is a *life-threatening condition,* which describes an extreme state of hyperthyroidism; excessive TH causes a rapid increase in metabolic rate requiring immediate treatment to avoid death
6. Signs and symptoms
  a. Hyperthyroidism (see Figure 9-1): note all symptoms are elevated or high except weight loss, sex drive, and fluid volume
  b. Symptoms are caused by excessive stimulation of:
    1) Sympathetic (adrenergic) branch of central nervous system (CNS): cardiac activity, reflexes
    2) Thyroxine: increased metabolism, weight loss, and psychological symptoms
  c. Thyroid storm: leads to extreme hyperthermia (102–106°F), tachycardia, agitation, seizures
  d. Classic symptoms are weight loss, nervousness, **exophthalmos** (protrusion of eyeballs), increased appetite, palpitations, and heat intolerance

C. Nursing assessment
1. Assessment for hyperthyroidism includes assessment of eyes, vital signs (VS), cardiac monitor for rhythm changes, nutrition assessment, integument assessment, weight, fluid status, goiter, muscle strength and appearance, reproductive history, signs of heart failure (HF), and reports of GI distress
2. Assessment findings for thyroid storm include elevated temperature, symptom analysis of pain, bowel or GI complaints, neurological status, (development of seizures), changes in VS, respiratory status
3. Diagnostic tests
  a. Serum thyroid antibodies (Serum TA): elevated
  b. Thyroid-stimulating hormone (TSH): decreased
  c. Serum thyroxine (T_4): increased; decreased in primary hyperthyroidism
  d. Serum triiodothyronine (T_3): increased
  e. T_3 uptake test (T_3RU): increased
  f. Radioactive iodine (RAI) uptake with thyroid suppression test: increased

D. Nursing management (see Table 9-1, p. 231)
1. Medications
  a. Antithyroid medications to reduce TH production: methimazole (Tapazole) and propylthiouracil (PTU)
  b. Propranolol (Inderal) to treat cardiac dysrhythmias
  c. Glucocorticoids: interfere with conversion of T_4 to T_3

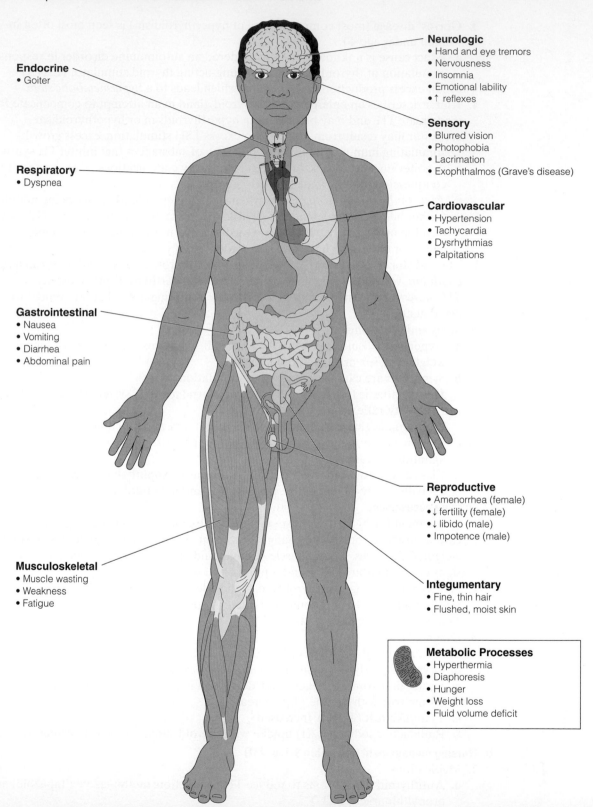

Neurologic
- Hand and eye tremors
- Nervousness
- Insomnia
- Emotional lability
- ↑ reflexes

Endocrine
- Goiter

Sensory
- Blurred vision
- Photophobia
- Lacrimation
- Exophthalmos (Grave's disease)

Respiratory
- Dyspnea

Cardiovascular
- Hypertension
- Tachycardia
- Dysrhythmias
- Palpitations

Gastrointestinal
- Nausea
- Vomiting
- Diarrhea
- Abdominal pain

Reproductive
- Amenorrhea (female)
- ↓ fertility (female)
- ↓ libido (male)
- Impotence (male)

Musculoskeletal
- Muscle wasting
- Weakness
- Fatigue

Integumentary
- Fine, thin hair
- Flushed, moist skin

Metabolic Processes
- Hyperthermia
- Diaphoresis
- Hunger
- Weight loss
- Fluid volume deficit

Figure 9-1

Body system effects of hyperthyroidism

Table 9-1	Comparison of Symptoms and Treatment of Hyperthyroidism and Hypothyroidism	
	Hyperthyroidism	**Hypothyroidism**
Etiology	Autoimmune responses, excess secretion of thyroid-stimulating hormone (TSH), neoplasms, excessive intake of thyroid medications	Congenital defects, antithyroid medications, iodine deficiency, damage to thyroid from surgery or radiation
Clinical Manifestations	Emotional lability, agitation, exophthalmos, increased reflexes, tachycardia, diarrhea, muscle weakness, fatigue, flushed skin, goiter, hyperthermia, weight loss, heat intolerance, diaphoresis *Hint:* Everything is elevated except weight	Memory impairment, confusion, decreased reflexes, periorbital edema, hypotension, bradycardia, constipation, muscle weakness, goiter, edema, weight gain, hypothermia, cold intolerance *Hint:* Everything is decreased except weight
Laboratory Values	• Elevated serum thyroid antibodies (Serum TA) • Decreased TSH in primary hyperthyroidism • Increased serum triiodothyronine (T_3) • Increased T_3 uptake	• Increased TSH in primary hyperthyroidism • Decreased serum thyroxine (T_4) • Decreased serum triiodothyronine (T_3) • Decreased T_3 uptake • Hyponatremia
Treatment	Pharmacologic agents: methimazole (Tapazole), propylthiouracil (PTU), propranolol (Inderal), glucocorticoids Lugol's solution Radioactive therapy Thyroidectomy	Pharmacologic agents Levothyroxine sodium (Synthroid) Liothyronine sodium (Cytomel) Liotrix (Euthroid) Vasopressor agents

    d. Lugol's solution (iodine) to decrease vascularity and size of thyroid prior to surgery

    e. Antipyretics if needed

2. Educate client that it may take several weeks before therapeutic effects of antithyroid medications are noticed

    a. Instruct to take medication as prescribed and to not abruptly discontinue medication

    b. Educate about signs of hypothyroidism, which may occur if too much medicine is taken or dose needs adjusting

3. Monitor for cardiac dysrhythmias, tachycardia

4. Implement antipyretic measures

5. Elevate head of bed to decrease eye pressure

6. Teach eye care and monitor for vision changes if exophthalmos occurs, since it will not change even after medications have been started

 7. Monitor dietary intake: client may require up to 4,000–5,000 calories a day during hypermetabolic state

8. Monitor intake and output

9. Monitor weight

10. Keep environment cool and quiet because of symptoms

11. Radioactive therapy may be recommended to destroy thyroid cells in order to reduce production of TH

    a. Give radioactive iodine orally; results are expected in 6–8 weeks

    b. Does not require hospitalization or radiation precautions

    c. Contraindicated in pregnant women

    d. Monitor for signs of *hypothyroidism*

12. Preoperative and postoperative care for surgery to remove all or part of thyroid (thyroidectomy)

    a. Subtotal thyroidectomy leaves part of thyroid gland intact in order to produce adequate amounts of TH

    b. If a total thyroidectomy is performed (usually for treatment of cancer), *life-long* thyroid hormone replacement is necessary; educate client about importance of compliance with medication regime

    c. Preoperative care includes administering antithyroid medications to promote a euthyroid state, and iodine preparations to decrease vascularity of gland; teach client how to support neck with both hands while sitting up, moving, or coughing following surgery to reduce strain on suture line

    d. Postoperative care includes monitoring for complications such as hemorrhage, respiratory distress, laryngeal nerve damage, and tetany (positive Chvostek's and Trousseau's signs); assess for pain and treat accordingly

  13. Priority nursing diagnoses for thyroid hyperfunction disorders: Activity Intolerance, Imbalanced Nutrition: Less than Body Requirements, Hyperthermia, Risk for Injury

III. THYROID HYPOFUNCTION DISORDERS

A. Overview

  1. Hypofunction of thyroid leads to an insufficient amount of thyroid hormone (TH), known as **hypothyroidism**; classified as primary or secondary

  2. Decreased TH results in a *hypometabolic state* manifested by a decrease in metabolic function, a decrease in O_2 consumption by tissue, and a decrease in heat production

  3. Thyroid hypofunction disorders include hypothyroidism, myxedema, and myxedema coma

  4. Causes of primary and secondary hypothyroidism

    a. Causes of primary hypothyroidism include congenital defects, loss of thyroid tissue from surgery or radiation, antithyroid medications, endemic iodine deficiency, or thyroiditis

    b. Causes of secondary hypothyroidism include peripheral resistance to thyroid hormones or pituitary TSH deficiency

B. Pathophysiology

  1. *Hypothyroidism* describes an insufficient amount of thyroid hormone (TH), which leads to a decrease in metabolic rate; manifestations develop slowly over months to years

  2. **Myxedema** describes a generalized hypometabolic state occurring with untreated hypothyroidism; accumulation of proteins in interstitial spaces results in an increase in interstitial fluids, causing mucinous edema (myxedema), a non-pitting edema is often found in pretibial and facial areas

  3. **Myxedema coma** (also known as *hypothyroid crisis*) results from extreme or prolonged hypothyroidism; though rare, it is a life-threatening condition

    a. Characterized by a severe hypometabolic state: lactic acidosis, hypoglycemia, hyponatremia, hypotension, bradycardia, cardiovascular collapse, hypothermia, hypoventilation, and coma

    b. Precipitated by inadequate thyroid replacement, infection, trauma, exposure to cold temperatures, central nervous system depressants

  4. *Iodine deficiency*: iodine is necessary for TH synthesis and secretion

    a. Iodine deficiency occurs as a result of antithyroid drugs, lithium intake or inadequate iodine intake

    b. In the United States, thyroid deficiency because of inadequate iodine intake is less frequent because of use of iodized salt

  5. *Hashimoto's thyroiditis* is an autoimmune disorder generally affecting women aged 30–50, in which antibodies develop and destroy thyroid tissue

    a. TH levels decrease because fibrous tissue replaces functional thyroid tissue

    b. Goiter develops as thyroid enlarges to compensate for decreasing TH levels

  6. Signs and symptoms

    a. Hypothyroidism (see Figure 9-2): note that most symptoms are decreased except weight and fluid volume

    b. Myxedema coma: hypothermia, cardiovascular collapse, coma, hyponatremia, hypoglycemia, lactic acidosis

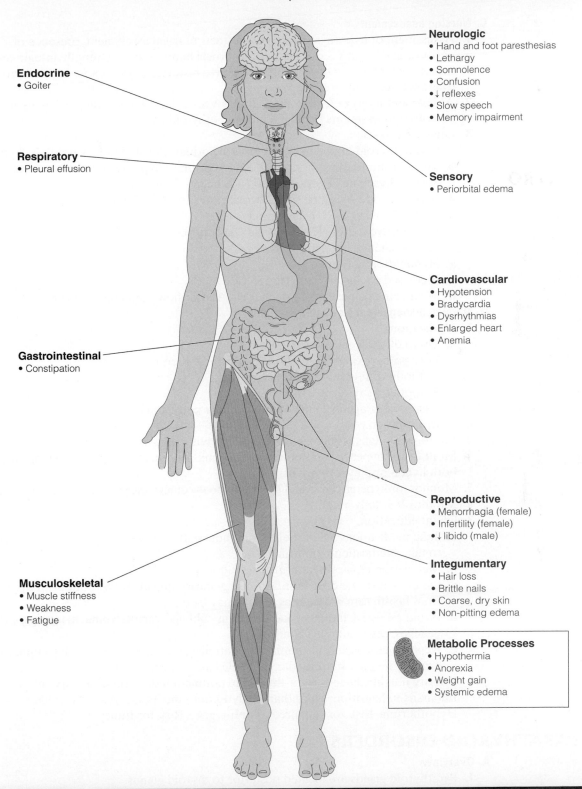

Neurologic
- Hand and foot paresthesias
- Lethargy
- Somnolence
- Confusion
- ↓ reflexes
- Slow speech
- Memory impairment

Endocrine
- Goiter

Respiratory
- Pleural effusion

Sensory
- Periorbital edema

Cardiovascular
- Hypotension
- Bradycardia
- Dysrhythmias
- Enlarged heart
- Anemia

Gastrointestinal
- Constipation

Reproductive
- Menorrhagia (female)
- Infertility (female)
- ↓ libido (male)

Integumentary
- Hair loss
- Brittle nails
- Coarse, dry skin
- Non-pitting edema

Musculoskeletal
- Muscle stiffness
- Weakness
- Fatigue

Metabolic Processes
- Hypothermia
- Anorexia
- Weight gain
- Systemic edema

Figure 9-2

Body system effects of hypothyroidism

C. **Nursing assessment**

1. Assessment of hypothyroidism includes neurological assessment, presence of periorbital edema, VS, cardiac rhythm, bowel habits, muscle strength, integument assessment, presence of goiter, reproductive history, fluid status, weight, activity tolerance, respiratory status

2. Assessment in myxedema coma includes VS, cardiac and neurological assessments, and other assessments performed for hypothyroidism

3. Diagnostic tests

   a. Serum thyroid antibodies (serum TA): normal; elevated in Hashimoto's thyroiditis
   b. Thyroid stimulating hormone (TSH) in primary hypothyroidism: increased
   c. Serum thyroxine (T_4): decreased (normal 5–12 ng/dL)
   d. Serum triiodothyronine (T_3): decreased (normal 80–200 ng/dL)
   e. T_3 uptake test (T_3RU): decreased
   f. Radioactive iodine (RAI) uptake test (thyroid scan) with thyroid suppression test: no change or decreased
   g. Hyponatremia (dilutional)
   h. Increased cholesterol and triglyceride levels
   i. Myxedema coma: glucose decreased, ABGs show metabolic acidosis

D. **Nursing management (see Table 9-1 again)**

1. Medications
   a. Thyroid replacement medications
      1) Levothyroxine sodium (T_4) (Synthroid, others)
      2) Liothyronine sodium (T_3) (Cytomel)
      3) Liotrix (Thyrolar)
   b. Vasopressor agents to maintain adequate perfusion

2. Intravenous glucose

3. Monitor for signs of digoxin toxicity if receiving digoxin (Lanoxin)

 4 Monitor for hyperthyroidism with excess medication; teach signs and symptoms of both hyper- and hypothyroidism

5. Monitor for hyperglycemia and also for hypoglycemia (since myxedema can lead to this)

 6 Monitor VS, daily weight

7. Client education

   a. Take medications 1 hour before or 2 hours after meals for optimal absorption and to take medication in morning
   b. Medication replacement is *lifelong*
   c. Do not substitute drug brands or use generic equivalents without prior approval from health care provider as dosing may be different
   d. Avoid excessive intake of foods such as cabbage, carrots, spinach, turnips, and peaches, which inhibit TH utilization
   e. Report nervousness, insomnia, palpitations, excess weight loss or leg cramps to primary health care provider (possible excess medication)

8. Priority nursing diagnoses for thyroid hypofunction disorders: Activity Intolerance, Imbalanced Nutrition: More than Body Requirements, Decreased Cardiac Output, Hypothermia, Risk for Impaired Skin Integrity, Risk for Injury

IV. PARATHYROID DISORDERS

A. **Overview**

1. Parathyroid glands are located posterior to thyroid glands
   a. Their major function is to maintain normal serum calcium levels by secreting parathyroid hormone (PTH), which increases bone resorption of calcium
   b. PTH responds to decreased calcium levels by increasing calcium absorption from bone, kidneys, and intestines

Practice to Pass

The nurse is providing teaching to a client newly diagnosed with hypothyroidism. Her family is also included in the teaching process. What instructions should the nurse provide to the client and the client's family?

    2. Hyperparathyroidism is an *increase* in PTH, which leads to hypercalcemia, hypophosphatemia, bone damage, and renal damage

    3. Hypoparathyroidism is a *decrease* in PTH, which leads to hypocalcemia, hyperphosphatemia, hyperreflexia, and an altered sensorium

    4. Most common cause of hypoparathyroidism is damage to or removal of parathyroid glands during thyroidectomy

    5. Causes of hyperparathyroidism

        a. *Primary hyperparathyroidism* results from an adenoma or hyperplasia of one of parathyroid glands

        b. *Secondary hyperparathyroidism* occurs as a response of parathyroid glands to chronic hypocalcemia (usually caused by renal failure)

        c. *Tertiary hyperparathyroidism* results from hyperplasia of parathyroid glands and a resulting loss of response to serum calcium levels

B. Pathophysiology

    1. Hyperparathyroidism

        a. Increased PTH causes an increased resorption of calcium by kidneys, leading to *hypercalcemia,* and an increased excretion of phosphate by kidneys, leading to hypophosphatemia

        b. Increased PTH causes an increased release of phosphorus and calcium by bones, leading to bone decalcification and formation of renal calculi

        c. Increased PTH causes an increased bicarbonate excretion and decreased acid excretion, leading to hypokalemia and metabolic acidosis

    2. Hypoparathyroidism

        a. Decreased PTH causes a decrease in bone and renal resorption of calcium, leading to *hypocalcemia,* and a decrease in renal excretion of phosphate, elevating serum phosphate levels (hyperphosphatemia)

        b. Calcifications may form on eyes, causing cataracts, and on basal ganglia, causing brain calcifications

        c. Decreased serum calcium levels cause muscular excitability, tetany, and laryngeal spasms

    3. Signs and symptoms

        a. Hyperparathyroidism

            1) Neurological: depression, psychosis, paresthesias, decreased neuromuscular irritability, impaired vision, altered level of consciousness (LOC)

            2) Cardiovascular: hypertension, dysrhythmias

            3) Gastrointestinal: nausea, abdominal pain, constipation, peptic ulcers, gastric bleeding, thirst, anorexia, pancreatitis

            4) Renal: renal calculi, hypercalciuria, hyperphosphaturia

            5) Musculoskeletal: muscle atrophy and weakness, bone pain, pathologic fractures, back pain, osteoporosis, demineralization of bone

            6) Metabolic: metabolic acidosis, weight loss, polyuria, polydipsia, dehydration

        b. Hypoparathyroidism

            1) Neurological: hyperactive reflexes; increased intracranial pressure; irritability; anxiety; depression; paresthesias of lips, hands, and feet; laryngeal spasms; seizure activity

            2) Cardiovascular: dysrhythmias

            3) Gastrointestinal: malabsorption syndromes, abdominal cramps

            4) Musculoskeletal: carpopedal spasms, facial grimacing, muscle spasms, tetany, seizures, positive Chvostek and Trousseau signs, hyperactive deep tendon reflexes, calcification of bones

            5) Renal: renal colic

            6) Integumentary: dry and scaly skin, hair loss, brittle nails

C. Nursing assessment

1. Assessment of hyperparathyroidism includes neurological assessment including LOC, VS, heart rhythm, GI assessment, complaints of pain, muscle strength, weight, I & O

2. Diagnostic tests for hyperparathyroidism
   a. Serum calcium level: hypercalcemia: normal 9–11 mg/dL
   b. Serum phosphorus level: hypophosphatemia; normal 2.5–4.5 mg/dL
   c. ABGs: metabolic acidosis
   d. Serum potassium level: hypokalemia
   e. Urine calcium and urine phosphates: increased (leads to stones):
   f. Parathyroid hormone (PTH): increased
   g. Alkaline phosphate: increased
   h. Radiological examinations reveal deposits of calcium in soft tissues and renal structures, osteoporotic changes, demineralization of bone

3. Nursing assessment of hypoparathyroidism includes reflexes and other neurological assessments, VS, cardiac rhythm, GI complaints, Chvostek and Trousseau signs, signs of tetany, any integumentary or renal complaints

4. Diagnostic tests for hypoparathyroidism
   a. Serum calcium levels (hypocalcemia)
   b. Serum phosphate levels (hyperphosphatemia)
   c. Parathyroid hormone (PTH): decreased
   d. Urine calcium: decreased
   e. Radiologic examination reveals calcification of skull

D. Nursing management

1. Hyperparathyroidism
   a. Medications
      1) Bisphosphonate regulator: alendronate sodium (Fosamax) or pamidronate disodium (Aredia)
      2) Furosemide (Lasix) (oral or intravenous [IV]) to promote diuresis
      3) Phosphates (oral or IV) for replacement
      4) Calcitonin (Calcimar): IV to decrease release of calcium by bones
      5) Gallium nitrate (Ganite) to inhibit bone resorption of calcium
      6) Glucocorticoids to decrease GI absorption of calcium

   b. Educate client to consume diet low in calcium and vitamin D, and increase oral intake of fluids as prescribed
   c. Intravenous saline fluids to increase excretion of calcium

   d. Preoperative and postoperative care for surgical removal of parathyroid gland (parathyroidectomy) for primary hyperparathyroidism
   e. Strain urine for stones, monitor I & O
   f. Monitor EKG rhythm, VS

2. Hypoparathyroidism
   a. Medications
      1) Calcium gluconate (Kalcinate) IV initially, then supplemental oral calcium replacement
      2) Oral vitamin D
      3) Administer parathyroid hormone (PTH)

   b. Educate client to consume a diet high in calcium and low in phosphate
   c. Monitor for seizure activity and laryngeal spasms; provide protective environment if seizures occur

   d. Perform Chvostek and Trousseau signs for hypocalcemia
   e. Keep tracheostomy set at bedside for respiratory emergencies caused by laryngeal spasm
   f. Monitor neuromuscular function

Practice to Pass

The nurse is providing care to a client who has recently had a thyroidectomy. What clinical manifestations and abnormal laboratory values should the nurse expect to observe if the client was experiencing symptoms related to damage of the parathyroid gland?

3. Priority nursing diagnoses for parathyroid disorders: Impaired Physical Mobility, Risk for Injury, Pain

V. ADRENAL CORTEX HYPERFUNCTION DISORDERS

A. Overview

1. Adrenal glands are located above each kidney and are composed of adrenal medulla (inner layer) and adrenal cortex (outer layer)
   a. Adrenal medulla secretes catecholamines: epinephrine, norepinephrine, and dopamine
   b. Adrenal cortex secretes mineralocorticoids (aldosterone), glucocorticoids (cortisol), androgens and estrogens (sex hormones)
2. Epinephrine and norepinephrine (catecholamines) increase metabolic rate, increase alertness, increase insulin levels, and are responsible for "fight-or-flight" response
3. Glucocorticoids (cortisol) assist body's response to stress; suppress inflammation; increase serum glucose by acting as an insulin antagonist; regulate metabolism of carbohydrates; fat; and protein; enhance protein synthesis; increase breakdown of protein and fatty acids, and decrease pain
4. Adrenocorticotropic hormone (ACTH) aids growth and development
5. Mineralocorticoids (aldosterone) aid in sodium (Na^+) and water retention, and potassium (K^+) excretion
6. Androgens and estrogens contribute to growth and development
7. Adrenal cortex hyperfunction disorders result in excess production of
   a. Cortisol: **Cushing's syndrome**—or hypercortisolism
   b. Aldosterone: **Conn syndrome—hyperaldosteronism**
8. Causes of hypercortisolism include adrenal tumors, adrenal hyperplasia, or exogenous glucocorticoids
9. Causes of hyperaldosteronism include an adrenal lesion or any condition that stimulates overproduction of aldosterone: heart failure, cirrhosis of liver, dehydration, renal disease

B. Pathophysiology

1. Cushing's disease (also known as hypercortisolism)
   a. Functions of glucocorticoids (cortisol, ACTH) include promoting gluconeogenesis, maintaining serum glucose levels, adaptation to stress, and augmenting release of catecholamines to increase blood pressure (BP)
   b. *Primary Cushing's disease* is caused by a benign or malignant adrenal tumor, which stimulates an increased production of cortisol
   c. *Secondary Cushing's disease* results from disorders of pituitary or hypothalamus, which causes an increased release of ACTH, or from an ectopic disorder that produces ACTH
   d. *Iatrogenic Cushing's disease* (most common form) results from use of long-term glucocorticoid therapy, which results in excess cortisol levels
   e. Signs and symptoms of hypersecretion of cortisol include:
      1) Neurological: psychosis, emotional liability, loss of memory, depression, poor concentration
      2) Cardiovascular: hypertension, dysrhythmias
      3) Gastrointestinal: peptic ulcers
      4) Musculoskeletal: muscle weakness, muscle wasting, osteoporosis, "buffalo" hump, truncal obesity
      5) Integumentary: ecchymosis, hirsutism, purple striae on abdomen, poor wound healing, skin infections, thin skin, acne
      6) Renal: glycosuria, polyuria, polydipsia, renal calculi

7) Reproductive: decreased libido, impotence, amenorrhea, masculine characteristics in females

       8) Metabolic: hypokalemia, hypernatremia, edema, "moon face," weight gain

       9) Classic symptoms of Cushing's disease: "moon face," dorsocervical fat pad at back of neck and upper back, purple striae, truncal obesity

2. Conn syndrome (primary hyperaldosteronism)

    a. Role of aldosterone (a mineralocorticoid) is sodium and water retention

    b. Aldosterone affects tubular resorption of sodium (Na^+) and water; also has role in excretion of potassium (K^+) and hydrogen ions (H^+)

    c. In *primary hyperaldosteronism* excessive secretion of aldosterone causes increases in Na^+ and water retention, and an increase in K^+ excretion

       1) As BP increases, renin production is suppressed

       2) BP continues to rise to dangerous levels, potentially leading to renal damage and cerebral infarcts

       3) Despite water and Na^+ retention, edema is *rarely* a complication because water is generally excreted with K^+ ions in urine

    d. In *secondary hyperaldosteronism* hypertension is uncommon

    e. Signs and symptoms include visual disturbances, paresthesias, hypertension, dysrhythmias, fluid retention, renal damage or failure, polyuria, muscle weakness, tetany, and electrolyte and acid–base imbalance

C. Nursing assessment

1. Assessment of Cushing's disease includes VS; cardiac rhythm; neurological assessment; history of GI, renal, and reproductive problems; muscle strength; integument assessment; weight; presence of edema; I & O

2. Diagnostic tests for Cushing's disease

    a. Serum cortisol levels: increased

    b. Serum Na^+ levels: increased (hypernatremia)

    c. Serum K^+ levels: decreased (hypokalemia)

    d. Serum glucose levels: increased (hyperglycemia)

    e. Serum ACTH levels in secondary Cushing's disease: increased

    f. Serum ACTH levels in primary Cushing's disease: decreased

    g. 24-hour urine collection for 17-ketosteroids and 17-hydroxycorticosteroids: increased

    h. ACTH suppression test is performed in order to identify cause; dexamethasone suppression test is done to determine if cause is pituitary or adrenal

    i. White blood cell count (WBC) greater than 10,000/mm^3

    j. Radiological examinations reveal pituitary tumor or adrenal tumor

3. Assessment of Conn syndrome includes neurological assessment, eye exam, VS, cardiac rhythm, fluid status, I & O, muscle strength, electrolytes, and renal status

4. Diagnostic tests for Conn syndrome

    a. Serum Na^+ levels: increased (hypernatremia)

    b. Serum K^+ levels: decreased (hypokalemia)

    c. ABGs: metabolic alkalosis (elevated HCO_3^-)

    d. Serum and urine aldosterone levels: elevated

    e. Serum renin levels (primary hyperaldosteronism): decreased

    f. Serum renin levels (secondary hyperaldosteronism): increased

    g. Radiological examinations reveal tumor

D. Nursing management

1. Cushing's disease

    a. Medications

       1) Mitotane (Lysodren): cytotoxic antihormonal agent that inhibits corticosteroid synthesis without destroying cortical cells

       2) Metyrapone (Metopirone) or the antiinfective ketoconazole (Fluconazole) to inhibit corticosteroid synthesis

Practice to Pass

The nurse is providing care to a client with Cushing's disease. What nursing interventions should be implemented for a diagnosis of Fluid Volume Excess?

3) Cyproheptadine (generic), somatostatin (Octreotide), or bromocriptine (Parlodel): interferes with ACTH production
4) Lifelong steroid replacement if bilateral adrenalectomy is performed and short-term steroid replacement if unilateral adrenalectomy is performed until client adjusts to loss of gland
5) Somatostatin analog (Octreotide) to suppress ACTH
b. Preoperative and postoperative care for adrenalectomy if performed
c. Assist in monitoring effects of radiation therapy if performed
d. Monitor for Addisonian crisis caused by drug therapy
e. Priority nursing diagnoses for Cushing's disease: Excess Fluid Volume, Risk for Infection, Risk for Injury, Activity Intolerance, Anxiety, Deficient Knowledge, Risk for Impaired Skin Integrity

2. Conn syndrome
   a. Medications
      1) Spironolactone (Aldactone) to treat hypertension and hypokalemia for nonsurgical clients
      2) Amiloride (Midamor) for clients unable to tolerate spironolactone
      3) Administer glucocorticoids preoperatively as prescribed to prevent adrenal hypofunction
   b. Preoperative and postoperative care for unilateral or bilateral adrenalectomy
   c. Educate client that if bilateral adrenalectomy is performed, lifetime replacement of glucocorticoids is necessary; unilateral surgery may require temporary replacement until remaining gland adjusts hormonal output
   d. Monitor BP, urine output (UO), electrolytes
   e. Educate client about low-Na$^+$ diet
   f. Teach side effects of medications
   g. Priority nursing diagnoses for Conn syndrome: Excess Fluid Volume, Risk for Injury

VI. ADRENAL CORTEX HYPOFUNCTION DISORDER: ADDISON'S DISEASE

A. Overview
   1. **Addison's disease** is a chronic adrenocortical insufficiency because of destruction of adrenal glands; also known as adrenal insufficiency
   2. Adrenal cortex hypofunction results in decreased production of cortisone and aldosterone
   3. Causes include destruction of adrenal gland because of trauma, infection, hemorrhage into gland, or sudden stress

B. Pathophysiology
   1. Gradual destruction of adrenal cortical tissue leads to hypofunction of adrenal glands
   2. Insufficient hormonal secretion of mineralocorticoids and glucocorticoids results in deficient aldosterone, cortisol, and androgens
   3. Insufficient levels of aldosterone lead to decreased Na$^+$ absorption and increased Na$^+$ excretion
   4. Water follows Na$^+$, leading to increased water excretion and hypovolemia
   5. Hypotension occurs as a result of hypovolemia
   6. K$^+$ is retained (moves opposite direction of Na$^+$), resulting in hyperkalemia

   7. **Addisonian crisis** can occur, which is an acute insufficiency of adrenocortical hormone from a lack of cortisol during stress, such as surgery or pregnancy, or when exogenous corticosteroid therapy is abruptly discontinued
      a. If not treated immediately, circulatory collapse, shock, and death may occur

b. Signs and symptoms include severe nausea and vomiting (N/V), diarrhea, dehydration, sudden pain in lower back, abdomen and legs, hypotension, tachycardia, confusion, restlessness, fatigue, shock, headache

 8. Signs and symptoms of Addison's disease include:

   a. Neurological: neurosis, depression

   b. Cardiovascular: hypotension, EKG changes such as tall, peaked T waves because of hyperkalemia

   c. Musculoskeletal: muscle weakness, fatigue

   d. Integumentary: skin hyperpigmentation (bronzing)

   e. Gastrointestinal: diarrhea, N/V, anorexia

   f. Reproductive: decreased libido, scant pubic hair

   g. Metabolic: hyperkalemia, hyponatremia, hypoglycemia, weight loss

C. Nursing assessment

   1. Assessment includes neurological assessment, VS, cardiac monitoring, activity tolerance, muscle strength, GI symptoms, libido, electrolyte balance, weight

   2. Diagnostic tests

   a. Serum cortisol levels: low

   b. Serum ACTH levels: high

   c. Serum Na^+ levels: low (hyponatremia)

   d. Serum K^+ levels: high (hyperkalemia)

   e. Serum aldosterone levels: decreased

   f. Urinary cortisol levels: decreased

   g. ABGs: metabolic acidosis (decreased HCO_3^-)

   h. Electrocardiogram

D. Nursing management

 1. Medications include mineralocorticoid and glucocorticoid replacement

   a. Addison's disease: administer cortisone, prednisone, or fludrocortisone acetate (Florinef) as prescribed

   b. Addisonian crisis: immediate IV glucocorticoid replacement and fluids with Na^+

   2. Monitor for signs of dehydration

   3. Maintain high-Na^+, low-K^+ diet

   4. Prepare client for surgical intervention if tumor is causative factor

   5. Priority nursing diagnoses for Addison's disease: Deficient Fluid Volume, Risk for Injury

   6. Teach client about need to carry medical alert identification

Practice to Pass

The nurse is educating a client with Addison's disease about nutritional requirements for the management of this disease. What instructions should be provided?

VII. ADRENAL MEDULLA HYPERFUNCTION DISORDER: PHEOCHROMOCYTOMA

A. Overview

 1. Pheochromocytoma is a rare catecholamine-secreting tumor (usually benign) of adrenal medulla that causes severe hypertension as well as hyperglycemia and hypermetabolism

   2. Cause is usually linked to individual with other multiple endocrine neoplasia syndromes

B. Pathophysiology

   1. A tumor in chromaffin cells of sympathetic nervous system arises, in most cases, in adrenal medulla

   2. Tumor causes secretion of excessive amounts of catecholamines (epinephrine and norepinephrine)

   3. The effects of excessive amounts of epinephrine and norepinephrine can lead to a risk of cerebral hemorrhage, cardiac failure, and death if left untreated

4. Signs and symptoms
   a. Neurological: agitation, emotional outbursts, emotional instability, dilated pupils, severe headache, nervousness
   b. Cardiovascular: hypertension (may be persistent, intermittent, or fluctuating; may occur rapidly and abruptly cease), tachycardia, palpitations
   c. Gastrointestinal: N/V, diarrhea
   d. Renal: glucosuria, polyuria
   e. Musculoskeletal: tremors
   f. Metabolic: hyperglycemia, cold extremities, excessive perspiration

C. Nursing assessment
1. Nursing assessment includes VS, emotional stability, reports of neurological symptoms or headache, GI distress, I & O, skin temperature
2. Diagnostic tests
   a. Urine catecholamines (metanephrines and vanillylmandelic acid [VMA]): positive
   b. Serum catecholamines: elevated
   c. Serum and urine glucose: elevated (hyperglycemia and glycosuria)
   d. Radiologic examinations reveal tumor

D. Nursing management
1. Medications
   a. Phenoxybenzamine (Dibenzyline) preoperatively for hypertension control
   b. Metyrosine (Demser) to inhibit synthesis of norepinephrine
   c. IV antihypertensive agents for hypertensive crisis

2 Preoperative and postoperative care for unilateral or bilateral adrenalectomy
3. Monitor for heart failure, cerebrovascular accident, myocardial infarction, shock, renal failure
4 Monitor BP, UO, and neurological status (maintain seizure precautions)
5. Priority nursing diagnoses: Risk for Injury, Pain

VIII. ANTERIOR PITUITARY DISORDERS

A. Overview
1. Pituitary gland, referred to as "master gland," is located at base of brain adjacent to hypothalamus; it regulates endocrine function by producing hormones that affect body systems and stimulate other endocrine glands to secrete hormones
2. Hormones produced by anterior pituitary gland include growth hormone (GH), thyroid-stimulating hormone (TSH), adrenocorticotropic hormone (ACTH), follicle-stimulating hormone (FSH), luteinizing hormone (LH), and prolactin (PRL)
3. Disorders of anterior pituitary gland result in excessive or insufficient pituitary hormones, but are not as common as other endocrine disorders
4. *Growth hormone* (GH) is a hormone necessary for growth that regulates cell division and synthesis of protein; exerts other metabolic effects on endocrine organs, skin, skeletal muscle, cardiac muscle, and connective tissue
5. *Hyperfunction* of anterior pituitary (hyperpituitarism) results in excess production and secretion of one or more hormones: GH, PRL, or ACTH, leading to manifestations such as tissue overgrowth seen in hyperpituitarism
6. Most common cause of hyperpituitarism is benign adenoma
7. *Hypofunction* of anterior pituitary (hypopituitarism) results in a deficiency of one or more of pituitary hormones: GH, FSH, TSH, LH, and ACTH
8. Causes of hypopituitarism include surgical removal of pituitary gland, congenital defects, radiation, and pituitary tumors, infection, or trauma

9. Common disorders
   a. Hyperpituitarism: gigantism and acromegaly
   b. Hypopituitarism: dwarfism

B. **Pathophysiology**
   1. Gigantism
      a. Gigantism results from GH hypersecretion that begins *before closure of epiphyseal plate*; person becomes abnormally tall, often reaching 7–8 feet in height; body proportions are generally normal
      b. Most common cause of gigantism is tumor of pituitary gland
      c. Early detection, diagnosis, and treatment has made this disorder rare in occurrence
      d. Signs and symptoms include excessive height and acromegaly as an adult
   2. Acromegaly
      a. Acromegaly is a result of GH hypersecretion beginning *during adulthood*; bone and connective tissue continue to grow, leading to *disproportionate* enlargement of tissues
      b. Most common cause of acromegaly is a tumor of pituitary gland
      c. Signs and symptoms include large hands and feet; protrusion of lower jaw; coarse facial features; signs of osteoporosis; change in hand, shoe, and glove size that slowly progresses; systemic symptoms: hypertension; coronary heart disease; heart failure; enlarged adrenal, thyroid, and parathyroid glands; amenorrhea; headache; sweating; weakness
   3. Dwarfism
      a. Dwarfism results from deficient secretion of anterior pituitary hormones, which leads to growth retardation and accompanying metabolic disorders
      b. Signs and symptoms include short stature, obesity, high-pitched voice, slow-maturing skeletal system, hyperlipidemia, hypercholesterolemia

C. **Nursing assessment**
   1. Assessment of gigantism includes growth chart for height and weight by age and visual exam
   2. Assessment of acromegaly includes VS, visual disturbances, growth and development, symptom analysis of any pain, signs of heart failure or diabetes mellitus
   3. Assessment of dwarfism includes growth chart for height and weight by age, development of sex organs
   4. Diagnostic tests: bone scan, cholesterol, lipid panel, and hormone levels

D. **Nursing management**
   1. Medications include cortisol and thyroid replacement drugs; growth hormone for dwarfism
   2. Assist client in obtaining proper counseling to facilitate psychosocial adjustment to altered body image
   3. Monitor for diabetes insipidus since posterior pituitary gland may be affected simultaneously
   4. Priority nursing diagnoses for anterior pituitary disorders: Activity Intolerance, Anxiety, Disturbed Body Image, Sexual Dysfunction, Anticipatory Grieving, Ineffective Coping, Risk for Disproportionate Growth

IX. POSTERIOR PITUITARY DISORDERS

A. **Overview**
   1. Posterior pituitary gland secretes hormones oxytocin and **antidiuretic hormone (ADH),** also known as vasopressin; purpose of ADH is to control serum osmolality and water balance

2. Disorders of posterior pituitary gland primarily result from excessive or deficient ADH secretion

    a. Diabetes insipidus (DI) results from ADH insufficiency, leading to excess fluid excretion

    b. Syndrome of inappropriate antidiuretic hormone (SIADH) results from excessive excretion of ADH and excessive water retention

3. Causes

    a. DI: unknown etiology in most cases; tumor or head trauma with damage to pituitary

    b. SIADH: occurs most often because of ectopic production of ADH by malignant tumors, but may also occur as a result of pituitary surgery, head injury, or certain drugs such as diuretics, anesthetics, and barbiturates

B. Pathophysiology

    1. Diabetes insipidus

        a. Normally, fluid balance is maintained by actions of hypothalamus, kidneys, and pituitary gland

            1) Hypothalamus detects dehydration, sends a message to pituitary, which in turn releases ADH and sends it to kidney

            2) In kidney it acts on collecting and distal tubules to reabsorb water, promoting *retention* to restore fluid balance

            3) When excess fluid volume occurs, hypothalamus sends a message to pituitary to inhibit secretion of ADH, promoting *excretion* to restore fluid balance

        b. In DI, ADH *insufficiency* leads to excretion of large amounts of urine (polyuria), up to 12 liters a day

        c. Classifications

            1) *Neurogenic DI* occurs when there is a decrease in synthesis and excretion of ADH; may be idiopathic, or may result from trauma or dysfunction of hypothalamus and pituitary gland

            2) *Nephrogenic DI* occurs when renal tubules are not sensitive to ADH

        d. If DI results from cerebral injury or other trauma, it may resolve without further incident, however, if disorder is chronic, lifelong treatment is required

        e. Signs and symptoms include polyuria, excess thirst, polydipsia, dehydration (if client is unable to replace fluid loss), weakness

    2. Syndrome of inappropriate antidiuretic hormone (SIADH)

        a. Normal feedback mechanisms (as previously described) from hypothalamus, pituitary gland, and kidney fail despite low serum osmolality and increased fluid volume, resulting in *excessive secretion* of ADH, which leads to excessive water retention

        b. Excessive water retention results in dilute plasma, decreased serum Na$^+$ (dilutional hyponatremia), and water intoxication

        c. Signs and symptoms include lethargy, confusion, and/or other changes in neurological status, cerebral edema, muscle cramps, weakness, decreased UO, fluid retention, and weight gain

C. Nursing assessment

    1. Assessment of DI includes I & O, reports of thirst, signs of dehydration (poor skin turgor, dry skin and mucous membranes, sunken eyeballs, weakness, decreased UO)

    2. Diagnostic tests for DI

        a. Serum Na$^+$ level (hypernatremia)

        b. Urine specific gravity: low

        c. Serum osmolality: high

        d. Urine osmolality: decreased

        e. Serum ADH levels: decreased

Practice to Pass

In providing discharge instructions to a client with chronic diabetes insipidus, what information should be included?

      f. Vasopressin test and water deprivation test: increased (hyperosmolality); diagnostic for DI

  3. Assessment of SIADH includes: LOC and other neurological indicators, I & O, weight

  4. Diagnostic tests for SIADH: low serum Na⁺ (hyponatremia), low serum osmolality, and increased urine specific gravity

D. Nursing management

  1. Diabetes insipidus

    a. Medications include vasopressin (Pitressin) for treatment of neurogenic DI; desmopressin acetate (DDAVP) to reduce urine volume

    b. Administration of hypotonic IV fluids

    c. Increase oral fluid intake

    d. Treatment is lifelong for chronic DI

    e. Monitor I & O

    f. Monitor daily weight at same time on same scale in same amount of clothing

    g. Provide dietary instructions for low-Na⁺ diet and teach to avoid caffeine, which increases UO

    h. Educate client about need for MedicAlert bracelet

  2. Syndrome of inappropriate antidiuretic hormone

    a. Medications include diuretics, antibiotics such as demeclocycline (Declomycin)

    b. Administration of hypertonic saline IV fluids

    c. Oral fluid restriction

    d. Monitor I & O

    e. Monitor daily weight at same time on same scale in same amount of clothing

    f. Monitor for neurological changes and other signs of water intoxication

    g. Educate client about need for MedicAlert bracelet

  3. Priority nursing diagnoses for posterior pituitary disorders: Excess Fluid Volume, Deficient Fluid Volume, Risk for Injury, Deficient Knowledge

X. DIABETES MELLITUS

A. Overview

  1. **Diabetes mellitus (DM)** is defined as a lack of or inadequate secretion of insulin, or insulin resistance resulting in hyperglycemia (elevated serum glucose)

    a. Is the most common chronic disorder of endocrine system

    b. Pancreas (beta cells of islets of Langerhans) fails to secrete an adequate amount of **insulin** (hormone responsible for glucose metabolism)

    c. Lack of adequate insulin secretion results in inappropriate *hyperglycemia*

    d. Obesity, especially when centralized in abdomen, may lead to insulin resistance

  2. Types

    a. *Type 1 diabetes* results from destruction of pancreatic beta cells, which leads to insulin dependence (no insulin is produced from beta cells of pancreas); insulin *must* be received exogenously

    b. *Type 2 diabetes* results from a decrease in beta cell weight and number or insulin resistance; may be managed with diet and exercise, and/or oral antidiabetic agents; situations increasing stress on body (surgery, illness, trauma) may create a need for supplemental insulin temporarily because of rise in glucose levels because of adrenal cortex response to stress

    c. Gestational DM: results from glucose intolerance during pregnancy

  3. Causes

    a. Type 1 DM: occurs as a result of genetic, environmental, or immunological factors that damage the pancreatic beta cells (the insulin-secreting cells)

   b. Type 2 DM: etiology is unknown; however, obesity is the single most important risk factor
   c. Other types may be caused by genetic defects, drugs or chemicals, infections or pancreatic disorders, or stress of pregnancy
B. Pathophysiology
   1. Type 1 DM
      a. Damage to pancreatic beta cells leads to hyperglycemia
      b. Renal threshold for glucose is approximately 180–200 mg/dL; glucose spills into urine once it exceeds renal threshold
         1) Because glucose is highly osmotic, fluids "follow" glucose and are excreted from body in large amounts of urine (called *osmotic diuresis*), causing an excessive loss of fluids and electrolytes (*polyuria*)
         2) Loss of fluids leads to *polydipsia* (excessive thirst)
      c. Because of lack of insulin, body is unable to utilize carbohydrates, its primary source of energy; therefore, it must use proteins and fats for energy, leading to unexplained weight loss
         1) This use of fat results in *ketones* (acid end-products of fat metabolism)
         2) As ketones build in body, *acidosis* occurs
         3) Breakdown of nutritional stores leads to excessive hunger, known as *polyphagia*
      d. Polyuria, polydipsia, and polyphagia are classic signs of diabetes and are known as the "3 Ps"
      e. Failure to receive adequate amounts of insulin results in continued fat metabolism, which produces ketone bodies leading to acidosis
      f. **Diabetic ketoacidosis (DKA)** results in severe metabolic, fluid, and electrolyte disturbances, and is a life-threatening condition of hyperglycemia and metabolic acidosis requiring immediate action
   2. Type 2 DM
      a. Results from a decrease in beta cell weight and number or from insulin resistance
      b. There is an *inadequate secretion of insulin* or *insensitivity* (resistance) to insulin, which leads to hyperglycemia
      c. Symptoms are generally same as for type 1 diabetes, but type 2 has a gradual onset and may be undetected for years (later adulthood); additionally, ketones are not usually present and excess weight rather than weight loss is noted
   3 Signs and symptoms
      a. Early manifestations of type 1 DM: polyuria, polydipsia, polyphagia, glucosuria, fatigue, weight loss, N/V, abdominal pain
      b. Early manifestations in type 2 DM: polyuria, polydipsia, blurred vision, weight gain
      c. General multisystem findings (see Figure 9-3)
         1) Sensory and neurological: diabetic retinopathy, cataracts, glaucoma, paresthesias, loss of sensation, peripheral neuropathy
         2) Cardiovascular assessment: coronary heart disease, peripheral vascular disease, hypertension
         3) Gastrointestinal assessment: constipation or diarrhea
         4) Musculoskeletal assessment: contractures
         5) Integumentary assessment: atrophy, foot ulcers, poor wound healing, chronic skin infections
         6) Renal assessment: edema, chronic renal failure, albuminuria, urinary tract infections
         7) Reproductive assessment: sexual dysfunction, vaginitis
         8) Metabolic: hyperglycemia, hypokalemia, metabolic acidosis

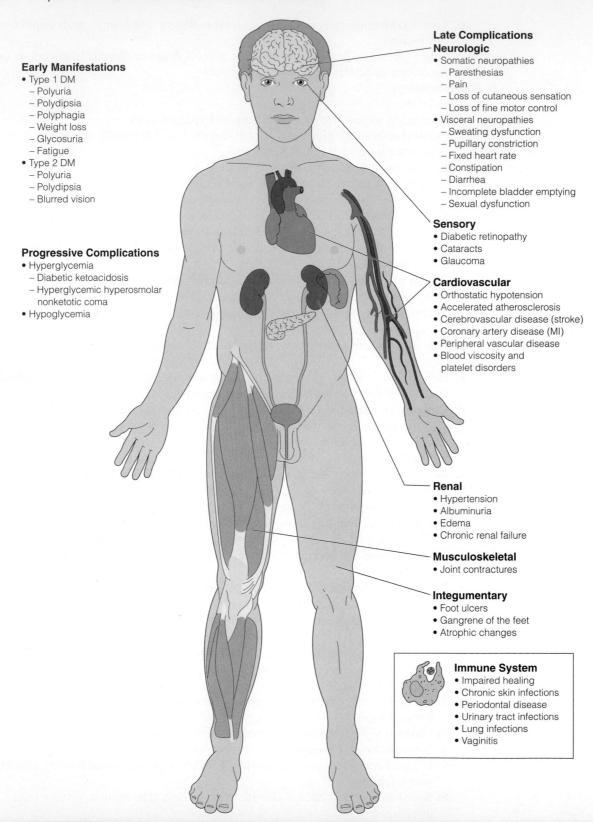

Early Manifestations
- Type 1 DM
  – Polyuria
  – Polydipsia
  – Polyphagia
  – Weight loss
  – Glycosuria
  – Fatigue
- Type 2 DM
  – Polyuria
  – Polydipsia
  – Blurred vision

Progressive Complications
- Hyperglycemia
  – Diabetic ketoacidosis
  – Hyperglycemic hyperosmolar nonketotic coma
- Hypoglycemia

Late Complications
Neurologic
- Somatic neuropathies
  – Paresthesias
  – Pain
  – Loss of cutaneous sensation
  – Loss of fine motor control
- Visceral neuropathies
  – Sweating dysfunction
  – Pupillary constriction
  – Fixed heart rate
  – Constipation
  – Diarrhea
  – Incomplete bladder emptying
  – Sexual dysfunction

Sensory
- Diabetic retinopathy
- Cataracts
- Glaucoma

Cardiovascular
- Orthostatic hypotension
- Accelerated atherosclerosis
- Cerebrovascular disease (stroke)
- Coronary artery disease (MI)
- Peripheral vascular disease
- Blood viscosity and platelet disorders

Renal
- Hypertension
- Albuminuria
- Edema
- Chronic renal failure

Musculoskeletal
- Joint contractures

Integumentary
- Foot ulcers
- Gangrene of the feet
- Atrophic changes

Immune System
- Impaired healing
- Chronic skin infections
- Periodontal disease
- Urinary tract infections
- Lung infections
- Vaginitis

Figure 9-3

Body system effects of diabetes mellitus

      d. Symptoms of diabetic ketoacidosis (DKA): abdominal pain, N/V, metabolic acidosis, fruity breath odor, Kussmaul respirations, decreased LOC, coma, and death if untreated

    4. Complications include DKA, hypoglycemia, atherosclerosis, stroke, PVD, diabetic retinopathy, paresthesias (especially feet), diabetic neuropathy, renal failure, carpal tunnel syndrome, periodontal disease, gangrene, amputation, and inability to heal

C. Nursing assessment

    1. Assessment includes symptom analysis, fluid status, I & O, nutritional status, weight, energy level, GI symptoms, neurological assessment, history of recent infections with difficulty healing

    2. Diagnostic tests

        a. Serum fasting glucose: increased (hyperglycemia greater than 126 mg/dL)

        b. Serum glycosylated hemoglobin levels: increased (greater than 7%)

        c. Urine for glucose and ketones: positive

        d. Urine for protein: positive

        e. Serum K^+: decreased (hypokalemia)

        f. 2-hour-plasma glucose (after meal) greater than 200 mg/dL

        g. Cholesterol and triglyceride levels: elevated

D. Nursing management

    1. Medications include insulin or oral antidiabetic agents

        a. Type 1 diabetes: short-acting (regular) insulin, intermediate-acting (NPH) insulin, long-acting (Lantus) insulin, or combination insulins such as Novolin 70/30; insulins are usually "U 100" with 100 units of insulin per mL; but may be U 500

        b. Type 2 diabetes: oral agents

            1) Sulfonylureas: glimepiride (Amaryl), glipizide (Glucotrol), glyburide (Micronase or DiaBeta), tolazamide (Tolinase), tolbutamide (Orinase)

           2) Meglitinides: repaglinide (Prandin)

           3) Biguanides: metformin (Glucophage)

           4) Alpha-glucosidase inhibitors: acarbose (Precose), miglitol (Glyet)

           5) Thiazolidinediones: rosiglitazone (Avandia), pioglitazone (Actos)

           6) D-phenylalanine derivative: netaglinide (Starlix)

    2. Monitor I & O, serum glucose, electrolytes

    3. Client education

        a. Teach signs and symptoms of hypoglycemia (irritability, fatigue, weakness, tremors, headache, possible coma) and hyperglycemia with appropriate interventions for each

        b. Teach self-administration of insulin or oral antidiabetic agents

        c. Teach onset and peak actions of insulin (see Table 9-2)

        d. Teach self-monitoring of glucose

        e. Teach proper dietary management of diabetes (will need nutritionist consult): include need for balanced meal plan, food groups, food exchanges and need to correlate diet with serum glucose levels

        f. Teach proper diabetic foot care, need for proper shoe fit, and wound care

        g. Teach sick day rules: maintain or increase insulin when a common sickness occurs (virus, colds, etc.), and monitor glucose more often (every 2 to 4 hours) and maintain fluid intake

        h. Teach proper exercise to aid in management of diabetes

    4. Priority nursing diagnoses for diabetes mellitus: Imbalanced Nutrition, Risk for Self-Care Deficit, Risk for Deficient Fluid Volume, Risk for Impaired Skin Integrity, Risk for Deficient Knowledge

Table 9-2	Reaction Time of the Most Common Insulin Preparations	
	Onset (hours)	**Peak (hours)**
Rapid-acting insulin Regular (R) Regular Humulin	0.5–1	2–3
Intermediate-acting NPH (N) Lente (L)	1–2	6–8
Long-acting Lantus Ultralente	not defined 2	not defined 16–20
Combinations Humulin 70/30 Novolin 70/30	0.5	4–8

Case Study

A 16-year-old female is admitted for a workup because of symptoms of excessive weight loss, fatigue, inability to maintain her grades in school, and complaints of constant hunger. These symptoms began rather suddenly, and her mother did not recognize how severe her weight loss had become until she tried on bathing suits. Her admitting lab work was all within normal limits except glucose 425 mg/dL, and her urine test was positive for glucose and ketones. There is no family history of diabetes mellitus (DM). The doctor orders glucose monitoring before meals and at bedtime with regular insulin according to sliding scale along with NPH 30 units subcutaneous every morning.

1. When the health care provider confirms the diagnosis of DM, how should the nurse explain the disease so she can understand?

2. What are the most important symptoms she should be taught?

3. The mother is frantic and doubts the diagnosis because no one in the family has DM. How should the nurse handle this situation?

4. What should the client be taught about the possible problems associated with administration of both NPH and regular insulin?

5. What instructions should the client and her mother be given about hypoglycemia and hyperglycemia and why does she need instructions on both?

For suggested responses, see pages 464–465.

POSTTEST

1 A client with exophthalmos from Graves' disease has expressed a wish for the medications to "hurry up and work so that my eyes will go down." The nurse's response to the client will be based on which of the following?

1. Reversal of exophthalmos will occur after antithyroid medication has achieved a therapeutic level.
2. Reversal of exophthalmos occurs after treatment with ophthalmic medications.
3. Changes in the eyes as a result of Graves' disease are not reversible, even after treatment of the disease.
4. Exophthalmos as a result of Graves' disease is only a temporary symptom and should resolve spontaneously.

2 The nurse is providing care to a client with myxedema coma. Priority nursing care would include which of the following measures?

1. Reducing fever to achieve normal body temperature
2. Decreasing heart rate from tachycardic state
3. Maintaining circulating volume with intravenous fluids
4. Decreasing blood pressure to prevent hypertensive crisis

3 A client diagnosed with primary hyperparathyroidism demonstrates to the nurse an understanding of the teaching plan by making which statement?

1. "I know I must have surgery to remove my parathyroid gland."
2. "I must take diuretics the rest of my life."
3. "I must eat a diet low in potassium."
4. "I must limit my daily fluid intake."

4 The nurse would select which of the following as the priority nursing diagnosis for a client with hypoparathyroidism?

1. Risk for Excess Fluid Volume
2. Risk for Injury
3. Anxiety
4. Deficient Knowledge

5 A client with hyperfunction of the adrenal gland is receiving mitotane (Lysodren). When assessing the client's response to the medication, the nurse would expect therapeutic effects to be the result of which of the following?

1. Halting utilization of glucocorticoids in the tissues
2. Suppression of adrenocorticotropic hormone (ACTH)
3. Direct suppression of activity of the adrenal cortex
4. Destruction of the pituitary gland

6 The nurse has provided preoperative teaching for a client with Conn syndrome who is scheduled for a bilateral adrenalectomy. The nurse concludes that the client understands the information presented after the client makes which statement?

1. "I will need to be on lifetime replacement of glucocorticoids."
2. "I will need to increase my salt intake."
3. "I need to avoid salt the rest of my life."
4. "I will need temporary replacements of glucocorticoids."

7 A client with a history of Addison's disease is admitted to the unit with Addisonian crisis manifested by severe hypotension and unresponsiveness. Which statements provided by the client's spouse provide information to the nurse as to possible precipitating factors to the crisis? Select all that apply.

1. Client stopped taking prescribed hydrocortisone several days ago.
2. Client began eating a reduced salt diet.
3. Client is taking fludrocortisone (Florinef).
4. Client has type 1 diabetes mellitus.
5. Client has recently experienced stressors including an infection and an accident.

8 The nurse administering desmopressin (DDAVP) to a client with diabetes insipidus anticipates implementing which of the following actions for this client? Select all that apply.

1. Maintaining fluid restriction
2. Monitoring urine output and specific gravity
3. Administering oral fluids or hypotonic intravenous fluids
4. Monitoring blood glucose levels
5. Administering drug by route ordered, which may be oral, nasal, or parenteral

9 The nurse would monitor which of the following as the highest priority for a client with pheochromocytoma?

1. Blood pressure
2. Urine output
3. Neurological status
4. Serum glucose levels

10 The nurse concludes that a client newly diagnosed with type 1 diabetes mellitus has understood discharge instructions after the client makes which statement? Select all that apply.

1. "I will notify my health care provider if my glucose levels run higher or lower than the target range."
2. "I will take my insulin as prescribed, and I will not miss a dose."
3. "I will check my glucose level 30 minutes before I eat and at bedtime."
4. "I will not take my insulin if I am sick and cannot eat."
5. "I should call my health care provider if my blood glucose reaches 250 while I am ill."

➤ *See pages 252–253 for Answers and Rationales.*

ANSWERS & RATIONALES

Pretest

1 **Answer: 2** **Rationale:** Hyperthyroidism is an excess of thyroid hormone (TH), which places the body in a hypermetabolic state manifested by increases in appetite, body temperature, and oxygen consumption. Hypothyroidism manifestations are the opposite of those seen in hyperthyroidism. The manifestations of hypoparathyroidism and hyperparathyroidism are related to a decrease or increase in calcium level, respectively. **Cognitive Level:** Analyzing **Client Need:** Physiological Adaptation **Integrated Process:** Nursing Process: Diagnosis **Content Area:** Adult Health **Strategy:** Note that the options contain 2 pairs of opposites. To choose between the pairs, recall that the symptoms listed relate to metabolism, which is a function of the thyroid gland. Next consider that the signs are consistent with hyperthyroidism to choose this over the hypothyroid option. **Reference:** LeMone, P., Burke, K., & Bauldoff, G. (2012). *Medical-surgical nursing: Critical thinking in patient care* (5th ed.). Upper Saddle River, NJ: Pearson Education, pp. 496–497.

2 **Answer: 1** **Rationale:** Although fluid volume status, neurological status, and pain are all important assessments, the immediate priority for postoperative thyroidectomy is airway management. Respiratory distress may result from hemorrhage, edema, laryngeal damage, or tetany. Assessment of respiratory status should include rate, depth, rhythm, and effort. **Cognitive Level:** Analyzing **Client Need:** Reduction of Risk Potential **Integrated Process:** Nursing Process: Assessment **Content Area:** Adult Health **Strategy:** The critical words in the question are *immediate priority*. This indicates that more than one or all are correct but that one is better than the others. Use the ABCs—airway, breathing, and circulation—to make the correct selection. **Reference:** LeMone, P., Burke, K., & Bauldoff, G. (2012). *Medical-surgical nursing: Critical thinking in patient care* (5th ed.). Upper Saddle River, NJ: Pearson Education, p. 499.

3 **Answer: 3** **Rationale:** For best absorption, thyroid medications should be taken 1 hour before meals or 2 hours after meals. Lifelong treatment of hypothyroidism is necessary. Foods that inhibit thyroid hormone (TH) synthesis, such as cabbage, spinach, and carrots, should not be consumed in excessive amounts. Thyroid medications should be taken in the morning to reduce the possibility of insomnia. **Cognitive Level:** Applying **Client Need:** Pharmacological and Parenteral Therapies **Integrated Process:** Nursing Process: Evaluation **Content Area:** Adult Health **Strategy:** The wording of the question indicates the correct option is an incorrect statement by the client. Use specific medication knowledge and the process of elimination to make a selection. **Reference:** LeMone, P., Burke, K., & Bauldoff, G. (2012). *Medical-surgical nursing: Critical thinking in patient care* (5th ed.). Upper Saddle River, NJ: Pearson Education, pp. 502–503.

4 **Answer: 2 Rationale:** Hypercalcemia is the primary complication of hyperparathyroidism, and manifestations of the disorder are directly related to the effects of hypercalcemia. Administering large amounts of IV saline promotes renal excretion of calcium. A strict fluid restriction is unnecessary and could promote retention of calcium from decreased urine output. Calcium gluconate would increase serum calcium levels, and tetany is a symptom of hypocalcemia. **Cognitive Level:** Applying **Client Need:** Physiological Adaptation **Integrated Process:** Nursing Process: Implementation **Content Area:** Adult Health **Strategy:** First recall that the calcium level is high in hyperparathyroidism. Next note that 2 options are opposites, making it more likely that 1 of them is correct. Consider that if the calcium level is high then increased fluid therapy will be needed to dilute the electrolyte. **Reference:** LeMone, P., Burke, K., & Bauldoff, G. (2012). *Medical-surgical nursing: Critical thinking in patient care* (5th ed.). Upper Saddle River, NJ: Pearson Education, pp. 505–506.

5 **Answer: 9 Rationale:** The normal serum calcium level is 9 to 11 mg/dL. The therapeutic response of supplemental calcium is demonstrated by normal calcium levels. **Cognitive Level:** Analyzing **Client Need:** Reduction of Risk Potential **Integrated Process:** Nursing Process: Evaluation **Content Area:** Adult Health **Strategy:** Specific knowledge of normal serum electrolyte levels (specifically calcium) is needed to answer the question. If needed, review the upper and lower limits of the normal reference range for calcium. Note the question asks for a whole number. **Reference:** Kee, J. (2010). *Laboratory and diagnostic tests with nursing implications* (8th ed.). Upper Saddle River, NJ: Pearson Education, Inc, pp. 96–97.

6 **Answer: 2 Rationale:** Cushing's disease is manifested by sodium retention, which leads to edema and hypertension. Excess Fluid Volume is the highest priority nursing diagnosis. Treatment is aimed at restoring normal body fluid balance. Anxiety and Knowledge Deficit should be addressed after fluid volume excess. Weight gain is possible with Cushing's syndrome because of weight gain, but the gain is due to fluid retention, not additional calories. **Cognitive Level:** Applying **Client Need:** Physiological Adaptation **Integrated Process:** Nursing Process: Diagnosis **Content Area:** Adult Health **Strategy:** Use Maslow's hierarchy

to determine that physiological needs take priority over psychosocial needs. Link the term *edema* in the stem with *excess fluid* in the correct option to make the correct selection. **Reference:** LeMone, P., Burke, K., & Bauldoff, G. (2012). *Medical-surgical nursing: Critical thinking in patient care* (5th ed.). Upper Saddle River, NJ: Pearson Education, pp. 507–509.

7 **Answer: 4 Rationale:** Hyperaldosteronism promotes increased renal sodium and water reabsorption causing hypervolemia and hypertension, and renal excretion of potassium. Surgical removal of the adrenal gland(s) is the treatment of choice; however, when surgery is not performed then spironolactone (Aldactone), a potassium-sparing diuretic, is used to treat both hypertension and hypokalemia. It would be counterproductive to reduce the serum potassium level further or to promote additional fluid retention. The disease is lifelong and cannot be reversed by medication. **Cognitive Level:** Applying **Client Need:** Pharmacological and Parenteral Therapies **Integrated Process:** Teaching and Learning **Content Area:** Adult Health **Strategy:** Consider the function of aldosterone and what problems would come with an excess of the hormone. What does the drug do to reverse the response? **Reference:** Huether, S. E., & McCance, K. L. (2012). *Understanding pathophysiology* (5th ed.). St. Louis, MO: Elsevier, p. 470.

8 **Answer: 1, 2, 4, 5 Rationale:** Corticosteroids are immuno-suppressants; therefore, careful monitoring for infection is necessary. Additionally, an increase in the medication may be required for stressors such as infection. A MedicAlert bracelet is recommended to inform health-care providers of Addison's disease and cortisol treatment. Safety measures are encouraged to prevent injuries. The treatment is lifelong. Weight must be monitored *daily*; any increase indicates fluid retention and should be reported immediately. **Cognitive Level:** Analyzing **Client Need:** Physiological Adaptation **Integrated Process:** Nursing Process: Evaluation **Content Area:** Adult Health **Strategy:** First recall that Addison's disease is hypofunction of the adrenal gland, and therefore medication therapy must replace corticosteroids and mineralocorticoids. With this in mind, use the process of elimination and knowledge of possible adverse medication effects to make a selection. **Reference:** LeMone, P., Burke, K., & Bauldoff, G. (2012). *Medical-surgical nursing: Critical thinking in patient care* (5th ed.). Upper Saddle River, NJ: Pearson Education, p. 471.

9 **Answer: 3 Rationale:** Syndrome of inappropriate antidiuretic hormone secretion (SIADH) results in fluid retention, possible water intoxication and hyponatremia. Correction is aimed at restoring fluid and electrolyte balance. Anxiety and Risk for Injury should be addressed following excess fluid volume. Deficient Fluid Volume would not be expected to occur. **Cognitive Level:** Analyzing **Client Need:** Physiological Adaptation **Integrated Process:** Nursing Process: Diagnosis

Content Area: Adult Health Strategy: Consider that fluid status is part of the circulation part of ABCs. With this in mind, consider fluid imbalance to be a higher priority using Maslow's hierarchy, followed by injury, and then anxiety. Use specific knowledge of syndrome of inappropriate antidiuretic hormone secretion (SIADH) to make a final selection, perhaps thinking of the "I" in SIADH as meaning *increased* instead of *inappropriate* will help to recall the direction of change. Reference: LeMone, P., Burke, K., & Bauldoff, G. (2012). *Medical-surgical nursing: Critical thinking in patient care* (5th ed.). Upper Saddle River, NJ: Pearson Education, pp. 516–518.

10 Answer: 1 Rationale: Type 1 diabetes mellitus requires lifelong exogenous replacement of insulin, because no insulin is produced from the beta cells of the pancreas. Insulin therapy is not short-term, nor is insulin therapy required because oral drugs are merely less effective than injections. The pancreas will not be able to resume production of insulin. Cognitive Level: Applying Client Need: Physiological Adaptation Integrated Process: Teaching and Learning Content Area: Adult Health Strategy: Compare the differences between drug therapy for type 1 diabetes to type 2 diabetes mellitus. Which type does the client have? Reference: LeMone, P., Burke, K., & Bauldoff, G. (2012). *Medical-surgical nursing: Critical thinking in patient care* (5th ed.). Upper Saddle River, NJ: Pearson Education, pp. 522–524.

Posttest

1 Answer: 3 Rationale: The treatment of Graves' disease may stabilize the manifestations but generally does not reverse changes to the eyes. Exophthalmos occurs as a result of accumulation of fat deposits and by-products in the retro-orbital tissues and is not reversible by medication therapy. The client should receive instructions on proper eye care to prevent drying and injury. Cognitive Level: Analyzing Client Need: Physiological Adaptation Integrated Process: Communication and Documentation Content Area: Adult Health Strategy: Recall that exophthalmos is permanent. With this in mind, you will be able to eliminate many of the answer choices. Reference: LeMone, P., Burke, K., & Bauldoff, G. (2012). *Medical-surgical nursing: Critical thinking in patient care* (5th ed.). Upper Saddle River, NJ: Pearson Education, pp. 490, 494.

2 Answer: 3 Rationale: Myxedema coma is a life-threatening hypothyroid crisis manifested by hypothermia (not fever), hyponatremia, hypoglycemia, lactic acidosis, cardiovascular collapse and coma. Pulse and blood pressure are not elevated. Maintaining airway and circulation (with fluid volume) are the priority interventions along with replacement hormone because they are life sustaining. Cognitive Level: Applying Client Need: Physiological Adaptation Integrated Process: Nursing Process: Implementation

Content Area: Adult Health Strategy: One option stands out as different from the others. Use Maslow's hierarchy helps in prioritizing. Reference: LeMone, P., Burke, K., & Bauldoff, G. (2012). *Medical-surgical nursing: Critical thinking in patient care* (5th ed.). Upper Saddle River, NJ: Pearson Education, pp. 500–502.

3 Answer: 1 Rationale: The treatment for primary hyperparathyroidism is a parathyroidectomy (surgical removal of parathyroid glands). Primary hyperparathyroidism leads to an increased calcium level, so a low potassium diet is not indicated. Increasing fluid intake, not limiting it, would help with the hypercalcemia that occurs with primary hyperparathyroidism. Diuretic therapy for life is not a treatment measure for primary hyperparathyroidism. Cognitive Level: Applying Client Need: Physiological Adaptation Integrated Process: Nursing Process: Evaluation Content Area: Adult Health Strategy: Review the normal function of the parathyroid gland. Then eliminate the options that relate to other endocrine problems. Reference: LeMone, P., Burke, K., & Bauldoff, G. (2012). *Medical-surgical nursing: Critical thinking in patient care* (5th ed.). Upper Saddle River, NJ: Pearson Education, pp. 505–506.

4 Answer: 2 Rationale: Risk for Injury related to hypocalcemia is the priority diagnosis as injury may occur as a result of low calcium levels and tetany. In severe cases of tetany, death may occur. The client is at risk for Deficient Fluid Volume, not excess, and Anxiety and Deficient Knowledge would not take priority over Risk for Injury. Cognitive Level: Applying Client Need: Physiological Adaptation Integrated Process: Nursing Process: Diagnosis Content Area: Adult Health Strategy: First determine the pathophysiology and risks for a client with hypoparathyroidism. Next choose the nursing diagnosis that focuses on a physiological need and addresses the problem. Reference: LeMone, P., Burke, K., & Bauldoff, G. (2012). *Medical-surgical nursing: Critical thinking in patient care* (5th ed.). Upper Saddle River, NJ: Pearson Education, pp. 505–506.

5 Answer: 3 Rationale: The therapeutic effects of mitotane are the results of direct suppression of activity of the adrenal cortex to block hormone synthesis and decreasing (not halting) peripheral metabolism of corticosteroids. Octreotide suppresses ACTH, and radiation destroys the pituitary gland. Cognitive Level: Applying Client Need: Pharmacological and Parenteral Therapies Integrated Process: Nursing Process: Evaluation Content Area: Adult Health Strategy: Consider what the action of an "antiadrenal" agent might be. Find clues in the stem to help select an answer if guessing. Reference: LeMone, P., Burke, K., & Bauldoff, G. (2012). *Medical-surgical nursing: Critical thinking in patient care* (5th ed.). Upper Saddle River, NJ: Pearson Education, p. 508.

6 Answer: 1 Rationale: Since the client will have a bilateral adrenalectomy, lifetime corticosteroid replacement is necessary. The surgery creates a state of permanent hypofunction of the gland because there is no hormone production. After the adrenalectomy, the client's aldosterone levels should return to normal; therefore, no dietary restrictions will be necessary. **Cognitive Level:** Analyzing **Client Need:** Physiological Adaptation **Integrated Process:** Teaching and Learning **Content Area:** Adult Health **Strategy:** Note that 2 sets of opposites appear as options. Ask if salt or hormone is used to manage the problem to help make the appropriate distinctions among the various options. **Reference:** LeMone, P., Burke, K., & Bauldoff, G. (2012). *Medical-surgical nursing: Critical thinking in patient care* (5th ed.). Upper Saddle River, NJ: Pearson Education, pp. 507–510.

7 **Answer: 1, 2, 5** **Rationale:** Hydrocortisone is given to replace cortisol in the client with adrenal insufficiency. Abrupt withdrawal of the hormone can precipitate Addisonian crisis. Hyponatremia is caused by aldosterone deficiency, which affects the renal tubules' ability to conserve sodium; therefore adding salt to the diet is recommended. Major stressors are a common precipitating factor in Addisonian crisis. Diabetes mellitus requiring insulin therapy is a complication of Addison's disease; however, there is no indication that diabetes precipitated the crisis. **Cognitive Level:** Analyzing **Client Need:** Physiological Adaptation **Integrated Process:** Nursing Process: Assessment **Content Area:** Adult Health **Strategy:** Choose the events or behaviors that contribute to electrolyte imbalance or require corticosteroids for homeostasis. Remember which hormone is deficient in Addison's disease. (Think of the "d" in *Addison* and the "d" in *down* to recall this is a hypofunction of the adrenal gland.) **Reference:** LeMone, P., Burke, K., & Bauldoff, G. (2012). *Medical-surgical nursing: Critical thinking in patient care* (5th ed.). Upper Saddle River, NJ: Pearson Education, pp. 512–513.

8 **Answer: 2, 3, 5** **Rationale:** Diabetes *insipidus* results in massive diuresis and dehydration. Desmopressin (DDAVP) is a synthetic analog of human ADH that acts on the kidneys to increase the reabsorption of water. It is used to control the acute symptoms of diabetes *insipidus* in clients who have insufficient ADH secretion. Oral fluids are encouraged and hypotonic fluids are administered via IV if necessary. The nurse must monitor urine output to evaluate the therapeutic effect of the DDAVP to determine fluid

needs. Glucose levels are monitored for diabetes *mellitus*. **Cognitive Level:** Analyzing **Client Need:** Physiological Adaptation **Integrated Process:** Nursing Process: Implementation **Content Area:** Adult Health **Strategy:** Distinguish between diabetes *insipidus* and diabetes *mellitus*. What is the pathophysiology in this client? **Reference:** Adams, M. P., Holland, L. N., & Urban, C. Q, (2011). *Pharmacology for nurses: A pathophysiologic approach* (3rd ed.). Upper Saddle River, NJ: Pearson Education, Inc., pp. 661–662.

9 **Answer: 1** **Rationale:** Pheochromocytoma is life threatening. Hypertension with systolic blood pressures that may rise to 200–300 mmHg and diastolic to 150–175 mmHg is possible; therefore, monitoring blood pressure is a priority. Urine output and neurological status would follow blood pressure, and there is no indication to monitor glucose levels. The treatment of choice for this disorder is an adrenalectomy. **Cognitive Level:** Applying **Client Need:** Physiological Adaptation **Integrated Process:** Nursing Process: Implementation **Content Area:** Adult Health **Strategy:** What is the life-threatening complication for this client? Monitor for that first. **Reference:** LeMone, P., Burke, K., & Bauldoff, G. (2012). *Medical-surgical nursing: Critical thinking in patient care* (5th ed.). Upper Saddle River, NJ: Pearson Education, p. 514.

10 **Answer: 1, 2, 3, 5** **Rationale:** The client should inform the health care provider of illness, and then should follow "sick-day rules" as prescribed by health care provider, which include taking insulin as prescribed, or increasing insulin as prescribed, consuming extra fluids, resting, and self-monitoring glucose every 2–4 hours. Notifying the provider of blood glucose levels outside the target range, adherence to insulin therapy, and routine monitoring of blood glucose levels are correct elements of self-management of diabetes mellitus. **Cognitive Level:** Analyzing **Client Need:** Physiological Adaptation **Integrated Process:** Teaching and Learning **Content Area:** Adult Health **Strategy:** The wording of the question indicates that more than one option is correct. Recall the elements of client teaching for diabetes, including sick day management, to choose correctly. **Reference:** LeMone, P., Burke, K., & Bauldoff, G. (2012). *Medical-surgical nursing: Critical thinking in patient care* (5th ed.). Upper Saddle River, NJ: Pearson Education, pp. 527–528, 538.

References

Adams, M., Holland, L., & Bostwick, P. (2011). *Pharmacology for nurses: A pathophysiologic approach* (3rd ed.). Upper Saddle River, NJ: Pearson Education.

Ignatavicius, D., & Workman, M. (2013). *Medical-surgical nursing:*

Critical thinking for collaborative care (7th ed.). Philadelphia: W. B. Saunders Company.

Kee, J. L. (2009). *Laboratory and diagnostic tests* (8th ed.). Upper Saddle River, NJ: Pearson Education.

Lehne, R. (2010). *Pharmacology for nursing care* (7th ed.). St. Louis, MO: Saunders.

LeMone, P., Burke, K., & Bauldoff, G. (2011). *Medical-surgical nursing: Critical thinking in patient care* (5th ed.). Upper Saddle River, NJ: Pearson Education.

ANSWERS & RATIONALES

Lewis, S., Dirksen, S. Heitkemper, M., Bucher, L., & Camera, I. (2011). *Medical surgical nursing: Assessment and management of clinical problems* (8th ed.). St. Louis, MO: Elsevier.

McCance, K., & Huether, K. (2010). *Understanding pathophysiology: The biologic basis for disease in adults and children* (6th ed.) St. Louis, MO: Elsevier.

Porth, C., & Matfin, G. (2010). *Pathophysiology: Concepts of altered health states* (8th ed.). Philadelphia, PA: Lippincott Williams & Wilkins.

Osborn, K. S., Wraa, C. E., & Watson, A. (2010). Medical surgical nursing: *Preparation for practice.* Upper Saddle River, NJ: Pearson Education.

Ralph, S., & Taylor, C. (2010). *Sparks and Taylor's nursing diagnosis reference manual* (8th ed.). Philadelphia, PA: Lippincott William & Wilkins.

Wilson, B.A., Shannon, M.T., & Shields, K.M. (2012). *Pearson nurse's drug guide 2012.* Upper Saddle River, NJ: Pearson Education.

Renal and Urinary Health Problems

10

Chapter Outline

Risk Factors Associated with
    Renal and Urinary Health
    Problems
Urinary Tract Infection (UTI)

Urinary Calculi
Polycystic Kidney Disease
Pyelonephritis
Glomerulonephritis

Acute Renal Failure
Chronic Renal Failure
Bladder Cancer
Kidney Cancer

Objectives

➤ Define key terms associated with renal and urinary health
  problems.
➤ Identify risk factors associated with the development of renal and
  urinary health problems.
➤ Explain the common etiologies of renal and urinary health problems.
➤ Describe the pathophysiologic processes associated with specific
  renal and urinary health problems.
➤ Distinguish between normal and abnormal renal and urinary
  findings obtained from nursing assessment.
➤ Prioritize nursing interventions associated with specific renal and
  urinary health problems.

NCLEX-RN® Test Prep

Use the accompanying online resource,
NursingReviewsandRationales, to test
yourself with hundreds of NCLEX®-style
practice questions.

Review at a Glance

acute renal failure (ARF) sudden
decrease, over days to weeks, in renal
function, resulting in retention of urea,
nitrogen, and creatinine in blood
azotemia increased blood levels of
nitrogenous waste products
calculi masses of crystals composed
of minerals normally excreted in urine
chronic renal failure (CRF)
progressive inability of kidneys, over
months to years, to respond to changes
in body fluid and electrolyte composition,
GFR below 20% of normal, serum
creatinine above 5 mg/dL

cystitis inflammation of urinary
bladder
glomerulonephritis inflammation
of capillary loops of glomeruli
hematuria blood in urine
nephrolithiasis stones in kidney
oliguria urine output less than 400 mL
in 24 hours
polycystic kidney disease
a hereditary disease characterized
by cyst formation and massive
kidney enlargement
prostatitis inflammation of prostate

pyelonephritis inflammatory
disorder affecting renal pelvis and
functional portion of kidney
pyuria presence of pus in urine
uremia syndrome of renal failure
that includes increased blood urea and
creatinine levels accompanied by
fatigue, anorexia, nausea, vomiting,
pruritis, and neurologic changes
urethritis inflammation of urethra
urinary tract infection (UTI)
infection of urinary bladder, kidney,
urethra, or prostate
urolithiasis stones in urinary bladder

PRETEST

1 A 25-year-old male college student is diagnosed with an upper urinary tract infection (UTI). The nurse anticipates that which diagnosis is likely to be documented on the medical record?

1. Cystitis
2. Pyelonephritis
3. Urethritis
4. Prostatitis

2 The nurse would expect to see which pathogen on the urine culture and sensitivity (C&S) report of a female client with an uncomplicated urinary tract infection (UTI)?

1. *Streptococcus*
2. *Staphylococcus*
3. *E. coli*
4. *Klebsiella*

3 The nurse would consider that a urinary tract infection (UTI) is complicated when it is present in which of the following clients?

1. Adolescent girl who has recently become sexually active
2. 2-year-old child
3. Elderly, bedridden client
4. Male client

4 The client with cystitis has a routine urinalysis (UA) and pyuria is noted on the report. The nurse concludes the client has which of the following?

1. Kidney damage
2. A host response to the infection
3. Infection with a gram negative organism
4. Foul-smelling urine

5 An adult client has passed a kidney stone and wants to prevent a recurrence. The nurse would include which measures in a teaching plan to prevent recurrence of stones? Select all that apply.

1. Limit fluids, coffee, and milk to concentrate the urine.
2. Limit foods high in dietary oxalate such as spinach, cocoa, and peanuts to prevent calcium oxalate stones.
3. Lower pH of the urine to acidify the urine and reduce stone formation.
4. Provide adequate fluids to reduce risk of crystals forming.
5. Take vitamin D and calcium tablets to strengthen bones and kidneys.

6 Which laboratory finding should alert the nurse to the presence of glomerular injury and the increased risk of renal failure for a client?

1. Cystitis with a urine culture positive for *E. coli*
2. Presence of red blood cell casts in the urine
3. Blood urea nitrogen (BUN) level of 15 mg/dL
4. Hypotension and increased volume of very dilute urine

7 The nurse would conclude that which of the following is an iatrogenic factor that may apply as a cause of acute renal failure in an adult client? Select all that apply.

1. Alcohol
2. Diet
3. Nephrotoxic medications
4. Exercise
5. Severe postoperative hypotensive episode

8 A client has been told that the glomerular filtration rate (GFR) is less than 20% of normal. The nurse's discussion with this client will take into account that this level of filtration is seen in which health problem?

1. Urinary tract infection
2. Kidney cancer
3. Renal failure
4. Polycystic kidney disease

9 The nurse is reviewing laboratory results for an adult client. The nurse would look to the results of which laboratory test as indicators of the client's renal function? Select all that apply.

1. Complete blood count (CBC)
2. Blood urea nitrogen (BUN)
3. Serum glucose
4. Alanine aminotransferase (ALT)
5. Serum creatinine

10 In intershift report the nurse hears that a client is in end-stage renal disease (ESRD). The nurse should anticipate that what treatment will be planned?

1. Postmortem care since death is near
2. Dialysis or kidney transplantation
3. No treatment is indicated until renal function deteriorates further
4. Loop diuretics and measures to lower the potassium

➤ *See pages 272–274 for Answers and Rationales.*

PRETEST

I. RISK FACTORS ASSOCIATED WITH RENAL AND URINARY HEALTH PROBLEMS

A. Urinary tract infection: female, geriatric clients; strictures; impaired bladder innervation; chronic disease such as diabetes, prostatic hyperplasia, and prostatitis; diaphragm use; instrumentation; and impaired immune response

B. Urinary calculi: male, Caucasian race, young and middle adulthood; prior personal or family history of calculi; diseases such as gout, hyperparathyroidism, urinary stasis, repeated infections; medications such as vitamins (A, C, and D), loop diuretics, calcium-containing antacids; frequent cola ingestion

C. Polycystic kidney disease: genetics; dialysis

D. Pyelonephritis: pregnancy; urinary tract obstruction; congenital malformation; urinary tract trauma; scarring; calculi; other kidney disorders; vesicoureteral reflux (urine moves from bladder back toward kidney); diabetes; and sickle cell disease

E. Glomerulonephritis: systemic diseases; poststreptococcal infections; staphylococcal or viral infections

F. Acute renal failure: major trauma or surgery; African Americans; predominantly males; infection; hemorrhage; diseases such as severe heart failure; severe liver disease; lower urinary tract obstruction; nephrotoxic medications; radiologic contrast dye; and shock

G. Chronic renal failure: African Americans, Native Americans, Asians, and European Americans; circulatory failure; urinary tract obstruction; analgesic abuse; diseases such as untreated hypertension (HTN) and diabetes; and cigarette smoking

H. Bladder cancer: geographic (heavily industrialized areas and northern regions); men; cigarette smoke; chemicals and dyes used in plastics, rubber, and cable industries; substances in work environment of textile workers, leather finishers, spray painters, hairdressers, petroleum workers; and chronic use of phenacetin-containing analgesics

I. Kidney cancer: males, over age 50; smoking; obesity; chronic irritation caused by renal calculi; urban environment; industrial chemicals; phenacetin or analgesic abuse

II. URINARY TRACT INFECTION (UTI)

A. Overview
  1. **Urinary tract infection (UTI)** is defined as an infection of bladder, kidney, urethra, or prostate
  2. Urinary tract is normally sterile above urethra, maintained by a free flow of urine from kidneys to meatus and by emptying bladder completely

      3. UTIs are classified according to region and primary site affected

          a. Lower UTIs include **urethritis** (inflammation of urethra), **prostatitis** (inflammation of prostate) and **cystitis** (inflammation of urinary bladder); cystitis is most common form of UTI

          b. Upper UTIs include **pyelonephritis** (inflammation of kidney and renal pelvis)

      4. Causes include bowel incontinence, procedures requiring instrumentation, sexual activity, urinary obstruction or calculi, and improper cleaning (especially in children)

B. Pathophysiology

      1. Pathogens enter urinary tract by 1 of 2 routes

          a. Ascending from mucous membranes of perineal area to lower urinary tract (most common type); gram-negative bacteria, usually *E. coli*, is present in 90% of cases; is most frequent in adult females because of short, straight female urethra

          b. Hematogenously from blood; this type is rare and usually associated with previous damage or scarring of urinary tract

      2. A UTI can be categorized as:

          a. *Uncomplicated*: isolated incidence of UTI

          b. *Complicated*: more than 2 UTIs per year, related to functional, anatomic, metabolic, or neurological disorders, related to an antibiotic-resistant pathogen or pregnancy

      3. Any UTI in a male client is considered complicated

      4. Signs and symptoms include dysuria (painful or difficult urination), urinary frequency and urgency (sudden, compelling need to urinate) and nocturia (2 or more awakenings at night to urinate); urine may have a foul odor and appear cloudy; presence of **pyuria** (excess mucus and white cells in urine) or **hematuria** (bloody urine) caused by bleeding of inflamed bladder wall; older clients may not experience classic symptoms, but instead present with nocturia, incontinence, confusion, behavior change, lethargy, anorexia, or "just not feeling right"

C. Nursing assessment

      1. Assessment

          a. Subjective data: duration of symptoms, history of kidney stones, previous urinary, kidney or prostate problems, history of diabetes or hypertension; inquire about last menstrual period (LMP), pregnancy, and birth control methods; question client regarding allergies, medications, and recent antibiotic use; review diet such as increased caffeine, carbonated drinks, and water intake; ask about pain and tenderness (see Box 10-1)

          b. Objective data: vital signs (VS), observe urine (color, consistency, odor), associated symptoms

          c. Older adults may present with atypical signs, such as behavior changes, confusion, incontinence, or general deterioration

      2. Diagnostic tests

          a. Dipstick urinalysis (UA) is usually adequate for diagnosis of isolated acute UTI

          b. A culture and sensitivity (C&S) of urine should be performed if UTI is thought to be complicated, caused by recent instrumentation, antibiotic sensitivities, or previous treatment failures

Practice to Pass

A client tells the nurse that she has had frequency and burning on urination. What assessment should the nurse make? What instructions should the nurse give her?

Box 10-1	• Dysuria
Common Signs and Symptoms of Urinary Tract Infection	• Urinary frequency
	• Pyuria
	• Hematuria
	• Nocturia
	• Suprapubic tenderness

      c. Urinalysis (UA) may show presence of blood cells or bacteria in urine; bacteria counts of 100–100,000 (normal is none) are indicative of infection; many red blood cells (RBCs) are often present as well as casts

D. Nursing management

    1. Medications

      a. Short term (3- to 5-day) antibiotic therapy for uncomplicated UTI; first-line therapy is trimethoprim-sulfamethoxazole (Bactrim), ciprofloxacin (Cipro) or ofloxacin (Floxin), and nitrofurantoin (Macrobid); alternate first-line therapy includes amoxicillin (Amoxil) and cephalexin (Keflex)

      b. Second-line quinolones are more expensive, however, and can promote resistant strains of bacteria

      c. Phenazopyridine hydrochloride (Pyridium) may be prescribed for comfort measures only (no antibacterial activity); clients should be warned that this drug can stain semen or urine orange

    2. Instruct to take antibiotics at nighttime if possible as drug will remain in bladder longer

    3. Instruct to increase fluid intake unless contraindicated

    4. Assess pain levels and note any change, which may indicate additional disease processes

    5. Teach client to avoid caffeinated drinks and alcoholic beverages that can increase bladder spasms and mucosal irritation

    6. Teach preventive measures such as emptying bladder every 2–4 hours while awake and maintaining fluid intake of 8–10 glasses of fluid per day

    7. Teach women to cleanse the perineal area front to back, void before and after intercourse; avoid bubble baths, feminine hygiene sprays, douching, and whirl pools and spas; and to wear cotton briefs

    8. Unless contraindicated, teach client measures to maintain acidic urine (pH = 5 or less) such as drinking cranberry juice or taking vitamin C daily; avoid excess intake of milk products, fruit juices, and sodium bicarbonate; acidity of urine inhibits bacterial growth by preventing adherence to bladder wall

    9. Stress importance of taking all prescribed medication and keeping follow-up appointments

III. URINARY CALCULI

A. Overview

    1. **Calculi** are defined as masses of crystals composed of minerals that are normally excreted in urine; majority are composed of calcium; other calculi may be made up of magnesium ammonium phosphate, uric acid, or cystine

    2. Stones may develop and cause obstruction at any point in urinary system

    3. Termed **urolithiasis** (stones in urinary tract) or **nephrolithiasis** (stones formed within kidney)

    4. Causes include dehydration, immobility, excess dietary intake of calcium, oxalate, or protein

B. Pathophysiology

    1. Urolithiasis involves precipitation of a poorly soluble salt around a mucoprotein to form a crystalline structure

    2. Ingesting an increased amount of involved mineral or decreasing fluid intake (such as during night), allows an increased concentration where precipitation occurs and stones are formed; when fluid intake is adequate, no stone growth occurs

    3. Stone formation is also affected by acidity or alkalinity of urine and presence or absence of calculus-inhibiting compounds such as pyrophosphate and nephrocalcin in urine

   4. Most kidney stones are composed of calcium oxalate or calcium phosphate, which may be associated with increased calcium levels in blood or urine

   5. Signs and symptoms vary with their location and size

   a. Renal calculi may be associated with a dull, aching flank pain

   b. Bladder calculi may cause a dull, suprapubic pain

   c. Renal colic causes an acute, severe, intermittent pain of flank and upper outer abdomen on affected side; pain may radiate to suprapubic region, groin, and external genitalia; renal colic may be associated with nausea and vomiting (N/V), pallor, and cool, clammy skin

C. Nursing assessment

   1. Assessment includes symptom analysis, pain (severity, quality, onset, duration, location, and intensity); UA for presence of blood, protein, or leukocytes; previous history of stones and treatments and family history of calculi; review dietary intake, milk, calcium-rich foods, and antacids; question client about hematuria, recent injury or trauma; assess VS; inspect, palpate, and auscultate abdomen and inspect external genitalia; and assess for vaginal discharge and pelvic pain

   2. Diagnostic tests

   a. A UA is useful in diagnosis; gross or microscopic hematuria is generally present

   b. Other diagnostic tests may be necessary including urine calcium, uric acid studies, urine oxalate, culture and sensitivity, serum calcium, and phosphorus

   c. Radiographic studies include kidney, ureter, and bladder (KUB), intravenous pyelography (IVP), ultrasound, CT scan, and cystoscopy

D. Nursing management

   1. Medications include pain medications as needed; antiemetics to control nausea

   2. Increase fluid intake to increase urine output (UO), which facilitates movement of stone

   3. Monitor UO and strain urine for stones; document presence of hematuria

   4. Maintain patency and functioning of catheter system if in place

   5. Teach client about all diagnostic tests and interventions, such as lithotripsy, and to strain urine, saving all stones for analysis

   6. Maintain frequent telephone contact with client until stone passes if discharged

   7. Instruct client on preventive measures: fluid intake 2,500–3,000 mL/day, dietary modifications (low purine, limiting vitamin D and calcium [see Table 10-1]), promote activity level to prevent urinary stasis and to take all medications as prescribed

   8. Teach client that presence of a stone increases risk for developing UTIs; teach client signs and symptoms of infection and preventive measures

Practice to Pass

What self-management instructions should be given to the client with urolithiasis?

Table 10-1	Foods to Avoid with Urolithiasis
Food Group	**Samples of Foods**
Acidic	Cheese, cranberries, eggs, grapes, plums, prunes
Alkaline	Green vegetables, fruit except those listed above, legumes, milk products
High calcium	Beans, chocolate, dried fruits, canned fish except tuna, milk products
High purine	Organ meats, sardines, venison, chicken, crab, pork, salmon, veal
High oxalate	Asparagus, beer, colas, celery, cabbage, green beans, nuts, tea, tomatoes

Adapted from: LeMone, R. E., Burke, K., & Bauldoff, G. *Medical-surgical Nursing: Critical Thinking in Patient Care*, 5th ed., © 2011. Reprinted and Electronically reproduced by permission Pearson Education Inc., Upper Saddle River, NJ.

IV. POLYCYSTIC KIDNEY DISEASE

A. Overview

1. **Polycystic kidney disease** (PKD) is defined as a hereditary disease (genetic predisposition) characterized by cyst formation and massive kidney enlargement
2. There are 2 forms: autosomal dominant (affects adults) and autosomal recessive (typically affects children)
3. Genetics is the primary cause

B. Pathophysiology

1. Adult PKD is a slow, progressive disease that is relatively common, accounting for 10% of clients with end-stage renal disease (ESRD) who require dialysis and/or kidney transplant; clients with PKD often develop cysts elsewhere in body, including liver, spleen, and pancreas
2. Of those affected, 9–10% experience subarachnoid brain hemorrhage from a congenital aneurysm; there is also an increased incidence of incompetent cardiac valves in clients with PKD
3. Renal cysts are fluid-filled sacs affecting nephrons of kidneys, which may vary in size; as cysts fill and enlarge, kidneys will enlarge; renal blood vessels and nephrons become obstructed and functional tissue is destroyed

4. Signs and symptoms include flank pain, hematuria, proteinuria, polyuria, and nocturia; UTI and calculi are common as cysts interfere with urine drainage; most clients develop hypertension due to obstruction of blood vessels; kidneys become palpable, enlarged, and knobby as fluid-filled cysts replace functional tissue

C. Nursing assessment

1. Assessment includes presence, location, and duration of symptoms; fluid intake; VS; urination practices; polyuria and nocturia; family history and/or previous history of kidney disease and hypertension; review present and past medications and allergies; assess pain levels and intensity
2. Diagnostic tests: renal ultrasound, IVP, CT scan of kidney, UA

Practice to Pass

A client has just been diagnosed with polycystic kidney disease. How should the nurse explain this disorder to the client?

D. Nursing management

1. Medications include angiotensin-converting enzyme (ACE) inhibitors to control hypertension
2. Instruct and teach client about diagnostic testing
3. Instruct client on signs and symptoms of UTIs and obstruction to avoid further damage to kidney
4. Encourage fluid intake of 2,000–2,500 mL/day as a preventive measure
5. Stress importance of monitoring BP to identify hypertension for pharmacological intervention
6. Instruct client to avoid nephrotoxic medications and to check with a health care provider before taking any over-the-counter (OTC) medications
7. Discuss genetics and optional screening of family members especially if renal transplantation is contemplated

V. PYELONEPHRITIS

A. Overview

1. Pyelonephritis is defined as an inflammatory disorder affecting renal pelvis and functional portion of kidney tissue
2. Classification

   a. *Acute pyelonephritis*, a bacterial infection of kidney
   b. *Chronic pyelonephritis*, associated with nonbacterial infections and processes that may be metabolic, chemical, or immunological
3. Causes include an ascending bladder infection, blood-borne infections, frequent calculi, or other obstructions

B. Pathophysiology

1. The ascending route from lower urinary tract is most common pathway; infection develops in patchy areas spreading to cortex with WBC infiltration and inflammation
2. Kidney becomes grossly edematous and localized abscesses may form; tissue damage may occur primarily to tubules; scar tissue replaces infected/inflamed areas
3. *E. coli* is responsible in 85% of cases; other common pathogens are *proteus* and *klebsiella*
4. Onset of pyelonephritis is typically rapid with chills and fever, malaise, and vomiting along with flank pain, costovertebral tenderness, urinary frequency, and dysuria
5. As with UTIs, older clients may present with behavior changes, confusion, incontinence, or general deterioration
6. Chronic renal failure and ESRD may develop with chronic pyelonephritis; hypertension may develop as renal tissue is destroyed

C. Nursing assessment

1. Assessment includes onset and duration of symptoms and any associated symptoms including pain (description, severity, frequency); rule out pregnancy; review previous history of urinary tract problems, treatments and testing; review present medications and allergies; VS; inspect respiratory and cardiac status; hydration status; inspect external genitalia and abdomen for tenderness, masses, or pain; evaluate UA (preferably a midstream specimen); I & O, urinary frequency, urgency, and nocturia; assess urine for blood, odor, and appearance; question client about family history of kidney disease, infections, diabetes, and hypertension
2. Diagnostic tests: UA (midstream, clean-catch or catheterization), gram stain of urine, urine C&S, WBC, IVP, voiding cystourethrography (after contrast medium instilled into bladder), cystoscopy (direct visualization of urethra and bladder), pelvic/prostate exam

D. Nursing management

1. Medications
   a. Analgesics
   b. 7 to 10 days of oral antimicrobial therapy: sulfonamides, trimethoprim-sulfamethoxazole (TMP-SMZ, Bactrim, Septra), ciprofloxacin hydrochloride (Cipro), or ofloxacin (Floxin)
   c. Urinary anti-infectives: methenamine (Hiprex), nalidixic acid (Neg Gram), nitrofurantoin (Macrodantin)
   d. Urinary analgesics: phenazopyridine (Pyridium)
2. Alleviate pain using medication and nonpharmacologic measures such as heating pads or warm baths, rest, and balanced activity
3. Unless contraindicated, increase fluid intake to 8–10 glasses/day to dilute urine, lessening irritation of mucosa
4. Teach preventive measures of UTI such as emptying bladder every 2–4 hours and increased fluids; for women, proper perineal hygiene, voiding before and after intercourse, avoiding bubble baths, douching, spas, hot tubs, and whirlpools
5. Teach client on obtaining a midstream clean-catch specimen
6. Teach to maintain acidic urine (inhibits bacterial growth) by drinking cranberry juice, taking vitamin C, avoiding excess milk products, and avoiding sodium bicarbonate
7. Instruct to complete full course of prescribed medications even if symptoms have resolved
8. Instruct to keep follow-up appointments as scheduled
9. Referral to urologist may be necessary
10. Teach about common side effects of antibiotics: nausea and superinfections (candidiasis); also teach about others specific to that medication, such as photosensitivity with sulfa medications

VI. GLOMERULONEPHRITIS

A. Overview

1. **Glomerulonephritis** is defined as an inflammation of capillary loops of glomeruli
2. It is classified as acute, rapidly progressive, or chronic glomerulonephritis

3. Acute poststreptococcal glomerulonephritis is most common form
4. Rapidly progressive glomerulonephritis may either be *idiopathic* or *secondary* to an acute infection or a multisystem disease with a greater incidence in males than females
5. Chronic glomerulonephritis is end stage of glomerular disorders
6. Causes

   a. Acute: systemic diseases such as systemic lupus erythematosus (SLE) or primary glomerular disease, but a *beta hemolytic strep* infection of pharynx or skin is most common precipitating factor; *staphylococcal* or viral infections can also lead to postinfectious acute glomerulonephritis

   b. Rapidly progressive: unknown, vasculitis, SLE, or acute glomerulonephritis

   c. Chronic: unknown, lupus nephritis, diabetic nephropathy, rapid, progressive glomerulonephritis

B. Pathophysiology

1. In *acute* glomerulonephritis, circulating antigen-antibody immune complexes are formed and trapped in glomerular membrane; these cause an inflammatory response activating complement system and releasing vasoactive substances and inflammatory mediators; edema and inflammation increase porosity of glomerular capillaries allowing plasma proteins and blood cells to escape into urine; renin-angiotensin-aldosterone (RAA) system is disrupted, which could lead to hypertension

   a. Symptoms usually subside in 10–14 days and 60% completely recover

   b. The remaining 40% may have persistent impaired renal function, continued proteinuria and/or hematuria leading to chronic glomerulonephritis or renal failure

2. In *rapidly progressive* glomerulonephritis, glomerular cells proliferate along with macrophages forming crescent-shaped lesions that obstruct Bowman's space

   a. More than 70% of glomeruli are affected with a rapid decrease in glomerular filtration rate (GFR)

   b. Up to 50% of clients will require maintenance dialysis and/or kidney transplant

3. *Chronic* glomerulonephritis involves a slow, progressive destruction of glomeruli with impaired renal function; kidneys decrease in size symmetrically and become granular or roughened; eventually, all nephrons are destroyed

4. Signs and symptoms (see Figure 10-1)

   a. Acute: hematuria-brown tinged, proteinuria, salt and water retention, red blood cell casts, hypertension, **azotemia**, fatigue, anorexia, N/V, and headache

   b. Rapidly progressive: weakness, N/V, flulike symptoms, oliguria, abdominal or flank pain

   c. Chronic: develops insidiously and is often unrecognized until renal failure is evident

C. Nursing assessment

1. Assessment includes VS (increased fluid volume increases cardiac workload); weight and presence of edema; I & O; assess energy, activity and fatigue status; signs of infections including skin, throat, and lungs; client's knowledge of disease, coping abilities, support system, lifestyle changes, and need for additional interventions or support

2. Diagnostic tests: throat or skin cultures, antistreptolysin (ASO) titer, erythrocyte sedimentation rate (ESR), antinuclear antibody (ANA), blood urea nitrogen (BUN), creatinine, electrolytes, UA, 24–hour urine for creatinine clearance, abdominal x-rays, kidney scan, and biopsy

Practice to Pass

A client recovering from hepatitis B begins to exhibit signs and symptoms of rapid, progressive glomerulonephritis. What is the significance of this disease on the GFR?

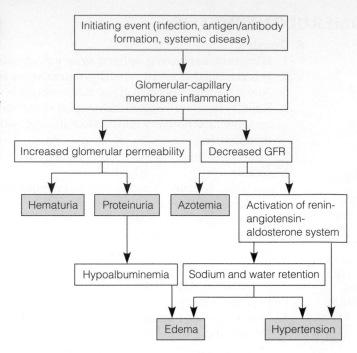

Figure 10-1

Critical pathway of glomerulonephritis.

Lemone, Priscilla; Burke, Karen M.; Bauldoff, Gerene, *Medical-Surgical Nursing: Critical Thinking in Patient Care*, 5th Edition, © 2011. Printed and Electronically reproduced by permission of Pearson Education, Inc., Upper Saddle River, New Jersey.

D. Nursing management

1. Medications (treat symptoms since no cure exists)
   a. Immunosuppressive therapy (to decrease risk of ESRD): cyclophosphamide (Cytoxan), azathioprine (Imuran), chlorambucil (Leukeran)
   b. Glucocorticoids (to enhance remission of nephrotic syndrome): prednisone—these may worsen certain types of glomerulonephritis, such as poststreptococcal
   c. ACE inhibitors and nonsteroidal anti-inflammatory drugs (NSAIDs) that decrease protein loss
   d. Antibiotics: penicillin
   e. Antihypertensives
2. Monitor IV fluids and monitor diuretic effect
3. Assess urinary catheter system if indicated
4. Educate client and family regarding disease process
5. Instruct client on the following:
   a. Prescribed medications and side effects of immunosuppressive or steroid drugs
   b. Activity level and dietary restrictions; arrange for a dietary consultation if necessary
   c. Weigh self daily on same scale, at same time, and with same amount of clothing; report weight gains to provider
   d. Fluid restriction if ordered and importance of measuring I & O
   e. Signs and symptoms of improving or declining renal function
   f. Signs and symptoms of infectious processes
6. Assist with problem solving and support services as needed

VII. ACUTE RENAL FAILURE

A. Overview

1. **Acute renal failure (ARF)** is defined as a rapid decrease in renal function
2. ARF is generally recognized by a fall in UO and increase in BUN and/or creatinine; oliguria is common but high output failure is possible

3. Most common causes of ARF are ischemia and nephrotoxins; a fall in BP or volume can cause ischemia of kidney tissue; exposure of renal tissue is great when nephrotoxins (such as contrast media) are present in blood (see Figure 10-2)

4. ARF may have iatrogenic causes such as nephrotoxic drugs, radiologic contrast dye, and surgical shock

5. Causes are categorized as prerenal, intrarenal, and postrenal (see Box 10-2)

6. A newer term, *acute kidney injury* (AKI) or *acute renal injury* (ARI) is being popularized to indicate milder degrees of renal impairment in clients developing ARF

   a. In ARI, UO is less than 0.5 mL/kg/hr for at least 12 hours, while in AFR the UO is less than 0.3 mL/kg/hr for at least 24 hours and anuria is present for at least 12 hours

   b. There are different criteria for GFR; serum creatinine (often used as an indirect indicator of GFR) may not reliably distinguish ARF from ARI because of variables such as nutrition, volume, and lag time to steady state

   c. Treatment considerations for ARI follow the same principles as for ARF

B. **Pathophysiology**

1. Ischemia is primary cause of ARF; if allowed to continue longer than 2 hours, ischemia leads to severe and irreversible damage to tubules with patchy necrosis; GFR is decreased due to ischemia; activation of renin-angiotensin system occurs and tubular obstruction is caused by debris

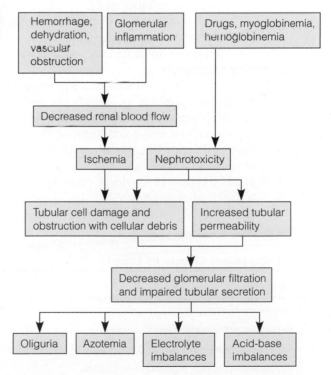

Figure 10-2

Critical pathway of acute renal failure

Box 10-2

Categories of Acute Renal Failure

- Prerenal: hypovolemia, cardiovascular failure, and altered vascular resistance
- Intrarenal: vascular disease, glomerulonephritis, nephritis, and tubular necrosis
- Postrenal: interstitial nephritis, extrarenal obstruction, and intrarenal obstruction

2. Nephrotoxins destroy tubular cells allowing for increased permeability caused by necrosis and sloughing; nephrons then have decreased ability to eliminate waste
3. ARF follows 3 phases: initiation, maintenance, and recovery
   a. *Initiation phase*: begins with onset of event causing tubular necrosis; this phase ends when tubular injury occurs
   b. *Maintenance phase*: begins within hours of initiation phase and typically lasts 1–2 weeks; it is characterized by persistent reduction in GFR and tubular necrosis
   c. *Recovery phase*: begins when GFR and tubular function have recovered and there is no further elevation of BUN and creatinine; renal function improves rapidly during first 5–25 days and continues up to 1 year
4. Signs and symptoms
   a. Initiation: has few manifestations and often is identified after later manifestations have occurred

   b. Maintenance:
      1) **Oliguria** (decreased UO) is usually present early in this phase; kidney cannot eliminate waste products, leading to azotemia, fluid retention, electrolyte imbalance, and metabolic acidosis; salt and water retention leads to edema and increased risk for heart failure and pulmonary edema; impaired renal elimination leads to hyperkalemia, hyperphosphatemia, and hypocalcemia; infection is a leading cause of death but other complications include hypertension, neurologic symptoms, GI manifestations, and **uremia**, a syndrome of renal failure (see Table 10-2)
      2) End of maintenance phase in oliguric clients is characterized by a progressive increase in urine volume; damaged tubules are repaired; diuresis indicates nephrons are sufficiently recovered

C. Nursing assessment

1. Assessment includes weight; VS (note orthostatic hypotension due to diuretics); hydration status; I & O; identify any underlying causes; assess client's knowledge of disease process, coping methods, and needs; pain status and effect of medications; question client about symptoms of illness as well as past medical history, present and past medications, and family history of kidney disease; common signs and symptoms of renal failure include:
   a. Skin: yellow skin, edema, ecchymosis, uremic frost
   b. ENT: urinous breath
   c. Pulmonary: crackles, effusion, tachypnea

Table 10-2	The Multisystem Effects of Uremia
System	**Symptoms**
Respiratory	Pulmonary edema, pleuritis, respiratory distress
Urinary	Hematuria, proteinuria, oliguria, nocturia
Gastrointestinal	Anorexia, nausea, vomiting, abdominal pain, GI bleeding, uremic fetor
Endocrine	Hyperparathyroidism, intolerance to glucose
Musculoskeletal	Bone pain, fractures
Neurologic	Apathy, lethargy, headache, impaired cognition, insomnia, paresthesias, decreased level of consciousness
Cardiovascular	Elevated blood pressure, cardiac dysrhythmias, congestive heart failure
Hematologic	Anemia, difficulty clotting
Reproductive	Females experience amenorrhea, males experience impotence
Integumentary	Pallor, uremic frost, dry skin, pruritis, ecchymosis

      d. Cardiovascular: hypertension, S_3 or S_4 heart sound, cardiac dysrhythmia

      e. Gastrointestinal: GI bleeding

      f. Neurologic: change in LOC

      g. Neuromuscular: tremors, hyperreflexia

    2. Diagnostic tests: electrolytes (hyperkalemia, hyponatremia, hyperphosphatemia), BUN and creatinine (elevated), ABGs (metabolic acidosis), CBC (anemia), UA (fixed specific gravity, protein, casts), bladder catheterization, renal ultrasonography, tomography, IVP, renal biopsy

   3. Creatinine is more accurate than BUN because it is not affected by dietary protein or fluid status; BUN to creatinine ratio should be 10:1; creatinine does not increase unless 25% of nephrons are not functioning

D. Nursing management

   1. Medications

      a. Renal blood flow enhancer: dopamine (Intropin)

      b. Diuretics: furosemide (Lasix) or mannitol (Osmitrol)

      c. Antihypertensives if necessary: ACE inhibitors

      d. Antacids and H_2-receptor blockers to prevent GI ulcer

      e. Potassium-binding exchange resin: polystyrene sulfonate (Kayexelate)

      f. Specific antacid: calcium carbonate (Tums) to control hyperphosphatemia

   2. Weigh client at same time daily to document fluid volume status; restrict fluids as ordered

   3. Treat infections as soon as possible

   4. Record VS and monitor for onset of heart failure or pulmonary edema; use semi-Fowler's position to enhance cardiac and respiratory function

   5. Monitor lab values

   6. Monitor skin status since edema can decrease tissue perfusion and increase risk for skin breakdown

   7. Administer medications cautiously as ordered and document effectiveness; avoid any drugs that are nephrotoxic or contraindicated in ARF, such as metformin (Glucophage)

   8. Document food intake and arrange for a dietary consultation to incorporate requirements (low protein, high carbohydrate [CHO]), restrictions, and client's preferences

   9. Explain and answer questions regarding disease process and concerns

  10. Teach client to monitor weight, BP, and pulse to assess fluid status

  11. Teach client about drugs that are nephrotoxic such as NSAIDs, some antibiotics, x-ray contrast, and heavy metals; instruct to avoid magnesium-containing antacids; explain that alcohol may increase nephrotoxic effects drugs

  12. Stress importance of follow-up visits, UA, and bloodwork

VIII. CHRONIC RENAL FAILURE

A. Overview

   1. Chronic renal failure (CRF) is defined as a progressive inability, over months to years, of kidneys to respond to changes in body fluids and electrolyte composition and an inability to produce sufficient urine; GFR is less than 20% of normal and serum creatinine is greater than 5 mg/dL

   2. There are four stages of chronic renal failure (see Box 10-3)

      a. *Early stage* (decreased renal reserve): unaffected nephrons compensate for lost nephrons

      b. *Second stage* (renal insufficiency): more than 25–50% of functional renal tissue is destroyed

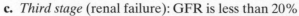

Box 10-3	• First: decreased renal reserve (BUN and creatinine are normal)
	• Second: renal insufficiency (BUN 20–50 mg/dL)
Stages of Chronic Renal Failure	• Third: renal failure (BUN > 100 mg/dL; Cr > 4 mg/dL)
	• Fourth: end-stage renal disease (BUN > 200 mg/dL; Cr > 5 mg dL)

> c. *Third stage* (renal failure): GFR is less than 20%
> d. *Fourth stage* (end-stage renal disease [ESRD]): GFR is less than 5%
>
> 3. Ideally, conservative treatment is used; educate client and family and explore options for long-term management; when conservative treatment is no longer effective, dialysis or renal transplantation is considered
> 4. Most common causes of CRF are diabetic nephropathy, hypertension, glomerulonephritis, cystic kidney disease, and urologic disease

B. Pathophysiology

1. Pathophysiologic process of CRF appears as a gradual loss of entire nephron units
2. As functional capacity of entire nephron is lost and renal mass is reduced, there is progressive deterioration of glomerular filtration, tubular secretion and reabsorption; eventually, kidneys are unable to excrete metabolic waste and regulate fluid and electrolyte balance
3. Signs and symptoms
   a. Early stage: clients remain free of symptoms and BUN and creatinine are normal
   b. Second stage: there is a slight rise in BUN and creatinine; few symptoms may be present including oliguria or polyuria, hypertension, and azotemia
   c. Third stage: there is a sharp increase in BUN and creatinine; symptoms of oliguria and uremia are present; there are usually multisystem effects of renal failure such as uremia, metabolic acidosis, and increasing azotemia
   d. Fourth stage: there is extreme elevation in BUN and creatinine; client has overt uremia; survival depends on dialysis or transplant

C. Nursing assessment

1. Assessment includes VS, I & O, edema, daily weight, measurement of abdominal girth daily; fluid and dietary restrictions; client's knowledge of disease, treatment options, and support systems; activity level and fatigue; medication effects and any side effects; question client about end-of-life care
2. Diagnostic tests: BUN and creatinine (elevated), electrolytes (hyponatremia [may be normal], hyperkalemia, hyperphosphatemia, hypocalcemia), CBC (severe anemia and thrombocytopenia), UA (fixed specific gravity, proteins, blood cells, casts), urine C&S, creatinine clearance (decreased), ABGs (metabolic acidosis), renal ultrasonography, and kidney biopsy

D. Nursing management

1. Medications
   a. Diuretics: usually loop diuretics
   b. Antihypertensives: ACE inhibitors: minoxidil (Loniten), clonidine (Catapres)
   c. Sodium bicarbonate, calcium carbonate (Tums), phosphate-binding agents, calcium supplements, vitamin D
   d. Iron and folic acid supplements; epoetin alfa (Epogen) for anemia
   e. Potassium-binding exchange resin: polystyrene sulfonate (Kayexelate)
2. Maintain fluid and dietary restrictions; refer for dietary consultation if necessary; limit Na^+ and protein, high CHO
3. Administer and document medication effects and side effects; meds should be administered cautiously
4. Monitor lab values

Practice to Pass

A client with CRF asks why he cannot have a drink with his meal tray and why proteins are limited. How should the nurse respond?

5. Use standard precautions and good hand hygiene at all times to decrease transfer of organisms to client
6. Provide oral hygiene at least every 4 hours
7. Monitor activity level and fatigue
8. Arrange mealtime and activities around procedures and per client preferences
9. Encourage expression of feelings or concerns and assist client in developing realistic goals and coping strategies; refer to mental health counselor if necessary
10. Whether client has arteriovenous fistula or peritoneal dialysis, assess site for signs and symptoms of infection, patency (bruit and thrill with fistula), and check tubing for kinks

IX. BLADDER CANCER
A. Overview
1. Defined as a tumor of bladder; majority of tumors affecting urinary tract arise from epithelial tissue and most common site is urinary bladder
2. Bladder cancer is fifth most common malignancy and tenth leading cause of cancer deaths
3. Causes include cigarette smoke, exposure to chemicals and dyes, chronic use of phenacetin-containing analgesic agents
B. Pathophysiology
1. Two major factors are implicated in bladder cancer: presence of carcinogens in urine and chronic inflammation or infection of bladder mucosa
2. Urinary tract tumors begin as nonspecific cellular alterations that develop either as flat or papillary lesions that may be invasive or superficial; papillary lesions are characterized by a polyp-like structure attached by a stalk to bladder mucosa; papillomas are superficial noninvasive tumors that frequently recur; carcinoma in situ is a poorly differentiated flat tumor that invades directly and has a poor prognosis
3. Signs and symptoms include painless hematuria (most common), which is gross or microscopic, constant or intermittent; symptoms of UTI, and colicky pain
C. Nursing assessment
1. Assessment includes urinary pattern, history of hematuria, pain
   a. Preoperative assessment: assess client's coping mechanisms and concerns; UO and change in color; fluid intake to keep urine dilute; activity level; urinary catheters, tubing, and drainage system for patency and obstruction; signs of infection
   b. Postoperative assessment: I & O; color and consistency of urine (bright red blood may indicate hemorrhage); stoma and surrounding skin (with cystectomy); and pain level
2. Diagnostic tests: UA, urine cytology, IVP, renal ultrasound, CT scan, cystoscopy, and ureteroscopy
D. Nursing management
1. Medications and treatment
   a. Chemotherapy agents may be used either as primary treatment or prophylactically to prevent recurrence; doxorubicin (Adriamycin), mitomycin C (Mutamycin), bacille calmette guerin (BCG Live)
   b. Radiation can reduce tumor size prior to surgery
   c. Surgical procedures range from simple resection to removal of bladder
2. Teach client about disease process, interventions, and postoperative care
3. Monitor I & O carefully, notify health care professional if UO less than 30 mL/hr; irrigate catheter as ordered
4. Monitor lab values, electrolyte, and renal function tests
5. Encourage fluid intake to 3,000 mL/day to dilute urine and decrease irritation

6. Teach family and client about stoma care and catheter care
7. Discuss family/client concerns about activity, sexual relations, and employment; initiate support group or counseling if necessary
8. Teach client/family about signs and symptoms of infection and preventive measures
9. Instruct client on toiletry care after receiving bacille Calmette Guerin (BCG live)

X. KIDNEY CANCER

A. Overview

1. Defined as a tumor of kidney; renal cell cancer is most common primary tumor; another primary tumor occurs in renal pelvis; these tumors arise in epithelium of proximal convoluted tubules
2. Causes include metastasis from lung and breast cancer, melanoma, and malignant lymphoma

B. Pathophysiology

1. Renal cell tumors metastasize most commonly to lungs, mediastinum, bone, lymph nodes, liver, and central nervous system
2. Tumor may produce hormones or hormone-like substances, including parathyroid hormones, prostaglandins, prolactin, renin, gonadotropins, and glucocorticoids
3. Classic triad of symptoms (gross hematuria, flank pain, and a palpable abdominal mass) are seen in only 10% of those with renal cell cancer
4. Signs and symptoms include microscopic or gross hematuria, flank pain, palpable abdominal mass, fever, fatigue, weight loss, and anemia and/or polycythemia

C. Nursing assessment

1. Assessment includes pain (level, location, intensity, and character); client's knowledge of disease and procedures to be performed; lab values; VS; UO; fluid intake (oral and IV); activity level and fatigue
2. Postoperative assessment includes incision site for signs/symptoms of inflammation or infection; drainage catheters and tubes for patency; respiratory status and GI function to prevent major complications; potential complications of surgery such as paralytic ileus, thrombosis, and embolus
3. Diagnostic tests: renal ultrasound (first diagnostic evidence of a kidney tumor); CT scans (provide information about tumor density, extension of tumor and regional lymph node or vascular involvement); chest x-ray, bone scan, and liver function studies are done prior to intervention to evaluate potential metastasis of disease

D. Nursing management

1. Medications and treatment
   a. Chemotherapy: immunotherapy such as interferon alpha (Roferon-A)
   b. Radiation therapy
   c. Radical nephrectomy (usual treatment); transabdominal approach
2. Instruct on signs and symptoms of infection
3. Teach client to maintain fluid intake 2,000–2,500 mL/day and increase during hot weather or exercise
4. Instruct client to void when urge is experienced, and before and after intercourse
5. Teach client to avoid trauma to remaining kidney
6. Continue to encourage family and client to discuss feelings and concerns
7. Instruct about home medications, wound care, diet, and activity
8. Refer to support services if appropriate
9. Stress importance of follow-up visits and scheduled bloodwork; instruct to report decreased UO, fever, or abdominal pain

Case Study

L. J. is a 45-year-old construction worker who experienced a large myocardial infarction with cardiovascular complications. On day 3 of his hospital stay, the nurse notices his urine output is being maintained at 20 to 25 mL/hr. Another symptom is edema. His potassium (K^+) is 5.2 mg/L, sodium (Na^+) is 125 mEq/L, ABGs show pH 7.25, PCO_2 38, HCO_3^- 21. The BUN is 28, Cr is 2.5 mg/dL, and lung sounds reveal soft crackles. He is diagnosed with acute renal failure (ARF).

1. What do L. J.'s ABGs show and is this common with ARF? Why or why not?

2. What is significant about his electrolytes in relation to his cardiac condition?

3. What phase of ARF is L. J. in, and what can the nurse tell him is the expected time frame until the kidneys are hopefully working properly again?

4. Considering his initial diagnosis, presenting signs and symptoms, and the known complications of ARF, what is the greatest cardiovascular concern for L. J.?

5. Should L. J. be given a low-sodium or high-sodium diet? Why or why not?

For suggested responses, see page 465.

POSTTEST

POSTTEST

1 A urinalysis is ordered for a client with urinary calculi. The nurse anticipates that which of the following is usually positive on the urinalysis report in clients with this diagnosis?

1. Leukocytes
2. Nitrite
3. Protein
4. Blood

2 The nurse considers that a 40-year-old male client is at high risk for which disorder if his father also experienced this problem?

1. Glomerulonephritis
2. Renal failure
3. Polycystic kidney disease
4. Urinary tract infection

3 The client has a temperature of 102°F and urinalysis reveals a white blood count of 14,000/mm³. Further diagnostic testing pinpoints the origin in the kidney. The nurse concludes the client most likely has which disorder?

1. Acute pyelonephritis
2. Renal failure
3. Chronic pyelonephritis
4. Urinary calculi

4 A client is diagnosed with chronic pyelonephritis. The nurse explains to the client that it will be important to have ongoing monitoring for which associated problems? Select all that apply.

1. Severely high blood pressure
2. Elevated body temperature
3. Hyperlipidemia
4. Renal failure
5. Sexually transmitted infections (STIs)

5 A client with pharyngitis has had a throat culture done. After the health care provider prescribes oral penicillin, the nurse explains that this medication will help to prevent development of acute glomerulonephritis from which microorganism?

1. *Group-A beta Hemolytic-streptococcus*
2. *Staphylococcus*
3. *E. coli*
4. *Proteus*

6 The nurse interprets that which client is at highest risk for a urinary tract infection (UTI)?

1. 79-year-old female
2. 45-year-old male
3. 14-year-old female
4. 27-year-old male

7 During interdisciplinary rounds on a client with rapidly progressive glomerulonephritis, the health care provider describes that crescent-shaped lesions form and obliterate Bowman's space. During subsequent nursing care, what problems should the nurse be alert for?

1. Azotemia and hematuria
2. Renal colic and flank pain
3. Hypotension and tachycardia
4. Urinary urgency and frequency

8 A 19-year-old female client is diagnosed with an uncomplicated urinary tract infection. In addition to antibiotic therapy, the nurse will encourage which of the following?

1. Tub baths or saunas for relaxation and comfort
2. Increasing fluids to 2–2.5 liters per day
3. Avoiding sexual intercourse
4. Using acetaminophen (Tylenol) for pain

9 Because an older adult may not report dysuria with a urinary tract infection (UTI), the nurse should be alert for what other manifestations of infection? Select all that apply.

1. Incontinence
2. Cloudy urine
3. Diluted, clear urine
4. Foul-smelling urine
5. Ketonuria

10 The nurse would teach the client who has a urinary tract infection about which helpful self-care measures? Select all that apply.

1. Taking antiinfective medication until feeling better
2. Increasing fluids
3. Decreasing caffeine drinks and alcohol
4. Douching daily
5. Drinking at least two 8-ounce low-sugar cranberry juice servings per day

➤ *See pages 274–275 for Answers and Rationales.*

POSTTEST

ANSWERS & RATIONALES
Pretest

ANSWERS & RATIONALES

1 Answer: 2 Rationale: Pyelonephritis is an upper urinary tract infection, involving the pelvis of the kidney. Lower urinary tract infections include urethritis, prostatitis, and cystitis. The most common upper urinary tract infection is pyelonephritis. **Cognitive Level:** Applying **Client Need:** Physiological Adaptation **Integrated Process:** Nursing Process: Diagnosis **Content Area:** Adult Health **Strategy:** A critical word in the stem is *upper*. Review anatomy of the urinary tract and eliminate the options that apply to the lower urinary tract. **Reference:** LeMone, P., Burke, K., & Bauldoff, G. (2012). *Medical-surgical nursing: Critical thinking in patient care* (5th ed.). Upper Saddle River, NJ: Pearson Education, pp. 785–788.

2 Answer: 3 Rationale: *E. coli* from the lower GI tract is the infective organism in over 90% of first-time infections

due to the proximity of the anus. The nurse should check that the organism is sensitive to the antibiotic or notify the health care provider. *Staphylococcus* is the second most common pathogen seen in urinary tract infections (UTIs). *Klebsiella* is less common in UTIs, and *streptococcus* is not an expected microorganism. **Cognitive Level:** Applying **Client Need:** Reduction of Risk Potential **Integrated Process:** Nursing Process: Assessment **Content Area:** Adult Health **Strategy:** Consider the anatomy of a female and the proximity of the urinary meatus to the anus. **Reference:** Huether, S. E., & McCance, K. L. (2012). *Understanding pathophysiology* (5th ed.). St. Louis, MO: Elsevier Inc., pp. 785–786.

3 Answer: 4 Rationale: Because of the anatomic structure of the male urethra and bacteriostatic effect of prostatic fluid, all urinary tract infections (UTIs) in the male client should be considered complicated. UTIs are more likely to be uncomplicated in females. **Cognitive Level:** Applying **Client Need:** Physiological Adaptation **Integrated Process:** Nursing Process: Diagnosis **Content Area:** Adult Health **Strategy:** Consider the normal anatomy of the GU system. Which client is least likely to be infected? That client's infection has contributing factors. **Reference:** Huether, S. E., & McCance, K. L. (2012). *Understanding pathophysiology* (5th ed.). St. Louis, MO: Elsevier Inc., pp. 747–750.

4 Answer: 2 Rationale: The presence of leukocytes (pyuria) means the host has an immune response to the infection instead of just an asymptomatic bacterial colonization. A gram stain is needed to determine the type of bacteria (gram + or 2). Urine may have a foul odor and appear cloudy due to the presence of mucus and excess white cells; however, the presence of pyuria does not mean the urine will be foul smelling. **Cognitive Level:** Analyzing **Client Need:** Physiological Adaptation **Integrated Process:** Nursing Process: Diagnosis **Content Area:** Adult Health **Strategy:** First define *pyuria* (WBCs in the urine) and then determine what biological response is needed to get WBCs in the urine. Recognize that a clinical clue is in the diagnosis given in the question. **Reference:** LeMone, P., Burke, K., & Bauldoff, G. (2012). *Medical-surgical nursing: Critical thinking in patient care* (5th ed.). Upper Saddle River, NJ: Pearson Education, pp. 785–787.

5 Answer: 2, 3, 4 Rationale: Prevention requires analysis of the stone to determine the formation. Depending on the type, dietary changes to limit calcium oxalates and measures to acidify pH will lower the risk of recurrence. Adequate fluid makes the dilute urine less likely to form crystals. Concentrated urine and high doses of vitamin D increase the risk of renal calculi. **Cognitive Level:** Applying **Client Need:** Physiological Adaptation **Integrated Process:** Teaching and Learning **Content Area:** Adult Health **Strategy:** Recall that when there are opposite options, they both cannot be correct. Apply knowledge of saturated solutions and crystal formation to the question. **Reference:** Huether, S. E., & McCance, K. L. (2012). *Understanding pathophysiology* (5th ed.). St. Louis, MO: Elsevier Inc., pp. 742–743.

6 Answer: 2 Rationale: Red blood cell casts are not present in the normal urinalysis but are present in glomerular diseases, which are the leading causes of chronic renal failure. Cystitis does not indicate glomerular involvement. Glomerulonephritis presents with hypertension, cola-colored urine, azotemia, and water retention. A BUN of 15 mg/dL is within normal limits of 8–22 mg/dL. **Cognitive Level:** Applying **Client Need:** Physiological Adaptation **Integrated Process:** Nursing Process: Assessment **Content Area:** Adult Health **Strategy:** Recall that normal renal glomeruli do not allow proteins and blood cells to filter into the urine. Review normal lab values if needed. **Reference:** Kee, J. (2010). *Laboratory and diagnostic tests with nursing implications* (8th ed.). Upper Saddle River, NJ: Pearson Education, Inc, pp. 412–418.

7 Answer: 3, 5 Rationale: Iatrogenic causes of renal failure result from treatment from a health care provider. Examples include nephrotoxic medications and radiologic contrast dye as intrarenal causes of renal failure, and severe hypotension after surgery as a prerenal cause of renal failure. Alcohol is more likely to result in cirrhosis of the liver. Exercise and diet are not likely to cause renal function changes, and are lifestyle habits, not iatrogenic factors. **Cognitive Level:** Analyzing **Client Need:** Physiological Adaptation **Integrated Process:** Nursing Process: Assessment **Content Area:** Adult Health **Strategy:** Knowing the definition of *iatrogenic* helps to eliminate the incorrect options. Review medical terminology if this is a weak area. **Reference:** LeMone, P., Burke, K., & Bauldoff, G. (2012). *Medical-surgical nursing: Critical thinking in patient care* (5th ed.). Upper Saddle River, NJ: Pearson Education, p. 760.

8 Answer: 3 Rationale: In renal failure, 90% or more of the nephrons are destroyed and glomerular filtration rate (GFR) is less than 20% of normal with increased creatinine and BUN, edema, and hyperkalemia. Renal cancer and urinary tract infection do not involve a reduced GFR. Polycystic kidney disease can lead to renal failure, but by itself is not a cause of reduced GFR. **Cognitive Level:** Applying **Client Need:** Physiological Adaptation **Integrated Process:** Nursing Process: Assessment **Content Area:** Adult Health **Strategy:** Apply knowledge of glomerular filtration rate (GFR) to aid in deciding what the client's problem is. **Reference:** Huether, S. E., & McCance, K. L. (2012). *Understanding pathophysiology* (5th ed.). St. Louis, MO: Elsevier Inc., pp. 731–732.

9 Answer: 2, 5 Rationale: Although it can be influenced by hydration status and protein intake, the blood urea nitrogen (BUN) is a good indicator of kidney function because most renal diseases interfere with urea excretion and cause blood levels to rise. Creatinine is produced in relatively constant amounts, according to the amount of muscle mass, and is excreted entirely by the kidneys, making it an excellent indicator of renal function. Complete blood count (CBC), alanine aminotransferase (ALT), gamma-glutamyl transpeptidase (GGT), and glucose do not indicate renal function. **Cognitive Level:** Applying **Client Need:** Reduction of Risk Potential **Integrated Process:** Nursing Process: Diagnosis **Content Area:** Adult Health **Strategy:** Review the normal reference ranges for common laboratory tests if this question was difficult. What compounds do healthy kidneys eliminate, keeping the blood levels down? **Reference:** Kee, J. (2010). *Laboratory and diagnostic tests with nursing implications* (8th ed.). Upper Saddle River, NJ: Pearson Education, Inc, pp. 16–17, 84–86, 150, 412–418, 731–732.

10 Answer: 2 Rationale: In end-stage renal disease (ESRD) with signs and symptoms of uremia, dialysis or organ transplantation is needed for survival. Loop diuretics will not be effective at this stage. Since medical treatment is available, it is premature to anticipate the imminent need to provide postmortem care. **Cognitive Level:** Applying

Client Need: Physiological Adaptation **Integrated Process:** Nursing Process: Planning **Content Area:** Adult Health **Strategy:** Recall that end-stage renal disease (ESRD) is a step worse than renal failure, and very few nephrons are functioning. With this in mind, select the option that provides a replacement mechanism for renal filtration and excretion of fluid and metabolic wastes. **Reference:** Huether, S. E., & McCance, K. L. (2012). *Understanding pathophysiology* (5th ed.). St. Louis, MO: Elsevier Inc., pp. 757–760.

Posttest

1 **Answer: 4** **Rationale:** Hematuria, either gross or microscopic, is generally present in clients with urinary calculi. The presence of protein may be associated with disorders that disrupt the glomerular membrane of the kidney. Leukocytes and nitrites may be associated with urinary infection. **Cognitive Level:** Applying **Client Need:** Reduction of Risk Potential **Integrated Process:** Nursing Process: Assessment **Content Area:** Adult Health **Strategy:** Recall that calculi are not infections but cause trauma to the ureter. This trauma can cause bleeding, resulting in hematuria. **Reference:** Huether, S. E., & McCance, K. L. (2012). *Understanding pathophysiology* (5th ed.). St. Louis, MO: Elsevier Inc., pp. 742–743.

2 **Answer: 3** **Rationale:** Adult polycystic kidney disease is an autosomal dominant disorder. In children, it is caused by an autosomal recessive trait. Glomerulonephritis, renal failure, and urinary tract infections are not inherited disorders. **Cognitive Level:** Applying **Client Need:** Physiological Adaptation **Integrated Process:** Nursing Process: Assessment **Content Area:** Adult Health **Strategy:** The core issue of the question is an understanding of which disorder is inherited. Eliminate the ones that are not. **Reference:** Huether, S. E., & McCance, K. L. (2012). *Understanding pathophysiology* (5th ed.). St. Louis, MO: Elsevier Inc., p. 766.

3 **Answer: 1** **Rationale:** Acute pyelonephritis is a bacterial infection of the kidney. Infection is characterized by an elevation in WBC count and fever. Chronic pyelonephritis is associated with nonbacterial infections and noninfectious processes that may be metabolic, chemical, or immunological. Renal failure and urinary calculi are not infectious processes. **Cognitive Level:** Applying **Client Need:** Physiological Adaptation **Integrated Process:** Nursing Process: Diagnosis **Content Area:** Adult Health **Strategy:** Recall that elevated WBCs are seen with infection and that the suffix *-itis* refers to inflammation and/or infection. Note the high temperature to determine that this is an acute process rather than a chronic one. **Reference:** Huether, S. E., & McCance, K. L. (2012). *Understanding pathophysiology* (5th ed.). St. Louis, MO: Elsevier Inc., p. 749.

4 **Answer: 1, 4** **Rationale:** Severe hypertension may develop as renal tissue is destroyed (secondary hypertension). Chronic pyelonephritis is a significant etiology of renal failure. It is a condition of inflammation and scarring,

not bacterial infection, and will not have impact on body temperature. Sexually transmitted infections (STIs) and lipid abnormalities are not consequences. **Cognitive Level:** Applying **Client Need:** Physiological Adaptation **Integrated Process:** Teaching and Learning **Content Area:** Adult Health **Strategy:** Note the critical word *chronic*, which differentiates the client's problem from an acute problem. Recall the difference in pathophysiology between these to make an accurate selection. **Reference:** Huether, S. E., & McCance, K. L. (2012). *Understanding pathophysiology* (5th ed.). St. Louis, MO: Elsevier Inc., pp. 748–749.

5 **Answer: 1** **Rationale:** Infection of the pharynx or skin with *group-A beta Hemolytic-streptococcus* is the common precipitating factor for acute glomerulonephritis. *Staphylococcus*, *E. coli*, and *proteus* organisms do not lead to glomerulonephritis as a consequence of infection with these organisms. **Cognitive Level:** Applying **Client Need:** Physiological Adaptation **Integrated Process:** Teaching and Learning **Content Area:** Adult Health **Strategy:** Apply knowledge of microbiology in identifying the pathogen. This is a critical point and one that should be committed to memory if this question was difficult. **Reference:** LeMone, P., Burke, K., & Bauldoff, G. (2012). *Medical-surgical nursing: Critical thinking in patient care* (5th ed.). Upper Saddle River, NJ: Pearson Education, pp. 822–824, 829.

6 **Answer: 1** **Rationale:** Risk factors for urinary tract infections (UTIs) include female gender, older age, urinary obstruction or calculi, strictures, chronic disease, prostatic hyperplasia and prostatitis, diaphragm use, instrumentation, and impaired immune system. Although children and adolescents can contract a UTI, incontinence and disease conditions in older adults make them a population at higher risk. **Cognitive Level:** Analyzing **Client Need:** Physiological Adaptation **Integrated Process:** Nursing Process: Assessment **Content Area:** Adult Health **Strategy:** The differences among the options are ages of the client and the genders. Determine which age and/or gender is at highest risk. **Reference:** LeMone, P., Burke, K., & Bauldoff, G. (2012). *Medical-surgical nursing: Critical thinking in patient care* (5th ed.). Upper Saddle River, NJ: Pearson Education, pp. 783, 787.

7 **Answer: 1** **Rationale:** The pathophysiology of glomerulonephritis can lead to a rapid decline in glomerular filtration rate (GFR), which leads to azotemia and other complications of severe glomerular injury such as hypertension, oliguria, and hematuria. Renal colic and flank pain would occur with renal calculi. Hypertension, not hypotension, is more likely to affect a client with renal disease, and tachycardia is not specifically related to the disorder. Urinary urgency and frequency would accompany urinary tract infection. **Cognitive Level:** Analyzing **Client Need:** Physiological Adaptation **Integrated Process:** Nursing Process: Assessment **Content Area:** Adult Health **Strategy:** Recall the physiology of Bowman's space and the pathophysiology of glomerulonephritis.

With these concepts in mind, consider that the correct answer would reflect declining renal function as well as hematuria because of the suffix *-itis*. **Reference:** Huether, S. E., & McCance, K. L. (2012). *Understanding pathophysiology* (5th ed.). St. Louis, MO: Elsevier Inc., pp. 749–752.

8 Answer: 2 Rationale: Increasing fluid intake may relieve signs and symptoms of a UTI as an adjunct to the antibiotics. Tub baths may contribute to the infection. Although some data suggests sexual intercourse may contribute to UTIs, the risk can be lowered by emptying the bladder after intercourse. Antibiotic therapy and phenazopyridine, not acetaminophen, will be effective in relieving the pain associated with UTIs. **Cognitive Level:** Applying **Client Need:** Physiological Adaptation **Integrated Process:** Nursing Process: Planning **Content Area:** Adult Health **Strategy:** Consider what action helps to eliminate the bacteria from the bladder and what actions are contraindicated. **Reference:** Huether, S. E., & McCance, K. L. (2012). *Understanding pathophysiology* (5th ed.). St. Louis, MO: Elsevier Inc., pp. 747–748.

9 Answer: 1, 2, 4 Rationale: Immune responses diminish with aging, reducing the irritating symptoms of a UTI. The nurse must be alert for cloudy (not clear), malodorous urine or incontinence. Ketones would be present when there is fat breakdown, usually as a result of diabetic ketoacidosis, dieting with severe calorie restriction, or starvation. **Cognitive Level:** Applying **Client Need:** Physiological Adaptation **Integrated Process:** Nursing Process: Assessment **Content Area:** Adult Health

Strategy: Eliminate one of the options that represent opposites and choose findings consistent with a UTI. **Reference:** LeMone, P. Burke, K., & Bauldoff, G. (2012). *Medical-surgical nursing: Critical thinking in patient care* (5th ed.). Upper Saddle River, NJ: Pearson Education, Inc., pp. 786–787, 789.

10 Answer: 2, 3, 5 Rationale: Fluids should be increased unless contraindicated by another condition to help flush microorganisms from the urinary system. Because caffeine and alcohol can increase bladder spasms and mucosal irritation, they should be decreased to reduce the signs and symptoms of a urinary tract infection (UTI). Fluids should be increased rather than restricted, and douches will not help a UTI. Antibiotics should be taken completely for the full course of therapy to prevent development of resistant strains of organisms. Cranberry juice may help to acidify the urine, which may inhibit bacterial growth or ability to adhere to bladder mucosa. **Cognitive Level:** Applying **Client Need:** Health Promotion and Maintenance **Integrated Process:** Teaching and Learning **Content Area:** Adult Health **Strategy:** Recall the prime treatment for UTIs includes antibiotic therapy and that classic adjunct measures are increasing fluid intake, acidifying the urine, and preventing further irritation. Evaluate each option in light of these and use the process of elimination to make a selection. **Reference:** LeMone, P., Burke, K., & Bauldoff, G. (2012). *Medical-surgical nursing: Critical thinking in patient care* (5th ed.). Upper Saddle River, NJ: Pearson Education, pp. 786–787, 789.

References

Adams, M., Holland, L., & Bostwick, P. (2011). *Pharmacology for nurses: A pathophysiologic approach* (3rd ed.). Upper Saddle River, NJ: Pearson Education.

Corbett, J. V. (2013). *Laboratory tests and diagnostic procedures with nursing diagnoses* (8th ed.). Upper Saddle River, NJ: Pearson Education.

Kee, J. (2009). *Laboratory and diagnostic tests and nursing implications* (8th ed.). Upper Saddle River, NJ: Pearson Education.

LeMone, P., Burke, K. M., & Bauldoff, G. (2011). *Medical-surgical nursing: Critical thinking in patient care* (5th ed.). Upper Saddle River, NJ: Pearson Education.

Lewis, S., Dirksen, S., Heitkemper, M., Bucher, L., & Camera, I. (2011). *Medical surgical nursing: Assessment and management of clinical problems* (8th ed.). St. Louis, MO: Elsevier.

McCance, K., & Huether, K. (2010). *Understanding pathophysiology: The biologic basis for disease in adults and children* (6th ed.). St. Louis, MO: Elsevier.

Osborn, K. S., Wraa, C. E., & Watson, A. (2010). *Medical surgical nursing: Preparation for practice*. Upper Saddle River, NJ: Pearson Education.

Porth, C., & Matfin, G. (2010). *Pathophysiology: Concepts of altered health states* (8th ed.). Philadelphia, PA: Lippincott Williams & Wilkins.

Wilson, B. A., Shannon, M. T., & Shields, K. M. (2012). *Pearson nurse's drug guide 2012*. Upper Saddle River, NJ: Pearson Education.

ANSWERS & RATIONALES

11 Male and Female Reproductive Health Problems

Chapter Outline

Risk Factors Associated with Male and Female Reproductive Health Problems

Male Reproductive Health Problems

Female Reproductive Health Problems

Sexually Transmitted Infections (STIs)

NCLEX-RN® Test Prep

Use the accompanying online resource, NursingReviewsandRationales, to test yourself with hundreds of NCLEX®-style practice questions.

Objectives

➤ Define key terms associated with male and female reproductive health problems.

➤ Identify risk factors associated with development of male and female reproductive health problems.

➤ Explain the common etiologies of male and female reproductive health problems.

➤ Describe the pathophysiologic processes associated with specific male and female reproductive health problems.

➤ Distinguish between normal and abnormal male and female reproductive findings obtained from nursing assessment.

➤ Prioritize nursing interventions associated with specific male and female reproductive health problems.

Review at a Glance

adenomyosis condition in which endometrium is present between myometrial cells

balanitis infection or inflammation of foreskin

benign prostatic hyperplasia (BPH) enlargement of prostate gland from noncancerous hyperplasia

cryptorchidism undescended testicle

dysfunctional uterine bleeding (DUB) condition causing irregular menstrual bleeding from lack of progesterone

dysmenorrhea painful menstruation

dyspareunia painful intercourse

endometriosis condition in which endometrium implants are present outside uterus

epispadias condition in which urethral meatus is located on upper (dorsal) aspect of penis instead of tip of shaft; may be located just above penile tip or anywhere along shaft

hypospadias condition in which urethral meatus is located on lower (ventral) aspect of penis instead of tip of shaft; may be located just below penile tip or anywhere along shaft

menorrhagia excessive or heavy menstrual flow

metrorrhagia irregular, frequent menstrual bleeding of abnormal amounts

myoma uterine muscle tumor

orchiectomy removal of a testicle

pelvic inflammatory disease (PID) inflammation of uterus, fallopian tubes, and ovaries

phimosis unretractable foreskin that may impede or prohibit urine flow

prostate specific antigen (PSA) blood test to measure antigen produced by prostate cancer

PRETEST

1 The nurse would question a client with balanitis about the presence of which of the following symptoms?

1. Vaginal discharge
2. Pain with urination
3. Spontaneous urethral discharge
4. Back pain

2 The nurse would assess the client experiencing prostatitis for which of the following symptoms?

1. Urinary retention or incontinence
2. Painful blisters and crater-like lesions, enlarged groin nodes, fever
3. Brownish rash on palms, painful crater-like lesions, malaise, and fever
4. Rectal pain, pain with erection, low abdominal pain, and low back pain

3 A male client in the ambulatory clinic reports that a female sexual partner from about 5 months ago has been diagnosed with syphilis. If the client became infected during this relationship, the nurse would expect him to have which of the following at this time?

1. Painless sore that healed and a rash on the palms of his hands
2. Negative VDRL, negative rapid plasma reagin (RPR) and positive fluorescent treponemal antibody absorption (FTA-ABS)
3. Night sweats, cough, low-grade fever, and elevated white count
4. Penile discharge, dysuria, and urinary frequency

4 The nurse concludes that teaching has been effective when the mother of an infant born with hypospadias says which of the following about her son?

1. "He will need surgical correction so that he looks like the other boys."
2. "He will require circumcision now to prevent complications later."
3. "He needs to have surgical correction so he will be fertile as an adult."
4. "He will likely have other reproductive tract anomalies we can't see."

5 The nurse is preparing to teach a client who has dysfunctional uterine bleeding (DUB). Which medication would the nurse expect to include in the teaching plan?

1. Testosterone
2. Estrogen
3. Corticosteroid
4. Progesterone

6 In preparing to discharge a client with gonococcal pelvic inflammatory disease (PID), the nurse determines that teaching was successful if the client makes which statements? Select all that apply.

1. "I should douche after every episode of intercourse."
2. "Using latex condoms will decrease the risk of this happening again."
3. "My boyfriend and I should be monogamous."
4. "The sexual position I use won't prevent this infection."
5. "Voiding after intercourse will help prevent pelvic inflammatory disease (PID)."

7 A 23-year-old male client has been diagnosed with testicular cancer. Which information should the nurse include in his teaching plan?

1. Future fertility is not affected by treatment.
2. Impotence often results from needed treatments.
3. Sperm banking should be done prior to treatment.
4. Sexual interest is likely to increase as a result of successful treatment.

8 The nurse working with a female client who has fibrocystic breast disease expects the client to report a diet high in which of the following?

1. Bacon, sausage, and ground meat
2. Fresh fruits and whole grain cereal
3. Cheese and milk
4. Coffee and cola

9 A male client has been diagnosed with *Chlamydia trachomatis* infection. The nurse should include which of the following when developing the plan of care?

1. Instructions to take all of the doxycycline (Vibra-tabs) that was ordered
2. Encouragement to use condoms with most episodes of intercourse
3. Obtaining the names of sexual contacts if client desires
4. Teaching testicular self-exam (TSE) for self-diagnosis

10 The client has a diagnosis of primary dysmenorrhea. Which of the following would the nurse expect to find when obtaining the client's history?

1. Heavy flow and clots for at least 3 months
2. Irregular menses with breakthrough bleeding
3. Painful periods since menarche
4. No periods for the last 7 months

➤ *See pages 296–297 for Answers and Rationales.*

I. RISK FACTORS ASSOCIATED WITH MALE AND FEMALE REPRODUCTIVE HEALTH PROBLEMS

A. Multiple sexual partners increase risk of sexually transmitted infections (STIs) and subsequent problems

B. Smoking creates endothelial cell changes that predispose cells to more radical changes from viruses such as human papilloma virus (HPV) or precancerous conditions and cancer

C. Obesity increases amount of fat-soluble hormones (such as estrogen), chemicals, and illicit drugs in tissues, which increases risk of cellular changes in reproductive tract

D. Alcohol use is associated with increased numbers of sexual partners and sexual assault

E. Illicit drug use is also associated with increased numbers of sexual partners and sexual assault, and some drugs (marijuana, cocaine, heroin) are fat-soluble, leading to long-term storage of drugs in fatty tissues of body for weeks to months after last ingestion; this can lead to greater effects on reproductive tract such as decreased spermatogenesis

F. Ionizing radiation can disrupt normal cell division associated with oogenesis and spermatogenesis, leading to changes in genetic structure of gametes

G. Chemical exposure from occupational hazards or misuse of household chemicals can decrease sperm count, motility, and change morphology, as well as cause menstrual cycle changes

H. Specific conditions

1. Urethral disorders: congenital
2. Prostatitis: urinary catheterization or similar procedures, consumption of alcohol, caffeine, and spicy foods
3. Benign prostatic hyperplasia: age
4. Prostate cancer: age, ethnicity, chemical/environmental exposures

5. Testicular cancer: history of **cryptorchidism** (undescended testicle), trauma, estrogen administration to mother during pregnancy such as diethylstilbestrol (DES), decreased birth weight, prematurity, family history
6. Uterine bleeding: age, family history, stress, weight change, oral contraceptives, intrauterine device (IUD)
7. Dysmenorrhea: smoking, non-use of oral contraception, early menarche
8. Pelvic inflammatory disease (PID): use of IUD, oral contraceptives, and condoms, STIs, multiple sex partners, previous PID
9. Endometriosis: nulliparity, family history
10. Benign breast disease: age
11. Breast cancer: age, family history (first-degree relative with breast cancer), ethnicity (Caucasian or African American), previous chest area radiation (i.e., treatment for Hodgkin's disease), menarche before age 12 or menopause after age 50, use of hormone replacement therapy over 5 years, nulliparous or first pregnancy after age 30, never breastfed, daily alcohol use, obesity
12. STIs: unprotected sex, multiple sex partners, intravenous (IV) drug use, use of street drugs

II. MALE REPRODUCTIVE HEALTH PROBLEMS

A. Urethral disorders

1. Overview
   a. **Hypospadias**: urethral meatus is located on lower (ventral) aspect of penis instead of tip of shaft; may be located just below penile tip or anywhere along shaft
   b. **Epispadias**: urethral meatus is located on upper (dorsal) aspect of penis instead of tip of shaft; may be located just above penile tip or anywhere along shaft
   c. **Phimosis**: unretractable foreskin, which impedes or prohibits urine flow
   d. **Balanitis**: infection or inflammation of foreskin
   e. Urethritis: inflammation of urethra
   f. Causes
      1) Hypospadias and epispadias: congenital
      2) Phimosis: congenital or secondary to infection or injury
      3) Balanitis: improper hygiene
      4) Urethritis: insertion of an instrument/catheter, gonococcal infection
2. Pathophysiology
   a. Developmental anomalies
      1) Hypospadias and epispadias develop when urinary tract forms during embryological development; 8% of men have a father or brother with same condition; occurs in about 1 in 250 males
      2) Phimosis is an acquired stenosis of intact foreskin resulting in an inability to retract foreskin
   b. Inflammatory processes

      1) Balanitis occurs as a result of overgrowth of normal flora under intact foreskin caused by inadequate hygiene
      2) Urethritis is most common urinary tract infection (UTI)
   c. Signs and symptoms
      1) Hypospadias and epispadias: visual deformity noted
      2) Phimosis: secondary infections and scarring; edema and pain of glans penis (if constriction occurs); necrosis of glans
      3) Balanitis: redness, swelling, and pain of penis; foul odor and purulent drainage; dysuria
      4) Urethritis: painful urination; discharge from penis

3. Nursing assessment

   a. Physical exam of urethral meatus, color and retractability of foreskin; characteristics of urine; vital signs (VS, especially temperature); amount of urine; report of discomfort during voiding; presence of discharge

   b. Diagnostic tests: urinalysis (UA), preferably clean catch; culture and sensitivity (C&S)

4. Nursing management

   a. Medications

      1) Urethritis: oral antibiotics, analgesics

      2) Balanitis: topical or oral antibiotic or antifungal

      3) Phimosis: topical steroid application

   b. Teach client about cause of problem

   c. Teach client hygiene measures to prevent recurrence

   d. Teach males with intact foreskin to retract foreskin before voiding, wipe glans dry after voiding, and then replace foreskin; additionally, glans of penis should be retracted, cleansed, dried, and replaced after intercourse and during daily bathing

   e. Instruct client in proper use of medications, including route, amount, and frequency of use

   f. Surgical correction may be done in early childhood if urethral opening is along shaft of penis, primarily to promote fertility in adulthood

   g. Treatment of phimosis may consist of stretching under local anesthetic; circumcision may be required

Practice to Pass

The client with hypospadias asks if his sons will have the condition. How should the nurse respond?

B. Prostatitis

  1. Overview

   a. Most common form is acute prostatitis, a bacterial infection; chronic prostatitis can be bacterial or noninfectious

   b. Causes: trauma, autoimmune response, gonorrhea, and bacterial infection

  2. Pathophysiology

   a. Prostate gland (see Figure 11-1) secretes a thin, alkaline fluid that is part of seminal secretion

   b. Is not well understood; bacteria from rectum or infected urine invade prostate; is not considered sexually transmitted

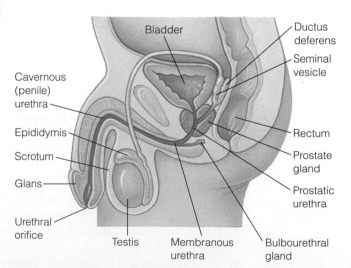

Figure 11-1

Components of the male reproductive system

Labels: Bladder · Ductus deferens · Seminal vesicle · Cavernous (penile) urethra · Epididymis · Scrotum · Glans · Urethral orifice · Testis · Membranous urethra · Rectum · Prostate gland · Prostatic urethra · Bulbourethral gland

c. Signs and symptoms

    1) Acute: chills, fever, urinary (dysuria, frequency, urgency, hematuria); pain (suprapubic, perineal, scrotal, lower back, rectal); discharge; enlarged prostate that is tender and warm; palpable seminal vesicles; blood and pus in urine; pain during ejaculation

    2) Chronic and nonbacterial: may be asymptomatic; low-grade fever; pain; nocturia; dysuria

3. Nursing assessment

    a. History of onset, severity, and precipitating factors of symptoms; inspection of urine; VS; symptom analysis of pain

    b. Diagnostic tests: urinalysis, physical examination, urine C&S

4. Nursing management

    a. Medications include antibiotics

    b. Educate client about cause and treatment plan

    c. Instruct client to avoid caffeine and alcohol (irritants)

C. Benign prostatic hyperplasia (BPH)

1. Overview

    a. Benign prostatic hyperplasia (BPH) is defined as a noncancerous enlargement of prostate gland because of hyperplasia or hypertrophy (see Figure 11-2)

    b. Begins around age 40 but usually not symptomatic until 60 years and older; is an age-related problem

2. Pathophysiology

    a. Results from decreased testosterone and increased estrogen levels

    b. Prostate cells increase in size and in number, which causes pressure on and decreases diameter of urethra

    c. Although androgen levels decrease as male ages, prostate gland is still sensitive to presence of dihydrotestosterone (DHT), which causes growth of prostate gland

    d. May be asymptomatic until acute onset inhibits opening of bladder sphincter; excess alcohol intake can be a trigger

    e. Signs and symptoms: incomplete bladder emptying, difficulty starting urine stream and weak stream; nocturia; feeling of fullness in bladder; increased urinary time; dribbling of urine

3. Nursing assessment

    a. Client history related to urinating; symptom analysis of urinary problems; characteristics of urine

    b. Diagnostic tests: biopsy of prostate, physical exam, ultrasonography, UA, serum creatinine (Cr) and blood urea nitrogen (BUN)

Practice to Pass

The client with benign prostatic hyperplasia with transurethral resection of the prostate (TURP) scheduled in 1 week calls to ask if there are any over-the-counter (OTC) medications that he shouldn't take. How should the nurse reply?

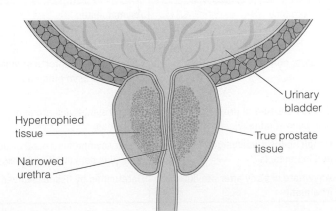

Figure 11-2

Benign prostatic hyperplasia

Urinary bladder

Hypertrophied tissue

True prostate tissue

Narrowed urethra

4. Nursing management
   a. Medications: finasteride (Proscar), which inhibits testosterone conversion to dihydrotestosterone; alpha-adrenergic antagonist; phytotherapy (newer treatment) with saw palmetto berry, echinacea, and hypoxis rooperi
   b. Instruct client to avoid alcohol use, and report increased urinary symptoms
   c. If transurethral resection of prostate (TURP) is indicated, educate client about the following:
      1) Nature of surgical procedure and regional anesthesia
      2) Recovery, including continuous bladder irrigation (to prevent clotting) and going home with an indwelling urinary catheter
      3) Potential for bladder spasms
      4) Avoidance of nonsteroidal anti-inflammatory drugs (NSAIDs) for 10 days preoperative
      5) Newer treatments that are less invasive: balloon urethroplasty, laser energy microwave hyperthermia, intraurethral stents

D. Prostate cancer
   1. Overview
      a. Usually slow growing, often asymptomatic in early stages; average age at diagnosis is 65
      b. African American men are 50% more likely to develop prostate cancer than Caucasian men; incidence is increased if first-degree relative has prostate cancer
      c. Causes include genetic disposition, history of STIs, high-fat diet; hormones; often unknown
   2. Pathophysiology
      a. Single or multiple areas within prostate gland develop proliferative cancer and enlarge gland both outward toward capsule and then inward toward urethra (see Table 11-1)
      b. Extension of cancer outside of prostate gland capsule may also occur, first into seminal vesicles

      c. Compression of urethra by tumor may cause urinary symptoms
      d. Cancer of prostate is testosterone-dependent early in course of disease
      e. Common sites of metastases: lymph nodes, bones, lungs, liver
      f. Signs and symptoms: increased urinary frequency, urgency, reduction in stream, nocturia, and hematuria; blood during ejaculation; back pain; pain of joints and bone if metastasis occurs; weight loss; fatigue; client may be asymptomatic

Table 11-1   **Stages of Prostate Cancer**

Stage	Location	Symptoms	Diagnosis
1	Prostate only	Asymptomatic	Accidental discovery (i.e., during transurethral resection of prostate for benign prostatic hyperplasia)
2	Prostate only	Mild urinary symptoms of enlarged prostate or asymptomatic	Prostate specific antigen (PSA) elevated or gland palpated during rectal exam
3	Outside capsule of prostate; may also be in seminal vesicles	Urinary symptoms, rectal or pelvic pain	PSA elevated or gland palpated during rectal exam
4	Lymph nodes involvement and metastasis	Urinary symptoms, rectal or pelvic pain; plus pain in affected tissue	PSA elevated or gland palpated during rectal exam
Recurrent	Anywhere in body after previous treatment	Determined by tissue involved	PSA elevated after treatment

3. Nursing assessment
    a. Symptom analysis of urinary status; question client for known risk factors; symptom analysis of pain (hips, low back, abdomen, pelvis); assess weight, energy level, and presence of sexual function problems
    b. Diagnostic tests
        1) Screening utilizes **prostate specific antigen (PSA)** blood tests (PSA should be less than or equal to 4.0)
        2) Digital rectal exams recommended yearly for men over 45
        3) Urinalysis
        4) Transrectal ultrasonography (TRUS) if PSA is elevated
        5) Tissue biopsy: diagnosis is through rectal or perineal fine-needle aspiration after increased PSA or rectal exam detects hard nodules on prostate; from tissue biopsy, a Gleason Score is derived
            a) Classic Gleason scoring diagram shows 5 basic tissue patterns technically referred to as tumor "grades," represented by a number ranging from 1 to 5 (5 being worst)
            b) Biopsy Gleason score is a sum of primary grade (representing majority of tumor) and a secondary grade (assigned to minority of tumor), and is a number ranging from 2 to 10; higher Gleason scores are associated with more aggressive tumor and a worse client prognosis
        6) Magnetic resonance imagery (MRI), bone scan, or computerized tomography (CT) for possible metastasis
4. Nursing management
    a. Medications: hormone therapy (via bilateral orchiectomy or monthly injections) and chemotherapy
    b. Other treatments: surgery (TURP or radical abdominal prostatectomy) and/or internal or external radiation
    c. Reinforce explanation that most men will be impotent after abdominal prostatectomy, and 40% will experience urinary incontinence, which can be treated in some men with an artificial urinary sphincter
    d. Age of client at diagnosis, concurrent medical conditions, and stage of cancer determine recommended treatment regimen
    e. If receiving chemotherapy or radiation therapy, assess mouth for stomatitis, skin condition at radiation site, and signs of dehydration
    f. Reinforce explanation of what cancer stage means and assess for suicidal tendencies
    g. Provide support for body image disturbance and sexual dysfunction issues, including referral to support groups for client and family

E. **Testicular cancer**
    1. Overview: most common cancer in males age 15 to 35; many forms exist and cause is unknown
    2. Pathophysiology
        a. Types:
            1) Germ cell (95%): originating in sperm-producing cells of testes
            2) Seminomas (40%): slow-growing and remain localized within a testis
            3) Nonseminoma (60%): are more aggressive
            4) Other forms may be leydig, sertoli, leiomyosarcoma, rhabdomyosarcoma, mesothelioma, or stromal cell
        b. Cancer cells grow within testicle, replacing parenchymal tissue
        c. Spread of disease is usually by lymphatic (lymph nodes) and vascular channels (to lungs, bone, or liver), even before any large mass appears in scrotum

Table 11-2	Stages of Testicular Cancer
Stage	**Location**
I	Confined to testicle
II	Retroperitoneal lymph nodes and testicle
III	Beyond lymph nodes; metastasis

  d. Signs and symptoms
    1) Painless, hard nodule or swelling (usually on only one side of testis), dull ache in testes
    2) Metastatic symptoms include respiratory problems (coughing, dyspnea), back or bone pain, or gastrointestinal problems
  e. There are 3 stages of testicular cancer (see Table 11-2)
  3. Nursing assessment
    a. Assessment
      1) History of testicular or groin pain, change in size, shape, or consistency of testis, and size and consistency of palpable lumps, presence of cryptorchidism with or without surgical correction
      2) Other: symptom analysis of any pain, respiratory or GI problems
    b. Diagnostic tests
      1) Radioimmunoassay studies for tumor markers (human chorionic gonadotropin [hCG] and alpha-fetoprotein [AFP])
      2) Serum lactic acid dehydrogenase (LDH)
      3) Metastasis: liver function tests, x-ray, and CT scan
      4) Diagnosis made via pathology exam following inguinal **orchiectomy** (removal of a testis) on affected side
  4. Nursing management
    a. Medications include chemotherapy
    b. Treatment after orchiectomy involves radiation and/or chemotherapy
    c. Monitor VS during chemotherapy or radiation therapy and fluid balance assessment because of nausea, vomiting, and diarrhea from treatment
    d. Provide client education on expected client experience with treatment
    e. If client desires fertility, explain option of sperm banking before chemotherapy
    f. Teach client monthly testicular self-examination (TSE) of remaining testis and to have annual visits to provider; education about TSE should begin at age 15

Practice to Pass

The client with a testicular lump is scheduled for an inguinal orchiectomy and asks why the doctor doesn't just remove the lump "like they do with breast lumps." How should the nurse respond?

III. FEMALE REPRODUCTIVE HEALTH PROBLEMS

  A. Uterine bleeding disorders
    1. Overview
      a. Dysfunctional uterine bleeding (DUB) is a nonspecific condition from lack of progesterone, where menstruation is irregular and frequent (**metrorrhagia**), excessive (**menorrhagia**), or both (metromenorrhagia)
      b. Occurs mostly in adolescents and in premenopausal women
      c. 25–50% of women will develop fibroid tumors (**myomas**, leiomyomas), usually in their 30s and 40s, which can also create bleeding disorders
      d. Causes
        1) Adenomyosis (a condition in which endometrium is present between myometrial cells) can also cause irregular or heavy menstrual bleeding
        2) Over 90% caused by anovulatory cycles
        3) Other: blood dyscrasias, endocrine problems, pelvic inflammatory disease, endometrial cancer or polyps, exogenous estrogen, pregnancy, menopause, athletic training or excessive athletic activity, or no known cause

2. Pathophysiology
   a. Dysfunctional uterine bleeding results from a lack of progesterone
      1) This causes proliferation of fragile endometrium that does not mature into secretory endometrium
      2) Endometrium sheds at irregular times
   b. If proliferative phase of menstrual cycle is shortened because of a defect in follicular phase, spotting and breakthrough bleeding may occur
   c. Excessive flow may be a result of defects during luteal phase
   d. Disorders of DUB
      1) Amenorrhea (absence of menstruation), which can be primary (by age 17) or secondary (absence in a previously menstruating woman)
      2) Oligomenorrhea (scant menses)
      3) Menorrhagia
      4) Metrorrhagia
      5) Postmenopausal bleeding
   e. Uterine myomas form in several areas (see Figure 11-3), including myometrial wall (intramural), pedunculated (having a stalk) and into uterine cavity (submucosal), and pedunculated and outwards into pelvis (subserosal)
   f. Adenomyosis is endometrium in myometrium, which enlarges each month under hormonal influence but is not shed because it is trapped between myometrial cells
   g. Signs and symptoms: change in menstrual cycle (repetitive or long history), fatigue, anemia, hemorrhage, sexual dysfunction, cramping, water retention, anxiety, problems with reproduction; large tumors or presence of more than 1 tumor tend to cause more symptoms (enlarged uterus, metrorrhagia, **dysmenorrhea** (painful menstruation), pelvic pressure or fullness, and increased urinary frequency)
3. Nursing assessment
   a. Obtain history of bleeding pattern
   b. BP and pulse sitting and standing
   c. Symptom analysis of pain or discomforts associated with problem
   d. Activity level
   e. Sexual and reproductive history
   f. Diagnostics include pelvic exam, pelvic ultrasound, pap smear, CT or MRI, hysteroscopy, and for adenomyosis—microscopic exam of myometrium after hysterectomy

Figure 11-3

Myomas of the uterus.
A. Intramural, B. Submucosal,
C. Subserosal.

4. Nursing management

    a. Medications: analgesics for discomfort, NSAIDs to inhibit prostaglandins, oral contraceptives to reduce bleeding if indicated, leuprolide acetate (Lupron) to decrease tumor size, and gonadotropin-releasing hormone (GnRH) agonists; antibiotics for secondary form

    b. Educate clients about cause of their dysmenorrhea

    c. Teach how to take prescribed or OTC medications correctly

    d. Instruct clients to drink plenty of fluids and have adequate calcium intake

    e. Application of heat to lower abdomen may help when discomfort occurs

B. Pelvic inflammatory disease (PID)

  1. Overview

    a. **Pelvic inflammatory disease (PID)**: inflammation of uterus and fallopian tubes (salpingitis), endometrium (endometritis), pelvic peritoneum, and ovaries (oophoritis) usually resulting from infection

    b. Highest incidence occurs in women who have had more than 1 sexual partner in their lifetime, increasing with numbers of partners

    c. 20% of women will be infertile after infectious PID; 20% will have chronic pelvic pain; ectopic pregnancy occurs 10 times as often after PID

    d. Most prominent in women ages 15–24 who are nulliparous

    e. May be acute or chronic

    f. Causes: use of IUDs, oral contraceptives, or condoms; secondary infections are caused by appendicitis, peritonitis, STIs, douching

  2. Pathophysiology

    a. Bacteria invade uterine and tubal tissues after migrating through cervix

    b. Migration occurs during ovulation, menstruation, forced through cervix with douching, childbirth, abortion, or surgery of reproductive tract

    c. Scar tissue is formed from infection, which obstructs uterine tubes

    d. Tubo-ovarian abscesses can form because of obstruction

    e. Bacterial infection causes inflammation, which in turn causes symptoms

    f. Common infecting organisms include *Neisseria gonorrhea*, *Chlamydia trachomatis*, *E. coli*, *Gardnerella vaginalis*, or *Mycoplasma hominis*

    g. Signs and symptoms include low abdominal pain, dysmenorrhea, **dyspareunia** (painful intercourse), dysuria, and fever; vaginal discharge may be noted (green-yellow, green-gray, or yellow); nausea, malaise

    h. Complications: infertility, ectopic pregnancy, pelvic abscess, and dysmenorrhea

  3. Nursing assessment

    a. Assessment

      1) History for onset of symptoms, precipitating factors, known exposure to STIs, number of sexual partners, and amount of douching

      2) Assess VS (fever), activity level, any discharges

      3) Symptom analysis of pain and GI symptoms

      4) History of menstrual cycle and pregnancies

    b. Diagnostic tests: ultrasound, laparoscopy, CBC for elevated white blood cell (WBC) count, review of client's symptoms, Pap smear, and culture of cervical discharge

  4. Nursing management

    a. Medications include analgesics for fever and at least 2 broad spectrum antibiotics (may require inpatient intravenous [IV] form)

      1) Tetracycline: doxycycline (Vibramycin)

      2) Cephalosporin: cefoxitin (Mefoxin) or ceftriaxone (Rocephin)

       3) Aminoglycoside: gentamicin (Garamycin)

       4) Fluoroquinolone: ofloxacin (Floxin)

       5) Antiprotozoal: metronidazole (Flagyl)

       6) Anti-infective: clindamycin (Cleocin)

    b. Client education: causes of PID; avoid douching; proper timing and use of oral antibiotics; measure temperature 3 times a day and call if elevated; report PID to provider if she becomes pregnant so ectopic pregnancy can be detected early

C. Endometriosis

  1. Overview

    a. Endometriosis is defined as a growth of endometrium outside of uterus

    b. Most likely sites of growth include bladder, ovaries, fallopian tubes, bowel, and broad ligament

    c. Most often occurs in European American women of childbearing age

    d. Major complication is infertility

    e. Causes include unknown, theorized to be caused from embryonic epithelial cells; backflow of menstrual fluid through uterine tubes during menstruation; and spread of endometrial implants by way of lymphatic or vascular system

  2. Pathophysiology

    a. Endometrial tissue is present outside of uterus, and responds to hormonal influence of menstrual cycle

    b. However, blood (normally shed from intrauterine endometrium) cannot escape and builds up causing scarring and further growth of endometriosis

    c. Bleeding results in inflammation and pain in tissues

    d. Infertility associated with endometriosis may be unexplained or occurs from mechanical blockage of tubes from endometrial implants

    e. Signs and symptoms: dysmenorrhea, dyspareunia, dysuria, constipation, painful bowel movements during menses, and tender palpable masses

  3. Nursing assessment

    a. Assessment: thorough history of symptoms and their onset and whether symptoms improve or worsen during menstrual cycle; assess bowel characteristics

    b. Diagnostic tests: laparoscopy, pelvic ultrasonography, CBC to identify low hemoglobin and hematocrit (H&H) and rule out infection (WBC)

  4. Nursing management

    a. Medications: analgesics for pain, NSAIDs (inhibit prostaglandin synthesis); hormone therapy such as leuprolide (Lupron); gonadotropin-releasing hormone (GnRH) to raise estrogen and progesterone levels to control bleeding; danazol (generic) to induce amenorrhea

    b. Educate client about endometriosis and treatment being utilized, including side effects of medications such as hot flashes

    c. Provide support and refer to support groups for infertility issues

D. Benign breast disorders

  1. Overview: fibrocystic disease is defined as presence of benign breast lesions; common in women 30–50 years of age; causes include hormonal changes, aging, and diet high in caffeine

  2. Pathophysiology

    a. Mammary tissue retains fluid and forms a cyst during latter half of menstrual cycle, which resolves spontaneously with menstruation

    b. Inflammation from repetitive filling causes wall of cyst to fibrose and become hard, blocking drainage of fluid

    c. Cyst remains even after menses

      d. Classification

        1) Nonproliferative lesion: may be cystic or fibrous and may result in a mass in upper outer breast quadrant after an inflammatory response to irritation of ducts

        2) Proliferative lesion: lesions without atypical cells

        3) Atypical hyperplasia: lesions that are "borderline," possible morphologic characteristics of cancer cells

      e. Signs and symptoms: painful, mobile, round or oval, smooth lump in breast tissue that enlarges or becomes more painful premenstrually; nipple discharge (clear, milky, straw-colored, green)

    3. Nursing assessment

      a. Assessment

        1) Obtain history on when the lump was first detected, with size, shape, location, mobility, tenderness, and cyclical changes

        2) Determine if ultrasound or mammogram has been previously performed

        3) Performance of breast self-exam (SBE) monthly

        4) Identify details of menstrual cycle and previous problems

      b. Diagnostic tests: mammogram, ultrasound examination, possible needle aspiration, excisional biopsy possible to rule out cancer, and breast exam

    4. Nursing management

      a. Medications include mild analgesics and vitamin E

      b. There is no cure, but limiting caffeine, smoking, and chocolate usually improves or eliminates condition

      c. Explain what is known about fibrocystic breast disease and vagueness of prevention and treatment

      d. Reassure client that fibrocystic breast lumps are not precancerous

      e. Educate on monthly SBE and yearly exam by provider; mammograms for women over 40

E. Breast cancer

    1. Overview

      a. Defined as growth of abnormal cells in breast tissue that is irregular

      b. Affects 1 out of 9 women over course of a lifetime; 10% of cases linked to mutations in BRCA1 or BRCA2 gene

      c. Involves mammary ducts, lobules, or both

      d. Cause: unknown, see risk factors

    2. Pathophysiology

      a. Two main locations: lobular (20%) and ductal (80%)

      b. Breast cancer is hormone dependent; must have functioning ovaries

      c. Termed

        1) Noninvasive (in situ): proliferation of cancer cells are either ductal or lobular but do not invade surrounding tissue

        2) Invasive (penetration of tumor into surrounding tissue); arise in terminal section of ductal tissue; 5 types

          a) Infiltrating ductal carcinoma: stony hardness when palpated; metastasizes to axillary lymph nodes; most common; poor prognosis

          b) Tubular carcinoma or "well-differentiated"; less common

          c) Medullary carcinoma: bulky, large tumor that is well circumscribed

          d) Mucinous carcinoma: bulky, slow-growing tumor with sharp edges

          e) Infiltrating lobular carcinoma: uncommon; thick, ill-defined area in breast

      d. May metastasize to bone, brain, lung, liver, skin, and lymph nodes

      e. Tumors are staged using TNM system according to size of tumor, involvement of lymph node, and metastasis to other sites (see Table 11-3)

Table 11-3	Staging of Breast Cancer		
Stage	**Tumor**	**Node**	**Metastasis**
0	Tis-Carcinoma in situ or Paget's disease of the nipple	N0-No regional lymph node metastasis	M0-No evidence of distant metastasis
I	T1-Tumor no larger than 2 cm	N0	M0
IIA	T0-No evidence of primary tumor	N1-Metastasis to movable ipsilateral axillary nodes	M0
	T1		
	T2-Tumor no larger than 5 cm	N0	M0
IIB	T2	N1	M0
	T3-Tumor larger than 5 cm	N0	M0
IIIA	T0	N2-Metastasis to ipsilateral fixed axillary nodes	M0
	T1		
	T2		
	T3	N1	M0
		N2	M0
IIIB	T4-Tumor of any size with direct extension to chest wall or skin	Any N	M0
	Any T	N3-Metastasis to ipsilateral internal mammary lymph nodes	M0
IVA	Any T	N0 and N1	M1-Distant metastasis

Source: LeMone, P., Burke, K., & Bauldoff, G. (2011). *Medical-surgical nursing: Critical thinking for patient care* (5th ed.). Upper Saddle River, NJ: Pearson Education, p. 1705.

    f. Metastasis occurs as small masses of cells break away from tumor, enter lymphatic system where they remain, causing swelling of node or traveling to another node; lymphatic drainage has 3 pathways
       1) Axillary (most common route of spread)
       2) Internal mammary
       3) Transpectoral
    g. Signs and symptoms: hard, irregular, painless, fixed lump or thickening of a breast area; red, scaly patch of skin on breast; development of nipple inversion or calcifications detected on mammogram; possibly no palpable or visible symptoms initially
    h. *Inflammatory carcinoma* is a systemic disease of breast and most malignant form of breast cancer
       1) Signs and symptoms: skin erythema, redness, warmth, and induration of breast; *peau d'orange* sign (edema of skin with orange peel look) is present
       2) Prognosis is poor

    i. *Paget's disease* is a rare type of breast cancer that involves epithelium of nipple
       1) Signs and symptoms: itching, burning of nipple; crusting or ulceration of nipple
       2) Excellent prognosis if confined to nipple
  3. Nursing assessment
    a. History of lump: size, shape, location, fixed or mobile, presence of pain, and when discovered; family history of breast cancer; date and location of last mammogram (if any); client's fear and knowledge of cancer

    b. Diagnostic tests: screening mammography, clinical breast exam, ultrasonography, MRI, biopsy (fine needle, excisional, or stereotactic needle) with cytologic examination of fluid, and ductal lavage and nipple aspiration

4. Nursing management

    a. Medications: estrogen-antagonist medication (Tamoxifen)—may be ordered if tumor has estrogen receptors; chemotherapy used with large tumors, age less than 50, if nodes are positive, or metastasis present

    b. Treatment: lumpectomy or mastectomy with axillary node dissection followed by radiation

    c. Breast reconstruction surgery, if desired by client, can be performed at time of mastectomy or later

    d. Provide education about the following:

        1) Results of screening and diagnostic tests (mammogram, ultrasound, biopsy, pathology report following lumpectomy or mastectomy)

        2) Expected client experience with procedures ordered and anesthesia required for them

        3) Appropriate use of home medications

        4) Side effects of radiation or chemotherapy if utilized

        5) Placement of drains after surgery and their care postdischarge

    e. Provide support to client and family, and encourage client to attend support groups such as Reach for Recovery

Practice to Pass

A 40-year-old client wants to know when she should start having mammograms. How should the nurse respond?

IV. SEXUALLY TRANSMITTED INFECTIONS (STIS)

A. Gonococcal infection

1. Overview

    a. Defined as infection of cervix and male urethra with *Neisseria gonorrhea*, a gram-negative anaerobic diplococci; can also affect mouth, throat, and anus

    b. Second most common STI; incidence is decreasing, highest incidence in urban areas among men and women 15–24 years old

    c. Also known as GC or "clap"

    d. Cause: direct sexual contact with infected person or by an infected mother to a fetus during delivery

2. Pathophysiology

    a. Bacteria present in semen, vaginal, and cervical secretions are distributed during unprotected sex to mucous membranes, causing damage to cells

    b. Damage to cells triggers inflammatory response, accounting for symptoms

    c. Infection occurs at site of contact (i.e., vagina, rectum, urethra, oropharynx)

    d. Incubation period is 2–8 days with symptoms appearing about day 10 after exposure

    e. Signs and symptoms

        1) Female: often asymptomatic; if symptomatic, presents with thick yellow or greenish-yellow vaginal discharge, new onset of dysmenorrhea and/or dyspareunia, pelvic pain, enlarged groin nodes, possible rectal pain or urethral discharge; pharyngitis; purulent exudate from urethra or Bartholin's duct

        2) Males: dysuria, thick yellow or greenish-yellow spontaneous penile discharge, pain with ejaculation, rectal pain if engage in rectal intercourse; (oropharynx)— extremely sore throat, reddened oropharynx with copious adherent yellow discharge, fever, enlarged neck nodes

    f. Complications: female—spontaneous abortion if pregnant, premature delivery, salpingitis, PID, infertility secondary to scarring and blockage of fallopian tubes or vas deferens, ectopic pregnancy or chorioamnionitis, abscess of Bartholin's gland

3. Nursing assessment
    a. Assessment
        1) Obtain sexual history including unprotected intercourse, onset and severity of symptoms, any known exposure to gonorrhea; menstrual history
        2) Assess VS, palpate lymph nodes, visually inspect any discharge, perform oral exam
        3) Symptom analysis of any pain
    b. Diagnostic tests: culture of cervix or urethra; urine specimen for polymerase chain reaction (PCR) testing
4. Nursing management
    a. Medications include antibiotic therapy
        1) Oral: ciprofloxacin hydrochloride (Cipro), a single or 7-day course of azithromycin (Zithromax), doxycycline (Vibra-tabs), or ceftriaxone sodium (Rocephin); note that resistance to azithromyin has been documented recently
        2) Intramuscular (IM): ceftriaxone sodium (Rocephin)
    b. Client education
        1) Bacterial cause of gonorrhea and transmission through unprotected intercourse
        2) Use of condoms correctly for each episode of intercourse
        3) Limit number of sexual partners or become abstinent
        4) Use of oral antibiotics including need to finish all medication
    c. Obtain names of sexual contacts for follow-up testing and treatment
B. **Nongonococcal infection**
    1. Overview
        a. Defined as an STI known as chlamydial infection, which causes an acute infection of reproductive tract
        b. *Chlamydia trachomatis*, a very small anaerobic, obligate intracellular bacteria; the most common STI among men and women 15–24 years of age
        c. Incidence is increasing across United States
        d. Majority of cases still go undiagnosed; fewer than one half of sexually active women are screened yearly as recommended
        e. Causes: direct sexual contact or perinatally (mother-to-child transmission in delivery)
    2. Pathophysiology
        a. Bacteria found in semen, vaginal, and cervical secretions are transported during sexual contact; bacteria replicate rapidly and can be spread within 24 hours of becoming infected
        b. Organism usually invades urethra in men and cervix in women
        c. Can cause conjunctivitis and blindness in newborn
        d. Incubation period is about 2 weeks after exposure
        e. Permanent tissue scarring can result from infection
        f. Symptoms: often asymptomatic, and may remain so for years
            1) Females: greenish or yellowish vaginal discharge that is visualized in cervical os, sudden onset of dysmenorrhea or dyspareunia, dysuria, or midcycle postcoital bleeding, pelvic pain, pain with orgasm
            2) Males: more likely to be symptomatic than females; dysuria, expressed yellowish penile discharge, pain with ejaculation
        g. Complications include pneumonitis if client is immunocompromised, endocarditis, and meningoencephalitis
            1) Females: PID, endometritis, salpingitis, infertility, ectopic pregnancy
            2) Males: epididymitis, prostatitis, sterility

Practice to Pass

When instructing the female client on taking doxycycline (Vibra-tabs) for her *Chlamydia trachomatis* cervicitis, the client states that she thinks she may be pregnant. What should the nurse do?

3. Nursing assessment

　a. Assessment

　　1) Obtain sexual history including unprotected intercourse, onset and severity of symptoms, known exposure to chlamydia, menstrual history

　　2) Assess VS, discharge, and complete a symptom analysis of pain

　b. Diagnostic tests: cultures of tissue, antibody tests such as direct fluorescent antibody test (DEA) or enzyme-linked immunosorbent assay (ELISA), urine specimen for polymerase chain reaction (PCR) testing

4. Nursing management

　a. Medications: oral antibiotics such as azithromycin (Zithromax), or doxycycline (Vibra-tabs)

　b. Client education

　　1) Bacterial cause of chlamydia and transmission through unprotected intercourse

　　2) Use of condoms correctly with each episode of intercourse

　　3) Limiting number of sexual partners or becoming abstinent

　　4) Use of oral antibiotics including need to finish all medication

　c. Obtain names of sexual contacts for follow-up testing and treatment

C. Syphilis

1. Overview

　a. Defined as a chronic form of STI caused by a spirochete bacteria, *Treponema pallidum*

　b. Four stages: primary, secondary, latent, and tertiary

　c. Often occurs with other STIs such as chlamydial infection or gonorrhea

　d. Highest incidence in African American men in southeast United States, especially men who have sex with men (MSM)

　e. Cause: transmission during sexual contact; through blood; mother-to-child transfer during childbirth

2. Pathophysiology

　a. Distinct stages, onset/timing, symptoms, and transfer are described in Table 11-4

　　1) Primary stage: initial chancre (typical lesion) appears

　　2) Secondary stage: development of a systemic illness

Table 11-4 Syphilis

Stage	Onset/timing	Symptoms	Transfer
Primary	10–90 days after exposure; average 21 days, lasts 3–6 weeks	Firm, round, small, crater-like chancre at site of bacterial entry that heals spontaneously, lymphadenopathy	Contact with lesion, sexual contact, or blood
Secondary	2 weeks to 6 months after chancre appears; may come and go up to 2 years	Brownish non-itchy rash especially on palms of hands and soles of feet; malaise; may have patchy hair loss; mild swollen glands, glomerulonephritis, nephrotic syndrome, oral mucous patches, arthralgia, alopecia	Contact with rash, sexual contact, blood
Latent	Disappearance of secondary stage symptoms; lasts for years	None	No
Tertiary	Onset may be several years from initial infection; can be fatal	Depends on site of invasion: heart valve or aortic stenosis. Neurosyphilis leads to CNS involvement, leading to dementia, blindness, paralysis	No

3) **Latent stage:** period until manifestations of tertiary stage begin; no clinical manifestations occur

4) **Tertiary stage:** systemic manifestations occur and complications in this stage may result in death

  b. Upon entering body, spirochete is spread by way of blood and lymphatic system; infestation can occur in any body tissue or organ

  c. Incubation period ranges from 10–90 days

  d. See Table 11-4 for signs and symptoms

  e. Complications: blindness, paralysis, mental illness, cardiovascular damage, encephalitis, and death; pregnant women with syphilis can transmit infection to fetus, resulting in congenital syphilis, causing intrauterine fetal death or numerous central nervous system (CNS) defects

3. Nursing assessment

  a. Assessment

   1) Obtain sexual history including unprotected intercourse, onset and severity of symptoms, and known exposure to syphilis

   2) Assess for IV drug use

   3) Assess VS, mental clarity, lung and heart sounds, and activity level

   4) Visual inspection for lesions

  b. Diagnostic tests

   1) Dark field microscopy of scraping from lesion

   2) Blood work: if venereal disease research laboratory (VDRL) or rapid plasma reagin (RPR) are positive, more specific fluorescent treponemal antibody absorption (FTA-ABS) is performed; VDRL will remain positive for life (serofast reaction) in most cases, but 15–25% of clients may revert to being serologically nonreactive after 2–3 years

   3) Immunofluorescent staining

4. Nursing management

  a. Medications include long-term IV and/or IM penicillin; weekly then monthly; dose depending on stage; doxycycline may also be used

  b. Explain cause of syphilis and potentially long duration of infection

  c. Encourage client to use condoms during every episode of intercourse and to avoid sharing needles

  d. Obtain names of sexual contacts for follow-up testing and treatment

  e. Explain need for compliance with follow-up testing and antibiotic treatment

  f. Assess if allergic to penicillin; educate on expected client experience with desensitization to penicillin in an intensive care unit if penicillin-allergic

D. Herpes

1. Overview

  a. A common STI involving transmission of herpes virus; is second most common viral STI (*human papilloma* virus [HPV] is most common)

  b. Two types: HSV1 (more likely to be present orally) and HSV2 (more likely to cause genital infection)

  c. Cause: sexual transmission, blood borne; and mother-to-fetus during delivery

2. Pathophysiology

  a. Retrovirus infection develops at site of viral entry into body; virus travels along dermatome to nerve root and remains dormant there until next outbreak, which occurs at same site as primary lesion

  b. Transmission can occur during genital contact, oral–genital contact, or digital contact after contact with lesions

  c. Asymptomatic viral shedding also occurs

  d. Incubation period ranges from 1 to 26 days

    e. Reactivation occurs at any time (often caused by physical or emotional stress, or hormone changes); vesicles will reappear

    f. Signs and symptoms

        1) Primary infection symptoms: extremely painful blisters that progress to crater-like lesions lasting up to 3 weeks, malaise, enlarged groin nodes, low-grade temperature

        2) Recurrent infection: extremely painful blisters progressing to crater-like lesions that heal within 10 days

    g. Complications: meningitis, encephalitis, arthritis, hepatitis, or prostatitis; neonatal transmission can occur transplacentally if primary infection occurs during pregnancy or birth while in primary stage or during recurrent infection, causing systemic neonatal herpes, which has high morbidity (from CNS involvement) and mortality

3. Nursing assessment

    a. Assessment

        1) Obtain sexual history including unprotected intercourse or oral-genital intercourse with partner having oral herpes lesions ("cold sores"), onset and severity of symptoms, and known exposure to herpes

        2) Assess VS and complete a symptom analysis of pain

    b. Diagnostic tests: cultures; diagnosed primarily by symptoms and physical exam

4. Nursing management

    a. Medications include oral antiviral medications: acyclovir (Zovirax) or valacyclovir (Valtrex) started with diagnosis for primary infection, or with onset of symptoms with recurrence; valacyclovir may be used for suppressive therapy; penciclovir (Danavir) and famcyclovir (Famvir) may be used

    b. Client education

        1) Transmission of herpes simplex virus infections

        2) Appropriate use of medications prescribed

        3) Encourage client with primary infection to report headache or stiff neck immediately

        4) Instruct client with urinary hesitancy to run water while trying to void or pour warm water over perineum or glans of penis

Case Study

T. J. is a 45-year-old client who has been diagnosed with prostate cancer. He will be having abdominal prostatectomy surgery next week for the condition.

1. How should the nurse describe the expected client experience with this surgery?

2. T. J. asks the nurse how the doctor determines if the cancer has spread beyond the prostate gland. How should the nurse reply?

3. T. J. asks why his surgery will be abdominal when his 82-year-old uncle had transurethral surgery. What is a correct answer?

4. Describe the treatments T. J. will most likely undergo after recovering from his surgery.

5. The pathology report indicates that T. J.'s cancer is stage 3. Describe what this means.

For suggested responses, see page 465.

POSTTEST

① The nurse who is triaging clients in the ambulatory clinic determines that the client with which health problem should be seen first?

1. Genital herpes infection diagnosed yesterday, with a severe headache
2. Recurrent herpes infections for 3 years, with burning during urination
3. Chlamydia diagnosed yesterday, now with worsening pelvic pain
4. Secondary syphilis diagnosed last month, due for penicillin injection

② Which statement should be presented by the nurse teaching in a breast cancer detection program for the community?

1. Mammograms should be started when women become age 50.
2. Self-breast exams should be performed weekly.
3. Birth control pills may prevent breast cancer.
4. Estrogen replacement may increase breast cancer risk.

③ The client with benign prostatic hyperplasia has undergone transurethral resection of the prostate (TURP) and is asking why he needs continuous bladder irrigation (CBI). What is the nurse's best response?

1. "The irrigation prevents blood from clotting and blocking the catheter."
2. "Your bladder needs to be kept full to promote healing after this surgery."
3. "The urine would be very concentrated without the irrigation."
4. "The saline running through the bladder helps keep you hydrated."

④ The nurse is caring for a female client who has endometriosis and wants to start a family. If she has the classic triad of symptoms, the nurse anticipates that which of the following will be the goal of treatment? Select all that apply.

1. Relief from dysmenorrhea
2. Less painful sexual intercourse
3. Menstrual periods regularly every 28 days
4. Restoration of fertility
5. Relief of headache and constipation

⑤ The nurse interprets that which male client is at the highest risk for developing balanitis?

1. 1-year-old with intact foreskin
2. Circumcised 40-year-old
3. 12-year-old with intact foreskin
4. Circumcised 6-year-old

⑥ The nurse conducting health screenings determines that which client is at lowest risk for developing breast cancer?

1. Client with BRCA1 gene mutation
2. Client who had Hodgkin's disease
3. First child at age 18, breastfed for 2 years
4. Smoker, age 74

⑦ The clinic nurse anticipates that female clients with *Chlamydia trachomatis* infections will most likely present with which signs and symptoms?

1. Painful perineal blisters and high fever of sudden onset
2. Painless, crater-like lesion on the labia that lasts 6 weeks
3. Rapidly progressing pruritic rash on labia and buttocks
4. Yellow-green vaginal discharge, dyspareunia, pelvic pain

8 The client with a new diagnosis of genital herpes simplex virus 2 (HSV2) wants to know how she contracted the infection. The nurse's best answer is based on which of the following?

1. Inanimate objects can harbor HSV for several hours.
2. Herpes simplex virus 1 (HSV1) is found only in the genital tract and not orally.
3. Sexual contact is the most common mode of transmission.
4. Immune system suppression is needed to contract the infection.

9 The nurse is assessing a client diagnosed with benign prostatic hyperplasia (BPH). What findings would the nurse expect to note? Select all that apply.

1. Forceful urinary stream
2. Frequency and urgency
3. Increased time to void
4. Incomplete bladder emptying
5. Nocturia

10 The nurse would assess the client with multiple subserosal uterine myomas for which of the following?

1. Uterine enlargement, urinary frequency, and pelvic pressure
2. Uterine enlargement, pain with urination, and vaginal discharge
3. Uterine atrophy, heavy and painful menses, and decreased libido
4. Uterine atrophy, pain with intercourse, and vaginal dryness

➤ *See pages 297–299 for Answers and Rationales.*

ANSWERS & RATIONALES

Pretest

1 **Answer: 2** **Rationale:** Balanitis, or inflammation of the foreskin and prepuce, would cause edema and pain of the penile glans, leading to dysuria. Balanitis affects males not females; a urethral discharge may occur in gonorrhea; and back pain could indicate many disorders, but not balanitis. **Cognitive Level:** Applying **Client Need:** Physiological Adaptation **Integrated Process:** Nursing Process: Assessment **Content Area:** Adult Health **Strategy:** Use nursing knowledge and the process of elimination to make a selection. If you need to make an educated guess, go with an option that fits an inflammatory problem: balan*itis*. **Reference:** Osborn, K. S., Wraa, C. E., & Watson, A. (2010). *Medical surgical nursing: Preparation for practice.* Upper Saddle River, NJ: Pearson Education, p. 1514.

2 **Answer: 4** **Rationale:** Prostatitis creates pain in the tissues surrounding the prostate gland, and it may manifest as rectal pain or pain with erection, as well as low back or rectal pain. Urinary retention or incontinence would indicate problems with control of the urinary bladder. Blisters, groin lesions, and fever are characteristic of infection with herpes virus; and a brownish palmar rash represents syphilis (secondary stage). **Cognitive Level:** Applying **Client Need:** Physiological Adaptation

Integrated Process: Nursing Process: Assessment **Content Area:** Adult Health **Strategy:** Differentiate prostatitis from sexually transmitted infections or other problems. Use nursing knowledge and the process of elimination to make a selection. **Reference:** LeMone, P., Burke, K., & Bauldoff, G. (2011). *Medical-surgical nursing: Critical thinking in patient care* (5th ed.). Upper Saddle River, NJ: Pearson Education, pp. 1659–1660.

3 **Answer: 1** **Rationale:** Secondary syphilis begins with the healing of the chancre, and ends when the rash disappears, which can take up to 6 months from time of infection. The latent stage of syphilis then starts, which can last for years. VDRL and rapid plasma reagin (RPR) would need to be positive for syphilis. Night sweats, cough, and fever could indicate tuberculosis (TB) or HIV; and penile discharge, dysuria, and urinary frequency suggest symptoms of a bacterial infection such as chlamydia. **Cognitive Level:** Applying **Client Need:** Physiological Adaptation **Integrated Process:** Nursing Process: Assessment **Content Area:** Adult Health **Strategy:** Review the manifestations of sexually transmitted infections. Which relate to syphilis? Note that the time frame given in the question is a clue. **Reference:** LeMone, P., Burke, K., & Bauldoff, G. (2011). *Medical-surgical nursing: Critical thinking in patient care* (5th ed.). Upper Saddle River, NJ: Pearson Education, pp. 1729–1730.

4 **Answer: 3** **Rationale:** Hypospadias repair is undertaken using the foreskin to create a channel through the penis to the tip of the glans so that he will deposit sperm near his partner's cervix. Although the anatomy will appear more "normal," this is not the purpose of the surgery. Circumcision is not required and other anomalies are not likely. **Cognitive Level:** Applying **Client Need:** Health Promotion and Maintenance **Integrated Process:** Teaching and Learning **Content Area:** Child Health **Strategy:** If the problem is unfamiliar, use clues to help choose the correct option. Note the age of the client, the gender, and the prefix *hypo-* in the question. **Reference:** McCance, K., & Huether, K. (2006). *Understanding pathophysiology: The biologic basis for disease in adults and children* (5th ed.). St. Louis, MO: Elsevier, p. 1339.

5 **Answer: 4** **Rationale:** Dysfunctional uterine bleeding (DUB) most commonly results from a progesterone deficiency that causes a fragile endometrium that fails to mature from proliferative stage to secretory. This causes irregular menstrual bleeding. Treatment is aimed at correcting the cause; thus, progesterone supplementation is prescribed. Testosterone, unopposed estrogen, and corticosteroids are unnecessary. **Cognitive Level:** Applying **Client Need:** Pharmacological and Parenteral Therapies **Integrated Process:** Nursing Process: Planning **Content Area:** Adult Health **Strategy:** Recall which hormone regulates uterine bleeding. If guessing, eliminate the hormones that are not predominantly female ones. **Reference:** LeMone, P., Burke, K., & Bauldoff, G. (2011). *Medical-surgical nursing: Critical thinking in patient care* (5th ed.). Upper Saddle River, NJ: Pearson Education, pp. 1685–1686.

6 **Answer: 2, 3, 4** **Rationale:** Douching should be avoided in order to prevent bacteria present in the lower reproductive tract from being forced upwards into the uterus, potentially causing pelvic inflammatory disease (PID). Condoms and monogamy help prevent reinfection. Position does not affect the spread of sexually transmitted infections (STIs). Voiding after intercourse will help prevent urinary tract infection. **Cognitive Level:** Applying **Client Need:** Physiological Adaptation **Integrated Process:** Teaching and Learning **Content Area:** Adult Health **Strategy:** The critical words in the question are *teaching* and *successful*. With this in mind, choose the options that prevent sexually transmitted infections (STIs). **Reference:** LeMone, P., Burke, K., & Bauldoff, G. (2011). *Medical-surgical nursing: Critical thinking in patient care* (5th ed.). Upper Saddle River, NJ: Pearson Education, pp. 1718–1719.

7 **Answer: 3** **Rationale:** Chemotherapy and radiation used in the treatment of testicular cancer often cause a radically decreased sperm count. If the client desires children, he should consider sperm banking prior to beginning treatment. Impotence is not a key concern, and the client's increase in sexual activity may return to normal, but not directly because of successful treatment. **Cognitive Level:** Applying **Client Need:** Health Promotion and Maintenance

Integrated Process: Nursing Process: Planning **Content Area:** Adult Health **Strategy:** Consider the age of the client, the type of cancer, and the side effects of cancer treatments. **Reference:** LeMone, P., Burke, K., & Bauldoff, G. (2011). *Medical-surgical nursing: Critical thinking in patient care* (5th ed.). Upper Saddle River, NJ: Pearson Education, pp. 1658–1659.

8 **Answer: 4** **Rationale:** Xanthines (caffeine) can precipitate or worsen fibrocystic breast disease, and elimination of coffee, tea, cola, and chocolate in the diet can decrease the symptoms. No other dietary factors have been identified. **Cognitive Level:** Applying **Client Need:** Health Promotion and Maintenance **Integrated Process:** Nursing Process: Assessment **Content Area:** Adult Health **Strategy:** If you were thinking high-fat diet was the answer, note that 2 options contain high-fat foods. Look for another food culprit since there is only one answer to this question. **Reference:** LeMone, P., Burke, K., & Bauldoff, G. (2011). *Medical-surgical nursing: Critical thinking in patient care* (5th ed.). Upper Saddle River, NJ: Pearson Education, p. 1703.

9 **Answer: 1** **Rationale:** Doxycycline (Vibra-tabs) is a commonly utilized treatment for chlamydia infections and, like all antibiotics, must be taken until completed. Use of condoms with every sexual encounter decreases the transmission of sexually transmitted infections. Sexual contacts should be notified of the infection so that appropriate testing can be obtained. This is especially important with chlamydia because it is often asymptomatic in women, and early detection can prevent complications such as pelvic inflammatory disease. Testicular self-exam is a screening measure for testicular cancer. **Cognitive Level:** Applying **Client Need:** Physiological Adaptation **Integrated Process:** Nursing Process: Implementation **Content Area:** Adult Health **Strategy:** Consider which action cures the infection or prevents reinfection. **Reference:** LeMone, P., Burke, K., & Bauldoff, G. (2011). *Medical-surgical nursing: Critical thinking in patient care* (5th ed.). Upper Saddle River, NJ: Pearson Education, p. 1726.

10 **Answer: 3** **Rationale:** Primary dysmenorrhea begins at menarche and is usually a lifelong condition. Heavy flow, clots, irregularity, and amenorrhea can occur with secondary dysmenorrhea or endometriosis. **Cognitive Level:** Applying **Client Need:** Physiological Adaptation **Integrated Process:** Nursing Process: Assessment **Content Area:** Adult Health **Strategy:** Note the critical words *primary* in the question and *since menarche* in the correct option and make an association between the options. Alternatively, eliminate at least 2 options after noting 3 months and 7 months as time frames. **Reference:** LeMone, P., Burke, K., & Bauldoff, G. (2011). *Medical-surgical nursing: Critical thinking in patient care* (5th ed.). Upper Saddle River, NJ: Pearson Education, pp. 1684–1685.

Posttest

1 **Answer: 1** **Rationale:** The primary genital herpes infection involves systemic viremia, and encephalitis is a possible complication. Headache and stiff neck may indicate

ANSWERS & RATIONALES

encephalitis, a life-threatening disorder that requires prompt treatment with an antiviral agent. Having herpes for 3 years and secondary syphilis suggest a longer-term infection and requires intervention, but not urgently. The client with chlamydia has a less-acute problem, as the client is probably already taking antibiotics. Pain control is a priority, but not more urgent than the client with a potentially life-threatening problem. **Cognitive Level:** Analyzing **Client Need:** Physiological Adaptation **Integrated Process:** Nursing Process: Planning **Content Area:** Adult Health **Strategy:** Consider which problem may be life threatening if prompt treatment is not given. Note the critical word *headache* in the correct option, which is an atypical or nonlocal symptom of a new genital herpes infection. **Reference:** LeMone, P., Burke, K., & Bauldoff, G. (2011). *Medical-surgical nursing: Critical thinking in patient care* (5th ed.). Upper Saddle River, NJ: Pearson Education, pp. 1720–1721, 1725–1726, 1729–1731.

2 **Answer: 4** **Rationale:** Breast cancer detection begins with monthly self-breast exams. Some groups suggest that mammograms should be done every 2 years for all women beginning at age 50; the American Cancer Society recommends that mammograms be performed yearly after age 40. Birth control pills do not increase nor decrease breast cancer risk, but the longer a woman is on estrogen replacement therapy, the greater her risk for developing the disease. **Cognitive Level:** Applying **Client Need:** Health Promotion and Maintenance **Integrated Process:** Nursing Process: Implementation **Content Area:** Adult Health **Strategy:** Read the question and the options carefully. Some options are incorrect because one word or number changes the meaning. **Reference:** LeMone, P., Burke, K., & Bauldoff, G. (2011). *Medical-surgical nursing: Critical thinking in patient care* (5th ed.). Upper Saddle River, NJ: Pearson Education, pp. 1640, 1704–1705.

3 **Answer: 1** **Rationale:** Continuous bladder irrigation serves to flush out the blood that will be oozing from the raw edges of the transurethral resection of the prostate (TURP) site before the blood can clot. Clots in the bladder would obstruct the urine flow through the catheter. The resulting bladder distention increases the risk of bleeding. **Cognitive Level:** Applying **Client Need:** Physiological Adaptation **Integrated Process:** Communication and Documentation **Content Area:** Adult Health **Strategy:** Rationales for nursing actions are often tested in NCLEX®. Review "why" as well as "how" procedures are done. **Reference:** LeMone, P., Burke, K., & Bauldoff, G. (2011). *Medical-surgical nursing: Critical thinking in patient care* (5th ed.). Upper Saddle River, NJ: Pearson Education, p. 1663.

4 **Answer: 1, 2, 4** **Rationale:** The classic triad is dysmenorrhea (painful menses), dyspareunia (painful intercourse), and infertility. The treatment goals are pain management and restoration of fertility. Headache and constipation are not symptoms of endometriosis. The length of the

menstrual cycle is not relevant. **Cognitive Level:** Analyzing **Client Need:** Physiological Adaptation **Integrated Process:** Nursing Process: Planning **Content Area:** Adult Health **Strategy:** A clue in the question is the client's goal of pregnancy. The other correct answers relate to relieving symptoms of the disease. **Reference:** LeMone, P., Burke, K., & Bauldoff, G. (2011). *Medical-surgical nursing: Critical thinking in patient care* (5th ed.). Upper Saddle River, NJ: Pearson Education, pp. 1692–1693.

5 **Answer: 3** **Rationale:** Balanitis, inflammation of the foreskin, occurs in uncircumcised males with phimosis or poor hygiene, which predisposes them to bacterial growth in the secretions. It occurs after the foreskin becomes retractable (at about age 3). **Cognitive Level:** Analyzing **Client Need:** Physiological Adaptation **Integrated Process:** Nursing Process: Assessment **Content Area:** Adult Health **Strategy:** If the name of the problem is unfamiliar, look for a clue in the root or suffix (-itis means inflammation). Rule out options that are not clients with higher risk of inflammatory process. **Reference:** McCance, K., & Huether, K. (2006). *Understanding pathophysiology: The biologic basis for disease in adults and children* (5th ed.). St. Louis, MO: Elsevier, pp. 805–806.

6 **Answer: 3** **Rationale:** Early childbearing with breastfeeding for a total of 2 years or more decreases a woman's lifetime risk of developing breast cancer. BRCA1 or BRCA2 gene mutations increase risk. Hodgkin's disease treatment usually involves chest radiation, which increases breast cancer risk and breast cancer mortality. Aging is another factor: The older a woman becomes, the more likely she is to develop breast cancer. **Cognitive Level:** Analyzing **Client Need:** Physiological Adaptation **Integrated Process:** Nursing Process: Diagnosis **Content Area:** Adult Health **Strategy:** Consider the risk factors for breast cancer and select the option that has the fewest risks. **Reference:** LeMone, P., Burke, K., & Bauldoff, G. (2011). *Medical-surgical nursing: Critical thinking in patient care* (5th ed.). Upper Saddle River, NJ: Pearson Education, pp. 1703–1704.

7 **Answer: 4** **Rationale:** Chlamydia, although often silent and asymptomatic, will eventually present symptoms including new occurrence of dyspareunia, dysmenorrhea, and low abdominal and pelvic pain, with yellow or yellow-green vaginal discharge. The other answers describe symptoms of different sexually transmitted infections. **Cognitive Level:** Applying **Client Need:** Physiological Adaptation **Integrated Process:** Nursing Process: Diagnosis **Content Area:** Adult Health **Strategy:** Eliminate options that describe other diseases. **Reference:** LeMone, P., Burke, K., & Bauldoff, G. (2011). *Medical-surgical nursing: Critical thinking in patient care* (5th ed.). Upper Saddle River, NJ: Pearson Education, pp. 1724–1725.

8 **Answer: 3** **Rationale:** Herpes simplex virus 1 (HSV1) is transmitted by oral secretions and may be spread to the genital area by autoinoculation after poor handwashing or by oral intercourse. Herpes simplex virus 2 (HSV2) is spread by sexual contact or to the newborn passing through an infected birth canal. Sexual partners may not know that the client is infected and could be spreading the virus. The virus is inactivated by room temperature and drying so inanimate objects are seldom the means of transmission. Persons with intact immune systems can contract the infection. **Cognitive Level:** Applying **Client Need:** Safety and Infection Control **Integrated Process:** Nursing Process: Diagnosis **Content Area:** Adult Health **Strategy:** Watch for words that are absolute (e.g., *only*) since they allow no exceptions. **Reference:** LeMone, P., Burke, K., & Bauldoff, G. (2011). *Medical-surgical nursing: Critical thinking in patient care* (5th ed.). Upper Saddle River, NJ: Pearson Education, pp. 1720–1721.

9 **Answer: 2, 3, 4, 5 Rationale:** Manifestations are secondary to obstruction and may include weak urinary stream, incomplete bladder emptying, and increased time to void. Manifestations from the resulting irritation include frequency, urgency, dysuria, and nocturia. Chronic retention can lead to overflow incontinence. **Cognitive Level:** Applying **Client Need:** Physiological Adaptation **Integrated Process:** Nursing Process: Assessment **Content Area:** Adult Health

Strategy: Choose symptoms of obstruction and irritation. **Reference:** LeMone, P., Burke, K., & Bauldoff, G. (2011). *Medical-surgical nursing: Critical thinking in patient care* (5th ed.). Upper Saddle River, NJ: Pearson Education, pp. 1660–1661.

10 **Answer: 1 Rationale:** Subserosal uterine myomas are located on the outer surface of the uterus and tend to cause fewer menstrual disorders than submucosal or intramural myomas. However, they do cause mechanical pressure on the pelvic contents from their size and weight, including bladder pressure that results in urinary frequency and urgency. **Cognitive Level:** Analyzing **Client Need:** Physiological Adaptation **Integrated Process:** Nursing Process: Assessment **Content Area:** Adult Health **Strategy:** If unfamiliar with the disorder in the question, try decoding the terms. *Subserosal* (just below the outer serous layer) tells where the *-oma* (tumor) is located on the uterus. Now determine what manifestations a growth in that location may cause. **Reference:** LeMone, P., Burke, K., & Bauldoff, G. (2011). *Medical-surgical nursing: Critical thinking in patient care* (5th ed.). Upper Saddle River, NJ: Pearson Education, pp. 1691–1692.

References

Endo-online, the Voice of the Endometriosis Association (2011). Retrieved December 29, 2011 from http://www.endometriosisassn.org/cndo.html.

Gonorrhea Fact Sheet. Centers for Disease Control and Prevention, National Center for Infectious Diseases, Bacterial STD Branch of the Division of AIDS, STD, and TB Laboratory Research. Retrieved December 29, 2011 from http://www.cdc.gov/std/Gonorrhea/.

Ignatavicius, D., & Workman, L. (2012). *Medical surgical nursing: Patient-centered collaborative care* (7th ed.). Philadelphia, PA: W. B. Saunders.

LeMone, P., Burke, K.M., & Bauldoff, G. (2011). *Medical-surgical nursing: Critical thinking in patient care* (5th ed.). Upper Saddle River, NJ: Pearson Education.

Lewis, S., Heitkemper, M., Dirksen, S., Bucher, L., & Camera, I. (2011). *Medical surgical nursing: Assessment and management of clinical problems* (8th ed.). St. Louis, MO: Elsevier Science.

Lowdermilk, D., Perry, S., & Boback, I. (2011). *Maternity and women's health care* (10th ed.). St. Louis, MO: Mosby.

McCance, K. & Huether, K. (2010). *Understanding pathophysiology: The biologic basis for disease in adults and children* (6th ed.) St. Louis, MO: Elsevier.

Porth, C., & Matfin, G. (2010). *Pathophysiology: Concepts of altered health states* (8th ed.). Philadelphia, PA: Lippincott Williams & Wilkins.

Prostate Cancer Research Institute. (2011). The Gleason Score: A significant biologic manifestation of prostate cancer aggressiveness on biopsy. Retrieved February 12, 2012, from http://www.prostate-cancer.org/pcricms/node/165.

U.S. Department of Health and Human Services, Public Health Service, Centers for Disease Control and Prevention Division of STD Prevention. *Sexually transmitted disease surveillance, 2010.* Atlanta, GA. Retrieved December 29, 2011, from http://www.cdc.gov/nchstpidstd/dsta/stats-trends/stats_and_trends.htm.

Wilson, B., Shannon, M., & Shields, K. (2012). *Pearson nurse's drug guide 2012.* Upper Saddle River, NJ: Pearson Education.

ANSWERS & RATIONALES

12 Immunological Health Problems

Chapter Outline

Risk Factors for Immunological
   Health Problems
Allergies

Latex Allergy
Anaphylaxis

Acquired Immunodeficiency
   Syndrome (AIDS)

NCLEX-RN® Test Prep

Use the accompanying online resource,
NursingReviewsandRationales, to test
yourself with hundreds of NCLEX®-style
practice questions.

Objectives

➤ Define key terms associated with immunological health problems.
➤ Identify risk factors associated with the development of
immunological health problems.
➤ Explain the common etiologies of immunological health problems.
➤ Describe the pathophysiologic processes associated with specific
immunological health problems.
➤ Distinguish between normal and abnormal immunological findings
obtained from nursing assessment.
➤ Prioritize nursing interventions associated with specific
immunological health problems.

Review at a Glance

**acquired immunodeficiency
syndrome (AIDS)** disease
syndrome characterized by infection with
human immunodeficiency virus (HIV) and
opportunistic infections or neoplasms
allergen substance, foreign protein,
or cell capable of causing alterations
in sensitivity
antibody immune or protective
protein, evoked by an antigen; capable
of reacting with a certain antigen
antigen substance that as a result
of coming in contact with certain
tissues induces a state of sensitivity
or resistance
autoimmune disorders disorders
resulting when one's own tissues are
subject to destructive effects of
immune system
**cell-mediated immune
response** an immune system
response to antigens, which do not evoke
antibody-mediated response because
they live inside body's cells (viruses and

mycobacteria are examples of
such antigens)
cytokines agents of lymphoid system
(interferons and interleukins) that act to
modify body's response to cancerous
cells; they may also be cytotoxic
**graft-versus-host disease
(GvHD)** frequent and potentially fatal
complication of bone marrow transplant;
grafted tissue recognizes host tissue as
foreign and mounts a cell-mediated
immune response
**humoral immune
response** antibody-mediated
immune response produced by
B-lymphocytes
hypersensitivity altered immune
response in a client that results in harm
to client
immunodeficiency a state in
which client's immune system is
incompetent or unable to
respond effectively

immunotherapy natural and/or
synthetic substances used to stimulate or
suppress response of immune system
latex allergy allergic response to
latex; common in health care workers
and others who routinely use latex gloves
as barrier protection
lymphocytes small, nondescript
cells that account for 20–40% of circulating leukocytes; are principal effector and
regulator cells of specific immune
response
macrophage mature monocytes
that actively phagocytize large foreign
particles and cell debris
opportunistic disease any
infection resulting from a deficient
immune system
viral load number of circulating
human immunodeficiency virus (HIV)
particles per milliliter

PRETEST

1 An adult male client is admitted to the hospital with symptoms of pneumonia. He has not improved clinically and has not responded well to antibiotics. When the sputum culture and sensitivity (C&S) and chest x-ray (CXR) results are available, a diagnosis of *pneumocystis jerovici* pneumonia is made. The nurse should conclude that this client has which of the following?

1. Recent infection by HIV
2. AIDS
3. Tuberculosis
4. An infection of unknown origin

2 A child who was breastfed as an infant receives the varicella vaccine at age 18 months. The mother states, "But I've had the chickenpox." The nurse explains to the mother that the child will require a booster even though the child has experienced which types of immunity since birth? Select all that apply.

1. Active acquired, natural
2. Passive acquired, natural
3. Passive acquired, artificial
4. Active acquired, artificial
5. Passive artificial, permanent

3 A person who is HIV-positive starts to exhibit signs of AIDS. The nurse would accurately interpret that the client now has an AIDS-defining illness after noting which of the following? Select all that apply.

1. Low viral load and a high white blood cell (WBC) count
2. Low CD4 count and symptoms of immunodeficiency
3. High white blood cell (WBC) count and anemia
4. High viral load and CD4 count below 200 cells/mm^3
5. Diagnosis of *pneumocystis jerovici* pneumonia

4 The health care provider tells a sexually active 16-year-old female with flulike symptoms that a negative enzyme-linked immunosorbent assay (ELISA) will need to be repeated in several weeks. When the client asks the nurse why the second test is necessary, what is the best explanation by the nurse?

1. The first test may be inaccurate.
2. Antibodies do not always show up initially.
3. The test is sensitive and can give false positives.
4. It is standard practice.

5 A client experiences an anaphylactic reaction after taking the first dose of a newly prescribed antibiotic. The client history reveals that the client had taken the antibiotic once before without a problem. The nurse's explanation to the client will be based on what knowledge about the hypersensitivity response?

1. Histamine precursor causes anaphylaxis and a life-threatening situation.
2. IgE antibodies destroy mast cells, releasing substances that cause hypotension and vascular collapse.
3. Cell-mediated response, or delayed hypersensitivity, is caused by sensitized T lymphocytes and can lead to tissue injury.
4. Massive numbers of red blood cells are lysed because of an incompatibility with the medication that requires discontinuing the medication.

6 A female client who has recently been diagnosed with type 1 diabetes mellitus (DM) asks the nurse how she developed this because no one in her family is a diabetic. The nurse should respond that DM is an autoimmune disease characterized by which of the following?

1. Failure of the immune system to recognize self
2. Exacerbations and remissions
3. Accelerated production of killer T-cells
4. Immunosuppression and altered cortisol levels

7 A mother of twins calls the office and speaks to the nurse about a rash that has developed on both children since taking an antibiotic prescribed 7 days ago. The twins also have edema of the face and neck, joint pain, and fever. What conclusion does the nurse draw about the problem and what is the appropriate nursing action?

1. Type I hypersensitivity reaction—get an order for diphenhydramine (Benadryl) and stop the medication.
2. Type II hypersensitivity reaction—monitor renal function after stopping the drug.
3. Type III hypersensitivity reaction (serum sickness)—stop the drug and notify the pediatrician.
4. Type IV hypersensitivity reaction—get order to change to another drug and recommend calamine lotion for the rash.

8 The nurse is working with a client who has been asymptomatic with HIV until recently, when he developed *pneumocystis jerovici* pneumonia. The CD4 T-cell counts have dropped to below 200/mm^3 (Diagnostic Category 3). The nurse then assesses the client for the presence of what clinical problem that would also place this client in Clinical Category C? Select all that apply.

1. HIV encephalopathy
2. Persistent generalized lymphadenopathy
3. Chlamydia
4. Flulike symptoms of fever, sore throat, myalgia, and headache
5. Kaposi's sarcoma

9 The ambulatory care nurse concludes that the client who does which of the following is at highest risk of contact with the HIV virus?

1. Counsels HIV victims and their families
2. Works with athletes who perspire a lot
3. Collects blood donations via a mobile blood unit
4. Gives flu shots in a health care provider's office

10 A client is brought to the emergency department with anaphylaxis after taking a dose of penicillin. The nurse delivers care based on which nursing diagnosis that has highest priority?

1. Ineffective Breathing Pattern
2. Decreased Cardiac Output
3. Risk for Injury
4. Anxiety

➤ *See pages 319–320 for Answers and Rationales.*

I. RISK FACTORS FOR IMMUNOLOGICAL HEALTH PROBLEMS

A. Overview
1. Immunity is a specific bodily response to invasion by microorganisms and foreign protein and, with other defenses of body, constitutes an essential protective mechanism
2. Immune system is a complex network of specialized cells and organs that defend body against attack from foreign pathogens
3. The major **lymphocytes** (a white blood cell [WBC] accounting for 20–30% of total count) involved in protecting body against potential infections are B and T cells, which also play an important role in combating tumor growth
4. Cells of immune system patrol tissues and organs through both blood and lymphatic vessels
5. Immune system functions
   a. Defend and protect body from infection by bacteria, viruses, fungi, and parasites
   b. Remove and destroy damaged or dead cells
   c. Identify and destroy malignant cells, thereby preventing their development into tumors

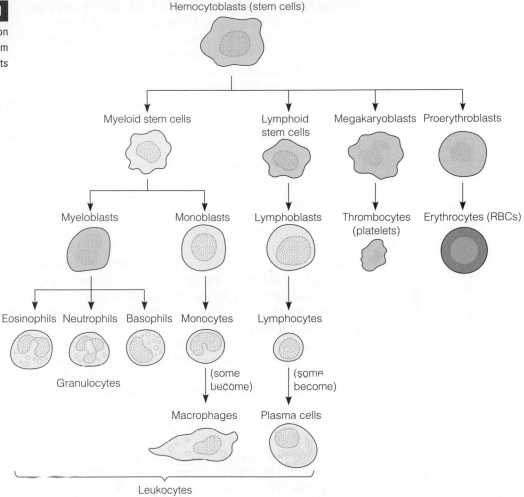

Figure 12-1

Production and differentiation of leukocytes from hemocytoblasts

6. Immune system components
   a. Human blood is made up of red blood cells (RBCs or erythrocytes) that transport oxygen, platelets (thrombocytes) that trigger clotting, and WBCs (or leukocytes); WBCs are an important element of immune system that defends human body against attack from foreign pathogens
   b. WBCs originate in bone marrow from hemocytoblasts (stem cells) that give rise to lymphoid and myeloid stem cells (see Figure 12-1)
      1) *Leukocytes* or WBCs are the principal cells involved in immune response; normal number is 4,500–10,000 cells/mm^3 of blood
      2) *Granulocytes* comprise 60–80% of total number of WBCs; have a relatively short life span (hours to days) and are key in defending body against harmful microorganisms during acute inflammation and infection; there are 3 types
         a) Neutrophils or polymorphonuclear leukocytes (or polys) comprise 55–70% of WBCs; are phagocytic (engulf and destroy pathogens) and arrive first at site of invasion (because of release of chemical triggers from damaged tissues and invading pathogens)
         b) Eosinophils (1–4% of WBCs) mature in bone marrow shortly before being released into circulation where they are very short-lived; are less efficient phagocytic cells than neutrophils; are commonly found in higher numbers in respiratory and gastrointestinal (GI) tracts

c) Basophils (0.5–1% of WBCs) are not phagocytic; granules within basophils contain proteins and chemicals such as heparin, histamine, bradykinin, serotonin, and a slow-reacting substance of anaphylaxis (leukotrienes); these are released into bloodstream during an acute **hypersensitivity** (abnormally sensitive to a stimulus) reaction or stress response

3) *Monocytes and macrophages*

   a) Monocytes are largest of WBCs and comprise 2–3% of total WBCs; released from bone marrow and circulate for 1–2 days before they attach to various tissues, where they remain for months to years before they are activated

   b) Monocytes mature into **macrophages** (mature monocytes that actively phagocytize large foreign particles and cell debris) after settling into tissues

   c) Both types are actively phagocytic with capacity to engulf large foreign particles and cell debris; are important in fight against chronic infections such as viral infections, tuberculosis, and certain intracellular parasitic infections

4) Lymphocytes (20–40% of WBCs) are small cells that are principal effectors and regulators of specific immune response (see Figure 12-2)

   a) Monitor body for cancerous cells in a process known as immune surveillance

   b) Lymphocytes constantly circulate, but in a homing pattern return to lymphoid tissues

   c) On contact with an **antigen** (substance capable of producing a specific immune response), lymphocytes are activated and mature into either effector cells (plasma cells or cytotoxic cells), which are instrumental in destruction of antigens, or memory cells

   d) Memory cells activate immediately upon subsequent exposure to same antigen; are responsible for providing acquired immunity

   e) There are 3 types of lymphocytes: T lymphocytes (T cells), B lymphocytes (B cells), and natural killer cells (NK cells)

   f) T and B cells are integral to specific immune response

   g) NK cells are large, granular cells found in spleen, lymph nodes, bone marrow, and blood that provide immune surveillance and resistance to infection and play an important role in destruction of early malignant cells

7. Lymphoid system

   a. Lymphocytes concentrate in lymphoid tissues, which include lymph nodes, spleen, thymus, tonsils, lymphoid tissue scattered in connective tissues and mucosa, and bone marrow

   b. Thymus and bone marrow, in which T and B cells mature, are considered primary lymphoid organs

   c. Spleen, lymph nodes, tonsils, and other peripheral lymphoid tissues are considered secondary lymphoid organs

   1) Lymph nodes are most numerous of lymphoid tissues and are distributed throughout body as small round or bean-shaped nodules that vary in size from 1 mm to 2 cm; they filter foreign products or antigens from lymph, and store and support proliferation of lymphocytes and macrophages

   a) Lymph, a clear, protein-filled fluid, is transported by lymph vessels

   b) Presence of a foreign protein stimulates lymphocytes and macrophages to proliferate in lymph nodes

   2) Spleen (largest lymphoid organ) is only part of system able to filter blood

   a) Located in upper left quadrant of abdomen

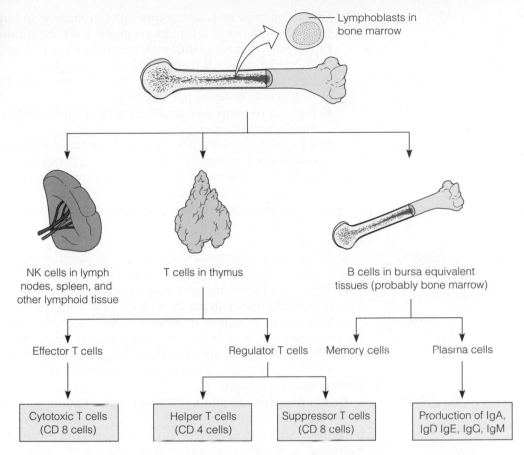

Figure 12-2

Development and differentiation of lymphocytes from lymphoblast in bone marrow

Lymphoblasts in bone marrow

NK cells in lymph nodes, spleen, and other lymphoid tissue

T cells in thymus

B cells in bursa equivalent tissues (probably bone marrow)

Effector T cells

Regulator T cells

Memory cells

Plasma cells

Cytotoxic T cells (CD 8 cells)

Helper T cells (CD 4 cells)

Suppressor T cells (CD 8 cells)

Production of IgA, IgD IgE, IgG, IgM

      b) Composed of white pulp (which serves as a site for B cell lymphocyte prolif-eration and immune surveillance) and red pulp (for blood filtration and storage of RBC breakdown products)

      c) Spleen is not essential for life; when removed or damaged, liver and bone marrow assume its functions

   3) Thymus gland is located in superior anterior mediastinal cavity beneath sternum

      a) It reaches maximum size at puberty and begins to atrophy slowly; in adult, it is difficult to differentiate from other tissue

      b) Main function is to serve as a site for maturation and differentiation of T cells

      c) Thymosin, an immunoregulatory hormone, stimulates lymphopoiesis (formation of lymphocytes or lymphoid tissue)

   4) Bone marrow is soft tissue found in hollow cavity of long bones, as well as flat bones of skull, sternum, ribs, and vertebrae; produces and stores stem cells (from which all cellular components of blood are derived)

   5) Lymphoid tissues are also located at key sites of potential invasion by microor-ganisms: the genitourinary, respiratory, and GI tracts

8. Bodily response

  a. Nonspecific inflammatory response: when first-line defenses are breached, a non-specific immune response (called inflammation) occurs

b. Specific immune response: occurs with introduction of foreign substances, or antigens, into body; specific immune response has these properties:
  1) Typically directed against materials recognized as foreign and is not usually directed against self (because of self-recognition)
  2) Response is specific; it is initiated by and directed against particular antigens
  3) Response is systemic, not localized
  4) Immune response has memory; repeated exposures to an antigen produce a more rapid response
  5) Recognition of self: effectiveness of immune system depends on its ability to differentiate normal host tissue from abnormal or foreign tissue
    a) Body's components have antigenic properties that are unique and are recognized by immune system as self
    b) External agents have antigenic properties which are identified by immune system as nonself

9. Antigens
  a. Antigens are substances recognized as foreign or nonself and provoke a specific immune response when introduced into body
  b. Typically, antigens are large protein molecules although other substances (polysaccharides, polypeptides, and nucleic acids) may be antigenic
  c. Other antigens include transplanted tissue or organs; incompatible blood cells, vaccines, pollen, egg white, and toxins such as snake or bee venom
  d. When an antigen is introduced into body, it is recognized by a specific receptor on a lymphocyte and an immune response is initiated

B. Humoral immune response
  1. Humoral immune response is defined as an antibody-mediated immune response produced by B lymphocytes
  2. Antigens such as bacteria, bacterial toxins, and free viruses usually activate B cells to produce **antibodies** (immune or protective protein evoked by an antigen)
  3. An antibody-mediated response is characterized by:
    a. Phagocytosis of antigen by neutrophils
    b. Precipitation: combining of soluble antigens to form insoluble forms (precipitates)
    c. Neutralization: combining with a toxin to neutralize its effects; followed by destruction by phagocytosis
    d. Lysis of antigen cell membrane
    e. Agglutination or clumping of antigens to form a noninvasive aggregate
    f. Opsonization: coating of antigen with antibodies and complement, making it more susceptible to phagocytosis

C. Cell-mediated immune response
  1. Cell-mediated immune response: immune system response to antigens that do not evoke antibody-mediated response because they live inside body cells (viruses and mycobacterium are examples of such antigens)
  2. Antigens, such as viral infected cells, cancer cells, and foreign tissue activate T cells, which are primary agents of cell-mediated (cellular) response
  3. T cells are antigen specific and are much more complex than B cells
    a. Killer T cells bind with cell surface antigens on infected or foreign cells and then either destroy cell membrane or release cytotoxic substances into cell
    b. Regulator T cells, (majority of which are T helper cells [CD4 cells]), play a key role in controlling immune response by:
      1) Stimulating proliferation of other T cells
      2) Amplifying cytotoxic activity of killer T cells

3) Activating B cells to proliferate and differentiate
4) Interacting directly with B cells to promote their conversion into plasma cells capable of producing antibodies

c. Other regulatory T cells (suppressor T cells) provide negative feedback, making immune response a self-limiting process; they are also important in preventing autoimmune disorders

d. T cells synthesize and release lymphokines, which stimulate:
  1) B cells to become plasma cells and produce antibodies
  2) Macrophages to become activated macrophages (most aggressive phagocyte)
  3) Proliferation of killer T cells

D. The processes of antibody-mediated and cell-mediated immunity result in development of acquired immunity or active immunity
  1. *Active immunity* occurs when body produces antibodies or develops immune lymphocytes against specific antigens
    a. Memory cells, which can produce an immediate immune response on re-exposure to an antigen, provide long-term immunity
    b. Active immunity can be *naturally acquired*, resulting from contact with a disease-producing antigen and subsequent development of disease; this is common for diseases such as chickenpox and hepatitis A
    c. Active immunity can be *artificially acquired* through immunization or vaccinations
  2. *Passive immunity* provides temporary protection against disease-producing antigens
    a. *Naturally acquired* passive immunity is provided by transfer of maternal antibodies via placenta and breast milk to infant
    b. *Artificially acquired* passive immunity is provided by immune globulins and serums

E. Risk factors
  1. Allergies: inherited or acquired sensitivity with repeated exposures; diseases (asthma, AIDS, immunodeficient states); contact with venomous animals; environment
  2. Latex allergy: acquired sensitivity with repeated exposures, employees required to use gloves often (health care professionals, rescue workers, firefighters, police officers, food service workers, housekeeping staff, etc.); clients identifying atopic conditions; spina bifida; clients with a history of multiple surgeries when young
  3. Anaphylaxis: history of known allergens; injection of antigenic material (allergy shots, serum from a sensitized animal); children receiving immunizations; blood transfusion; food; contrast media
  4. Acquired immunodeficiency syndrome (AIDS): health care professionals (contact, blood products, needle sticks); homosexual practice; homeless state; blood transfusion; IV drug abusers; link to sexually transmitted infections

II. ALLERGIES

A. Overview
  1. An allergy is defined as an abnormal response of immune system to an **allergen** (substance, foreign protein or cell, capable of causing alterations in sensitivity)
  2. When antigen is environmental or external it is called an allergy, and antigen is referred to as an allergen
  3. Hypersensitivity reactions are classified by type of immune response that occurs on contact and may also be classified by timing of response
    a. Anaphylaxis and transfusion reactions are examples of immediate hypersensitivity reactions
    b. Contact dermatitis is a typical delayed reaction

    4. Allergens are introduced by contact, inhalation, or ingestion

    5. Causes are numerous and include plants, animals, chemicals, molds, grasses, trees, pests, dust, food, drugs, latex, cosmetics, and perfumes

B. Pathophysiology

    1. An initial contact or exposure to an allergen is required to produce sensitization

    2. Following sensitization, subsequent contact with allergen produces symptoms; this may occur with next contact or years later

    3. Classified as 4 types of hypersensitivity responses

        a. *Type I* or *IgE-mediated hypersensitivity reaction*

            1) Produces an immediate reaction; local or systemic

            2) Examples are: immediate—allergic asthma, allergic rhinitis (hay fever), allergic conjunctivitis, and hives; rapid—anaphylactic

            3) Occurs when an allergen interacts with IgE bound to mast cells and basophils; this complex prompts release of histamine, complement, acetylcholine, kinins, and chemotactic factors

            4) Histamine is responsible for most inflammatory symptoms: peripheral vasodilation, increased vascular permeability, vascular congestion, and edema

            5) Leukotrienes and **cytokines** (agents of lymphoid system that modify body's response to cancerous cells) involve T lymphocytes, monocytes, eosinophils, and neutrophils, producing contraction of smooth muscle leading to bronchiolar constriction and edema

        b. *Type II* or *cytotoxic hypersensitivity* reaction

            1) Characterized by IgG or IgM type antibodies that react to foreign tissues or cells; are usually immediate responses

            2) Examples include hemolytic transfusion reaction of an incompatible blood type or a drug reaction (where drug forms an antigenic complex on surface of a blood cell)

            3) Lysis of blood cells (platelets, erythrocytes, and leukocytes) occurs because of activation of complement

            4) Transfusion reactions: antibodies in recipient's serum react against antigens in donor's RBCs

                a) Results in hemolysis of donor RBCs, unconjugated bilirubin from broken-down hemoglobin, and precipitation of large amounts of hemoglobin

                b) Symptoms include fever, chills, low back pain, hypotension, tachycardia, nausea and vomiting (N/V), urticaria, red-colored urine, shock, and renal failure

            5) Other conditions caused by a Type II reaction include erythroblastosis fetalis (Rh incompatibility in mother and child); autoimmune hemolytic anemia and drug induced hemolysis

        c. *Type III immune complex-mediated hypersensitivity* reaction

            1) Results from formation of IgG or IgM antibody-antigen complexes that circulate in blood; are usually immediate responses

            2) Complexes adhere to walls of vessels and cause inflammation and leads to intravascular, synovial, endocardial, or other organ complications

            3) Examples include serum sickness, arthus (joint) reactions, and autoimmune conditions

            4) Symptoms are specific to reaction: serum sickness—fever, joint and muscle pain, urticaria, rash; arthus (joint) reaction—acute, localized edema, tissue inflammation

        d. *Type IV delayed hypersensitivity reaction*

1) These reactions are cell-mediated, rather than antibody-mediated, involving T cells of immune system

2) Are delayed rather than immediate; with an onset 24–48 hours after exposure to antigen

3) Result from an exaggerated interaction between an antigen and normal cell-mediated mechanisms

4) Examples include contact dermatitis, infections, granulomatous inflammation, autoimmune diseases, transplant or graft rejection

5) Symptoms are specific to type of response

  a) Contact dermatitis such as poison ivy: redness, induration, lesions, urticaria, weeping

  b) Positive TB skin testing: reddening and induration of greater than 5 mm at 72 hours for people who are immunosuppressed or have close contact with a client positive for TB

  c) Granulomatous inflammation: leprosy, syphilis, cat-scratch disease

4. **Autoimmune disorders**

  a. Occur when immune system's ability to recognize self is impaired and immune defenses are directed against normal host tissue

  b. Can affect any tissue in body; some disorders are tissue- or organ-specific and some are systemic, with neither antibodies nor inflammatory lesions confined to any one organ

  c. Mechanism that causes immune system to recognize host tissue as a foreign antigen is not clear

  d. Known characteristics

    1) Genetics plays a role

    2) More prevalent in females than males

    3) Onset of an immune disorder is frequently associated with an abnormal stressor, either physical or psychological

    4) Are frequently progressive relapsing remitting disorders characterized by periods of exacerbation and remission

5. Tissue transplants

  a. Transplant success is closely tied to obtaining best match of tissue antigens to recipient; an autograft (transplant of client's own tissue) is most successful type of transplant

  b. *Hyperacute tissue rejections* occur immediately or 2–3 days after transplant and are due to preformed antibodies and T cells sensitized to antigens in donor organ; this type of rejection is most likely to occur in clients who have had previous organ or tissue transplants

  c. *Acute tissue rejection* is most common and treatable type of rejection episode; it occurs between 4 days and 3 months after transplant

    1) It is mediated primarily by cellular immune response and results in transplant cell destruction

    2) Client demonstrates signs of inflammatory process, with fever, redness, swelling, and tenderness over graft site

    3) Signs of impaired function of transplanted organ may be noted

  d. *Chronic tissue rejection* occurs from 4 months to years after transplantation of new tissues or organs

    1) It likely results from an antibody-mediated immune response

    2) Antibodies and complement deposit in transplanted tissue vessel walls, resulting in decreased blood flow and ischemia

Practice to Pass

The physician suggests weekly allergy shots for a child with asthma caused by seasonal allergies. How should the nurse explain how the shots will work to the mother?

Practice to Pass

Explain in simple terminology how the body develops an autoimmune disease or rejects organ tissue.

    e. Graft-versus-host disease (GvHD) is a frequent and potentially fatal complication of bone marrow transplant

        1) Defined as a disorder occurring when immunocompetent graft cells recognize host tissue as foreign and mount a cell-mediated immune response

        2) Host is usually immunocompromised and unable to fight graft cells, and host's cells are destroyed

        3) Other areas affected are skin, liver, and GI tract

C. Nursing assessment

    1. Assessment includes skin, vital signs (VS), lung sounds, respiratory status, level of consciousness (LOC), fluid status, peripheral perfusion (pulses, capillary refill, temperature of extremities); any reports of discomfort; mental status (anxiety); history of events leading to allergic reaction

    2. Diagnostic tests

        a. WBC, high eosinophil level

        b. Radioallergosorbent test (RAST), to determine presence of IgE

        c. Type and crossmatch

        d. Indirect Coombs' test; agglutination occurs if antibodies to an RBC antigen are present

        e. Direct Coombs' test; antibodies are present on client's RBCs

        f. Immune complex assays, circulating immune complexes present

        g. Complement assay; complement levels are decreased

        h. Skin testing

            1) Skin prick test, positive test produces a wheal and erythema

            2) Intradermal, wheal of 5 mm or greater and erythema

            3) Patch, mild to severe erythema with papules or vesicles

            4) Food allergy testing, presence of symptoms within hours of eating particular food thought to cause reaction

D. Nursing management

Practice to Pass

Why should the nurse explain to the client who is scheduled for a skin prick test for allergies to avoid antihistamines for 3 days prior to the test?

    1. Medications include **immunotherapy** (natural and/or synthetic substances used to stimulate or suppress response of immune system such as allergy shots), antihistamines, epinephrine for severe symptoms, budesonide (Rhinocort) or cromolyn sodium (Nasalcrom) for allergic rhinitis and asthma, glucocorticoids, over-the-counter (OTC) nasal decongestants such as pseudoephedrine tablets

    2. Goal is to minimize exposure, prevent a hypersensitivity response, and provide quick interventions if a response occurs

    3. Instruct clients to wear a MedicAlert bracelet

    4. Airway management is highest priority if laryngeal edema occurs; administer oxygen (O_2); intubate or use nasopharyngeal/oropharyngeal airway if necessary

    5. Other therapies consist of plasmapheresis (removal of components in plasma)

    6. Monitor VS

    7. Access an intravenous (IV) line and administer fluids as necessary; insert a urinary catheter and monitor intake and output (I & O) as indicated

    8. Administer blood products following hospital protocol

        a. Have a signed informed consent

        b. Check the blood for type, Rh factor (Rh− must have Rh− and Rh+ must have Rh+), expiration date; crossmatch with another licensed health care professional

        c. Monitor VS every 5 minutes for first 15 minutes and every 30 minutes or 1 hour thereafter until blood has been infused according to policy

        d. Administer blood with normal saline (NS) only

        e. Stop transfusion if any reaction occurs, send blood bag and tubing to lab for analysis; obtain urine specimen for urinalysis per protocol

    9. Educate client on having a bee sting kit or an Epi-pen available at all times

III. LATEX ALLERGY

A. Overview

1. A **latex allergy** is defined as a reaction to contact with latex, producing an allergic contact dermatitis, immediate hypersensitivity, or anaphylaxis
2. Latex is extracted from tissue beneath bark of rubber tree; it is a cloudy white liquid composed of rubber particles, protein, water, and other substances
3. The method used to process latex affects amount of protein left in finished product
4. Produces a type I or type IV reaction
5. Prevention of latex allergy reactions should focus on both client and staff
6. Causes of latex allergy include exposure through cutaneous route (gloves, tapes, masks); mucous membranes (anesthesia, rectal examinations, eye and ear droppers); intrauterine devices; intravascular (IV fluids, injectables, IV devices); internal contact through surgery

B. Pathophysiology

1. An allergic reaction is triggered upon contact with latex (see Section II, Allergies)
2. Reactions usually manifest in three ways
   a. Allergic contact dermatitis (type IV delayed hypersensitivity): most common
      1) An allergic reaction to residues of chemical agents used in latex and in manufacturing plastics
      2) Symptoms include dry, itchy red rash on hands and fingers; blistering and weeping of skin; swelling
   b. Immediate hypersensitivity (type I)
      1) Natural latex protein produces an IgE response
      2) Can cause severe, even fatal reactions
      3) Symptoms develop within 5–30 minutes from exposure and diminish quickly when exposure is removed
      4) Symptoms include immediate itching; intense swelling of fingers and hand; may proceed to anaphylaxis
   c. Anaphylaxis
      1) Occurs when there has been contact with latex through mucous membranes or body cavities such as in surgery
      2) Symptoms include local or generalized itching; urticaria; angioedema; rhinitis; conjunctivitis; asthma; extreme anxiety; GI complaints (N/V, abdominal pain); tachycardia; hypotension; faintness; coma; cardiac arrest

C. Nursing assessment

1. Color and moisture of skin; reports of itching; presence of wheals or urticaria; visual inspection of swelling; history of prior problems (especially if client is going to surgery); history of reaction to fruits (especially banana and kiwi fruit); if anaphylaxis suspected, assess respiratory and cardiac status; LOC; VS; mentation
2. Diagnostic tests
   a. Patch tests or skin prick test: positive for one or more latex accelerators
   b. Blood sample for specific IgE test

D. Nursing management

1. Medications include topical steroids, and those for anaphylaxis (see Section IV)
2. Primary treatment is removal of irritant
3. Teach client about cause of reaction and to avoid future contact
4. Instruct client to wear a MedicAlert bracelet
5. Instruct client to use a nonirritating soap substitute and emollient creams while affected area is red and irritated
6. Supervise housekeeping practices to reduce latex-containing dust from environment

Practice to Pass

What symptoms would be present in an environmental service worker who is allergic to latex and why? Why should the gloves not be snapped upon removal?

IV. ANAPHYLAXIS

A. Overview

1. Anaphylaxis is defined as an allergic response when an antigen is introduced to a highly sensitive individual
2. Response is a type I allergic reaction and is a medical emergency
3. Categorized as local or systemic
4. May lead to anaphylactic shock (see Chapter 17)
5. Multiple causes exist and are individualized: pollens, foods, drugs (antibiotics are common), venom, insect bites, diagnostic agents (contrast medium), antiserum, enzymes, hormones, vitamins, occupational agents, iodine

B. Pathophysiology

> **Practice to Pass**
>
> Why is an anaphylactic reaction considered an emergency?

1. An antigen is introduced and interacts with immunoglobulin E (IgE), which is bound to mast cells and basophils
2. This reaction causes mast cells to suddenly release histamines and other mediators throughout body or locally
3. Mast cells also release packets containing chemical mediators, which attract neutrophils and eosinophils
4. Local reactions include urticaria, vasodilation (warmth), edema, erythema
5. Systemic reactions include respiratory (bronchoconstriction, air hunger, stridor, wheezing, barking cough); cardiovascular (hypotension, tachycardia, impaired tissue perfusion); skin (same as local reaction); GI system (N/V); angioedema; anxiety
6. Systemic reactions can lead to anaphylactic shock when widespread vasodilation occurs

C. Nursing assessment

1. VS, lung sounds, heart sounds, skin assessment, analysis of symptoms, respiratory status, presence of edema or mottling, LOC, history of past allergies
2. Diagnostic tests
   a. Initial laboratory tests focus on acute symptoms: complete blood count (CBC), arterial blood gases (ABGs), type and crossmatch (if blood transfusion involved), RAST, direct and indirect Coombs' test, immune complex assay, complement assay
   b. Follow-up tests to determine cause of anaphylaxis once client is stabilized

D. Nursing management

1. Medications include antihistamines and epinephrine, vasopressors such as dopamine, and corticosteroids
2. Initial management and airway management are of highest priority
3. Client teaching
   a. Wear a MedicAlert bracelet
   b. Identify triggers and how to avoid these
   c. Know emergency management until client can be brought to an emergency room (bee sting kit, Epi-pen)
4. Initiate and maintain an IV access for fluids and emergency drugs
5. Administer O_2 as needed
6. Monitor VS frequently, as often as every 15 minutes if needed

V. ACQUIRED IMMUNODEFICIENCY SYNDROME (AIDS)

A. Overview

1. **Acquired immunodeficiency syndrome (AIDS)** is defined as last stage of infection with human immunodeficiency virus (HIV) (a retrovirus of lentivirus family)
2. **Immunodeficiency** is a state in which client's immune system is incompetent or unable to respond effectively

3. Adult classification of HIV disease is based on clinical manifestations and T4 cell counts
   a. Category A: asymptomatic, primary HIV or persistent generalized lymphadenopathy (PGL)
   b. Category B: symptomatic, not category A or C conditions
   c. Category C: AIDS-defining characteristics
4. Diagnosis is made on presence of all of the following
   a. CD4 count of less than 200 cells/mm^3
   b. Two opportunistic pathogens
   c. Presence of an AIDS-defining malignancy
5. Two primary human immunodeficiency viruses
   a. HIV-1: prototype virus, mostly in United States
   b. HIV-2: primarily limited to West Africa
6. Transmission
   a. Adult to adult: unprotected sexual activity and blood-to-blood contact
   b. Adult to child: perinatal transmission and blood-to-blood contact
7. Causes
   a. Unprotected sexual activity: vaginal, anal, and oral intercourse
   b. Blood to blood: needles, blood transfusions, exposure of health care workers
   c. Perinatal transmission: placental or intrapartum transmission and via breast milk

B. **Pathophysiology**
   1. HIV is a retrovirus, which carries its genetic information in RNA; on entry into body virus infects cells that have CD4 antigen [primarily T helper cells] (see Figure 12-3)
   2. As a virus, HIV is a parasite and must infect other cells in order to replicate
   3. Many target cells used by HIV to replicate are antigen-presenting cells needed for a normal immune response in body (CD4 lymphocytes, bone marrow CD4 precursor cells, monocytic T cell lines, etc.)
   4. Once inside cell, virus is transported to lymph nodes and attached by viral gp120 to host cell
   5. Once attached, virus enters host cell, reveals its RNA genome and uses an enzyme, reverse transcriptase, to convert viral RNA to viral DNA by using normal DNA
   6. This viral DNA insinuates itself into host cell DNA and is replicated during normal cell processes
   7. This process results in 2 major effects
      a. Viral number increases (viral load)
         1) **Viral load** is the number of circulating HIV particles per milliliter (should be zero)
         2) Viral loads of less than 10,000 = low risk; 10,000 to 100,000 = moderate risk; greater than 100,000 = high risk
      b. Infected CD4 cells die
         1) Competent immune system = T4 count of 650–1,200 cells/mm^3
         2) Suppressed immune system = T4 count of 500–200 cells/mm^3
         3) AIDS: indicator values = T4 count of less than 200 cells/mm^3
   8. Virus may lie dormant or become activated, producing new RNA and virions leading to destruction of host cells
   9. Although virus may remain inactive, antibodies are produced and detectable between 6 weeks and 6 months of infection; however, these antibodies are not able to fight HIV infection
   10. A client may show negative on antibody test for HIV but still have virus; a seroconversion time exists (6–12 weeks) that allows an HIV positive client who has no symptoms to start producing antibodies; after seroconversion, antibodies will continue to be produced

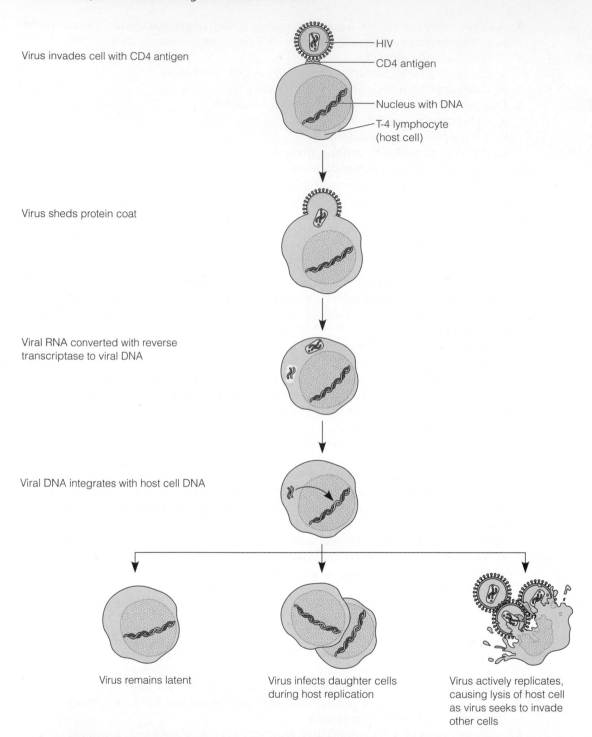

Virus invades cell with CD4 antigen

HIV

CD4 antigen

Nucleus with DNA

T-4 lymphocyte (host cell)

Virus sheds protein coat

Viral RNA converted with reverse transcriptase to viral DNA

Viral DNA integrates with host cell DNA

Virus remains latent

Virus infects daughter cells during host replication

Virus actively replicates, causing lysis of host cell as virus seeks to invade other cells

Figure 12-3

Pathophysiology of HIV

11. Although T helper cells are primarily infected with HIV, other cells (including macrophages and cells of central nervous system [CNS]) are also infected

12. Classification of HIV infection and AIDS
    a. *Category A*
       1) Primary HIV infection: negative HIV antibody tests; influenza-like symptoms; rash; symptoms cease after a few days
       2) Asymptomatic: positive antibody tests, no disease processes
       3) Persistent generalized lymphadenopathy (PGL): positive antibody tests, lymphadenopathy present for more than 3 months
       4) CD4 T cell counts: A1 = greater than or equal to $500/mm^3$; A2 = 200 to $499/mm^3$; A3 = less than $200/mm^3$
    b. *Category B*
       1) Positive antibody tests
       2) Symptomatic: oral thrush, candidiasis, cervical dysplasia, leukoplakia, herpes zoster, pelvic inflammatory disease (PID), fever, or diarrhea for more than 1 month
       3) CD4 T cell counts: B1 = greater than or equal to $500/mm^3$; B2 = 200 to $499/mm^3$; B3 = less than $200/mm^3$
    c. AIDS-indicator conditions
       1) Positive antibody tests
       2) AIDS-defining conditions: *Pneumocystis jerovici* pneumonia, candidiasis, cytomegalovirus (CMV), *Mycobacterium tuberculosis*, toxoplasmosis of brain, histoplasmosis, Kaposi sarcoma, lymphomas, AIDS dementia complex, and HIV wasting syndrome (unintentional weight loss of 10% or more body weight within a 6-month period)
       3) CD4 T cell counts: C1 = greater than or equal to $500/mm^3$; C2 = 200 to $499/mm^3$; C3 = less than $200/mm^3$

13. Signs and symptoms range from no symptoms to severe immunodeficiency with multiple severe **opportunistic disease** (any infection resulting from a deficient immune system) and neoplasm (such as cervical cancer); signs and symptoms include the following:
    a. Flulike or mononucleosis-like illness lasting days to weeks after contracting HIV
    b. Fever, sore throat, joint and muscle pain, headache, rash, and swollen lymph nodes (often first symptom); symptoms are commonly mistaken for influenza, upper respiratory infection, or gastroenteritis
    c. Progression from asymptomatic infection to AIDS is not clearly defined; client may report general malaise, fever, fatigue, night sweats, and unintentional weight loss; diarrhea is common, as are oral lesions of hairy leukoplakia, candidiasis/thrush, and gingival inflammation and ulceration
    d. Other symptoms include stiff neck; burning, numbness, and tingling of extremities; headache, lightheadedness, memory loss, mood swings; N/V; pain; dyspnea
    e. AIDS dementia complex (ADC) is a dementia with cognitive, behavioral, and motor deficits common in untreated HIV disease and affects CNS; it is thought to be caused by infection of HIV in brain cells and symptoms include impaired concentration, mental slowing, forgetfulness, apathy, confusion, hallucinations, personality changes, unsteady gait, leg tremors, and motor difficulties

14. There is a long asymptomatic period following initial infection; host is capable of infecting others during this latent period

15. Seroconversion occurs when an HIV-infected individual starts producing detectable HIV antibodies; seroconversion window is that time when infection has occurred but HIV antibodies are not detectable; individuals are able to pass virus to others unknowingly during this period

16. Mean length of time from infection to symptomatology is currently estimated to be 8–10 years

C. Nursing assessment

1. Assessment includes common symptoms, weight analysis, GI disturbances, neurological manifestations; gait; LOC; reports of pain; history of recurring infections; skin assessment; palpation of lymph nodes; VS; lung sounds; oral cavity; vaginal and rectal exam

2. Diagnostic tests

   a. Enzyme-linked immunosorbent assays (ELISA) to screen for HIV antibodies; usually will run 2 different tests

   b. Western-blot test (to confirm a positive ELISA finding)

   c. HIV viral load (high)

   d. CBC (anemia, leukopenia, thrombocytopenia)

   e. CD4 cell count (low)

   f. Immune complex dissociated p24 assay (shows active reproduction of HIV, used for progression of disease)

   g. Diagnostic tests for opportunistic infections include TB skin tests, Magnetic resonance imaging (MRI) of brain, lymphomas, cultures, Pap smears, Chest x-ray for *Pneumocystis jerovici* pneumonia

D. Nursing management

Practice to Pass

Explain why an initial ELISA test could be negative in an HIV-positive client and why 2 ELISA tests are usually conducted, followed by a Western blot?

1. Medications

   a. Antiretroviral agents

      1) Nucleoside reverse transcriptase inhibitors (NRTIs): inhibit viral reverse transcriptase (needed to introduce viral RNA into cells' DNA and replicate), resulting in an incomplete viral DNA; example: zidovudine (AZT)

      2) Protease inhibitors: inhibit protease, a viral enzyme necessary to produce mature viral particles; example: saquinavir (Invirase)

      3) Nonnucleoside reverse transcriptase inhibitors (NNRTIs): block manufacture of DNA by inhibiting reverse transcriptase enzyme; example: nevirapine (Viramune)

      4) Fusion inhibitor: interferes with entry of HIV-I into host cells by blocking fusion of virus and cell membranes: enfuvirtide (Fuzeon)

   b. Drug cocktails are a combination of above types in order to attack disease more aggressively; close monitoring is necessary

   c. Other agents include chemotherapy, antibiotics for infections, analgesics for pain and discomforts, antiemetics, antidiarrheals

   d. Consult Centers for Disease Control and Prevention (CDC) for most accurate information on new drug development

2. At present, there is a reasonable life expectancy that requires attention to prevention of transmission and avoidance of secondary infections

3. All persons should practice safe sex techniques and avoid contamination by body fluids or shared needles

4. For clients with advanced disease, information about community resources, nonjudgmental care, and health promotion activities are essential

5. Surgical treatments for abscesses and Kaposi's sarcoma may be indicated

6. Counseling for psychological and social effects should be initiated

7. Maintain clean perianal area if diarrhea is persistent

8. Instruct client about foods to avoid that are GI irritants; avoid spicy, acidic foods and those hard to chew

9. Instruct client on common side effects of medications
10. Offer and instruct on proper oral care; avoid toothbrushes; use mouthwash without alcohol
11. Educate client about symptoms of candida and herpes and when to seek help
12. If blood or body fluid spills occur, instruct client to use a 1:10 solution of bleach
13. Allow client and family to talk about illness and discuss concerns; offer touch
14. Monitor weight and nutritional status; assess caloric intake
15. Encourage ambulation and exercise as tolerated with planned rest periods
16. Offer O_2 as needed for dyspnea

Case Study

A 43-year-old man is brought to the emergency department after being stung multiple times by hornets while cutting grass. He has welts over most of his body, is itching all over, exhibits extreme anxiety, and shows tachycardia of 150 on the cardiac monitor and BP 108/65. His frantic wife states that he is allergic to penicillin and has reacted to bee stings in the past.

1. What immediate assessment should the nurse make?
2. What additional information is needed from the client or his wife?
3. What drug therapy would the nurse expect the emergency room physician to institute?
4. The client's wife asks the nurse to explain to her what is going on. How should the nurse respond?
5. What discharge instructions should be given to this client, once he is stabilized and able to return home?

For suggested responses, see pages 465–466.

POSTTEST

1 The nurse concludes that medications taken by a client with AIDS are effective if, in addition to a viral load of 25,000, the client exhibits which of the following?
1. Rare occurrence of symptoms
2. Negative enzyme-linked immunosorbent assay (ELISA)
3. CD4 T lymphocyte count of 490
4. White blood cell (WBC) count of 1,700 mm³

2 The nurse anticipates that a child with asthma caused by allergies will have which finding on a complete blood count (CBC) with differential report?
1. Eosinophils 21.9
2. White blood cells 10.9
3. Monocytes 4.0
4. Neutrophils 85.7

3 The mother of a child with swollen lymph nodes is extremely afraid that the swelling means cancer. What is the best statement that the nurse could make to calm the mother?
1. "The finding is very alarming and could be serious, but you must remember it may be insignificant also."
2. "The lymph nodes filter foreign products and may only be swollen because of an infection."
3. "The lymph nodes will swell quite often and we may not ever know it."
4. "The lymph nodes are the major organ indicating a problem with the immune system."

POSTTEST

4 A client in an allergy clinic asks the nurse why some allergic reactions affect only a small area while a reaction that occurred in the past involved "my whole body and my breathing." The nurse offers which of the following as examples of reactions that could cause systemic immune responses? Select all that apply.

1. Extreme redness and swelling to the arm after being bitten by ants
2. Anaphylaxis after ingesting a certain food such as shellfish
3. Developing symptoms of systemic latex allergy
4. Severe bronchoconstriction and wheezing after playing football in the grass
5. Sprained ankle becoming swollen, bruised, and painful

5 A client reports to the clinic with reports of itching and weeping along the back of her legs. Upon inspection, wheals are evident that appear to be poison ivy. The client states the symptoms developed 1 day after sitting in the car wearing shorts. She sat on the same seat as her husband, who had been working in a field of grass all day. The nurse concludes that the client is having which type of reaction?

1. Type I hypersensitivity
2. Type II hypersensitivity
3. Type III hypersensitivity
4. Type IV hypersensitivity

6 A family member of a client with type O negative blood is concerned about the risk of allergic reaction when the client receives a needed transfusion. The nurse explains that which type of blood will be transfused to avoid an allergic reaction?

1. O+
2. O–
3. AB+
4. AB–

7 In assessing a client with a suspected latex allergy, the nurse should ask which of the following questions?

1. "Are your hands usually moist or dry?"
2. "What drug allergies do you have?"
3. "Do the elastic bands in your underwear cause rash and itching?"
4. "What types of surgeries have you had?"

8 The nurse would immediately assess for which symptom in a client suspected of having an anaphylactic reaction?

1. Elevated blood pressure of 180/94
2. Decreased apical pulse rate of 56
3. Onset of lung crackles
4. Onset of stridor or wheezing

9 A 31-year-old female who has progressed to advanced AIDS is concerned about developing a secondary cancer. What diagnostic test should the nurse explain will probably be prescribed every 6 months?

1. Papanicolaou smear
2. Viral load
3. CD4 cell counts
4. CA 125 antigen level

10 The public health nurse considers that which of the following individuals is at increased risk of being infected with the HIV virus?

1. Police officer who works the streets and responds to emergencies
2. Sexually active teenager
3. School nurse who examines children
4. Nurse working on a telemetry unit

► *See pages 320–322 for Answers and Rationales.*

POSTTEST

ANSWERS & RATIONALES

Pretest

1 **Answer: 2** **Rationale:** *Pneumocystis jerovici* pneumonia is the most common opportunistic infection associated with AIDS. The fungus responsible is not pathogenic in individuals with a normal immune system. Opportunistic infections are likely to be seen when the CD4 cell count falls below 200/mm³ in the more advanced stages of AIDS. This infection would not occur in clients with tuberculosis, recent HIV infection, or infection of unknown origin. **Cognitive Level:** Analyzing **Client Need:** Physiological Adaptation **Integrated Process:** Nursing Process: Diagnosis **Content Area:** Adult Health **Strategy:** Analyze the signs and symptoms and decide what disease is being described. Note this infection is associated with immunocompromised individuals. Next determine whether this finding would occur in late or early stages. **Reference:** LeMone, P., Burke, K., & Bauldoff, G. (2011). *Medical-surgical nursing: Critical thinking in patient care* (5th ed.). Upper Saddle River, NJ: Pearson Education, p. 327.

2 **Answer: 2, 4** **Rationale:** Immunizations offer actively acquired artificial immunity. This child will need a booster vaccination at approximately age 5 because active artificial immunity can wane. Breastfeeding a child would offer passively acquired natural immunity, which also does not last. Active acquired natural immunity occurs when the body produces antibodies or develops immune lymphocytes against specific antigens—in this case, chickenpox (varicella), when the client contracts the disease. Immune globulins offer passively acquired artificial immunity. **Cognitive Level:** Applying **Client Need:** Health Promotion and Maintenance **Integrated Process:** Nursing Process: Planning **Content Area:** Child Health **Strategy:** Consider what immunologic mechanism occurs when a person recovers from a viral infection. **Reference:** LeMone, P., Burke, K., & Bauldoff, G. (2011). *Medical-surgical nursing: Critical thinking in patient care* (5th ed.). Upper Saddle River, NJ: Pearson Education, pp. 281–283.

3 **Answer: 2, 4, 5** **Rationale:** A client with Category 3 (AIDS) will have a low CD4 count (less than 200 cells/mm³) and a high viral load, and may have an opportunistic infection. What is desired is to have a high CD4 count and a low viral load (which should normally be zero). The white blood cell count is not used in classifying HIV. **Cognitive Level:** Analyzing **Client Need:** Reduction of Risk Potential **Integrated Process:** Nursing Process: Assessment **Content Area:** Adult Health **Strategy:** Recall that for an option to be correct, everything in the option must be correct. Analyze each option completely, eliminating first the options that contain WBC counts.

Reference: LeMone, P., Burke, K., & Bauldoff, G. (2011). *Medical-surgical nursing: Critical thinking in patient care* (5th ed.). Upper Saddle River, NJ: Pearson Education, pp. 324–327.

4 **Answer: 2** **Rationale:** The symptoms in the question are consistent with early HIV infection. The enzyme-linked immunosorbent assay (ELISA) test may be negative upon initial testing and positive at the time of seroconversion, which takes 6 weeks to 6 months after infection. This time period when the antibodies are negative is called the seroconversion window, and virally infected individuals may have negative antibody tests. **Cognitive Level:** Analyzing **Client Need:** Reduction of Risk Potential **Integrated Process:** Communication and Documentation **Content Area:** Adult Health **Strategy:** To answer this question accurately, it is necessary to know commonly performed diagnostic tests for the immune system. It is also helpful to know factors that will interfere with accurate diagnostic results—in this case, time after exposure to develop antibodies. **Reference:** LeMone, P., Burke, K., & Bauldoff, G. (2011). *Medical-surgical nursing: Critical thinking in patient care* (5th ed.). Upper Saddle River, NJ: Pearson Education, pp. 325, 330.

5 **Answer: 2** **Rationale:** Type I hypersensitivity reactions are caused by widespread antigen–antibody reactions such as anaphylaxis. This person has been sensitized by a prior exposure to the antigen and formed IgE antibodies, which reacted during a subsequent exposure. The anaphylactic response is usually immediate and leads to an antigen–antibody complex that causes the release of histamine and other substances. Lysis of massive numbers of red blood cells because of an incompatibility describes what occurs with a blood transfusion reaction and possibly some medications. The explanation that cell-mediated response is caused by sensitive T lymphocytes describes a Type IV delayed hypersensitivity. The statement that histamine precursor causes anaphylaxis is false. **Cognitive Level:** Applying **Client Need:** Physiological Adaptation **Integrated Process:** Nursing Process: Implementation **Content Area:** Adult Health **Strategy:** Review hypersensitivity reactions. This client situation clearly gives a history of past exposure to the antigen and an anaphylactic response this time. **Reference:** LeMone, P., Burke, K., & Bauldoff, G. (2011). *Medical-surgical nursing: Critical thinking in patient care* (5th ed.). Upper Saddle River, NJ: Pearson Education, pp. 308–311.

6 **Answer: 1** **Rationale:** Type 1 diabetes is caused by the autoimmune destruction of pancreatic beta cells. Recognition of self as foreign is the definition of any autoimmune disease. Further explanation may be needed to explain that the immune system usually recognizes self and identifies what is foreign, targets foreign cells, and destroys them. **Cognitive Level:** Applying **Client Need:** Physiological Adaptation **Integrated Process:** Nursing Process: Implementation **Content Area:** Adult Health **Strategy:** Eliminate the options that do not relate to an autoimmune process. The critical word is *autoimmune*, not diabetes mellitus. **Reference:** LeMone, P., Burke, K., & Bauldoff, G. (2011). *Medical-surgical nursing: Critical thinking in patient care* (5th ed.). Upper Saddle River, NJ: Pearson Education, pp. 315–316.

7 Answer: 3 Rationale: Serum sickness, a reaction a week after ingestion of a drug, is a Type III hypersensitivity reaction where formation of IgG or IgM antibody–antigen complexes occurs in the blood. The deposited immune complexes activate the inflammatory process causing focal tissue damage and edema. Urticaria, rash, extensive edema, and fever are usually temporary, resolving within a few days after the drug is stopped. Type I reactions occur within minutes of exposure to the antigen. Type II reactions involve IgG and IgM and cause hemolytic reactions. Type IV reactions are cell-mediated reactions and are delayed from the contact with the antigen. **Cognitive Level:** Analyzing **Client Need:** Physiological Adaptation **Integrated Process:** Nursing Process: Planning **Content Area:** Child Health **Strategy:** The core issue of the question is that the clients have developed an adverse drug reaction. Recall that antibiotics can cause hypersensitivity reactions to determine the correct option. **Reference:** LeMone, P., Burke, K., & Bauldoff, G. (2011). *Medical-surgical nursing: Critical thinking in patient care* (5th ed.). Upper Saddle River, NJ: Pearson Education, pp. 308–311.

8 Answer: 1, 5 Rationale: The classification system (1993 CDC recommendations) for HIV and AIDS lists several clinical problems that place an HIV-infected client into Clinical Category C. This is the most advanced category in which the client develops significant disease with neurological manifestations (HIV encephalopathy), opportunistic infections, cancers (Kaposi's sarcoma), and possibly HIV wasting syndrome. **Cognitive Level:** Applying **Client Need:** Physiological Adaptation **Integrated Process:** Nursing Process: Assessment **Content Area:** Adult Health **Strategy:** Select the problems seen in advanced AIDS. **Reference:** LeMone, P., Burke, K., & Bauldoff, G. (2011). *Medical-surgical nursing: Critical thinking in patient care* (5th ed.). Upper Saddle River, NJ: Pearson Education, pp. 324–328.

9 Answer: 3 Rationale: Fluids containing blood or blood cells have been identified as a mode of transmission for HIV. Collecting blood, especially in a mobile unit (where the population is more diverse) is a risk for any health care worker. Appropriate gloving is essential. Counseling may require touch, which is not a form of transmission; perspiration has not been identified as a form of contact. Using retractable syringes and disposing of used needles appropriately reduces the risk for nurses giving intramuscular (IM) injections.

Cognitive Level: Analyzing **Client Need:** Safety and Infection Control **Integrated Process:** Nursing Process: Assessment **Content Area:** Adult Health **Strategy:** Consider how the HIV virus is spread and which body fluid is known to contain the virus. **Reference:** LeMone, P., Burke, K., & Bauldoff, G. (2011). *Medical-surgical nursing: Critical thinking in patient care* (5th ed.). Upper Saddle River, NJ: Pearson Education, pp. 334–335.

10 Answer: 1 Rationale: Because laryngeal spasms and bronchial constriction can occur with anaphylaxis, assessing the client's airway is top priority. The nurse should maintain and establish a patent airway first. Remember the ABCs (airway, breathing, and circulation). Cardiac output would come next, followed by risk for injury, and finally anxiety. **Cognitive Level:** Analyzing **Client Need:** Physiological Adaptation **Integrated Process:** Nursing Process: Planning **Content Area:** Adult Health **Strategy:** Use the ABCs (airway, breathing, and circulation) and Maslow's hierarchy to prioritize. Recall that airway takes priority in life-threatening situations that do not involve cardiopulmonary resuscitation (which now uses CAB). **Reference:** LeMone, P., Burke, K., & Bauldoff, G. (2011). *Medical-surgical nursing: Critical thinking in patient care* (5th ed.). Upper Saddle River, NJ: Pearson Education, pp. 308–309.

Posttest

1 Answer: 3 Rationale: Positive results of medication are indicated by a reduced viral load and a CD4 count above 350 mm³. A client with AIDS will have exacerbations and remissions with opportunistic infections; therefore, symptoms may vary. With a diagnosis of AIDS, an enzyme-linked immunosorbent assay (ELISA) test would remain positive for antibodies. WBC of 1,700 shows neutropenia, which does not indicate improvement. **Cognitive Level:** Analyzing **Client Need:** Physiological Adaptation **Integrated Process:** Nursing Process: Evaluation **Content Area:** Adult Health **Strategy:** Compare the desired response to the options. Determine what factors will not change even with the treatment. **Reference:** LeMone, P., Burke, K., & Bauldoff, G. (2011). *Medical-surgical nursing: Critical thinking in patient care* (5th ed.). Upper Saddle River, NJ: Pearson Education, p. 330.

2 Answer: 1 Rationale: Eosinophils are usually elevated in an allergic response. WBC, monocytes, and neutrophils are not involved in an allergic response. **Cognitive Level:** Analyzing **Client Need:** Reduction of Risk Potential **Integrated Process:** Nursing Process: Assessment **Content Area:** Child Health **Strategy:** Specific knowledge of laboratory values is needed to answer the question. Review common lab values such as complete blood count (CBC) and differential if this question was difficult. **Reference:** LeMone, P., Burke, K., & Bauldoff, G. (2011). *Medical-surgical nursing: Critical thinking in patient care* (5th ed.). Upper Saddle River, NJ: Pearson Education, p. 270.

3 **Answer: 2** **Rationale:** The mother is already alarmed enough, and the nurse should be careful with wording of the response. Describe the function of the lymph nodes to reassure the mother, such as "The lymph nodes filter foreign products and may only be swollen because of an infection." The other statements are either inaccurate or alarming, or both. **Cognitive Level:** Applying **Client Need:** Physiological Adaptation **Integrated Process:** Communication and Documentation **Content Area:** Adult Health **Strategy:** The focus in this question is meeting the needs of the mother who is alarmed. Choose the response that best meets her needs for reassurance and yet gives correct information. **Reference:** LeMone, P., Burke, K., & Bauldoff, G. (2011). *Medical-surgical nursing: Critical thinking in patient care* (5th ed.). Upper Saddle River, NJ: Pearson Education, pp. 273–274.

4 **Answer: 2, 3, 4** **Rationale:** A nonspecific inflammatory response is evoked by any injury and is of short duration, occurring before the immune response is established. It is usually local and produces inflammation. In some cases, local injuries result in systemic manifestations that usually begin in hours or days generated by the release of cytokines causing fever, lethargy, and metabolic changes. Anaphylaxis, systemic allergies, and bronchoconstriction are indicative of system reactions; swelling to the arm and a sprained ankle are examples of localized inflammation. **Cognitive Level:** Analyzing **Client Need:** Physiological Adaptation **Integrated Process:** Nursing Process: Implementation **Content Area:** Adult Health **Strategy:** The critical word in the question is *systemic*. Separate local from systemic reactions and choose the options that are systematic. **Reference:** LeMone, P., Burke, K., & Bauldoff, G. (2011). *Medical-surgical nursing: Critical thinking in patient care* (5th ed.). Upper Saddle River, NJ: Pearson Education, pp. 308–311.

5 **Answer: 4** **Rationale:** This type of contact dermatitis is commonly a delayed reaction and indicates Type IV hypersensitivity. This reaction is cell-mediated rather than antibody-mediated and is delayed 24 to 48 hours. Type I hypersensitivity reaction are immediate, within minutes of exposure. A Type II reaction is cytotoxic and reacts to cell-bound antigens. Type III reactions result from the formation of antibody–antigen immune complexes in the circulation. **Cognitive Level:** Applying **Client Need:** Physiological Adaptation **Integrated Process:** Nursing Process: Diagnosis **Content Area:** Adult Health **Strategy:** The clue in the question is the timing of the reaction. Only one hypersensitivity type happens in a delayed time frame. **Reference:** LeMone, P., Burke, K., & Bauldoff, G. (2011). *Medical-surgical nursing: Critical thinking in patient care* (5th ed.). Upper Saddle River, NJ: Pearson Education, pp. 308–311.

6 **Answer: 2** **Rationale:** Remember the Rh (+ or −) must also match in addition to the type of blood (O in this case) matching. If antigens are present in the donor blood, which can interact with antibodies in the recipient's blood (a Type II hypersensitivity), hemolytic reaction follows. Type O negative blood can be given to any recipient (the "universal donor"). For all other types the blood given must match the client's blood type. **Cognitive Level:** Applying **Client Need:** Pharmacological and Parenteral Therapies **Integrated Process:** Nursing Process: Implementation **Content Area:** Adult Health **Strategy:** Recall principles of safely administering a blood transfusion including the type and crossmatch needed before transfusing. **Reference:** LeMone, P., Burke, K., & Bauldoff, G. (2011). *Medical-surgical nursing: Critical thinking in patient care* (5th ed.). Upper Saddle River, NJ: Pearson Education, pp. 309–310.

7 **Answer: 3** **Rationale:** Exposure to latex can be via skin, mucous membrane, inhalation, or internal tissue. The allergy can be a Type I or Type IV hypersensitivity reaction. Diagnosis is based on evidence of skin reaction after exposure. Most elastic bands contain latex, and would indicate dermal exposure to latex. The moistness or dryness of skin does not affect allergies to latex. Drug allergies do not affect latex allergy. If the client was previously exposed to latex during surgeries, this might be relevant, but is not a primary factor in determining latex allergy. **Cognitive Level:** Applying **Client Need:** Physiological Adaptation **Integrated Process:** Nursing Process: Assessment **Content Area:** Adult Health **Strategy:** Consider which option gives the best information in assessing for *latex* allergy. Do not be misled by options that sound good but assess for other problems. **Reference:** LeMone, P., Burke, K., & Bauldoff, G. (2011). *Medical-surgical nursing: Critical thinking in patient care* (5th ed.). Upper Saddle River, NJ: Pearson Education, p. 311.

8 **Answer: 4** **Rationale:** A barking cough, wheezing, and stridor are clinical manifestations of the bronchoconstriction and airway edema that accompanies anaphylaxis. Lung crackles are not part of the clinical picture. The blood pressure is usually low (hypotension) because of vasodilation, rather than high. The pulse would be rapid (tachycardia) rather than slow. **Cognitive Level:** Applying **Client Need:** Physiological Adaptation **Integrated Process:** Nursing Process: Assessment **Content Area:** Adult Health **Strategy:** Remember that anaphylaxis results in a type of shock, so choose the option that fits assessment findings of a client in shock. **Reference:** LeMone, P., Burke, K., & Bauldoff, G. (2011). *Medical-surgical nursing: Critical thinking in patient care* (5th ed.). Upper Saddle River, NJ: Pearson Education, pp. 308–309.

9 **Answer: 1** **Rationale:** Cervical dysplasia is present in 40% of women with HIV. Cervical cancer often develops and is aggressive. Younger women die from the cervical cancer rather than from AIDS. Papanicolaou (PAP) smears every 6 months are recommended with aggressive treatment of any cervical dysplasia. CD4 cell counts and viral loads monitor the progression of AIDS but do not check for cancer. The CA 125 antigen is useful for detecting ovarian cancer.

Cognitive Level: Analyzing **Client Need:** Health Promotion and Maintenance **Integrated Process:** Nursing Process: Planning **Content Area:** Adult Health **Strategy:** The question asks specifically for a diagnostic test for cancer, narrowing the options to 2. Recall which cancer is seen in women with AIDS. **Reference:** LeMone, P., Burke, K., & Bauldoff, G. (2011). *Medical-surgical nursing: Critical thinking in patient care* (5th ed.). Upper Saddle River, NJ: Pearson Education, p. 329.

10 **Answer: 2** **Rationale:** A sexually active teenager, especially if the act is unprotected, is at highest risk. The police officer and nurse on the telemetry unit should be using standard precautions, which include gloves any time body secretions are encountered. Although either of these may encounter blood accidentally, the percentage is low. A school nurse should not be coming into contact with body secretions that would increase the risk factor. **Cognitive Level:** Analyzing **Client Need:** Health Promotion and Maintenance **Integrated Process:** Nursing Process: Assessment **Content Area:** Adult Health **Strategy:** Consider the bloodborne transmission of the virus to analyze which person in the options is most likely to be exposed and unprotected. **Reference:** LeMone, P., Burke, K., & Bauldoff, G. (2011). *Medical-surgical nursing: Critical thinking in patient care* (5th ed.). Upper Saddle River, NJ: Pearson Education, pp. 334–335.

References

Centers for Disease Control and Prevention. Retrieved January 8, 2012, from http://www.cdc.gov/nchhstp/.

Kee, J. L. (2009). *Laboratory and diagnostic tests with nursing implications* (8th ed.). Upper Saddle River, NJ: Pearson Education.

NSW Health. Latex allergy policy. Retrieved January 8, 2012, http://www.health.nsw.gov.au/policies/pd/2005/pdf/PD2005_490.pdf.

LeMone, P., Burke, K. and Bauldoff, G. (2011). *Medical-surgical nursing: Critical thinking in patient care* (5th ed.). Upper Saddle River, NJ: Pearson Education.

Lilley, L., Collins, S., Harrington, S., & Snyder, J. (2011). *Pharmacology and the nursing process* (6th ed.). St. Louis, MO: Mosby, Inc.

McCance, K., & Huether, K. (2010). *Understanding pathophysiology: The biologic basis for disease in adults and children* (6th ed.) St. Louis, MO: Elsevier.

Porth, C., & Matfin, G. (2010). *Pathophysiology: Concepts of altered health states* (8th ed.). Philadelphia, PA: Lippincott Williams & Wilkins.

Wagner, K., Johnson, K., & Kidd, P. (2010). *High acuity nursing* (5th ed.). Upper Saddle River, NJ: Pearson Education.

Wilson, B., Shannon, M., & Shields, K. (2012). *Pearson nurse's drug guide 2012.* Upper Saddle River, NJ: Pearson Education.

Infectious Health Problems

13

Chapter Outline

Overview of Infectious Health
  Problems
Viral Infections
Bacterial Infections
Fungal Infections

Chlamydial Infections
Spirochete Infections
Rickettsial Infections
Protozoal Infections
Helminth Infections

Mycoplasma Infections
Mycobacterial Infections
Prion Infections

Objectives

➤ Define key terms associated with infectious health problems.
➤ Identify risk factors associated with the development of infectious
  health problems.
➤ Explain common etiologies of infectious health problems.
➤ Describe the pathophysiologic processes associated with specific
  infectious health problems.
➤ Distinguish between normal and abnormal infectious findings
  obtained from nursing assessment.
➤ Prioritize nursing interventions associated with specific infectious
  health problems.

NCLEX-RN® Test Prep

Use the accompanying online resource,
NursingReviewsandRationales, to test
yourself with hundreds of NCLEX®-style
practice questions.

Review at a Glance

chain of infection series of events
or conditions that lead to development of
a particular communicable disease
colonization establishment of an
infectious agent in a host
epidemiology study of distribution
of health and illness within a population
host organism capable of supporting growth and reproduction of
another organism

iatrogenic infection
disease acquired in a hospital or
health care setting; formerly called
nosocomial infection
opportunistic infection disease
that occurs only when host defenses
are impaired
pathogen microorganism capable
of causing disease
pathogenicity ability of a microorganism to cause pathologic changes
and process of developing disease

reservoir habitat in which a living
organism lives and multiplies
resident (normal) flora
relationship where parasites depend on
host's environment to grow and
reproduce but prevent colonization of
other microbes and may contribute to
synthesis of beneficial substances
virulence ease with which a
pathogenic organism can overcome
host defenses

PRETEST

1 A client has an opportunistic respiratory infection. The nurse considers that which of the following most likely represents the etiology of the client's infection?

1. Client consumed contaminated food or water.
2. Client encountered an extremely virulent microorganism.
3. Client's immune system is compromised.
4. Client has likely become infected in a health care facility.

2 A client presents to the emergency department with a fever of 102°F, malaise, and a productive cough. Which of the following should the nurse do first?

1. Administer prescribed antibiotic.
2. Obtain ordered sputum culture.
3. Administer dose of PRN acetaminophen to lower fever.
4. Teach client importance of hand hygiene.

3 The nurse is explaining why an antibiotic must be taken as directed to prevent the development of resistant bacterial strains. The nurse should use which items of information in explaining to the client the mechanisms of bacterial resistance? Select all that apply.

1. Production of enzymes, such as beta-lactamase, to inactivate antibiotics.
2. Stimulation of host's immune system, producing leukocytosis.
3. Genetic mutations altering bacterial binding sites.
4. Alternate metabolic pathways bypassing antibiotic activity.
5. Changes in bacterial cell wall preventing antibiotic from reaching intracellular target site.

4 The nurse is explaining infectious disease terminology to unlicensed assistive personnel (UAP) who are orienting to an infectious disease unit. One UAP asks what makes bacteria able to cause disease in a person. The nurse includes an explanation of what concept in a response?

1. Communicability
2. Pathogenicity
3. Toxigenicity
4. Latency

5 The nurse considers that a client with a fever and enlarged regional lymph nodes most likely has infection caused by which type of microorganism?

1. Bacterial
2. Fungal
3. Protozoal
4. Rickettsial

6 The public health nurse explains to a community group that which type of virus is most likely to be acquired through casual contact with an infected individual?

1. Influenza virus
2. Herpes virus
3. Cytomegalovirus (CMV)
4. Human immunodeficiency virus (HIV)

7 A young adult female who reports having unprotected sex with various partners enters the clinic for treatment of a sexually transmitted infection. The nurse anticipates preparing her and setting up equipment for culture and sensitivity testing for which of the following? Select all that apply.

1. Herpes virus
2. Chlamydia
3. Gonorrhea
4. Syphilis
5. Human papilloma virus (genital warts)

8 A woman is admitted to the hospital with hemorrhagic colitis. The etiology was found to be an exotoxin, produced by *Escherichia coli*. When the client asks the nurse what caused the problem, what information should the nurse include in a reply?

1. Eating food from a can that was damaged or bulging.
2. Kissing someone who was infected with the organism.
3. Eating undercooked hamburger meat or drinking unpasteurized fruit juices.
4. The toxic shock-like symptoms came from a tampon used incorrectly.

9 After taking a client history, the nurse explains to a client exhibiting symptoms of a rickettsia infection that it was probably acquired through which mechanism?

1. Respiratory droplets
2. Mosquito bites
3. Bites or feces of ticks, lice, or fleas
4. Direct skin contact with infected animals

10 The nurse is analyzing the development of an infectious disease in the community. The nurse incorporates each element of the chain of infection in the study because each gives information regarding which of the following?

1. The linkages between various forms of microorganisms.
2. The sequence required for transmission of disease.
3. The clustering of bacteria in a specific pattern.
4. Increasing virulence patterns among species of micro-organisms.

➤ *See pages 345–346 for Answers and Rationales.*

I. OVERVIEW OF INFECTIOUS HEALTH PROBLEMS

A. Introduction
1. **Epidemiology**: study of distribution and patterns of disease in populations
2. Infectious diseases are caused by invasion of **pathogens** (microorganisms capable of causing disease), including bacteria, viruses, fungi, protozoa, rickettsiae, and helminths
3. Types of pathogens
   a. Communicable (such as influenza, hepatitis, tuberculosis)
   b. Noncommunicable (such as cellulitis and endocarditis)
4. Injury of body cells can occur directly by microorganisms, by toxins released from microorganisms, or indirectly from body's inflammatory response

B. Risk factors
1. Age (very young or very old)
2. Health habits: poor nutrition, smoking, alcohol consumption
3. Impaired lines of defense: immune deficiency (congenital or acquired), impaired integrity of skin or mucous membranes
4. Health problems: circulatory disturbances, diabetes mellitus
5. Drug therapy: corticosteroids, chemotherapy, alteration of normal flora by antibiotic therapy

C. Transmission of infection
1. Occurs through **chain of infection** (series of events or conditions that lead to development of a particular communicable disease) (see Figure 13-1)
2. Causative agents include pathogens previously listed
3. **Reservoir** (or source): environment where an infectious agent can survive
   a. Human: individuals or groups of people
   b. Environment/fomites: contaminated food, water, air, or soil
   c. Animals: such as ticks, fleas, mosquitoes, or bats
4. Portal of exit is route by which an agent leaves a reservoir
   a. Gastrointestinal (GI), such as ingestion, vomiting, or diarrhea
   b. Respiratory, such as coughing or sneezing

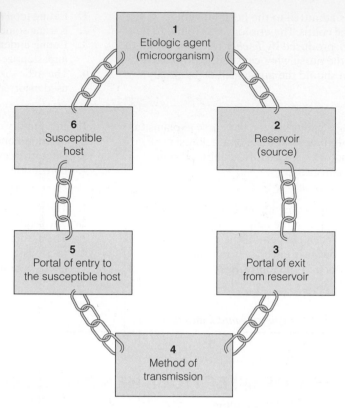

Figure 13-1

Steps in chain of infection

1 Etiologic agent (microorganism)

6 Susceptible host

2 Reservoir (source)

5 Portal of entry to the susceptible host

3 Portal of exit from reservoir

4 Method of transmission

    c. Genitourinary (GU), such as sexual contact
    d. Blood, such as insect bites, needles

   5. Mode of transmission is route of transmission of agent
    a. Contact transmission may be direct (person-to-person through body fluids or contaminated food or water) or indirect (through inanimate objects)

     b. Airborne or droplet transmission involves transfer through droplets (from coughing, sneezing, or talking) or droplet nuclei carried on air currents

    c. Vector transmission involves intermediaries such as flies, mosquitos, or other insects or rodents
  6. Portal of entry is location by which an agent enters body
  7. Susceptible **host** (organism capable of supporting growth and reproduction of another organism): person who lacks resistance to this infectious agent

D. Relationship of host to parasite (host-parasite interaction)
  1. Resident (normal) flora exemplify a symbiotic (balanced) relationship where parasites depend on host's environment to grow and reproduce but prevent **colonization** (establishment of an infectious agent in a host) by other microbes
  2. Opportunistic infection occurs when immunity is compromised and normal flora become unopposed and/or pathogenic

   3. Iatrogenic infections (formerly nosocomial infections) are hospital-acquired; typically caused by virulent or drug-resistant organisms and are often spread through poor hand hygiene

E. Factors affecting infection by pathogen
  1. Mechanism of action: pathogen can damage normal cells or interfere with cellular metabolism by producing toxins
  2. Infectivity: ability of pathogen to invade and multiply in host

Practice to Pass

Identify conditions that could lead to opportunistic infections.

   3. **Pathogenicity**: origin and process of developing disease
   4. **Virulence**: ease with which a pathogen can overcome host defenses; important components include invasiveness, adherence, and toxigenicity
   5. Toxigenicity refers to pathogen's ability to produce endotoxins or exotoxins
   6. Defense mechanisms of body
      a. Physical factors such as skin and mucous membranes
      b. Chemical factors such as pH of skin, urine, stomach, and so on
      c. Normal flora, which helps to prevent colonization by transient organisms by competing for nutrients and contributing to a low pH
      d. Immunity/inflammatory response
      e. Client factors such as nutrition, genetic makeup, and presence of other illnesses

F. **Stages of infectious process**
   1. Incubation stage: pathogen is present and reproduces, but host remains asymptomatic; could last from hours to years
   2. Prodromal stage: initial (mild) symptoms appear, which may be nonspecific
   3. Acute: pronounced symptoms are present; results from toxic by-products of microorganism's metabolic processes and tissue damage caused by inflammatory response
   4. Convalescent: diminished symptoms with infection contained
   5. Resolution: elimination of pathogen

G. **Clinical manifestations**
   1. General symptoms of systemic infection include malaise, weakness, headache, anorexia, and weight loss
   2. Infection may also produce acute inflammatory reactions; extent of tissue damage is determined by number and virulence of organisms, site of invasion, and host defenses
   3. General manifestations of specific types of infection
      a. Bacterial, viral, and mycoplasma infections: fever (may be low grade, especially with viral infection), body aches, regional lymph node enlargement, and site-specific signs (e.g., cough, earache, sore throat, and so on)
      b. Fungal infections: itching and redness of skin, nail thickening, thrush in mouth, and vaginal discharge (thick, white)
      c. Protozoa and helminthes: itching and rash (skin infections), diarrhea, fever (with malaria)
      d. Rickettsiae: skin rash, muscles aches, fever and chills, and headache

II. VIRAL INFECTIONS

A. **Overview**
   1. Viruses are tiny intracellular organisms (20–100 times smaller than bacteria) that totally depend upon host for survival and materials needed to replicate
   2. Intracellular development allows viruses to bypass many body defense mechanisms

B. **Pathophysiology**
   1. Viral particles are called virions and consist of a single strand of DNA or RNA contained within a protein shell called a capsid
   2. Viruses are classified as either DNA or RNA viruses according to genetic material, mechanism of replication, mode of transmission, or type of disease produced
   3. Viruses produce specific diseases in specific tissues
      a. Protein covering of virus is type-specific and attaches as a "lock and key" to host cell membrane
      b. Virus must be able to use host cell in production of nucleic acid in order to survive since they have no independent metabolism

      c. Mature virions are created within host cell and released through cell lysis, direct passage to adjacent cells, or through reverse endocytosis

  4. Viruses may damage or kill cells they infect, causing disease

  5. Viral replication cycle can be relatively brief (minutes or hours) or as long as several days; includes 6 phases of adsorption, penetration, uncoating, replication, assembly, and release

      a. Some viruses enter host cell and insert their genome into host chromosome, remaining in a latent, nonreplicating state for long periods of time; examples include the herpes viruses (varicella zoster, chickenpox, genital herpes) and cytomegalovirus

      b. Influenza virus is transmitted by respiratory droplets

  6. Viruses bind to cell membrane receptors, leading to endocytosis of virus; virus then uses cell's resources to synthesize new viral nucleic acids that are released from host cell to infect other cells

  7. Retroviruses replicate in a unique process

      a. Viral RNA is translated into DNA by an enzyme, reverse transcriptase, and is then integrated into host chromosome

      b. It then exists in a latent state until reactivated

      c. Replication requires reversal of the process

      d. HIV is an example of a retrovirus

  8. Bacteriophages are viruses that use bacteria as their hosts; these viruses attach to bacteria and inject their DNA into cell for replication

  9. Viral infections can be local or systemic and can be either acute or chronic; some viruses are thought to be agents of cancer (such as human papilloma virus [HPV] and cervical cancer), although role of viruses in human cancers is still not well understood

 10. Viral infection stimulates antibody production primarily through cell-mediated immunity and production of interferon

      a. Antibodies coat particles to make them better targets of macrophages

      b. This coating prevents viruses from entering target cells

      c. Macrophages also secrete cytokines that initiate inflammatory response

 11. Antiviral therapy is difficult to develop because of large number of variant viruses that cause same disease and inability of drugs to destroy viruses without destroying normal cells

 12. Common viral infections and antiviral agents are listed in Table 13-1

C. Nursing assessment

  1. Assessment includes identifying factors that increase risk for infection, vital signs, reports of pain, palpation of lymph nodes, signs and symptoms specific to type of virus

  2. Diagnostic tests

      a. Complete blood count (CBC)

         1) Lymphocytes increase in many viral infections; normal lymphocyte count is 25–35% of total white blood cell (WBC) count

         2) T-lymphocytes will decrease with HIV/AIDS virus, autoimmune disorders, and corticosteroids

         3) Neutrophil counts will decrease in most viral infections

      b. Enzyme-linked immunosorbent assay (ELISA) and Western Blot are positive in diagnosis of HIV

      c. Epstein-Barr nuclear antigen (EBNA) is used to confirm infectious mononucleosis

Table 13-1	Common Viral Infections		
Virus	**Transmission**	**Pathological Considerations**	**Therapeutic Management**
Hepatitis Viral Infections			
Hepatitis A (HAV)	Fecal–oral route and through contaminated food and water. Occurs in overcrowded and unsanitary conditions.	Acute onset with incubation of 2–6 weeks. Inflammation can result in destruction of hepatocytes. Signs and symptoms include anorexia, malaise, and jaundice. Liver enzymes likely elevated. ALT liver enzyme usually rises sharply at onset of fever. Serologic markers include anti-HAV (may persist for years) and IgM (short-lived and may disappear in about 2 weeks). Complete recovery is likely.	Disease can be avoided in most cases if immune globulins are administered within 7 days of exposure. Preventive vaccines Havrix and Vaqta are available for those traveling to areas endemic to disease.
Hepatitis B (HBV)	Transmitted through body fluids from sexual contact or parenterally. May also be transmitted to fetus during pregnancy.	Gradual onset with incubation 6–24 weeks. Infection may be acute and self-limiting or may lead to persistent viremia with chronic liver disease or chronic carrier state. There is a gradual and prolonged elevation of ALT liver enzyme. HbsAg is present in early infection. Anti-HBs is present in past infections and anti-Hbe is present in chronic carriers.	Hepatitis B hyperimmune globulin (HBIG) is recommended after exposure to hepatitis B virus. Recombivax HB and Engerix-B are used prophylactically for prevention in health workers and other high-risk populations. Liver enzymes should be monitored. Teach clients safe sex practices and to avoid sharing needles.
Hepatitis C (HCV)	Transmitted through sexual or parenteral routes.	Gradual onset with incubation of 5–12 weeks. May produce both acute and chronic hepatitis (most often chronic). Is associated with cirrhosis and liver cancer. Causes elevation of ALT. Can be detected with anti-HVC marker but is difficult to determine if infection is current or prior.	Vaccines do not currently exist for HCV. Treatment is symptomatic.
Hepatitis D (HDV)	Transmitted through blood and sexual contact.	Acute onset with incubation 3–13 weeks. Clinical manifestations similar to hepatitis B and those with HBV and carriers of HBV are susceptible to infection by HDV.	Vaccines do not currently exist for HDV. Treatment is symptomatic.
Hepatitis E (HEV)	Transmitted through fecal–oral route through contaminated food and water.	Rapid onset with incubation 3–6 weeks. Results in chronic hepatitis and cirrhosis. A serologic test for anti-HEV has been developed to detect virus in stool.	
Other Viral Infections			
Herpes simplex (HSV)	Transmitted through direct contact with skin and mucous membranes.	Replicates at site of entry, may pass through regional lymph nodes, enter blood, and proliferate in skin and mucous membranes. Most cases are subclinical. May remain latent at site of exposure and be activated by exposure to sunlight, fever, or stress. Is characterized by vesicular ulcerations on mouth or conjunctiva (HSV 1) or genital area (HSV 2); recurrence is common.	Acyclovir (Zovirax) is drug of choice. This drug reduces viral shedding, decreases local symptoms, and decreases severity and duration of acute episodes. It may be used topically, orally, or parenterally.

(continued)

Table 13-1	Common Viral Infections (continued)		
Virus	**Transmission**	**Pathological Considerations**	**Therapeutic Management**
Varicella zoster (shingles)	Transmitted primarily through respiratory tract, initially in form of chicken pox. Reactivated in form of shingles.	Primarily seen in older adults and immunocompromised clients; results from reactivation of latent virus that was dormant in sensory cells of dorsal root ganglion. Exact mechanism is unknown. Painful lesions appear to follow a specific dermatome, with lesions appearing on trunk, chest, forehead, face, and neck.	Acyclovir (Zovirax) and vidarabine (Vira-A) have been used for treatment. Vaccine zoster immunoglobulin (ZIG) may be useful for prevention in immunocompromised clients. High doses of interferon alfa (Roferon-A) have proven useful in reducing viral replication.
Cytomegalovirus (CMV)	Transmitted through saliva, urine, semen, breast milk, and vaginal secretions.	Latent infection usually seen in immunocompromised clients. Highly necrotizing to cells. Fluorescent antibody techniques are used for diagnosis.	Antiviral agents include gancyclovir (Cytovene) and foscarnet (Foscavir). CMV immunoglobulin used in combination with an antiviral has also proven useful.
Epstein-Barr	Transmitted through respiratory droplets or saliva.	Replicates in parotid gland and disseminates through blood. Incubation 4–7 weeks. Associated with mononucleosis. Signs and symptoms: lymphadenopathy, fever, chills, sore throat, and often a thick tonsillar exudate. Recovery may take up to 4 weeks. WBCs are markedly elevated. Antibodies to Epstein-Barr nuclear antigen appear during convalescence.	Disease is self-limiting and treatment is supportive.
Human immunodeficiency virus (HIV)	Transmitted through blood and body fluids.	Incubation may be 3–10 years in adults. CD4 protein of helper T lymphocytes is a receptor for virus, which attaches by means of its gp120 surface protein. Virus envelope fuses with cell membrane and virus enters cell. Virus makes a DNA copy of its own RNA using reverse transcriptase enzyme and DNA copy is inserted into genetic material of infected cell. Clients who are infected become immunocompromised and subject to opportunistic infections. A positive ELISA test for presence of antibodies is confirmed by Western Blot.	Antiviral agents used to treat HIV include nucleoside reverse transcriptase inhibitors (NRTIs), nonnucleoside reverse transcriptase inhibitors (NNRTIs), protease inhibitors (PIs) and a fusion inhibitor. PIs have been associated with reduction of viral loads to undetectable levels. Compliance with drug regimens is essential, and side effects often make compliance difficult.
Influenza	Transmitted through droplets of upper respiratory secretions.	Incubation period: 1–7 days. Viral replication occurs in epithelial cells of upper respiratory tract (does not typically enter blood). Endogenous pyrogens and interferon cause systemic symptoms (headache, body aches, chills, fever) and rhinitis. Complications: pneumonia or secondary bacterial infection; possibly Guillain-Barré and Reye syndromes.	Amantadine (Symmetrel) is the antiviral agent that prevents penetration of Influenza A into cells and limits replication if administered within 48 hours of onset. Vaccines are formulated each year that can be preventive for up to 6 months (recommended for older adult and high-risk clients).

D. **Nursing management**
1. Medications
   a. Antiviral agents (viruses are not sensitive to antibacterials since viruses have no cell wall or cytoplasm and virus is typically immersed in host cell); refer again to Table 13-1
   b. Acyclovir (Zovirax), a popular medication for treating herpes; amantidine (Symmetrel) for influenza; interferon alfacon–1 (Infergen) for hepatitis
   c. Anti-pyretic agents to reduce fever and analgesics for pain and discomfort

2. Instruct client/family concerning infection control measures (good hand hygiene, and so on)
3. Provide quiet environment, limiting visitors as needed
4. Provide comfort measures to ensure adequate rest; evaluate response to activity, noting weakness, fatigue, or dyspnea
5. Assist with self-care activities as needed
6. Monitor vital signs
7. Institute isolation precautions according to route of transmission
8. Document response to medication
9. Preventive vaccines should be encouraged when available

10. Instruct clients with genital herpes to avoid genital sexual contact during acute phase, especially during the breakout

Practice to Pass

What are the implications of the presence of latent or recurrent viruses?

III. BACTERIAL INFECTIONS

A. **Overview**
1. Bacteria are single-celled organisms that use human body as a source for nutrients and environment for growth; they contain a single chromosome and are capable of autonomous reproduction
2. Bacteria are classified according to shape, staining characteristics, and requirements related to oxygen

B. **Pathophysiology**
1. Bacterial growth depends on body's immune system function and ability of bacteria to resist body defenses
2. Bacteria may produce substances that enhance resistance to host defenses
   a. Production of adherins allows bacteria to strongly attach to structures and penetrate underlying tissues
   b. Development of carbohydrate or protein capsule or slime layers help to prevent phagocytosis
   c. Production of leukocidins helps destroy phagocytes
   d. Production of enzymes that break down fibrin clots or connective tissue (i.e., streptokinase, hyalurinidase, collagenase, elastase, and so on) allow bacteria to more easily spread into tissues; production of coagulase causes clotting of plasma and allows bacteria to form a fibrin layer of protection
3. Bacteria may produce toxins that cause damage to cells and tissues
   a. Exotoxins are proteins secreted from organisms into tissues; they have variable specificity and may cause fatal effects
      1) Exotoxins are produced by Gram-positive and Gram-negative organisms and most are denatured by extreme heat
      2) Common examples of effects of exotoxins are botulism and tetanus
   b. Endotoxins are lipopolysaccharides released from bacterial cell membranes with cell division or destruction
      1) They are produced only by Gram-negative bacteria and can withstand high heat

Practice to Pass

What are some examples of descriptions of bacteria in terms of shape? Staining characteristics? Requirements for oxygen?

      2) Endotoxins usually cause fever and induce production of cytokines that activate complement cascade and may cause septic shock

      3) They are generally less toxic than exotoxins

   4. Complement proteins may be activated by contact with bacterial cell wall or with release of endotoxins

      a. Activation results in opsonization of microorganisms (to enhance phagocytosis), activation of leukocytes, and destruction of bacterial cells

      b. Encapsulated bacteria are protected from phagocytosis unless coated with anticapsular antibody

      c. Antibiotics are often needed to assist immune system to destroy bacteria

   5. Common bacteria causing infectious diseases are identified in Table 13-2

C. Nursing assessment

   1. Assessment includes identifying organ system(s) affected by infection; signs and symptoms of infection (fever, malaise, and local or organ-specific indicators); VS; reports of pain; palpation of lymph nodes

   2. Diagnostic tests

      a. CBC

         1) WBC will be elevated (greater than 10,000/mm^3)

Table 13-2 **Common Bacteria That Cause Infectious Disease**

Bacteria/Disease Process	Type/ Morphology	Transmission	Pathological Effects	Nursing Management
Clostridium tetani (tetanus)	Gram-positive bacillus; spore-forming	Spores distributed in soil and human and animal GI tracts. Infects wounds from injury.	Clinical manifestations caused by spore generation of exotoxin with affinity for CNS. Manifestations include neck stiffness, dysphagia, muscle rigidity.	Treated with tetanus antitoxin or immune globulins. Prevention with tetanus toxoid. May require mechanical ventilation.
Clostridium botulinum (botulism)	Gram-positive bacillus; spore-forming	Inhabits soil; frequent contaminant of fruits, vegetables, and fish. Spores are highly heat resistant.	Life-threatening paralytic ileus is caused by neurotoxins. Prevents release of Ach from nerve terminals of myoneural junction. Damage to cranial nerves causes vision, hearing, and speech difficulties.	Treated with antitoxin from horse serum that only affects circulating toxin; has no effect on toxin bound to nerve cells. Recovery is very gradual over weeks to months.
Clostridium difficile (pseudomembranous colitis)	Gram-positive bacillus; spore-forming	Hospital acquired; acquired by antibiotic use.	Broad spectrum antibiotics are most common cause, altering normal flora and allowing *C. difficile* to colonize. Leads to abdominal cramping, severe foul-smelling diarrhea, and dehydration and/or electrolyte loss.	Treated with vancomycin and metronidazole (Flagyl).
Corynebacterium diphtheriae (diphtheria)	Gram-positive; non–spore-forming	Airborne droplets colonizing in upper respiratory system.	Produces toxin resulting in epithelial cell necrosis. Inflammatory response causes production of pseudomembrane that may lead to suffocation.	Administer antitoxin prior to cell penetration by toxin. Should test for hypersensitivity to horse serum proteins prior to administration. Prevention is through vaccine. Penicillin may be used but is rarely effective when used alone.

(continued)

Table 13-2   Common Bacteria That Cause Infectious Disease (continued)

Bacteria/Disease Process	Type/ Morphology	Transmission	Pathological Effects	Nursing Management
Coliform bacteria (Escherichia coli)	Gram- negative, non–spore- forming rod	Normal resident bacteria of intestines. May spread to urinary tract or wounds directly via blood or fecal contamination.	Frequent source of nosocomial infection. Manifestations include fever and chills. May develop shock from endotoxins. Also frequently cause urinary tract infections.	Prevent through good hand hygiene practices. Treat with cephalosporins, fluoroquinolones, or aminoglycosides. Monitor for nephrotoxicity and ototoxicity with aminoglycosides.
Klebsiella pneumoniae	Gram- negative rod, heavily encapsulated	Found in soil, water, food, and intestinal tract.	Also associated with hospital acquired infections. Responsible for severe respiratory tract infections in debilitated clients. Manifestations include productive cough and weakness.	Treated with aminoglycosides that bind to ribosomes and prevent protein synthesis in bacteria and with later generation cephalosporins, which interfere with cell wall synthesis.
Pseudomonas	Gram- negative rod	Common resident of skin and mucous membranes. Spreads by direct contact.	Major threat to hospitalized and debilitated clients.	Treated with aminoglycosides and later- generation cephalosporins.
Helicobacter pylori	Gram- negative spiral or straight rod	Penetrates gastric mucosa and colonizes gastric epithelium.	Produces enzyme urease that raises pH, allowing bacteria to survive in normally acidic environment. Urea in stomach is converted to ammonia, which is cytotoxic to gastric cells. Causes depletion of gastric mucus, allowing erosion of mucosa.	Treated with macrolides and metronidazole (Flagyl). Macrolides inhibit protein synthesis while metronidazole disrupts DNA synthesis. Avoid alcohol with metronidazole. Macrolides have frequent interactions with drugs.
Haemophilus influenza	Gram- negative bacillus	Occurs only in humans; more common in children than adults. Transmitted person to person via respiratory route.	Virulence enhanced by polysaccharide capsule; resists action of complement. Does not produce exotoxin; endotoxin does not seem to play significant role. Results in otitis media, sinusitis, and respiratory tract infections.	Prevention is through vaccine. Cephalosporins are drugs of choice for treatment.
Neisseria gonorrhoeae (gonorrhea)	Gram- negative diplococcus	Transmitted through sexual contact. Primary site of infection in women is cervix. Primary site in men is urethra.	Bacteria contain pili, which aid attachment to mucosa in humans and inhibit phagocytosis. Most strains produce extracellular proteases that inactivate immunoglobulins. They also produce a cytotoxic factor that damages ciliated epithelial cells. May be asymptomatic in women but result in salpingitis, pelvic inflammatory disease, and infertility; men generally have purulent discharge and dysuria and possible urethral stricture.	Drug of choice is a cephalosporin such as ceftriaxone (Rocephin). TMP/ SMX (Bactrim); ciprofloxacin (Cipro) may also be used. Ciprofloxacin inhibits DNA replication while TMP/SMX prevents synthesis of proteins and nucleic acid. Client should be instructed to avoid unprotected sexual contact.

(continued)

Table 13-2	Common Bacteria That Cause Infectious Disease (continued)			
Bacteria/Disease Process	**Type/ Morphology**	**Transmission**	**Pathological Effects**	**Nursing Management**
Staphylococcus	Gram-positive cocci that grow in clusters in short chains	Transmitted through hair follicles into bloodstream or through urinary or respiratory tracts.	Common resident of skin. Hardy non–spore-forming bacteria that are heat stable. Some forms produce coagulase, causing clots in citrated plasma. Pathogenic staph release a number of toxins including hemolysins, leukocidin, enterotoxins, and ex-foliatin. They have also been implicated in toxic shock syndrome.	Humans have high resistance to staph due to development of high antibody titers. Penicillinase-resistant penicillins and cephalosporins are drugs of choice; however, Vancomycin (Vancocin) is drug of choice for methicillin-resistant strains. Vancomycin-resistant strains may require drugs such as quinupristin and dalfopristin (Synercid) or linezolid (Zyvox) or combination therapy with mupirocin (Bactroban) and rifampin (Rifadin). Daptomycin (Cubicin) is a newer drug replacing vancomycin.
Streptococcus	Gram-positive cocci that grow in chains or as diplococci	Transmitted through respiratory droplets or direct contact with secretions.	*Group A beta-hemolytic streptococcus* produces erythrogenic toxin responsible for rash in scarlet fever. Two hemolysins and streptokinase are produced that promote lysis of blood clots. Diseases include pharyngitis, otitis media, peritonsillar abscesses, meningitis, and pneumonia. Glomerulonephritis and rheumatic fever are complications that can result.	Penicillin is the drug of choice, with erythromycin used for those allergic to penicillin. Instruct clients about importance of completing entire course of prescribed antibiotics.
Mycobacterium tuberculosis (tuberculosis)	Acid-fast and aerobic bacillus (due to large amounts of lipids in cell wall)	Transmitted via respiratory droplets from humans, cows, or birds. May also enter blood and lymph system and travel to other parts of body.	Grows slowly and often results in self-limiting lesion. Initial lesion appears as area of non-specific pneumonitis. The caseous lesion heals by fibrosis and calcification, and can be reactivated with low host resistance. Exotoxins or endotoxins are not produced. Mycobacteria primarily affect lungs but may also cause infection in kidney, liver, and GU tract.	Previous mycobacterial infection can be detected through a PPD skin test, but does not necessarily indicate active infection. Drugs of choice are antitubercular agents isoniazid (INH) and rifampin (Rifadin). Streptomycin and pyrazinamide (Tebrazid) are also used. Standard antibiotics are not effective against mycobacteria. Treatment usually continues for 3–6 months and requires client compliance.

    2) Neutrophil count: expressed as absolute neutrophil count (ANC) or percentage of total WBC; is elevated with most bacterial infections

        a) Both segmented neutrophils (mature) and bands (immature neutrophils) will likely be elevated with infection

        b) With severe or prolonged infection, percentage of bands will increase to a greater extent than segmented neutrophils (often referred to as a "shift to the left")

        c) Some bacterial infections (typhoid, brucellosis, and so on) may cause neutropenia

b. Culture and sensitivity: aids in identifying organism and determining antibiotic that can be most effective; collect prior to administering any antibiotics; complete cultures and first antibiotic administration according to agency protocol in a timely manner

c. Gram stain: allows presumptive identification of category of bacteria

D. Nursing management

1. Medications include antimicrobial agents, antipyretics, and nonsteroidal anti-inflammatory drugs (NSAIDs)

2. Teach and encourage good hand hygiene (single most effective way to prevent spread of infection)

3. Employ appropriate protective barriers (gloves, mask, goggles, gowns) when caring for clients with bacterial infections

4. Instruct client and family in methods to prevent spread of infection

5. Encourage balance of rest and activity

6. Encourage compliance with drug regimen; stress completion of all doses even though symptoms improve to avoid bacterial resistance

7. Encourage increased fluid intake with most antimicrobials

8. Document response to therapy

9. Collect lab specimens as needed to validate resolution of infection

IV. FUNGAL INFECTIONS

A. Overview

1. Fungi may be unicellular (yeasts) or multicellular (hyphae), or may alternate between forms

2. Fungi can cause allergic, toxic, and infectious disease in humans

3. Some fungi are part of normal flora of skin, mouth, intestines, and vagina

B. Pathophysiology

1. Fungi obtain nutrients by absorption and almost all are aerobic and reproduce by spores

    a. Spores germinate to produce different morphologic forms such as single-celled yeasts or multicelled molds

    b. Cell wall is rigid and composed primarily of polysaccharides external to cell membrane

2. Plasma membrane contains ergosterol rather than cholesterol, which is useful in antifungal therapy

3. Humans have a high level of innate immunity to fungi, and most infections are mild and self-limiting

4. Factors related to resistance include fatty acid content of skin, pH of skin and mucous membranes, normal flora, epithelial turnover, and cilia in respiratory tract

5. Infections are classified according to 3 levels

    a. Superficial: limited to outer layers of skin and hair (tinea versicolor)

    b. Cutaneous: extending deeper into keratinized layers of epidermis (caused by dermaphytes); tinea and candida are primary examples

     c. Subcutaneous: involves dermis, subcutaneous tissue, muscle, and fascia

      1) Most infections of this type are chronic and visualized as skin lesions

      2) They may be initiated by trauma and may require surgical excision

  6. Fungal infections can also be systemic; this form originates primarily in lung, but may appear as a secondary infection elsewhere; histoplasmosis is a common example

  7. Opportunistic mycotic infections are often seen in immunocompromised clients (those with AIDS, receiving chemotherapy, and so on) or those on long-term antibiotic therapy; most common forms are candidiasis, aspergillosis, and zygomycosis

  8. Transmission is through direct contact with persons or inanimate objects

  9. Moisture increases risk of growth and spread of fungal infection

C. Nursing assessment

  1. Assessment includes location, size, and characteristics of lesions of skin and mucous membranes; complaints of discomfort (itching); and specific assessment (vagina, mouth, nails)

  2. Diagnostic tests: cultures of skin, nails, or hair, microscopic exam of scrapings from lesions, and observation under ultraviolent light (spores fluoresce blue-green)

D. Nursing management

  1. Medications

    a. Superficial, cutaneous, and subcutaneous fungal infections are generally treated with topical antifungal agents such as clotrimazole (Lotrimin), ketoconazole (Nizoral), nystatin (Mycostatin), fluconazole (Diflucan), and terbinafine (Lamisil); most frequent side effects include burning, pruritis, and local irritation

    b. Antifungal agents used to treat fungal infections that are systemic (rather than superficial, cutaneous, or subcutaneous) include flucytosine (5-FC), fluconazole (Diflucan), ketoconazole (Nizoral), and nystatin (Mycostatin)

    c. Amphotericin B (Fungizone) is drug of choice for severe systemic mycoses; is often given along with flucytosine (5-FC) for a synergistic effect; is associated with many adverse effects including fever, chills, cardiac dysrhythmias, and nephrotoxicity

  2. Teach clients about method of transmission and conditions that increase risk

  3. Explain importance of using clean articles for personal hygiene each day

  4. Teach clients that antifungals often take 7–10 days to work

Practice to Pass

How would topical corticosteroids aggravate treatment of a fungal infection?

V. CHLAMYDIAL INFECTIONS

A. Overview

  1. Chlamydial organisms are obligate nonmotile intracellular parasites associated with many sexually transmitted infections (STIs)

  2. Chlamydia is most common bacterial STI in United States

  3. Originally considered a virus, it is now recognized as a bacteria since it contains both RNA and DNA and has a cell wall similar to Gram-negative bacteria

  4. Chlamydial infection can lead to pelvic inflammatory disease, infertility, ectopic pregnancy, and chronic pelvic pain

B. Pathophysiology

  1. Chlamydia are unicellular organisms that reproduce asexually in host cells of mammals and birds and transmit directly to humans

  2. Cell wall of chlamydia is similar in structure to Gram-negative bacteria with a lipid cytoplasmic membrane; DNA occurs as an irregular mass in cytoplasm, and cells lack flavoproteins and cytochromes

  3. Cell cycle begins with a highly infectious small cell taken into a host cell by phagocytosis; cell cycle varies from 24–48 hours

    a. Cell retains its integrity and is reorganized into a large cell that multiplies by binary fission

    b. Large cells then reorganize into small cells capable of infecting new host cells

4. They generally become parasites of epithelial cells, mainly targeting mucous membranes of eye or GU tract; some forms transmitted by birds can cause infection of lungs
5. There is generally low pathogenicity except in an immunocompromised host
6. Infection can remain latent or subclinical for years
7. Chlamydia has on its surface a peptide similar to one in heart myosin; this can trigger T cells that attack both chlamydia and heart cells, causing myocarditis
8. Many clients with chlamydial infection are asymptomatic initially; some may report vaginal discharge within 1–3 weeks of infection; later signs may include lower back pain, nausea, and fever

C. Nursing assessment
1. Assessment includes symptom analysis of pain, VS, inspection of vaginal discharge (females) or penile discharge (males)
2. Diagnostic tests
    a. Cell tissue culture is primary diagnostic tool
    b. Enzyme immunoassay (EIA) tests may be used for high-risk clients but result in a fairly high percentage of false positive results
    c. Nucleic amplification tests (usually along with urine tests and cervical swab) have been developed and have been found effective

D. Nursing management
1. Medications: single-dose or 7-day azithromycin (Zithromax) or doxycycline (Vibramycin) for 7 days
2. Instruct clients about transmission through sexual contact and need to treat sexual partners

VI. SPIROCHETE INFECTIONS

A. Overview
1. Spirochetes are spiral-shaped bacteria with great motility that live primarily as extracellular pathogens, rarely growing within a host cell
2. Spirochetes possess both DNA and RNA and can penetrate mucous membranes, entering blood and lymphatic system

B. Pathophysiology
1. Infections may remain latent for years
2. Humoral and cell-mediated immune responses are activated and may decrease spirochete load, but generally will not eliminate disease
3. Most common spirochetes are *Treponema pallidum* and *Borrelia burgdorferi*
4. *Treponema pallidum* causes syphilis, the third most common STI in United States
    a. First signs include indurated, circumscribed, painless ulcer at site of infection that lasts 10–14 days and heals spontaneously
    b. May experience headache, low-grade fever, and lymphadenopathy
    c. Enters period of latency where a certain percentage will develop tertiary symptoms with long-term effects in central nervous system (CNS), blood vessels, and perivascular areas
5. *Borrelia burgdorferi* causes Lyme disease, the most common tick-transmitted disease
    a. Lesion expands uniformly from site of bite that is clear in center, with redness at periphery
    b. Host response often leads to complications such as arthritis and neuropathies; if left untreated may lead to destruction of bone and joints
    c. Symptoms may include fever, neck stiffness, and neurological complications such as Bell's palsy

C. Nursing assessment
1. Assessment: appearance and location of lesions; VS; signs of lymphadenopathy; sexual history for suspicion of syphilis; discomfort

      2. Diagnostic tests: cultures (may take 8–12 weeks) and serologic testing for antibodies (may be negative in early stages); these include ELISA and indirect fluorescent antibody tests (IFA)

D. Nursing management

      1. Medications include penicillins and doxycycline (as drugs of choice)

       2. Teach clients to wear protective clothing and/or avoid tick-infested areas

      3. Encourage to seek early intervention for suspected tick bites

      4. Instruct in use of protective barriers during intercourse for prevention of syphilis

VII. RICKETTSIAL INFECTIONS

A. Overview

      1. Rickettsiae are similar to Gram-negative bacteria that can only reproduce within certain susceptible cells

      2. They are transmitted to humans by arthropod vectors through bites or feces of ticks, lice, or fleas

      3. Most common diseases caused by rickettsiae are typhus and Rocky Mountain spotted fever

B. Pathophysiology

      1. Rickettsiae are extremely small rod-shaped, coccoid, or pleomorphic bacteria that are intracellular parasites because of a highly permeable cytoplasmic membrane

      2. They typically consist of 3 layers: an inner cytoplasmic membrane, a rigid cell wall, and an outer layer, and they multiply by binary fission

      3. They are primarily found in endothelium of small blood vessels, particularly in brain, skin, and heart

        a. Hyperplasia of endothelial cells and localized thrombus formation lead to obstruction of blood flow, with escape of red blood cells into surrounding tissue

        b. Inflammation of blood vessels occurs (angiitis)

      4. Clinical manifestations are believed to be caused by production of endotoxin

      5. Untreated cases result in a 20–25% fatality

      6. Signs and symptoms include skin rash, headache, malaise, muscle aches, chills and nausea and vomiting; fever of sudden onset may last 2–3 weeks

C. Nursing assessment

      1. Assessment includes VS, skin, pain, and symptom analysis of complaints

      2. Diagnostic tests: complement fixation test (may be positive within 14 days) and indirect fluorescent antibody test (detects IgM and IgG antibodies)

D. Nursing management

       1. Medications include tetracycline (Doxycycline) and chloramphenicol (Chloromycetin); careful monitoring is required with chloramphenicol due to risk of possible bone marrow suppression

       2. Teach clients importance of prevention through avoidance of arthropod carriers and use of repellent in high-risk areas

      3. Sulfonamides should be avoided because they may stimulate rickettsial growth

VIII. PROTOZOAL INFECTIONS

A. Overview

      1. Protozoa are unicellular organisms that may be spherical-, spindle-, or cup-shaped

      2. Protozoal infections are among most common infections of humans world-wide

      3. They occur primarily as parasites of GI and GU systems and may result in pneumonia as an opportunistic infection in immunocompromised clients

B. Pathophysiology

1. Protozoans reproduce asexually by fission, schizogony (multiple fission), or budding
   a. Some also reproduce sexually by fusion of haploid sex cells
   b. Some protozoa produce cysts that enable them to survive outside their host
2. The most common infections caused by protozoa are amebiasis, giardiasis, malaria, toxoplasmosis, and *Pneumocystis jerovici* pneumonia
3. *Amoeba* are transmitted by fecal–oral route
   a. Cysts are excreted in feces of an infected client or carrier and ingested through contaminated food, water, or objects
   b. They penetrate walls of large intestines causing ulceration and may enter blood to cause damage to other organs
   c. Certain forms can also be transmitted through mucous membranes via contaminated water
   d. Many people serve as carriers without clinical symptoms
   e. Early clinical manifestations include diarrhea with mucus and blood, and flatulence, alternating with constipation
   f. Later manifestations of amebic disorders may include lesions of ulcerative colitis, secondary infection in other parts of body, and amebic liver abscess
4. *Giardiasis* is most common protozoan intestinal disease in United States and is also transmitted through fecal–oral route
   a. Cysts are ingested through contaminated food or water and result in gastroenteritis
   b. Clinical manifestations include epigastric pain and nausea
5. *Malaria* is caused by a particular genus of protozoa called *plasmodium* and is transmitted through bite of an infected mosquito
   a. Once infected, a primary exoerythrocytic cycle of asexual reproduction occurs in human liver and leads to synchronous lysis of large numbers of erythrocytes
   b. Extensive erythrolysis results in anemia and splenomegaly
   c. Since this activity occurs primarily in capillaries, small hemorrhages and ischemia from vascular plugging lead to tissue anoxia
   d. Early symptoms of malaria include headache, anorexia, nausea, vomiting, and photophobia; this may be followed by chills, high fever, and muscle pain
6. *Toxoplasmosis* is acquired through ingestion of cysts from cat feces, by ingesting uncooked meat or unpasteurized dairy products, or through blood transfusions
   a. While healthy people often remain asymptomatic, early symptoms may include chills, fever, headache, lymphadenitis, and extreme fatigue
   b. Reactivation toxoplasmosis has become a significant opportunistic infection in immunocompromised clients
7. *Pneumocystis jerovici* pneumonia results from a protozoan that produces cysts in lungs of several animal species and is increasingly common in immuno-compromised clients
   a. Protozoa line alveolar walls and block gas exchange
   b. Accumulations of lymphocytes, macrophages, and plasma cells, with almost no phagocytosis, results in aggregation of parasites, cellular debris, and plasma proteins that lead to interstitial plasma cell pneumonia
   c. Symptoms include a dry, nonproductive cough and absence of sputum; progressive dyspnea may lead to cyanosis

C. Nursing assessment

1. Assessment includes GI symptoms; risk for protozoal disorders; pain and/or nausea; VS; intolerance to light; lymph node enlargement; activity level; characteristics of sputum if present
2. Diagnostic tests
   a. Amoeba and giardiasis: note presence and morphology of cysts in fecal smear

   b. Malaria: observe erythrocytic stages on blood smears; CBC
   c. Toxoplasmosis: serologic tests (indirect fluorescent antibody, indirect hemagglutination assay, ELISA)
   d. Pneumocystitis: lung tissue biopsy or needle aspiration
D. Nursing management
   1. Medications
      a. Amebiasis and giardiasis: drug of choice is metronidazole (Flagyl); disrupts DNA synthesis and synthesis of nucleic acid
      b. Malaria: drugs of choice are chloroquine (Aralen Hydrochloride) and hydroxychloroquine (Plaquenil); interfere with protein synthesis and inhibit DNA and RNA replication as well as nucleic acid synthesis
      c. Toxoplasmosis: pyrimethamine (Daraprim) and pyrimethamine with sulfadoxine (Fansidar); folic acid antagonists
      d. Pneumocystitis: trimethoprim/sulfamethoxazole (Bactrim), a folic acid antagonist

   2. Instruct clients to boil water prior to drinking in areas with untreated water
   3. Instruct client on proper hand washing (not merely hand hygiene rubs) after defecating

IX. HELMINTH INFECTIONS
A. Overview
   1. Helminths (worms) gain entry into humans primarily through ingestion of fertilized eggs or penetration of larvae through skin or mucous membranes
   2. Helminths are classified as cestodes (tapeworms), nematodes (roundworms), or trematodes (flukes)
B. Pathophysiology
   1. Cestode infections are caused by tapeworms living in intestines
      a. Tapeworms are flat, segmented worms with structures that allow attachment to intestinal wall
      b. These usually cause little pathology and begin with ingestion of eggs or cysts from infected beef, pork, or fish
      c. Cyst lodges in intestinal mucosa and can cause symptoms including diarrhea, abdominal pain, nausea, fatigue, anorexia, and paresthesias
      d. The large size of an adult tapeworm results in irritation to mucosa, and infestations can result in intestinal obstruction
      e. Eggs can enter blood and migrate to various tissues (including brain)
   2. Nematodes are elongated, unsegmented, cylindrical worms
      a. Eggs develop in soil, and once ingested, they hatch and larvae undergo migration through lungs before localizing and maturing in small intestine
      b. Migration through walls of alveoli causes irritation and may result in transient pneumonitis, which may be asymptomatic
      c. This may result in fever, coughing, blood in sputum, and elevated eosinophil counts
      d. Intestinal nematodes may result in abdominal distention, fever, and obstruction
   3. Trematodes are unsegmented, flat, leaf-shaped worms that require asexual reproduction in a snail intermediate host
      a. Humans become infected by ingesting poorly cooked fish, crabs, or snails
      b. They usually have suckers for attaching to GI mucosa
      c. Flukes may infect various tissues including blood vessels, intestines, liver or lungs
      d. Flukes cover themselves with host antigens to avoid antibody response in order to exist in blood
      e. Inflammatory responses from migrating eggs often lead to scarring and fibrosis in affected organs

f. Early symptoms include fever, malaise, abdominal pain, itching (rectal), and gastroenteritis

g. Untreated infections can lead to chronic disorders in affected organs

C. Nursing assessment

1. Assessment includes discomfort, weight, bowel patterns, VS, and energy level
2. Diagnostic tests: examination of stool specimens for ova, cysts, and parasites; CT scan and CBC (eosinophilia)

D. Nursing management

1. Medications

Practice to Pass

What is the most severe and life-threatening complication of infestation with worms?

   a. All types helminths: mebendazole (Vermox), which inhibits uptake of glucose and other nutrients

   b. Other drugs for cestodes: albendazole (Albenza) and praziquantel (Biltricide)

   c. Other drugs for nematodes: diethylcarbamazine (Hetrazan), ivermectin (Stomectol), piperazine (Antepar) and pyrantel (Antiminth)

   d. Other drugs for trematodes: oxamniquine (Vansil) and praziquantel (Biltricide) cause loss of intracellular calcium and paralysis of parasites

2. Teach clients about importance of cooking meat; freezing meat for several days can also destroy infectious eggs

X. MYCOPLASMA INFECTIONS

A. Overview

1. Mycoplasma species are smallest known free-living organisms; are pleomorphic organisms with no cell wall (therefore resistant to cell wall–active antibiotics)
2. Mycoplasma pneumonia is also known as atypical or walking pneumonia

B. Pathophysiology

1. Mycoplasma are generally slow growing but vary widely in growth rates; they require fatty acids (sterol) and serum protein for growth and generally adhere to mucosal epithelium
2. Mycoplasma pneumonia occurs most often in children, young adults, and older adults

   a. It is transmitted by droplets, with an incubation period of 2–3 weeks

   b. Individuals may be asymptomatic, but common symptoms include headache, low-grade fever, malaise, anorexia, and hacking cough

C. Nursing assessment

1. Assessment includes VS, complaints of pain or discomfort, activity level, nutritional assessment, lung sounds, and presence of cough
2. Diagnostic tests: cold agglutin antibody titer (but is insensitive and nonspecific, positive enzyme immunoassay (EIA), and chest x-ray (CXR) will show infiltrates

D. Nursing management

1. Medications: antibiotic drug of choice is macrolides—azithromycin (Zithromax), clarithromycin (Biaxin), analgesics or NSAIDs for discomfort, and antipyretics for fever
2. Encourage balance of rest and activity; administer oxygen if needed

3. Offer fluids unless contraindicated

XI. MYCOBACTERIAL INFECTIONS

A. Overview

1. A group of acid-fast Gram-positive rods belonging to *Mycobacteriaceae* family
2. Common diseases include *M. tuberculosis* (tuberculosis); *M. leprae* (leprosy), and *M. avium-intracellulare* (an opportunistic infection)

B. Pathophysiology

1. Organisms are surrounded by a waxy capsule that is hard to penetrate; may form branches of a fungal nature
2. Are classified as common facultative intracellular parasites; able to survive and grow within a macrophage; humans are the only natural host
3. Response to cell includes tissue damage as a result of chronic inflammation
4. *M. tuberculosis* (tuberculosis) is an aerobic acid-fast rod
   a. Is transmitted by respiratory droplets, with incubation period of 4–8 weeks; can cause reinfection
   b. Signs and symptoms include lung involvement (can be seen on chest x-ray); fever, pleurisy; night sweats; cough; weight loss
5. *M. leprae* (leprosy), also known as Hansen's disease
   a. Is caused by an acid-fast rod-shaped bacillus; contracted by close contact or prolonged exposure; skin or nasal mucosa can be portal of entrance, with incubation period of 3–5 years
   b. Signs and symptoms include: lesions of skin that are destructive, involvement of peripheral nerves, upper respiratory passages, testes, hands, and feet; muscle weakness
   c. Erythema nodosum leprosum (ENL) reaction may develop during end of first year of therapy with red, painful nodules that become ulcerated and necrotic
6. *M. avium-intracellulare*
   a. An opportunistic acid-fast rod; contracted by respiratory transmission from soil, water, dairy products, birds, and mammals
   b. Signs and symptoms are pulmonary in nature

C. Nursing assessment

1. Assessment includes lung sounds; symptom analysis; VS; skin assessment; height and weight analysis; nutritional assessment; presence of cough
2. Diagnostic tests
   a. Sputum analysis: culture and sensitivity as well as acid-fast bacillus
   b. CXR
   c. Skin lesion biopsy
   d. Leprosy: lymphocyte transformation test and leukocyte migration inhibition test
   e. Tuberculosis: positive TB skin test (PPD or Mantoux), with induration of 10 mm or greater for clients not generally at risk, or 5 mm or greater for those with frequent exposure or greater risk (immunocompromised)

D. Nursing management

1. Medications
   a. Leprosy: dapsone (DDS), thalidomide (Thalomid)—drug of choice for ENL, and corticosteroids
   b. Tuberculosis: isoniazid (INH), pyrazinamide (PZA), rifampin (RMP) and others; combining INH and RMP is most effective
2. Teach client and family about exposure and incubation periods to avoid infecting others
3. Stress need to continue therapy even if feeling better; avoid alcohol with INH

XII. PRION INFECTIONS

A. Overview

1. Prions are mutant forms of protein on surface of some animal cells that are similar to viruses in ability to cause infection, although smaller in size
2. Prions lack nucleic acid found in viruses
3. They have been linked to chronic degenerative diseases of central nervous system

B. Pathophysiology

1. Although little is known about exact mechanism of action, characteristics of disorders have been identified; they are characterized by long incubation periods with a protracted course that usually results in death
2. Pathologic lesions are usually limited to a single organ or tissue system
3. Examples of prion disorders include spongiform encephalopathies such as Creutzfeldt-Jacob disease
    a. Transmission is thought to be through corneal transplants and contaminated growth hormone
    b. Begins with personality changes, memory loss, and altered visual acuity and results in progressive dementia, ataxia, and somnolence and eventually leads to death within 1–2 years after onset of symptoms
    c. CNS alterations occur primarily in cerebral cortex and cerebellum

C. Nursing assessment and management

1. Assess history and pattern of memory loss or changes in personality
2. Document progressive physical and behavioral changes

Case Study

A client has been hospitalized with an intestinal obstruction and undergoes surgery. While recovering from the surgery, she develops chills, fever, and malaise, and the surgical site is noted as red with purulent drainage. Because of a recent increase in the incidence of methicillin-resistant Staphylococcus aureus (MRSA) within the hospital unit, the physician suspects MRSA as the source of the wound infection.

1. What type of infection is this considered, and what is the most important nursing intervention concerning prevention?

2. What is the most appropriate diagnostic test to determine the causative organism?

3. What other relevant laboratory findings should be observed?

4. What is the drug of choice for treating MRSA, and what adverse effects should the nurse consider?

5. If the culture reveals vancomycin-resistant *Staphylococcus aureus* (VRSA), what medications are effective?

For suggested responses, see page 466.

POSTTEST

1 A client diagnosed with a bacterial infection that is resistant to penicillin asks the nurse, "Why can't penicillin be used to treat this infection?" The nurse's reply incorporates what pertinent information about the role of the bacterial capsule?

1. Protects the pathogenic bacteria from host defenses
2. Plays a major role in adherence of bacteria
3. Does not protect the organism from phagocytosis
4. Always composed of glutamic acid

2 The nurse reviews which client laboratory test result that is expected to be elevated with nematode infestation?

1. Neutrophils
2. Liver enzymes
3. Red blood cells
4. Eosinophils

3 A nurse researcher is interested in studying the type and incidence of risk behaviors for HIV in a given community, and a nursing student is assisting with the research. The student will expect to collect data related to which of the following?

1. Number of intravenous drug users
2. Exploration of money spent on treatment for known cases of HIV
3. Most effective treatment regimens and the CD4 cell counts of the study population
4. Distribution of the disease in the population being studied

4 A young male college student comes to the clinic after contracting genital herpes. Which intervention by the nurse would be most appropriate?

1. Encourage him to maintain bed rest for several days.
2. Monitor his temperature every 4 hours.
3. Instruct him to avoid sexual contact during acute phases of illness.
4. Encourage him to use antifungal agents regularly.

5 A client has been diagnosed with genital herpes and wants to reduce the length and severity of the outbreak. About which of the following drugs will the nurse plan to teach the client?

1. Penicillin (Bicillin)
2. Rifampin (Rifadin)
3. Acyclovir (Zovirax)
4. Podophyllin (Condylox)

6 A young adult male relates to the nurse that he has recently experienced signs and symptoms of infection. His neutrophil count is lower than normal. The nurse should draw which most appropriate conclusion?

1. He has a bacterial infection.
2. He has a viral infection.
3. He has an immune deficiency disorder.
4. He is recovering from the illness.

7 A young girl presents with fever and abdominal distention. Her mother states that she has also "coughed up blood" in recent days. The nurse considers that which health problem is compatible with these symptoms?

1. Mycoplasma pneumonia
2. Rickettsial infection
3. Infection with nematodes
4. Infection with spirochetes

8 The nurse is teaching a client recently diagnosed with Creutzfeldt-Jakob disease about the disease process. The nurse will base the teaching on what knowledge of the disease?

1. Prions are opportunistic organisms frequently seen in clients with human immunodeficiency virus (HIV).
2. Prions have been linked to chronic degenerative central nervous system disorders, called transmissible neurodegenerative diseases.
3. Lesions caused by the microorganisms associated with this disease are usually distributed throughout the body.
4. Prions are similar to viruses in their nucleic acid structure, but there is no drug to treat the infection.

9 A client has a white blood cell (WBC) count of 15,000, of which 60% are segmented neutrophils (segs), and 3% are bands. An antibiotic is prescribed. Three days later the WBC remains at 15,000, with 62% segs and 10% bands. The nurse concludes that this most likely indicates which of the following?

1. The infection is resolving.
2. The client is immunocompromised.
3. The infection is severe or prolonged and not responding to antimicrobial agents.
4. There is a shift to the right in the differential.

10 A client in the clinic asks why an antibiotic is needed to treat "a tick bite with a funny-looking ring around it." The nurse considers which facts about disease from tick bites when considering a response? Select all that apply.

1. Disease is caused by rickettsial pathogens.
2. Humoral and cell-mediated responses by the body will not generally be sufficient to eliminate the disease.
3. Disease is transmitted by ticks.
4. If untreated, it may lead to complications of arthritis and destruction of joints.
5. The most frequent time of onset is in the summer months.

➤ *See pages 346–348 for Answers and Rationales.*

ANSWERS & RATIONALES

Pretest

1 **Answer: 3** **Rationale:** Opportunistic infections occur when a normally nonpathogenic organism causes disease in an immunocompromised host. The route of entry does not imply whether the infection is opportunistic or not. An extremely virulent organism would cause infection in a health person. Although it is possible, opportunistic infections are not necessarily also nosocomial. **Cognitive Level:** Applying **Client Need:** Physiological Adaptation **Integrated Process:** Nursing Process: Diagnosis **Content Area:** Adult Health **Strategy:** The critical word in the question is *opportunistic*. Review medical terminology if needed. **Reference:** Lemone, P., Burke, K., & Bauldoff, G. (2011). *Medical-surgical nursing: Critical thinking in patient care* (5th ed.). Upper Saddle River, NJ: Pearson Education, Inc., pp. 323–324.

2 **Answer: 2** **Rationale:** Identifying the causative organism is critical for appropriate treatment and should be done as a priority action. After the infecting organism is identified, the appropriate antimicrobial therapy can be instituted. The fever is caused by the infection, so treating the infection will reduce the fever, although acetaminophen may help control this symptom. Hand hygiene is important to prevent the spread of disease, but the priority action is identifying the causative organism of this client's diseases. **Cognitive Level:** Analyzing **Client Need:** Physiological Adaptation **Integrated Process:** Nursing Process: Implementation **Content Area:** Adult Health **Strategy:** All options are correct actions but the question asks what to do *first*. Consider the importance of an accurate culture and sensitivity on the client's outcome to make your selection. **Reference:** Lemone, P., Burke, K., & Bauldoff, G. (2011). *Medical-surgical nursing: Critical thinking in patient care* (5th ed.). Upper Saddle River, NJ: Pearson Education, Inc., p. 296.

3 **Answer: 1, 3, 4, 5** **Rationale:** Production of enzymes, genetic mutations, alternate pathways, and changes in the bacterial cell wall are all examples of mechanisms of bacterial resistance. Leukocytosis is a positive host defense increasing the white blood cells to fight infection.

The prevalence of bacterial resistance is a great concern in the treatment of infectious diseases. **Cognitive Level:** Applying **Client Need:** Pharmacological and Parenteral Therapies **Integrated Process:** Nursing Process: Implementation **Content Area:** Adult Health **Strategy:** Differentiate between leukocytosis and leukopenia and read carefully. Recall that mechanisms of bacterial resistance are numerous. **Reference:** Lemone, P., Burke, K., & Bauldoff, G. (2011). *Medical-surgical nursing: Critical thinking in patient care* (5th ed.). Upper Saddle River, NJ: Pearson Education, Inc., pp. 295–302.

4 **Answer: 2** **Rationale:** A pathogen is any organism capable of causing disease. Pathogenicity refers to the ability of the organism to cause pathologic changes. Communicability is the ability to be transmitted from one person or organism to another. Toxigenicity is the ability of a microorganism to produce endotoxins or exotoxins. Latency is a period during which an organism has infected an individual but has not yet caused symptoms. **Cognitive Level:** Applying **Client Need:** Physiological Adaptation **Integrated Process:** Teaching and Learning **Content Area:** Adult Health **Strategy:** If the terms are unfamiliar, try decoding them for root word, suffix, and prefix. **Reference:** McCance, K., & Huether, K. (2006). *Understanding pathophysiology: The biologic basis for disease in adults and children* (5th ed.). St. Louis, MO: Elsevier, pp. 294–295.

5 **Answer: 1** **Rationale:** Bacterial infections are characterized by fever, body aches, possible regional lymph node involvement, and local signs of infection. Fungal infections are characterized by itching or rashes on skin, or thrush in mouth or vaginal discharge. Protozoal infections have skin manifestation such as itching or rash, diarrhea, and possibly fever if of malarial origin. Rickettsial infections are accompanied by skin rashes, muscle aches, headache, and possibly fever and chills. **Cognitive Level:** Applying **Client Need:** Physiological Adaptation **Integrated Process:** Nursing Process: Diagnosis **Content Area:** Adult Health **Strategy:** Familiarity with the types of infections caused by the different microorganisms is helpful in answering this question. Recall that the question is asking about the presence of both fever and regional lymph node involvement in making a selection. **Reference:** Lemone, P., Burke, K., & Bauldoff, G. (2011). *Medical-surgical nursing: Critical thinking in patient care* (5th ed.). Upper Saddle River, NJ: Pearson Education, Inc., p. 293.

6 **Answer: 1** **Rationale:** Influenza is spread by respiratory droplets, that is, by coughing or sneezing, and can be easily acquired through close casual contact. Herpes virus is transmitted by direct contact and HIV through blood and body fluids. Cytomegalovirus is an opportunistic infection. **Cognitive Level:** Analyzing **Client Need:** Safety and Infection Control **Integrated Process:** Nursing Process: Assessment **Content Area:** Adult Health **Strategy:** The critical words in the question are *casual contact*. Visualize each of the infections and recall the mode of transmission to make a selection. **Reference:** Lemone, P., Burke, K., & Bauldoff, G. (2011). *Medical-surgical nursing: Critical thinking in patient care* (5th ed.). Upper Saddle River, NJ: Pearson Education, Inc., p. 293.

7 **Answer: 2, 3** **Rationale:** Epidemiological studies indicate chlamydia as the most prevalent sexually transmitted infection (STI) in the United States. Cultures and sensitivity testing will be done for both chlamydia and gonorrhea. Syphilis is diagnosed by tissue scraping and microscopic analysis or by blood testing. Viruses can be cultured but do not undergo sensitivity testing, since this applies to antibiotics, which are utilized for bacterial infections. **Cognitive Level:** Analyzing **Client Need:** Physiological Adaptation **Integrated Process:** Nursing Process: Assessment **Content Area:** Adult Health **Strategy:** Note that 2 of the options are bacteria that cause STIs. Note that both will need to be cultured and undergo sensitivity testing. **Reference:** Lemone, P., Burke, K., & Bauldoff, G. (2011). *Medical-surgical nursing: Critical thinking in patient care* (5th ed.). Upper Saddle River, NJ: Pearson Education, Inc., pp. 1719–1727.

8 **Answer: 3** **Rationale:** Foods such as undercooked ground meat or unpasteurized fruit juices may be contaminated with *E. coli*, the organism that produces the toxin and disease. The organism typically found in damaged cans is *Clostridium botulinum*. *E. Coli* is not spread from oral secretions such as with kissing. Toxic shock syndrome (TSS) is caused by a *Staphylococcus aureus* infection. **Cognitive Level:** Applying **Client Need:** Health Promotion and Maintenance **Integrated Process:** Nursing Process: Implementation **Content Area:** Adult Health **Strategy:** Recall that this bacterial exotoxin is one that has received media attention, and nurses should be aware of the problem. **Reference:** Lemone, P., Burke, K., & Bauldoff, G. (2011). *Medical-surgical nursing: Critical thinking in patient care* (5th ed.). Upper Saddle River, NJ: Pearson Education, Inc., pp. 671–672.

9 **Answer: 3** **Rationale:** Rickettsiae are parasites of ticks, fleas, and lice and are transmitted from these vectors to humans. Influenza is an example of transmission by respiratory droplets. Mosquitoes are vectors for other infectious diseases, such as encephalitis, but do not transmit rickettsiae. Rickettsiae are transmitted from the *bites* of infected arthropods, not just direct skin contact. **Cognitive Level:** Applying **Client Need:** Safety and Infection Control **Integrated Process:** Nursing Process: Diagnosis **Content Area:** Adult Health **Strategy:** Recall that a vector is needed to transmit this infection. Knowing that narrows the answer choices to 2 options. **Reference:** Lemone, P., Burke, K., & Bauldoff, G. (2011). *Medical-surgical nursing: Critical thinking in patient care* (5th ed.). Upper Saddle River, NJ: Pearson Education, Inc., p. 293.

10 **Answer: 2** **Rationale:** Infection occurs in a predictable sequence commonly known as the steps in the chain of infection. The chain requires virulence of the organism, a reservoir or source, movement from a reservoir via a portal of exit, a method of transmission and entry into a susceptible host. Infection does not rely on linkages among different form of organisms or clustering of bacteria in a pattern. Increasing virulence patterns among microorganisms may lead to drug resistance, but not to transmission of infection. **Cognitive Level:** Applying **Client Need:** Physiological Adaptation **Integrated Process:** Nursing Process: Diagnosis **Content Area:** Adult Health **Strategy:** The critical words in the question are *chain of infection*. Eliminate the options that are not applicable to the chain. Read the question again if needed—it is asking about the development of an infectious disease in the community. **Reference:** Lemone, P., Burke, K., & Bauldoff, G. (2011). *Medical-surgical nursing: Critical thinking in patient care* (5th ed.). Upper Saddle River, NJ: Pearson Education, Inc., p. 292.

Posttest

1 **Answer: 1** **Rationale:** The development of resistant strains of bacteria is the reason penicillin will not treat this client's infection. The extracellular capsule is an added layer of protection for the bacteria from host defenses. Bacteria are not held together by the capsule. The capsule does not protect the bacteria from phagocytosis and is not always composed of glutamic acid. **Cognitive Level:** Applying **Client Need:** Physiological Adaptation **Integrated Process:** Nursing Process: Implementation **Content Area:** Adult Health **Strategy:** Beware of critical words such as *always*. Look for opposite options as a strategy and eliminate one of them using baseline nursing knowledge of how bacterial resistance occurs. **Reference:** Lemone, P., Burke, K., & Bauldoff, G. (2011). *Medical-surgical nursing: Critical thinking in patient care* (5th ed.). Upper Saddle River, NJ: Pearson Education, Inc., p. 293.

2 **Answer: 4** **Rationale:** Eosinophilia is present with allergies and infestation with parasites such as nematode infestation. Neutrophils are elevated with acute infections and bacterial organisms. Liver enzymes and red blood cells are not affected. **Cognitive Level:** Applying **Client Need:** Physiological Adaptation **Integrated Process:** Nursing Process: Assessment **Content Area:** Adult Health **Strategy:** First recall that white blood cells help to fight infection to eliminate 2 options. Next recall the role of neutrophils with acute infection and bacterial infections to eliminate a third option. **Reference:** Lemone, P., Burke, K., & Bauldoff, G. (2011). *Medical-surgical nursing: Critical thinking in patient care* (5th ed.). Upper Saddle River, NJ: Pearson Education, Inc., pp. 678–679.

3 Answer: 1 Rationale: High risk behaviors for HIV include multiple sexual partners, intravenous drug use, and exposure to blood and body fluids via childbirth. Cost of treatment, efficacy of various regiments, CD4 cell counts, and distribution of the disease do not address risk behaviors. **Cognitive Level:** Applying **Client Need:** Health Promotion and Maintenance **Integrated Process:** Nursing Process: Assessment **Content Area:** Adult Health **Strategy:** Apply the definition of epidemiology to this study of disease in a population. **Reference:** Lemone, P., Burke, K., & Bauldoff, G. (2011). *Medical-surgical nursing: Critical thinking in patient care* (5th ed.). Upper Saddle River, NJ: Pearson Education, Inc., p. 335.

4 Answer: 3 Rationale: Herpes is a virus spread through direct contact. Therefore the client should avoid sexual contact during the acute phases of illness and should use protection against transmitting the infection thereafter. An antifungal would not be useful; bedrest and temperature measurement are usually not necessary. **Cognitive Level:** Applying **Client Need:** Safety and Infection Control **Integrated Process:** Nursing Process: Implementation **Content Area:** Adult Health **Strategy:** Consider what instructions are needed to prevent the spread of the infection while it is active in this first outbreak. **Reference:** Lemone, P., Burke, K., & Bauldoff, G. (2011). *Medical-surgical nursing: Critical thinking in patient care* (5th ed.). Upper Saddle River, NJ: Pearson Education, Inc., p. 1721.

5 Answer: 3 Rationale: Acyclovir is the antiviral drug of choice for treating herpes virus. Penicillin products are used for a wide variety of bacterial infections. Rifampin is used for tuberculosis and podophyllin is used to treat genital warts. **Cognitive Level:** Applying **Client Need:** Pharmacological and Parenteral Therapies **Integrated Process:** Nursing Process: Implementation **Content Area:** Adult Health **Strategy:** Note that only one of the options is an antiviral. The name is a clue. **Reference:** Lemone, P., Burke, K., & Bauldoff, G. (2011). *Medical-surgical nursing: Critical thinking in patient care* (5th ed.). Upper Saddle River, NJ: Pearson Education, Inc., p. 1721.

6 Answer: 2 Rationale: Neutrophil counts are often decreased in viral infections and elevated in bacterial infections. Neutropenia can also occur because of chemotherapy and immunosuppression. However, with immunosuppression, the client's illness would not resolve untreated. The client's neutrophil count should be returning to normal if the infection has resolved, but more than one laboratory measurement of the neutrophil count would be needed to make this determination. **Cognitive Level:** Applying **Client Need:** Reduction of Risk Potential **Integrated Process:** Nursing Process: Diagnosis

Content Area: Adult Health **Strategy:** Specific knowledge is needed to answer the question. Learn the CBC differential values and what causes the various changes in values. Nurses must be able to interpret them. **Reference:** Lemone, P., Burke, K., & Bauldoff, G. (2011). *Medical-surgical nursing: Critical thinking in patient care* (5th ed.). Upper Saddle River, NJ: Pearson Education, Inc., p. 271.

7 Answer: 3 Rationale: Abdominal distention is caused from infestation of worms. Blood in sputum often results from migration of worms through alveoli. Mycoplasma pneumonia has similar side effects as bacterial pneumonia (cough, fatigue, crackles, and fever). Spirochetes cause rashes and tertiary disease; rickettsial infections cause headaches, nausea, vomiting, and muscle aches. **Cognitive Level:** Analyzing **Client Need:** Physiological Adaptation **Integrated Process:** Nursing Process: Assessment **Content Area:** Adult Health **Strategy:** Consider both the gastrointestinal and the pulmonary symptoms when selecting the answer. **Reference:** Lemone, P., Burke, K., & Bauldoff, G. (2011). *Medical-surgical nursing: Critical thinking in patient care* (5th ed.). Upper Saddle River, NJ: Pearson Education, Inc., p. 679.

8 Answer: 2 Rationale: Prions, related to the agent causing bovine spongiform encephalopathy or mad cow disease, are associated with degenerative encephalopathies. Prions do not cause opportunistic infections. Prion disease affects the central nervous system and is not distributed throughout the body. While similar to viruses, prions are protein particles lacking a nucleic acid structure. **Cognitive Level:** Applying **Client Need:** Physiological Adaptation **Integrated Process:** Teaching and Learning **Content Area:** Adult Health **Strategy:** First identify the agent causing the disease. Next determine the pathology. **Reference:** Lemone, P., Burke, K., & Bauldoff, G. (2011). *Medical-surgical nursing: Critical thinking in patient care* (5th ed.). Upper Saddle River, NJ: Pearson Education, Inc., p. 293.

9 Answer: 3 Rationale: With bacterial infection there is an increased need for neutrophils. When the percentage of immature neutrophils (bands) increases at a greater rate than mature neutrophils (segs), it is an indication that the infection is severe or prolonged. This is often referred to as a shift to the left. The infection is overcoming the client's immune system, not resolving. The client continues to mount an immune response, indicating a challenged but intact immune system. **Cognitive Level:** Analyzing **Client Need:** Physiological Adaptation **Integrated Process:** Nursing Process: Diagnosis **Content Area:** Adult Health **Strategy:** Learn the CBC differential values and the implications of abnormal values or changes. In this question, evaluate the trend of increasing bands. **Reference:** Lemone, P., Burke, K., & Bauldoff, G. (2011). *Medical-surgical nursing: Critical thinking in patient care* (5th ed.). Upper Saddle River, NJ: Pearson Education, Inc., p. 295.

10 Answer: 2, 3, 4, 5 Rationale: The lesion described is typical for Lyme disease. Lyme disease is a spirochete infection caused by *Borrelia burdorferi*. Lyme disease is carried by mice or deer, and ticks are vectors, usually in the summer months. Treatment of Lyme disease requires antibiotic therapy to eradicate the spirochete. Untreated Lyme disease can lead to rheumatic complications. Examples of rickettsial infections are typhus and Rocky Mountain spotted fever. **Cognitive Level:** Analyzing **Client Need:** Physiological Adaptation

Integrated Process: Nursing Process: Planning **Content Area:** Adult Health **Strategy:** First determine what the client's problem is. Then apply knowledge of that disease to select the correct options. **Reference:** Lemone, P., Burke, K., & Bauldoff, G. (2011). *Medical-surgical nursing: Critical thinking in patient care* (5th ed.). Upper Saddle River, NJ: Pearson Education, Inc., pp. 1380–1381.

References

Ignatavicius, D. D., & Workman, M. L. (2013). *Medical-surgical nursing: Critical thinking for collaborative care* (7th ed.). Philadelphia: W. B. Saunders Company.

Kee, J. L. (2010). *Laboratory and diagnostic tests* (8th ed.). Upper Saddle River, NJ: Pearson Education.

Lehne, R. (2010). *Pharmacology for nursing care* (7th ed.). St. Louis, MO: Saunders.

LeMone, P., Burke, K., & Bauldoff, G. (2011). *Medical-surgical nursing: Critical thinking in patient care* (5th ed.). Upper Saddle River, NJ: Pearson Education.

Lewis, S., Dirksen, S. Heitkemper, M., Bucher, L., & Camera, I. (2011). *Medical surgical nursing: Assessment and management of clinical problems* (8th ed.). St. Louis, MO: Elsevier.

Lilley, L., Collins, S., Harrington, S., & Snyder, J. (2011). *Pharmacology and the nursing process* (6th ed.). St. Louis, MO: Mosby, Inc.

McCance, K. L., & Huether, S. E. (2010). *Pathophysiology: The biologic basis for disease in adults and children* (6th ed.). St. Louis, MO: Mosby, Inc.

Osborn, K. S., Wraa, C. E., & Watson, A. (2010). *Medical surgical nursing: Preparation for practice*. Upper Saddle River, NJ: Pearson Education.

Porth, C., & Matfin, G. (2010). *Pathophysiology: Concepts of altered health states* (8th ed.). Philadelphia, PA: Lippincott Williams & Wilkins.

Wilson, B., Shannon, M., & Shields, K. (2012). *Pearson nurse's drug guide 2012*. Upper Saddle River, NJ: Pearson Education.

Integumentary Health Problems

14

Chapter Outline

Risk Factors for Integumentary
    Health Problems
Malignant Conditions of Skin
Benign Conditions of Skin

Bacterial Infections of Skin
Viral Infections of Skin
Fungal Infections of Skin
Infestations and Insect Bites

Allergic Conditions of Skin
Burns

Objectives

➤ Define key terms associated with integumentary health problems.
➤ Identify risk factors associated with integumentary health problems.
➤ Explain common etiologies of integumentary health problems.
➤ Describe the pathophysiological processes associated with
   integumentary health problems.
➤ Distinguish between normal and abnormal integumentary findings
   obtained from nursing assessment.
➤ Prioritize nursing interventions associated with integumentary
   health problems.

NCLEX-RN® Test Prep

Use the accompanying online resource,
NursingReviewsandRationales, to test
yourself with hundreds of NCLEX®-style
practice questions.

Review at a Glance

acne an androgenically stimulated, inflammatory disorder of sebaceous glands, resulting in comedones, papules, inflamed pustules, and occasionally scarring

atopic dermatitis an inflammation of skin from an unknown source in an individual with irritable skin; also known as eczema

basal cell carcinoma malignant tumor of skin originating from basal cells of epidermis

burn tissue injuries caused by application of heat, chemicals, electricity, or radiation to tissue

candidiasis a fungal infection caused by *Candida albicans*, a yeastlike fungus that most often causes superficial cutaneous infections

carbuncle (carbunculosis) aggregates of infected follicles coalesced together to form one large lesion

cellulitis a diffuse inflammation of skin and subcutaneous layers with various presenting lesions including vesicles (small sacs of fluid), bullae (large blisters), abscesses, and plaques

contact dermatitis an eruption of skin related to contact with an irritating substance or allergen

dermatophyte a group of fungi that are able to infect and survive only on keratin, classified as tinea infections

exfoliative dermatitis an inflammation of skin characterized by erythema involving loss of exfoliated (peeling) skin

folliculitis an inflammation of hair follicle usually caused by organism *Staphylococcus aureus* or *Pseudomonas aeruginosa*

furuncle (furunculosis) also known as an abscess or boil, a deep folliculitis consisting of a pus-filled mass that is painful and firm

herpes simplex a viral infection that occurs within keratinolytics and manifests as painful vesicles that often occur in clusters on skin

herpes zoster a viral infection (also known as shingles) that manifests as a cluster of vesicles on skin; a reactivation of varicella virus in dorsal root ganglia that remained in latent form after primary infection

impetigo a superficial skin infection initially seen as an erythemic vesicle, later changing to a honey-colored crusted lesion

lentigo a brown macule resembling a freckle except border is usually regular

malignant melanoma a skin cancer arising from melanocytes

molluscum contagiosum a benign, viral infection of skin caused by poxvirus, inducing epidermal cell proliferation

pediculosis an infestation of skin or hair by species of blood-sucking lice capable of living as external parasites on human host

psoriasis a genetically determined, chronic epidermal proliferative disease characterized by erythematous, dry scaling patches, usually with a heavy, silvery surface

seborrheic dermatitis an acute inflammation of skin from an unknown cause that usually begins on scalp and has rounded, irregular lesions and yellow scales

seborrheic keratosis benign plaques, beige to brown or maybe black in color, ranging in size from 3–20 mm with a velvety or warty surface

squamous cell carcinoma a slow-growing cancer of atypical squamous cells that originates in epidermis and may metastasize

tinea versicolor common noninflammatory fungal infection caused by lipophilic yeast

urticaria an itchy rash (hives)

warts virus-induced epidermal tumors

PRETEST

1 The nurse is teaching self-care to a client with psoriasis. The nurse should encourage which of the following for his scaled lesions? Select all that apply.

1. Petroleum-based emollients and moisturizers to soften the scales.
2. Critical importance of follow-up appointments.
3. Use of a clean razor blade each time he shaves.
4. Discussing all medications with the provider.
5. Keeping occlusive dressings on lesions 24 hours a day.

2 The nurse teaches a client that the first step in self-management of contact/irritant dermatitis is to do which of the following?

1. Take antihistamines to control the itch.
2. Identify and remove the causative agent.
3. Use over-the-counter (OTC) hydrocortisone cream.
4. Refer for allergy testing.

3 A mother asks how her 2nd-grade child got head lice. The nurse responds by telling the mother which information related to head lice?

1. Only occur in socioeconomically deprived people
2. Were probably spread by person-to-person contact in the classroom
3. Are an airborne infestation
4. Are due to improper washing of her hair

4 The nurse conducting a health fair teaches attendees that which groups of people are most at risk for developing malignant melanoma? Select all that apply.

1. Light-skinned people who work indoors and vacation in sunny climates.
2. Dark-skinned people who work indoors and have intermittent sun exposure.
3. People who are treated with medications that suppress the immune system.
4. Dark-skinned people who work outdoors getting regular sun exposure.
5. People with close relatives who have had melanoma.

5 A client is admitted to the emergency department with 50% burns to the chest and arms. The skin is white, dry, and there is no pain. The nurse assesses the type of burn the client has as which of the following?

1. Superficial thickness
2. Superficial partial thickness
3. Deep partial thickness
4. Full thickness

6 A young boy is brought to the trauma unit with a chemical burn to the face. What would be the nurse's priority assessment?

1. Skin integrity of the face
2. Blood pressure and pulse
3. Airway patency
4. Amount of pain

7 The mother of 10-year-old girl tells the pediatric office nurse that her child has dandruff. On examination, the nurse notices the whitish flakes don't brush off the hair, and there is a papular rash on the child's neck. The nurse suspects which disorder?

1. Tinea capitis
2. Dandruff
3. Seborrheic dermatitis
4. Pediculosis capitis

8 The nurse is most concerned about a wasp sting for a client with which of the following characteristics?

1. Has never been stung before
2. Has a history of fever or chills when bitten
3. Had hives and shortness of breath with the last sting
4. Had a rise in blood pressure to 140/90 when stung

9 A client who has been on 2 antibiotics reports burning on the tongue and not wanting to eat. Inspection of the tongue reveals a white, milky plaque that does not come off with rubbing. The nurse suspects which condition?

1. Impetigo
2. Candidiasis
3. Burns
4. Herpes

10 The nurse would include which items of information in health teaching for a client with warts on the fingers? Select all that apply.

1. Common warts grow above the skin with a rough surface and ragged borders.
2. Warts resolve spontaneously when immunity to the virus develops but this may take up to 5 years.
3. Warts can be transmitted through skin contact.
4. Warts only appear in childhood.
5. The causative agent is a virus.

➤ *See pages 372–374 for Answers and Rationales.*

I. RISK FACTORS FOR INTEGUMENTARY HEALTH PROBLEMS

A. Malignant conditions
  1. Skin pigmentation or fair-skinned complexions
  2. Preexisting lesions
  3. Exposure to chemicals, radiation, or excessive sun
  4. Trauma
  5. Viruses
  6. Ethnicity (Caucasian)

B. Individuals with fair skin and light-colored hair and those with heavy (even intermittent) sun exposure are more at risk for malignant melanoma
C. Benign conditions: exposure to sun, local trauma, infections, stress, physical disorders, and drugs
D. Bacterial conditions: clients with a compromised immune system, other disorders such as diabetes mellitus (DM), or lack of proper hygiene and nutrition
E. Viral infections: depressed immune system, infection with human immunodeficiency virus (HIV), radiation therapy, chemotherapy, or major organ transplants
F. Fungal infections: debilitating disease, poor nutrition, poor hygiene, tropical climates, contact with infected persons or animals, communal showers and pools, occlusive footwear,

excessive sweating, sharing of footwear, excessive moisture from clothing, or use of incontinence undergarments with older adults

G. Bites and infestations: living in overcrowded conditions or developing countries, unsanitary conditions, and certain geographic regions

H. Allergic conditions: immunosuppressed states (such as acquired immunodeficiency syndrome [AIDS]), drug therapy, and heredity

I. Burns: small children and older adults, high-risk occupations, decreased sensation to extremities or certain parts of body

II. MALIGNANT CONDITIONS OF SKIN

A. Overview
1. Defined as skin cancer from a malignant tumor or neoplasm of skin
2. There are 3 types of malignant conditions: basal cell carcinoma, melanoma, and squamous cell carcinoma
3. Causes include ultraviolet exposure, extremes in weather, radiological treatment, chemicals, trauma, burns, or chronic infections; fair-skinned people, older adults, and those who live in warm climates are at increased risk

B. Pathophysiology
1. **Basal cell carcinoma** is an abnormal growth of cells in basal layer of epidermal skin; it is least aggressive type and rarely metastasizes to other organs; it is most common form of skin cancer and may invade surrounding tissue, destroying parts of body; tumor takes many forms
   a. Nodular basal cell carcinoma is most common and appears on neck, face, and head; it is a pearly colored nodule with well-defined margins and a depressed center or rolled edge
   b. Superficial basal cell carcinoma is second most common tumor that is located on trunk and extremities
   c. Other forms include pigmented basal cell (head, neck, and face), rare morpheaform basal cell (head and neck), and keratotic basal cell (pre- and postauricular groove)
2. **Squamous cell carcinoma** is a more aggressive, slow-growing cancer of atypical squamous cells that originate in epidermis and may metastasize via lymphatic system
   a. Proliferation of keratinizing cells of epithelium causes tumor, forming keratin "pearls"
   b. It is most common on sun-exposed areas such as nose, lips, and hands
   c. Lower lip is a frequent location, especially in smokers
   d. It appears as a firm, irregular, flesh-colored papule with a scaly, keratotic surface
   e. It may be erythemic, sore, and/or bleed if touched
3. **Malignant melanoma** is a cancerous tumor arising from melanocytes (melanin-producing cells in deepest epithelial layer), which has ability to metastasize to any organ
   a. Melanoma initially grows superficially and laterally continuing to epidermis and dermis
   b. It then grows vertically with penetration of reticular dermis and subcutaneous fat
   c. This type of melanoma frequently affects young people with common sites being back and legs
   d. Melanomas tend to have **a**symmetry, **b**order irregularity, **c**olor variation, **d**iameter greater than 6 mm, and **e**levation of skin or **e**volving (ABCDE); see Box 14-1; key signs include irregular, circular-bordered lesion with hues of tan, black, or blue
   e. Precursor lesions of a malignant melanoma include dysplastic nevi (atypical mole), congenital nevi (present at birth), and lentigo maligna (tan or black patch that has appearance of a freckle)
   f. Classification of tumors includes superficial-spreading melanoma (about 70%) that arises from preexisting nevus, lentigo maligna melanoma, nodular melanoma, and acral lentiginous melanoma

Box 14-1	**A**symmetry
ABCDEs of Malignant Melanoma	**B**order irregularity
	Color variegation
	Diameter greater than 6 mm
	Elevation of skin or **E**volving (changing)

C. Nursing assessment

1. Assessment
   a. A symptom analysis of skin changes or new growths and a history of amount of sun exposure or sunburn
   b. Family history of skin disorders, and past history of burns, injury, trauma, or cigarette smoking
   c. Assessing any area/preexisting lesion for change in color, size, or shape, noting any local soreness, oozing or bleeding lesions, pruritis, lymph node enlargement, liver, and spleen
2. Diagnostic tests: shave biopsy (for diagnosis), punch biopsy, incisional biopsy (remove part of tumor), or excisional biopsy (remove all of tumor); for malignant melanoma, a liver profile, complete blood count (CBC), electrolytes, CT scan of liver and brain, chest x-ray (CXR), bone scan, magnetic resonance imaging (MRI) of liver, and biopsy of lymph nodes

D. Nursing management

1. Assess all lesions over entire body; encourage yearly exams for a client with excessive moles
2. Teach self-monitoring and examination of existing skin lesions and for any new lesions; early diagnosis and intervention are crucial
3. Instruct client to avoid contact with chemical irritants
4. Teach client about importance of sun exposure protection, wearing layered clothing while outdoors, avoiding midday sun (between 10 a.m. and 2 p.m.), and using sunscreen with a sun protection factor (SPF) over 15
5. Encourage verbalization of client concerns and changes in body image
6. Educate clients about harmful effects of tanning beds

III. BENIGN CONDITIONS OF SKIN

A. Overview

1. Defined as cutaneous growths with no malignant potential and include acne, lentigo, psoriasis, and seborrheic keratosis
2. Causes
   a. Acne: oversecretion of sebum and dysfunction of hormones
   b. Lentigo: prolonged exposure to sun
   c. Psoriasis and seborrheic keratosis: genetics

B. Pathophysiology

1. **Acne** is an androgen-stimulated, inflammatory disorder of sebaceous glands resulting in comedones (open form—blackhead; closed form—whitehead), papules (pimples), inflammatory pustules, cysts, and occasional scarring
   a. There are 3 stages of acne
      1) Mild: few to several papules, no nodules, and occurring on face or neck only
      2) Moderate: several to many papules or pustules and few to several nodules on the face, back, chest, or upper arms
      3) Severe: numerous and/or extensive papules or pustules, many nodules with acne-induced atrophic scarring

---

Practice to Pass

A client who regularly suntans states she is not worried about skin cancer. How should the nurse respond?

    b. Acne involves several factors including increased sebum production, abnormal keratinization of follicular epithelium, proliferation of propriobacterium acnes, and inflammation

    c. Rate of sebum production is determined genetically; it is increased by presence of androgens with earliest changes occurring in prepubescent years

    d. There are 3 types of acne: *acne vulgaris* (common adolescent type), *acne conglobata* (causes scarring), and *acne rosacea* (chronic form)

    e. Acne is graded as follows: *Grade 1*—comedonal (open or closed); *Grade 2*—papular with over 25 lesions on face and trunk; *Grade 3*—pustular with over 25 lesions, mild scarring; and *Grade 4*—nodulocystic, inflammatory nodules, and cysts with extensive scarring

2. Lentigo is a brown macule resembling a freckle except border is usually regular

    a. There are 3 types of lentigo: benign, maligna, and senile

    b. *Benign lentigo* may first appear on young children with ultraviolet light exposure and fade in color during winter months

    c. *Lentigo maligna* is a brown- or black-mottled, irregular bordered, slowly enlarging lesion with an increased number of melanocytes; it is considered premalignant in that one-third may progress to a melanoma, usually 10–15 years later

    d. *Senile lentigo*, also known as liver spots, occurs on skin exposed to ultraviolet light, especially in older Caucasians

3. Psoriasis is a genetically determined, chronic epidermal proliferative disease that is characterized by erythematous, dry scaling patches and a heavy, silvery surface; there are often recurring remissions and exacerbations

    a. Psoriasis is principally caused by altered cell kinetics of keratinocytes where cell cycle is shortened from 311 hours to 36 hours with an increase in epidermal cells

    b. It is often triggered by an infection, most often a *streptococcal* pharyngitis or a viral upper respiratory infection

    c. There are 2 types: *Type 1*, which affects young people who have strong family history of disease and is the more aggressive type, and *Type 2*, which affects older persons who generally have no family history

    d. Type 2 is a more stable type of disease

    e. It is a lifelong process without a cure

4. Seborrheic keratosis is characterized by benign plaques, beige, brown, or maybe black in color, ranging in size from 3–20 mm with a velvety or warty surface

    a. Seborrheic keratosis is caused by a proliferation of immature keratinocytes and melanocytes occurring totally within dermis that is generally seen beginning in middle age

    b. They appear as "stuck on" spots usually present on face, neck, scalp, back, and upper chest and may bleed when irritated by clothing or picked

C. Nursing assessment

    1. Acne

        a. Assessment

            1) Conduct a symptom analysis regarding onset, type of lesions, and distribution

            2) Types of cleansers, lubricants or moisturizers, and previous treatments and results

            3) In females, flare-ups of acne around menstrual cycle and use of oral contraceptives

            4) Skin exams to determine type of acne (mild, moderate, or severe) and document areas of involvement

            5) Determine grade of acne present

        b. Diagnostic tests: there are no diagnostic tests for acne; a culture may be taken to differentiate acne from other conditions if pustules are present

   2. Lentigo
      a. Assessment includes symptom analysis regarding onset, location, duration, color changes, and enlargement; ask client about sun exposure and use of sunscreens
      b. Diagnostic tests: may not require any tests, but a biopsy is suggested for any suspicious lesion
   3. Psoriasis
      a. Determine location, onset, and duration of plaques; inquire about previous treatments and results obtained; assess for any triggering factors such as emotional stress, trauma, or seasonal changes
      b. Diagnostic tests: skin biopsy may be needed to differentiate psoriasis from other conditions, or ultrasonography to measure skin thickness
   4. Seborrheic keratosis
      a. Determine location, onset, and duration of plaques; inquire about changes in lesion, erythema, or bleeding at site; assess client's sun exposure history and any treatments or interventions used in past
      b. Diagnostic tests: none specific

D. Nursing management
   1. Acne
      a. Medications
         1) Benzoyl peroxide preparations (over-the-counter, or OTC), which have an antibacterial, keratolytic, and drying effect
         2) Topical solutions such as clindamycin (Cleocin T solution), erythromycin (A/T/S or EryDerm), tetracycline (Topicycline), isotretinoin (Accutane), azelaic acid (Azelex), and tretinoin (Retinoic acid, Retin-A)
         3) Topical antibiotics may assist in decreasing formation of new lesions even though it is not an infection
         4) Many of these topical solutions are drying to skin; a small amount should be tested on a hidden area of skin first, before applying to entire face
         5) Most of these agents have side effect of photosensitivity; sun protection should be used
      b. Management is aimed at controlling disease and is not curative
      c. Instruct client to use a mild antibacterial soap, avoid cosmetics containing oil, and confine moisturizing lotions to dry patches of skin
      d. Instruct client not to pick at lesions, which could cause scarring
      e. Educate client that improvement may not be seen until treatment is used for 6–8 weeks
      f. Dietary factors have not been shown to affect sebum production, but client should be counseled on a well-balanced diet
   2. Lentigo
      a. Medications include tretinoin (Retinoic acid, Retin-A); however, no meds are necessarily required; cosmetics or bleaching solutions may be preferred by clients
      b. Instruct client on ABCDE method of assessing skin lesions: asymmetry, border, color, diameter, and elevation
      c. Teach client to inspect skin regularly and seek medical advice for any noted changes
      d. Instruct to use layered clothing while in sunlight and to use sunscreens with a sun protection factor (SPF) over 15
   3. Psoriasis
      a. Medications include topical corticosteroids and tar preparations to decrease inflammation and suppress mitotic activity of psoriasis, anthralin (Dithranol), and calcipotriene (Dovonex)

b. Photochemotherapy that involves drug methoxsalen and exposure to ultraviolet-A (UVA) rays has been effective in severe forms and promoting remission; hyper-keratosis is decreased with exposure to UVA and ultraviolet-B (UVB) light

c. Aveeno baths, tar shampoos, and wet dressings may help alleviate itching

d. Instruct client on use of moisturizing soaps, emollients, and scalp oils to soften scales followed by soft brushing while bathing

e. Instruct client about medication treatments and side effects

f. Emphasize that disorder is not contagious

g. Provide client with opportunity to discuss feelings regarding impact of disorder on client's life

h. Counsel client on importance of maintaining a healthy lifestyle, which includes a well-balanced diet, exercise, moderate alcohol intake, and avoidance of tobacco products

i. Discuss role of stress in relation to flare-ups of lesions

4. Seborrheic keratosis

a. Medication is usually not required; treatment is per client preference for cosmetic purposes

b. Educate client to use sunscreen with an SPF of 15 or higher, decrease sun exposure, avoid tanning, and wear hat and protective clothing while in sun

c. Provide assurance that lesions are benign in nature

d. Teach client ABCDE of skin lesions; assure client that treatment is not necessary unless requested for cosmetic purposes

Practice to Pass

A client has been diagnosed with acne. What self-care strategies should the nurse explain?

IV. BACTERIAL INFECTIONS OF SKIN

A. Overview

1. Defined as a break in skin integrity and invasion of a pathogenic organism

2. Disorders include impetigo, cellulitis, folliculitis; other lesions are furuncles (furunculosis) and carbuncles (carbunculosis)

3. May be primary (caused by one organism) or secondary (caused by disease process or trauma to skin)

4. Causes include poor hygiene, deficient nutrition, skin trauma, and excess moisture to skin; systemic diseases such as DM and malignancies may contribute to furuncles

B. Pathophysiology

1. **Impetigo** is a superficial skin infection initially seen as an erythemic vesicle and later changes to a honey-colored crusted lesion

   a. It is most commonly seen in 2- to 6-year-olds and may be enhanced by crowded living conditions, poor hygiene, and warm climates

   b. *Staphylococcus aureus* and *Streptococcus pyogenes* (beta-hemolytic) are most common organisms causing infection

   c. Impetigo is most often found on face, arms, legs, and buttocks

   d. Signs and symptoms include extreme itching and red, macular lesions

   e. Impetigo spreads quickly; therefore treatment should be started early

2. **Cellulitis** is a diffuse inflammation of skin and subcutaneous layers with various presenting lesions including vesicles (small sacs of fluid), bullae (large blisters), abscesses, and plaques

   a. Involved organisms usually are *Streptococcus*, *Haemophilus influenzae*, or *Staphylococcus aureus* (including methicillin-resistant strain called MRSA)

   b. There is usually a preceding wound or trauma to skin, even a minor skin scrape, and is most common in adults

   c. Signs and symptoms include erythema, warmth, edema, and pain; also frequently present are fever, chills, malaise, and lymphadenopathy

3. **Folliculitis** is an inflammation of hair follicle usually caused by *Staphylococcus aureus* or *Pseudomonas aeruginosa*
   a. It can occur at any age, occurs more in males, and is aggravated by shaving
   b. A stye is a folliculitis on eyelid
   c. Signs and symptoms include red lesions or erythemic pustules that can be painful
4. **Furuncles (furunculosis)**: a furuncle (abscess or boil) is a deep folliculitis consisting of a pus-filled mass that is painful and firm
   a. It is common in children, teens, and young adults
   b. It is caused by *Staphylococcus aureus* (including MRSA), and common sites of infection are nares, neck, axilla, and genital area
   c. Furunculosis is a condition resulting from multiple boils
   d. Signs and symptoms are deep, firm, red nodules that are painful and usually drain purulent secretions
5. **Carbuncles (carbunculosis)** are aggregates of infected follicles convalesced to form one large lesion
   a. Carbunculosis is a condition of several carbuncles
   b. Signs and symptoms include painful nodes with pus, chills, fever, and leukocytosis

C. **Nursing assessment**
1. Includes location, appearance (erythema, swelling, drainage), onset, and duration of lesions; symptom analysis of associated symptoms of fever, chills, and previous outbreaks; vital signs (VS); palpate surface of lesion and adjacent lymph nodes for fluctuance (fluid-filled); assess tetanus prophylaxis status
2. Diagnostic tests: wound culture and sensitivity (C&S) to identify organism and verify antibiotic choice

D. **Nursing management**
1. Medications include topical antibiotic ointments or oral antibiotics for 10–14 days; instruct on frequent use of antibacterial soaps for preventive therapy
2. Cleanse site with warm soapy water 2–3 times per day; avoid irritating lotions or creams
3. Use warm compresses for comfort
4. Instruct client to use a clean razor each time he or she shaves
5. Incision and drainage of lesion may be necessary

Practice to Pass

A client is being discharged home after hospitalization for cellulitis. What specific discharge instructions should be given?

V. VIRAL INFECTIONS OF SKIN

A. **Overview**
1. Conditions of skin resulting in a break in skin integrity and invasion of a virus or intracellular pathogen
2. Disorders include herpes simplex type 1 (HSV1), type 2 (HSV2), herpes zoster, molluscum contagiosum, and warts
3. Causes include drugs with immunosuppressive action such as corticosteroids, birth control pills, and antibiotics; stress and sunlight have been attributed to herpes simplex

B. **Pathophysiology**
1. **Herpes simplex** is a viral infection that occurs within keratinolytics and is manifested by painful vesicles that occur in clusters on skin (HSV1), also known as fever blister, or genital mucosa (HSV2)
   a. Virus transverses afferent nerves to host ganglion: trigeminal ganglia are target of HSV1 and usually affect lips, face, buccal mucosa, and throat
   b. Sacral ganglia is target for HSV2; it affects genital area and is considered a sexually transmitted infection (STI)
   c. Herpes simplex virus occurs in 3 stages: *primary*—initial outbreak of virus occurs as blisters; *latency*—virus remains dormant in ganglia; and *recurrent stage*—virus is reactivated, travels along peripheral nerves to site of initial infection, causing characteristic symptoms

      d. Transmission is by direct contact with active lesions or by virus-containing fluid such as saliva or cervical secretions with no evidence of active disease; incubation period is 2–14 days; recurrent infections may be triggered by skin trauma, stress, or illness

      e. Signs and symptoms include erythema, vesicles, discomfort (burning, tingling, or pain), fever, and sore throat; tenderness, pain, and burning may occur prior to eruption of lesions and may be associated with fever, myalgia, malaise, or cervical lymphadenopathy; HSV1 infections in infants and children usually appear as a gingivostomatitis with symptoms of pain in mouth and/or throat and may be accompanied by fever and malaise

  2. **Herpes zoster** is a viral infection (also known as shingles) that is manifested as a cluster of vesicles on skin that usually follows along a dermatome and is unilateral; vesicles may have purulent fluid in 3–4 days, then form crusts that fall off in 2–3 weeks

      a. It is a reactivation of varicella virus in dorsal root ganglia that remained in latent form after primary infection of chickenpox

      b. Signs and symptoms include erythematous lesions, itching, burning, and pain (may be severe); a complication is visual loss and severe pain along one of nerves; fever, headache, and malaise may precede rash

      c. It is commonly seen in older adults but can also affect children

  3. **Molluscum contagiosum** is a benign viral infection of skin characterized by white to flesh-colored, shiny dome-shaped papules with a firm, waxy appearance

      a. Is caused by poxvirus inducing epidermal cell proliferation, spreads by direct contact and has an incubation period of 2–7 weeks, and lasts as long as 6 months

      b. It is a common cutaneous manifestation in human immunodeficiency virus (HIV) infection

      c. Humans are the only known source; lesions occur in groups and are more common in children and adolescents but may affect all age groups

      d. Signs and symptoms include small, waxy, epithelial tumors that may be solid or semiliquid

  4. **Warts** are virus-induced epidermal tumors and are commonly seen in children and young adults

      a. Wart virus is located within epidermal layer proliferating from a mass

      b. They are transmitted by touch and often appear on hands, periungual regions, and plantar surfaces

      c. Most warts resolve in 12–24 months without treatment and are asymptomatic except for plantar warts, which may be very painful

      d. There are several types of warts: common (dome-shaped, above skin, scaly, irregular surface), filiform (thin projections on a narrow stalk usually on face), flat (flat-topped, skin-colored papules located on face and extremities), plantar (occur on weight-bearing surfaces of feet), and genital (considered an STI on glans of penis, anal region, and vulva)

      e. Signs and symptoms include lesions (round, raised, rough, and gray); genital warts are cauliflower in appearance

C. Nursing assessment

  1. Herpes simplex virus

      a. Assessment includes identifying clinical stage of disease; primary stage usually occurs 2–14 days after inoculation; lesions are usually grouped vesicles that may rupture, leaving erosions that form crusts; crusts signal end of viral shedding; ask about previous occurrences and exposures to infected persons

      b. Diagnostic tests: viral culture for most definitive diagnosis

2. Herpes zoster
   a. Assessment includes inquiring about prior varicella infection and immunocompromised status, examining skin for characteristic lesions, and determining ophthalmic involvement
   b. Diagnostic tests: Tzanck smear to identify herpes virus, culture of vesicles, and immunofluorescence to identify varicella
3. Molluscum contagiosum
   a. Assessment includes inquiring about location, appearance, onset, and duration of lesion, past medical history including HIV infection, examination of skin for lesions, and palpating lesions for firm or fluid-filled consistency
   b. No diagnostic tests are recommended
4. Warts
   a. Assessment includes identifying type of wart, onset, location, and duration of lesion, and about any previous treatments used
   b. No diagnostic tests are recommended
D. Nursing management
1. Herpes simplex
   a. Medications during primary stage of HSV1 include oral viscous xylocaine, Orabase, use of OTC products such as Blistex to prevent drying and acetaminophen (Tylenol) for pain; applying ice may help to reduce swelling
   b. Medications during recurrent stage of HSV1 or HSV2 include topical antiviral agents such as penciclovir (Denavir), which is not recommended for children, or acyclovir (Zovirax) ointment applied every 2 hours to speed healing and relieve pain; oral antivirals, such as acyclovir (Zovirax), valacyclovir (Valtrex), or famciclovir (Famvir), may be used in severe cases or for client who is immunocompromised and has persistent lesions
   c. Instruct client to use sunscreen to reduce number of outbreaks
   d. Instruct client about how to decrease spread of HSV to others
   e. Educate client to avoid sexual activity when active lesions are present and to use condoms with each sexual contact
2. Herpes zoster
   a. Medications include nonsteroidal anti-inflammatory drugs (NSAIDs) or acetaminophen (Tylenol) for pain and fever; wet compresses of Burow's solution or tap water for comfort; systemic therapy with acyclovir (Zovirax), vidarabine (Vira-A), and corticosteroids for clients when outbreak is less than 72 hours old or when over 72 hours old with newly developing lesions, when clients are over age 50, and for clients who are immunocompromised
   b. Suppression of pain, inflammation, and infection is goal of therapy
   c. Teach client about possibility of postherpetic pain (pain that persists more than one month after lesions have healed)
   d. Instruct on signs and symptoms of secondary bacterial infections, usually caused from scratching lesions, which are itchy
   e. Ophthalmic involvement requires emergency referral to an ophthalmologist
   f. Instruct to avoid clients who may be at risk for infection; such as neonates, pregnant women, and immunosuppressed persons, as well as those who have not previously had chickenpox
   g. Stress that follow-up in 1–3 days and then again in 7–10 days is necessary
   h. Educate client about disease and measures to maintain health
   i. Inform client that scarring at site of infection may occur
3. Molluscum contagiosum
   a. Medications include liquid nitrogen therapy (client preference), and Duofilm or tretinoin (Retin-A, Avita) for removal of lesions

Practice to Pass

A client has been diagnosed with herpes simplex type 2 (HSV2). What explanation should be given about this disease?

   b. Instruct client that these medications are to be used at bedtime; area should be exfoliated before reapplication and petroleum jelly applied to surrounding skin
   c. For a small number of asymptomatic lesions of molluscum contagiosum, observation for several months is indicated
4. Warts
   a. Medications include liquid nitrogen and topical preparations (acid therapy) to be used nightly for 6–8 weeks; instruct to apply petroleum ointment on surrounding skin to prevent irritation; OTC products for freezing warts are now available
   b. Most clients request treatment/removal of wart lesion; filiform wart is usually removed by curettage, cryotherapy, or electrodessication
   c. Instruct client about signs of infection after removal and pain relief measures if applicable
   d. Educate client that warts (because they are viral) may reappear in same site or on other areas of skin

VI. FUNGAL INFECTIONS OF SKIN

A. Overview
1. Defined as infections caused by fungi (dermatophytes), which are living organisms found on stratum corneum, hair, and nails
2. Include candidiasis, tinea versicolor, and dermatophyte infections; are named for area of body involved, including tinea capitis, tinea corporis, tinea cruris, tinea pedis, and tinea unguium
3. Causes include excess moisture, contact with an infected person or animal, use of broad-spectrum antibiotics, disorders such as DM, malnutrition, iron deficiency anemia, immunosuppressed states, pregnancy, and aging process

B. Pathophysiology
1. **Candidiasis** is an infection caused by *Candida albicans*, a yeast-like fungus that most often causes superficial cutaneous infections
   a. *Candida albicans* fungi are part of normal flora of skin and mucous membranes; overgrowth is caused when conditions such as moisture, warmth, and breaks in epidermal barrier occur
   b. Includes oral (thrush), vagina (vulvovaginitis), diaper area (perineal), glans and prepuce of penis (balantitis), nail folds (paronychia), perineal area, axilla, umbilical area, and under breasts
   c. Candida organisms may also be a causative agent in otitis externa and scalp disorders
   d. Signs and symptoms include lesions that are bright red, smooth macules with a macerated appearance and a scaling, elevated border
   e. Characteristic "satellite" lesions are small, similar-appearing macules outside main lesion; specific areas of body manifest as:
      1) Oral thrush: white, milky, nonremovable plaques on oral mucosa that may be associated with a burning sensation or decreased taste
      2) Vagina (vulvovaginitis): excessive itching and a thick, white, curdy vaginal discharge
      3) Perineal area (or diaper area in infant or young toddler): erythema, papules, pustules, and a scaling border
      4) Balanitis: flattened pustules, edema, scaling, erosion, burning, and tenderness on penis
      5) Paronychia: erythema, edema and tenderness with possible creamy, purulent discharge with pressure on nail bed; nails usually become discolored and have ridging

2. **Tinea versicolor** is a common noninflammatory fungal infection caused by lipophilic yeast and *Pityrosporum orbiculare* (part of normal flora of skin)
   a. Overgrowth occurs for unknown reasons; infection is not contagious
   b. Signs and symptoms include multiple small, circular macules of various colors (white, pink, or brown) usually on upper trunk, which are usually asymptomatic
3. **Dermatophyte** infections are caused by a group of fungi that are able to infect and survive only on keratin; they can affect all age groups
   a. These infections include tinea capitis (ringworm of scalp), tinea corporis (ringworm of body), tinea cruris (ringworm of groin and upper thighs), tinea pedis (ringworm of foot or athlete's foot, and tinea unguium (ringworm of nails or onychomycosis)
   b. Dermatophyte infections (tineas) have 3 causative agents: *Microsporum*, *Trichophyton*, or *Epidermophyton*
   c. Signs and symptoms
      1) Tinea capitis: erythema and scaling of scalp with patchy hair loss
      2) Tinea corporis: circular, erythematous, well-marginated lesions with a raised, scaly vesicular border
      3) Tinea cruris: lesions are sharply demarcated, scaling patches and usually extremely pruritic
      4) Tinea pedis: lesions are fine, vesiculopustular, or scaly areas that are usually itchy
      5) Tinea unguium: usually involves only 1–2 nails; toenails are affected more often than fingernails; characteristic features include distal thickening and yellowing of nail plate

C. **Nursing assessment**
1. Assessment
   a. Symptom analysis about onset, duration, distribution, and presence of symptoms
   b. Possible contact with others (including animals) with similar lesions
   c. Previous treatments used and results
   d. Any underlying chronic conditions and past or present medications
   e. Examination of skin to determine type and distribution of lesions and associated symptoms

2. Diagnostic tests: a culture of scraping (skin, hair, or nails) or microscopic exam of scaling using a 10% potassium hydrogen (KOH) preparation; a Wood's lamp, which uses ultraviolet (UV) light; area fluoresces blue-green in presence of a fungal infection

D. **Nursing management**
1. Medications

   a. Antifungals in various forms (creams, powders, shampoos, vaginal suppositories, and oral tablets): clotrimazole (Mycelex), nystatin (Mycostatin, Nilstat), miconazole (Monistat), undecylenic acid (Desenex), ketoconazole (Nizoral), fluconazole (Diflucan), and amphotericin B (Fungizone)
   b. Topical treatment is preferred, but some cases require oral medications such as miconazole (Monistat), nystatin (Nilstat), ketoconazole (Nizoral), and fluconazole (Diflucan)
   c. Systemic therapy is necessary for moderate to severe infection that occurs in immunocompromised persons
2. Instruct clients to avoid sharing linens or personal items
3. Instruct clients to dry all skin folds and use a clean towel and washcloth daily
4. For tinea pedis, put socks on before underwear to prevent spread of infection from feet; wear light cotton socks and change frequently; wear sandals or open-toed shoes when possible but avoid plastic footwear and occlusive shoes
5. Apply drying or dusting powders and topical antiperspirants to decrease moisture
6. For vaginal candida, avoid tight clothing and pantyhose, bathe frequently and dry genital area thoroughly; treatment of sexual partner may be necessary to avoid

Practice to Pass

A client returns to the clinic with recurrent tinea pedis. What should the client be told regarding preventive measures?

reinfection, or have partner use condoms until resolved; avoid douching and change perineal pads frequently

7. Reducing risk of fungal infections can occur with weight loss by clients who are obese and maintaining normal serum glucose levels in clients with diabetes to decrease risk of infection

8. Instruct clients that relief of symptoms may occur quickly with topical medication, but stress need to continue use for 7–10 days
9. Follow-up visits should be scheduled every 2–4 weeks for clients receiving long-term oral antifungal treatment to monitor liver function and complete blood count (CBC)

VII. INFESTATIONS AND INSECT BITES

A. Overview
1. Defined as an invasion of the skin by an insect or parasite
2. Disorders include common insect bites (stings) and pediculosis
3. Causes include living in infested areas and contact with an infected person or clothing/material

B. Pathophysiology
1. An insect sting or bite occurs when is secreted into skin by an insect or spider; arthropods affect many by being pests, inoculating poison, invading tissues, or transmitting disease
   a. Honeybees, wasps, hornets, and yellow-jackets embed a firm, sharp stinger in skin that injects venom, a protein with enzyme activity that causes local or general reactions classified as toxic or allergic (0.4% of reactions are allergic)
   b. There are many species of spiders, but brown recluse spider and black widow are 2 species capable of producing severe reactions
      1) Brown recluse spider is small, light brown, and lives in dark areas such as closets, basements, and under porches; bite can cause local or general reactions, even death; venom is equivalent to that of a rattlesnake
      2) Black widow bite resembles a pinprick, injecting a neurotoxin that causes an ascending motor paralysis; the potent toxin is rapidly absorbed, causing necrosis at site
   c. IgE-mediated hypersensitivity to insect venom may be confirmed by skin testing with suitable dilutions of available venom—usually done by an allergist
   d. Signs and symptoms
      1) Brown recluse spider: a large area of necrosis at site, pain, itching and swelling; after a week, area has extreme swelling with a raised white or black center (volcano appearing)
      2) Black widow spider: pain at site, which lasts only briefly, rigid abdominal muscles with extreme abdominal pain, and motor paralysis
      3) General reactions to insect bites: redness, itching, swelling, warmth, and extreme pain
      4) Systemic symptoms such as fever, chills, nausea, vomiting, and weakness may occur
      5) Anaphylactic reactions such as shortness of breath and wheezing may appear if client is allergic to sting
2. **Pediculosis** is an infestation of skin or hair by species of blood-sucking lice capable of living as external parasites on human host
   a. Pediculosis capitis is head louse, size of a sesame seed ranging in color from clear to red/brown
   b. Pediculosis pubis ("crabs") infests genital area and is a common STI; pubic lice can be spread by sexual contact

   c. Head lice are common among schoolchildren of all socioeconomic backgrounds and are spread by close contact as well as sharing combs, hats, and scarves

        d. *Scabies* is infestation of skin by mite Sarcoptes scabier hominis

            1) In scabies, fertilized female mite burrows into skin and remains there, laying 2–3 eggs per day

            2) Eggs hatch in 3–4 days, reach maturity in 4 days, migrate to skin surface, mate, and repeat cycle

            3) Scabies is more common among people who don't have access to bathing or laundry facilities; lice can live in clothing and be transmitted also by contact with infected clothing or bed linens

        e. Signs and symptoms

            1) Pediculosis corporis: macules, wheals, and papules, pruritus, excoriation from scratching; lines in skin folds are common, representing burrowing of mite; lesions may be erythematous papules or purplish nodules accompanied by raised burrows (threadlike linear ridges with a tiny black dot at one end)

            2) Pediculosis pubis: pruritus, irritation of genital area, and blue- or slate-colored macules

            3) Pediculosis capitis: itching, eczematous dermatitis, inflammation caused by scratching, pustules, crusts, matted, odorous hair

C. Nursing assessment

    1. Insect stings and bites

        a. Assessment includes symptom analysis regarding type of bite or sting, when it occurred, and location of bite or sting; assess for anaphylactic reactions and refer for immediate treatment; assess site for symptoms specific to type of bite

        b. Diagnostic tests: there are no tests indicated unless a severe allergic reaction is noted; a CBC and IgE may be performed if necessary

    2. Pediculosis

        a. Assessment

            1) Questions about intense pruritis (most common symptom)

            2) Appearance: head lice may resemble dandruff flakes; however, they are not easily brushed off because nits cling to hair shafts

            3) A papular urticaria, which may be present at neck or pubic area

            4) Severity of itching: nocturnal itching, which is a classic symptom of scabies, as well as itching during exposure to hot water or steam

            5) Inquire about onset of symptoms; client becomes itchy approximately 10–14 days after exposure

        b. Diagnostic tests: skin scraping of scabies nodule may reveal portions of mite, but clinical diagnosis is usually made by presentation

D. Nursing management

    1. Insect stings and bites

        a. Medications include local analgesics such as ibuprofen and antihistamines such as diphenhydramine (Benadryl) that are used for mild reactions; epinephrine 1:1000 or an Epi–pen may be used for mild symptoms also

        b. Outpatient or inpatient treatment for stings and bites depends on client response

            1) First aid treatment may include removal of stinger by scraping; do not squeeze or use tweezers; then clean wound

            2) Apply ice packs to bite, 10 minutes on/10 minutes off

            3) Elevate affected part, maintain adequate airway, and transport to emergency facility if warranted

            4) Wound from a brown recluse spider should not be opened but cleansed daily and allowed to erupt on its own

        c. If history suggests a severe anaphylactic reaction, initiate emergency treatment immediately and transport to local emergency department; if client is stable, assess client's vital signs and examine site for erythema and edema

   d. Educate client to prevent reexposure and about risks of increasing severity of responses in future

   e. Instruct client to use insect repellants when outdoors or in infected areas

   f. For clients allergic to insect bites, an Epi-pen should be available at all times; educate on its proper use if prescribed

   g. Client may need referral for allergy testing if a mild to severe anaphylactic reaction occurs

   h. For sensitive individuals, a medical alert tag should be obtained and worn at all times

2. Pediculosis

   a. Medications to kill nits include lindane (Kwell), gamma benzene hexachloride, malathion (Prioderm lotion) or permithrin (NIX), corticosteroids for itching, and antibiotics as needed for infections

   b. Nits on hair must be mechanically removed

   c. Instruct client as to proper way to treat condition; some medications such as NIX take only 1 treatment, while others (Lindane) take 2 treatments, 7 days apart in order to kill eggs; advise that olive oil or a solution of 50 parts white vinegar to 50 parts water may loosen nits

   d. Educate clients about mode of transmission (person to person) and preventive measures such as not sharing personal items

   e. Instruct client/family to machine wash all washable clothing and dry in a hot dryer at least 20 minutes; upholstered furniture, pillows, and stuffed animals may be ironed with a hot iron or vacuumed

   f. Stress importance that all family members must be treated at same time

VIII. ALLERGIC CONDITIONS OF SKIN

A. Overview

1. Allergic conditions cause inflammation (dermatitis) as a result of contact with an allergen, infection, or disease; these can be acute or chronic

2. Disorders include contact dermatitis, atopic dermatitis, seborrheic dermatitis, exfoliative dermatitis, and urticaria

3. Causes include plants such as poison oak, poison sumac, or poison ivy; harsh chemicals; dyes; perfumes; latex gloves; metals; insecticides; soaps; detergents; foods; drugs such as methyldopa for hypertension, diseases such as AIDS, leukemia, and lymphoma; transfusion reactions; insect bites or stings; heat; cold; stress; sunlight; and serum sickness

B. Pathophysiology

1. **Contact dermatitis** is an eruption of skin related to contact with an irritating substance or allergen (see Box 14-2); it is a type IV hypersensitivity reaction

   a. *Irritant contact dermatitis* affects clients exposed to specific irritants producing an immediate response

   b. *Allergic contact dermatitis* is an allergic reaction mediated by IgE and affects only those previously sensitized to irritant, thus it is a delayed hypersensitivity reaction; a sensitizing antigen is formed on initial contact, which is taken to T cells; these T cells become sensitized; on subsequent exposures, skin reactions will occur (see Figure 14-1)

   c. Location of rash helps provide clues about offending agent

   d. Signs and symptoms of acute contact dermatitis may include papules, vesicles, bullae with surrounding erythema; crusting, oozing, and pruritis; chronic contact dermatitis may present with an erythematous base, thickening of skin, scaling, and fissuring

Box 14-2	
Common Causes of Contact Dermatitis	• Acids

Box 14-2

Common Causes of Contact Dermatitis

- Acids
- Alkalis: soaps, detergents, household ammonia, lye, cleaners
- Bromide
- Chlorine
- Coloring agents
- Cosmetics: perfumes, dyes, oils
- Dusts of lime, arsenic, wood
- Hydrocarbons: crude petroleum, lubricating oil, mineral oil, paraffin, asphalt, tar
- Iodine
- Insecticides
- Fabrics: wool, polyester, dyes, sizing
- Metal salts: calcium chloride, zinc chloride, copper, mercury, nickel, silver
- Plants: ragweed, poison oak, poison ivy, poison sumac, pine
- Rubber products
- Soot

Source: LeMone, Priscilla; Burke, Karen M.; Bauldoff, Gerene, *Medical-Surgical Nursing: Critical Thinking In Patient Care*, 5th Ed., © 2011. Reprinted and Electronically reproduced by permission of Pearson Education, Inc., Upper Saddle River, New Jersey.

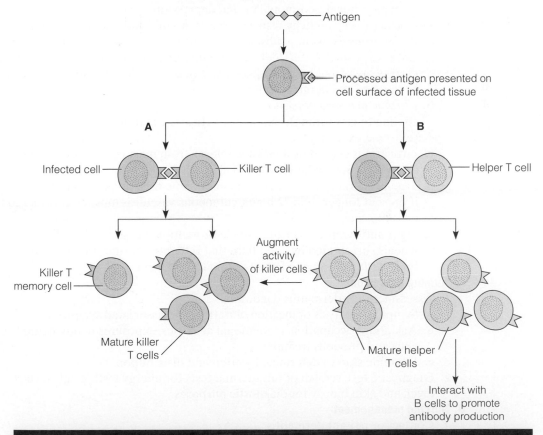

Figure 14-1

An antigen binds with a killer T cell or helper T cell in order to remember the event through the development of memory T cells or antibody production through B cells

2. **Atopic dermatitis** (eczema) is a common inflammatory skin disorder of unknown cause and is seen frequently with children and adults
   a. A cell-mediated immunity, excess sensitivity to histamine, and increased levels of IgE are related to this disorder; initiation of immune response triggers an inflammatory reaction
   b. Condition has allergic, heredity, and/or psychological components
   c. A complication is secondary infection
   d. Signs and symptoms include erythema, scaling, pruritis, and lesions on hands, feet, arms, and legs
3. **Seborrheic dermatitis** is an acute inflammatory condition with an unknown cause
   a. It affects scalp (cradle cap), forehead, postauricular regions, eyebrows, eyelashes, nasolabial folds, axillary, and genital areas; all ages can be affected
   b. Signs and symptoms include yellow or white plaques that may scale, crusts with a greasy appearance, pruritus, oozing, and loss of hair
4. **Exfoliative dermatitis** is an inflammation of skin characterized by erythema involving loss of exfoliated (peeling) skin
   a. Local and systemic effects may occur and have either an unknown cause or may be associated with other diseases or causes
   b. A complication of the generalized form is debilitation, dehydration, and secondary infection
   c. Signs and symptoms
      1) Local effects: scaling, erythema, pruritus, loss of hair and nails
      2) Systemic effects: weakness, malaise, hypothermia or fever, lymphadenopathy, hepatomegaly, eosinophilia, and depression
5. **Urticaria** (hives): an itchy rash with raised wheals that may be recurrent
   a. *Acute urticaria* usually subsides over several hours; examples include solar urticaria (exposure to sun), delayed pressure urticaria (produced by pressure, occurs after delay of 1–4 hours), aquagenic urticaria (ordinary water), and occurs because of an allergic reaction
   b. *Chronic urticaria* persists over 6 weeks; examples include cold urticaria (from cooling to rewarming), cholinergic urticaria (heat urticaria), and induced urticaria (extreme exercise)
   c. Urticaria is caused by a massive release from mast cells in superficial layers of skin and is a vascular reaction of skin
   d. True urticaria lesions do not remain in same area longer than 24 hours; if present longer than 72 hours, cutaneous vasculitis must be considered a possible cause
   e. Signs and symptoms include single or multiple areas of raised, blanched central wheals surrounded by a red flare that is highly pruritic; it may occur anywhere on body with size ranging from 1–2 mm to 15–20 cm

C. **Nursing assessment**
   1. Assessment for dermatitis conditions
      a. Symptom analysis of location, duration, and associated symptoms
      b. Ask about occupation, recreational activities, exposures to any irritants or allergens and previous treatments
      c. Examine skin to determine location and distribution
   2. Diagnostic test: scratch or intradermal tests for allergy testing, IgE level, eosinophil level, and skin biopsy for diagnostic purposes

D. **Nursing management**
   1. Contact or irritant dermatitis
      a. Medications include aluminum acetate for drying, antihistamines or calamine lotion for pruritus, cortisone if needed, and topical emollients

b. First step in managing contact or irritant dermatitis is to identify and remove causative agent
   c. Wet dressings and oatmeal baths may aid in alleviating oozing and pruritic lesions
   d. Instruct client on signs and symptoms of secondary bacterial infections
2. Atopic dermatitis
   a. Medications include antihistamines, softening lotions, cortisone lotion, and oral antibiotics if needed
   b. Instruct client to avoid soaps, ointment, and excessive bathing; bath oils may help soften skin
   c. Clothing should be of a soft texture and wool should be avoided
   d. Clip fingernails to decrease damage while scratching
3. Seborrheic dermatitis
   a. Medications include selenium containing shampoos, keratolytic agents, topical and systemic cortisone lotions
   b. Frequent shampooing is suggested if on scalp
   c. Scrupulous skin hygiene and keeping skin dry is imperative
4. Exfoliative dermatitis
   a. Medications include corticosteroids, emollients, and antihistamines
   b. Treatment is same as for contact dermatitis
5. Urticaria
   a. Medications include antihistamines to reduce itching and prevent prolonged symptoms; corticosteroids may be used for pressure urticaria and topical sunscreens are recommended for solar urticaria
   b. If urticaria occurred as a result of an allergic reaction, stress that possible life-threatening reactions may occur on reexposure
   c. Recommend cool moist compresses to help control itching, increasing fluids and use of skin lubricants, and avoidance of harsh soaps, frequent bathing, and products with alcohol
   d. Referrals to an allergist or dermatologist should be considered for unresolved itching

IX. BURNS

A. Overview
1. **Burns** are defined as interruptions in skin integrity resulting in tissue loss or injury caused by heat, chemicals, electricity, or radiation
2. A superficial-thickness burn involves a minimal depth of skin and is limited to outer skin layer (epidermis)
3. Superficial- and deep partial-thickness burns involve damage extending through epidermis and into dermis; regeneration of epidermis is not impaired
4. A full-thickness burn involves epidermis and dermis with damage into underlying tissue
5. Causes include thermal, chemical, electrical, and radiation
   a. *Thermal burns* result from dry heat (flames) or moist heat (steam or hot liquids) and are the most common type of burn; they cause cellular destruction that results in vascular, bony, muscle, or nerve complications
   b. *Chemical burns* are caused by direct contact with either acidic or alkaline agents; they destroy tissue perfusion, leading to necrosis
   c. *Electrical burns* follow path of least resistance (muscles-bones-blood vessels-nerves); severity of burn depends on type and duration of current and amount of voltage; electrical burns include sources such as direct current, alternating current, and lightning

 d. A *radiation burn* is usually associated with sunburn or radiation treatment for cancer; it is usually superficial; extensive exposure may lead to tissue damage and multisystem involvement

B. Pathophysiology

1. A burn from any source is a major insult to body, interrupting skin integrity (which could lead to infection) as well as causing many systemic effects
2. Within several hours, capillary integrity is lost due to release of several mediators of inflammation, primarily histamine and prostaglandin, which are vasodilators
3. Fluid passes from intravascular system (causing hypotension) to interstitial system (causing massive edema)
4. Fluid begins to shift back within 24–48 hours and intravascular overload then becomes a concern
5. Loss of intravascular volume causes an increased blood viscosity (with a risk for clots), decreased cardiac output (possibly leading to shock or pulmonary congestion), decreased renal blood flow (causing hypoxia and decreased urinary output), and renin-angiotensin-aldosterone (RAA) system activation to increase volume, which leads to retention of sodium and water and further edema
6. Cells cannot maintain adequate electrolyte shifts and results in excess intracellular sodium, excess extracellular potassium, and shifts in magnesium and phosphorus, which can lead to cardiac dysrhythmias and altered central nervous system function
7. Cortisol is released because of stress and depresses immune system, which intensifies risk for infection
8. Sympathetic nervous system is activated, increasing metabolic rate and oxygen demands; this hypermetabolism, increased energy needed for healing, and release of cortisol and epinephrine lead to a breakdown of tissue, protein metabolism, and fat wasting
9. Glucose is released as a result of stress and causes hyperglycemia
10. Complications are numerous (see Table 14-1)
11. Signs and symptoms
    a. Superficial-thickness burn: skin erythema; may be tender and blanches under pressure
    b. Partial-thickness burn: skin is red and blistered and very tender or painful; appearance may vary depending on whether burn is superficial partial thickness or deep partial thickness; deeper burns begin to resemble full-thickness burns
    c. Full-thickness burn: skin is tough and leathery but not tender; may also appear waxy or pearly white

Table 14-1   **Complications of Burns**

System	Major Complication
Immune	Infection with *Staphylococcus aureus* or methicillin resistant *staphylococcus aureus* (MRSA), septic shock
Cardiovascular	Blood clots leading to stroke or myocardial infarction, heart failure, cardiac arrest, pulmonary edema
Gastrointestinal	Peptic ulcer (decreased blood flow to gut), impaction
Respiratory	Acute respiratory distress syndrome (ARDS), lung damage if inhalation, hypoxia
Hematological	Burn shock, disseminated intravascular coagulopathy (DIC), anemia
Renal	Oliguria, renal failure
Fluids and electrolytes	First 24–48 hours: hyponatremia, hypokalemia, hypoproteinemia, hypochloremia After 24–48 hours: hypernatremia, hyperkalemia, hypovolemic shock, and dehydration

C. Nursing assessment
  1. Assessment
     a. A symptom analysis of cause of burn, time occurred, past medical history, and present medications and allergies
     b. Overall general appearance for distress and amount of pain
     c. Depth of burn
     d. Extent of the burn (% total body surface area or TBSA) using Rule of Nines (see Figure 14-2)
     e. Cardiac status, respiratory status, airway patency, and hydration status; airway status is essential whenever burn has capability of compromising airway because of edema (note singed eyebrows, nasal hair, or eyelashes; note soot; edema will peak 24–48 hours postinjury)
     f. Keep in mind possibilities of abuse and neglect; inquire about past injuries and burns
  2. Diagnostic tests: Rule of Nines to estimate burn size; blood urea nitrogen (BUN), creatinine clearance, urine output, urinalysis to avoid shock; CBC, electrolytes, albumin, bilirubin, alkaline phosphatase, arterial blood gases (ABGs), type and cross-match, CXR, electrocardiogram; C&S (if indicated); pulmonary function tests

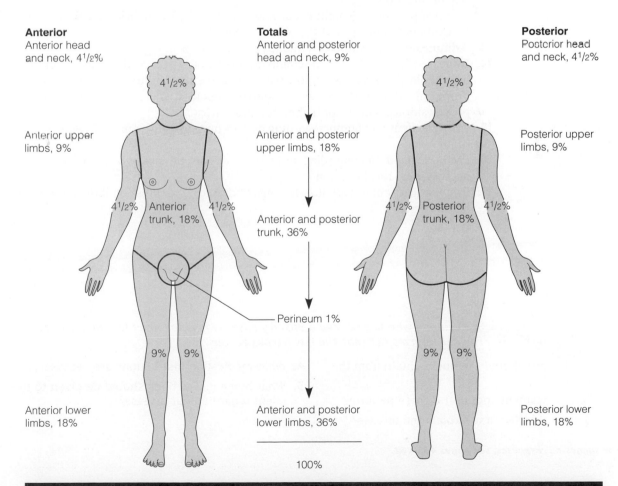

Anterior
Anterior head and neck, 4^1/$_2$%

Anterior upper limbs, 9%

Anterior trunk, 18%

Anterior lower limbs, 18%

Totals
Anterior and posterior head and neck, 9%

Anterior and posterior upper limbs, 18%

Anterior and posterior trunk, 36%

Perineum 1%

Anterior and posterior lower limbs, 36%

100%

Posterior
Posterior head and neck, 4^1/$_2$%

Posterior upper limbs, 9%

Posterior trunk, 18%

Posterior lower limbs, 18%

Figure 14-2

The "Rule of Nines" is a method of quickly estimating the percentage of total body surface area of the burn injury

D. Nursing management

1. Medications include opioid and/or nonopioid analgesics for pain, sedatives, tetanus booster (if not current), antibiotics, antacids or H_2-receptor blockers, topical antimicrobials such as silver nitrate, silver sulfadiazine, polysporin, and so on
2. Remove all rings and jewelry to avoid a tourniquet effect on affected site
3. Flush a chemical burn copiously with water and apply cool compresses; remove affected clothing and cover area with a dry sheet
4. Administer oxygen if necessary for any type of burn
5. Maintain proper hydration; encourage high-protein, high-calorie diet; monitor intake and output
6. For superficial-thickness burns, topical anesthetic creams or spray may be used several times a day to relieve pain and no dressings are needed
7. For partial-thickness burns, leave blisters intact
8. Small burns may be covered with antibiotic ointment and a nonadherent dressing to absorb drainage
9. For larger burns, cover area with silver sulfadiazine 1% as prescribed, and apply a nonadherent dressing covered by a bulky dressing to absorb any drainage
10. Full-thickness burns will not heal on their own and require skin grafting
11. Use meticulous sterile technique (and possibly protective isolation) to decrease risk of infection
12. Monitor pain management needs and treat pain before debriding episodes or hydrotherapy, and around-the-clock if needed
13. Administer tetanus toxoid if tetanus prophylaxis is not up to date
14. Educate client on use of sunscreens, accessing electrical cords/outlets, isolating household chemicals, use of low temperature setting for hot water heater, use and proper maintenance of household smoke detectors, risks of smoking in bed, and proper storage and use of flammable substances
15. Instruct client and family regarding care of burn at home, and signs and symptoms of infection
16. Evaluate need for counseling and family support, physical, vocational, or occupational rehabilitation
17. Encourage client to verbalize feelings of despair or depression if disfigurement has occurred

Case Study

The client is an 80-year-old woman who has noticed a blistery rash on her abdomen for the past several days. The health care provider informs her that she has herpes zoster.

1. What history should the nurse obtain from the client?
2. What assessment should the nurse perform?
3. How should the nurse explain the disease?
4. What medication instructions are necessary?
5. What home instructions should be given to the client regarding her disease?

For suggested responses, see pages 466–467.

POSTTEST

1. A 19-year-old female noticed severe itching under her waistband and in her axillae for several days. She thinks she has been bitten by something because she can feel a line of small bumps at the sites. The nurse suspects which condition based on this assessment data?
   1. Insect bites
   2. Herpes zoster
   3. Scabies
   4. Pediculosis capitis

2. A 23-year-old male presents with a pustular inflammation of his anterior neck and under his chin. Which of the following would the nurse recommend as an important management strategy?
   1. Squeeze the pustules periodically.
   2. Keep the area moist.
   3. Change razors each time he shaves.
   4. Decrease fat in the diet.

3. A client asks the nurse in the dermatologist's office about what characteristics folliculitis, furunculosis, and carbunculosis all have in common. The nurse makes which reply regarding all 3 disorders?
   1. "They are viral infections involving the epidermal layer of the skin."
   2. "They are fungal infections caused by poor hygiene."
   3. "They are bacterial infections that are highly contagious."
   4. "They are bacterial infections involving the hair follicles."

4. A 2-year-old child developed crusted lesions on her chin within the past 3 days. They started as a single blister that broke, discharging a honey-colored liquid that became a "stuck-on" crust. New blisters and crusts have been forming in the adjacent skin area. The nurse determines that this clinical picture is consistent with which of the following?
   1. Impetigo
   2. Scabies
   3. Herpes simplex
   4. Contact dermatitis

5. The nurse would include which of the following in client teaching regarding psoriasis? Select all that apply.
   1. The disease cannot be transmitted by skin-to-skin contact.
   2. It is important to keep the skin areas dry.
   3. Medications can be tried, but none bring about any improvement.
   4. Topical emollients, coal tar products, and corticosteroids soften and help remove the plaques.
   5. There is no cure for psoriasis; the goal of treatment is to suppress the symptoms.

6. A client presents to the clinic with thick, silver-white scaly patches over reddened skin. The client expresses fear of skin cancer, since it appears as skin sores that do not heal. What is the nurse's best therapeutic response?
   1. "You can stop worrying right away. You just have psoriasis."
   2. "You do not have cancer. You have herpes zoster, also called shingles, which can be treated with medications."
   3. "Impetigo can look like that. Try to manage your anxiety until the biopsy and cultures confirm a diagnosis."
   4. "It looks more like psoriasis. Can you tell me what you know about psoriasis?"

7 The nurse is staffing a booth on skin assessment at a community health fair and has provided a handout with the ABCDE acronym for early diagnosis of malignant melanoma. The nurse concludes that an attendee is not reading the handout correctly after the attendee states which acronym?

1. A — Area of sun-exposed skin — check the face, hands, arms, and back
2. B — Border irregular — not round
3. C — Color variegated — black and brown
4. D — Diameter greater than 6 mm — ¼ inch

8 A man sustained burns to the arms and chest when a fire got out of control in a campground. A fellow nurse camper immediately removes jewelry from the affected burn site to accomplish which priority objective?

1. Be able to assess the fingers more accurately
2. Prevent a tourniquet effect at the site
3. Prevent infection
4. Avoid interference with first aid treatment of the burn

9 The nurse working at a summer camp on a hot, humid day notes that a group of 9- and 10-year-old children are playing a baseball game. The nurse determines that the children are at risk for dehydration and which of the following conditions?

1. Skin cancer
2. Formation of nevi
3. Full-thickness skin burns
4. Superficial-thickness skin burns

10 When evaluating a client with a new pigmented skin lesion, the nurse would place highest priority on asking the client about which of the following?

1. Whether any new foods have been introduced into the diet
2. What cosmetics or skin products are being used
3. Sun tanning habits
4. History of food or environmental allergies

➤ *See pages 374–375 for Answers and Rationales.*

POSTTEST

ANSWERS & RATIONALES

Pretest

1 **Answer: 1, 4** **Rationale:** Emollients will ease the problem of dry skin that increases pruritus and causes the psoriasis to be worse. Certain medications, such as beta-blockers, indomethacin, and lithium, are known to precipitate exacerbations of psoriasis. Follow-up appointments are not crucial to management. Clients with psoriasis should be encouraged to use only electric razors. Constant occlusion may increase the effects of the medication and increase the risk of infection. **Cognitive Level:** Applying **Client Need:** Health Promotion and Maintenance **Integrated Process:** Nursing Process: Implementation **Content Area:** Adult Health **Strategy:** This is not a life-threatening problem needing close medical supervision. Choose the option that best strengthens the self-care, which is what the question is asking. **Reference:** LeMone, P., Burke, K., & Bauldoff, G. (2011). *Medical-surgical nursing: Critical thinking in patient care* (5th ed.). Upper Saddle River, NJ: Pearson Education, Inc., pp. 408–409.

2 **Answer: 2** **Rationale:** In order to plan the appropriate management of contact/irritant dermatitis, the cause of the inflammation should be identified. Removal of the cause may be all the treatment needed. Antihistamines and hydrocortisone creams are treatment options. Skin testing may be helpful to determine the allergen if not evident in the history. **Cognitive Level:** Applying **Client Need:** Physiological Adaptation **Integrated Process:** Teaching and Learning **Content Area:** Adult Health **Strategy:** The critical word in the question is *first step*. This is an allergic condition and the problem is contact with the skin. The answer is almost common sense. **Reference:** LeMone, P., Burke, K., & Bauldoff, G. (2011). *Medical-surgical nursing: Critical thinking in patient care* (5th ed.). Upper Saddle River, NJ: Pearson Education, Inc., pp. 419–420.

3 **Answer: 2** **Rationale:** Lice are transmitted by direct contact with infested persons or by sharing hats, brushes, or combs of infected persons. Classrooms are excellent areas for close contact, and children often do not know when other classmates have lice. Head lice can occur across socioeconomic boundaries, are not an airborne infestation, and is not the result of improper hair washing. **Cognitive Level:** Applying **Client Need:** Safety and Infection Control **Integrated Process:** Nursing Process: Assessment

ANSWERS & RATIONALES

Content Area: Child Health **Strategy:** Apply knowledge of the spread and incidence of pediculosis by recalling that direct contact is needed or through fomites such as inanimate objects. **Reference:** LeMone, P., Burke, K., & Bauldoff, G. (2011). *Medical-surgical nursing: Critical thinking in patient care* (5th ed.). Upper Saddle River, NJ: Pearson Education, Inc., pp. 414–415.

4 Answer: 1, 3, 5 Rationale: Melanoma is more common in light-skinned persons who work indoors and have sun exposure on weekends and vacations. Severe blistering sunburn as a child and intermittent sun exposure increases the susceptibility as adults. Sun exposure is a significant risk, but other risk factors such as atypical moles, immunosuppression, and tanning salons contribute to the problem. Episodic intense sun exposure is more damaging than constant exposure. Having a close relative with the disease is a risk factor. **Cognitive Level:** Applying **Client Need:** Health Promotion and Maintenance **Integrated Process:** Teaching and Learning **Content Area:** Adult Health **Strategy:** The choices are between light- and dark-skinned persons and regular or intermittent sun exposure. With options that contain 2 or more parts, all parts must be correct for the answer to be right. **Reference:** LeMone, P., Burke, K., & Bauldoff, G. (2011). *Medical-surgical nursing: Critical thinking in patient care* (5th ed.). Upper Saddle River, NJ: Pearson Education, Inc., p. 428.

5 Answer: 4 Rationale: There is no sensation of pain to light touch in full-thickness burns because the pain and touch receptors have been destroyed. There may not be pain with some deep partial thickness burns, but the appearance described is characteristic of full thickness. Superficial-thickness burns resemble sunburn and are painful, while superficial partial-thickness burns are likely to be reddened and accompanied by blistering and pain. **Cognitive Level:** Applying **Client Need:** Physiological Adaptation **Integrated Process:** Nursing Process: Assessment **Content Area:** Adult Health **Strategy:** Determine the classification of the burn from the assessment data given. Specific nursing knowledge is needed to answer the question, so review this material if the question was difficult. **Reference:** LeMone, P., Burke, K., & Bauldoff, G. (2011). *Medical-surgical nursing: Critical thinking in patient care* (5th ed.). Upper Saddle River, NJ: Pearson Education, Inc., pp. 449–450.

6 Answer: 3 Rationale: A burn involving the face, neck, or chest may cause airway closure because of the edema that occurs within hours. For this reason the nurse needs to assess the patency of the client's airway. The nurse will also assess skin integrity, blood pressure and pulse, and pain, but these are not the highest priority assessments when the airway is threatened. **Cognitive Level:** Analyzing **Client Need:** Physiological Adaptation **Integrated Process:** Nursing Process: Assessment **Content Area:** Child Health **Strategy:** Prioritize and assess for the most life threatening problem first. Remember the ABCs: airway, breathing, and circulation. Airway always comes first,

even before pain. **Reference:** LeMone, P., Burke, K., & Bauldoff, G. (2011). *Medical-surgical nursing: Critical thinking in patient care* (5th ed.). Upper Saddle River, NJ: Pearson Education, Inc., p. 455.

7 Answer: 4 Rationale: Pediculosis capitis is head lice, and nits are cemented to the hair shaft. They are most commonly seen on hair on the back of the head near the nape of the neck. A papular excoriation may be present at the nape of the neck secondary to scratching. Tinea capitis is a fungal infection of the scalp. Dandruff flakes come off the hair easily. Seborrheic dermatitis manifests with dandruff and erythema of the scalp, as well as of the eyebrow and eyelids. **Cognitive Level:** Applying **Client Need:** Physiological Adaptation **Integrated Process:** Nursing Process: Diagnosis **Content Area:** Child Health **Strategy:** The data described is characteristic of a common parasitic infestation. Read the question again carefully for clues. **Reference:** LeMone, P., Burke, K., & Bauldoff, G. (2011). *Medical-surgical nursing: Critical thinking in patient care* (5th ed.). Upper Saddle River, NJ: Pearson Education, Inc., pp. 415–420.

8 Answer: 3 Rationale: Hives and shortness of breath suggest a systemic response to the sting, and this client should be watched very carefully for anaphylaxis, and immediate treatment should be administered. The client who has never been stung should be monitored closely. Fever and chills suggest infection, not hypersensitivity reaction. Pain often causes the blood pressure to rise. **Cognitive Level:** Analyzing **Client Need:** Physiological Adaptation **Integrated Process:** Nursing Process: Diagnosis **Content Area:** Adult Health **Strategy:** Remember that insect venom can cause a type I hypersensitivity reaction. Sometimes these are life threatening. Look for an option with this potential. **Reference:** LeMone, P., Burke, K., & Bauldoff, G. (2011). Medical-surgical nursing: Critical thinking in patient care (5th ed.). Upper Saddle River, NJ: Pearson Education, Inc., pp. 308–309.

9 Answer: 2 Rationale: Candidiasis (oral thrush) often develops as a result of the overgrowth of fungal organisms after a client has been on an antibiotic. This side effect is a "superinfection" growth of nonsusceptible organisms. Impetigo is a bacterial infection of the skin. Burns do not produce plaque. Herpes is a viral infection that presents with blistering lesions. **Cognitive Level:** Applying **Client Need:** Physiological Adaptation **Integrated Process:** Nursing Process: Assessment **Content Area:** Adult Health **Strategy:** The history of 2 antibiotics is a clue to the new problem. **Reference:** LeMone, P., Burke, K., & Bauldoff, G. (2011). Medical-surgical nursing: Critical thinking in patient care (5th ed.). Upper Saddle River, NJ: Pearson Education, Inc., p. 413.

10 Answer: 1, 2, 3, 5 Rationale: Viral infections cause warts, which appear in many types. Common warts grow above the skin surface and have rough, ragged borders. Warts may resolve spontaneously; this may take up to 5 years. Warts can be transmitted through skin contact and any age person can get them (not only during childhood).

Cognitive Level: Applying Client Need: Physiological Adaptation Integrated Process: Teaching and Learning Content Area: Adult Health Strategy: Read the options carefully. An absolute word (*only*) makes one possibility incorrect. Reference: LeMone, P., Burke, K., & Bauldoff, G. (2011). *Medical-surgical nursing: Critical thinking in patient care* (5th ed.). Upper Saddle River, NJ: Pearson Education, Inc., pp. 415–416.

Posttest

1 **Answer: 3** **Rationale:** Scabies, a parasitic infection caused by a mite, presents with small red-brown burrows (bumps in a line) that produce intense itching. Insect bites do not generally fall in a line. Herpes zoster lesions follow the dermatome; they do not appear at the waistband or axillae. Head lice do not cause "lines" of bumps, and infect only the scalp area. **Cognitive Level:** Analyzing **Client Need:** Physiological Adaptation **Integrated Process:** Nursing Process: Diagnosis **Content Area:** Adult Health **Strategy:** Analyze all the data given and consider the expected manifestations with each of the options. One infestation fits the description. **Reference:** LeMone, P., Burke, K., & Bauldoff, G. (2011). *Medical-surgical nursing: Critical thinking in patient care* (5th ed.). Upper Saddle River, NJ: Pearson Education, Inc. pp. 414–415.

2 **Answer: 3** **Rationale:** Folliculitis is an inflammation of the hair follicle caused by infection, chemical irritants, or injury, including shaving. It is most commonly caused by *Staphylococcus aureus*. Using a clean razor each time he shaves will decrease the risk of reinfection. Pustules should not be squeezed. Moist areas are a place for folliculitis to develop. Poor nutrition, but not fat specifically, is a contributing factor. **Cognitive Level:** Applying **Client Need:** Health Promotion and Maintenance **Integrated Process:** Nursing Process: Implementation **Content Area:** Adult Health **Strategy:** Pustules indicate infection. Choose an option that fits the gender given in the question. **Reference:** LeMone, P., Burke, K., & Bauldoff, G. (2011). *Medical-surgical nursing: Critical thinking in patient care* (5th ed.). Upper Saddle River, NJ: Pearson Education, Inc., p. 410.

3 **Answer: 4** **Rationale:** All 3 diagnoses are a bacterial infection of the skin arising from the hair follicle, where bacteria can accumulate, grow, and cause a localized infection. They are not highly contagious and they are not associated with viral or fungal infections. **Cognitive Level:** Applying **Client Need:** Physiological Adaptation **Integrated Process:** Teaching and Learning **Content Area:** Adult Health **Strategy:** Determine the causative agent, and eliminate the options that have the incorrect etiology. **Reference:** LeMone, P., Burke, K., & Bauldoff, G. (2011). *Medical-surgical nursing: Critical thinking in patient care* (5th ed.). Upper Saddle River, NJ: Pearson Education, Inc. pp. 410–411.

4 **Answer: 1** **Rationale:** Impetigo is an infection of the skin typically beginning with a vesicle or pustule. The lesion ruptures, leaving an open area that discharges a honey-colored serous liquid that hardens into a crust. Impetigo spreads quickly if not treated. Scabies presents as pruritic, red-brown burrows. Herpes simplex presents with clusters of open lesions. Contact dermatitis results from contact with an allergen. **Cognitive Level:** Applying **Client Need:** Physiological Adaptation **Integrated Process:** Nursing Process: Diagnosis **Content Area:** Child Health **Strategy:** Recall the definitions of the various disorders listed. Note that the data given is a classic description of a common, superficial problem seen mostly in infants and young children. **Reference:** Lemone, P., & Burke, K. (2004). *Medical-surgical nursing: Critical thinking in client care* (3rd ed.). Upper Saddle River, NJ: Pearson Education, Inc., pp. 1461.

5 **Answer: 1, 4, 5** **Rationale:** Psoriasis is a chronic disease with factors such as stress precipitating an exacerbation. The disease is not contagious. Keeping the skin moist with an emollient lotion relieves the itching, and medications can be effective. Although there is no cure, treatment can suppress the symptoms of hyperkeratosis and inflammation. **Cognitive Level:** Applying **Client Need:** Physiological Adaptation **Integrated Process:** Nursing Process: Implementation **Content Area:** Adult Health **Strategy:** Note that some of the options contradict each other. Eliminate one of the opposing pairs. **Reference:** LeMone, P., Burke, K., & Bauldoff, G. (2011). *Medical-surgical nursing: Critical thinking in patient care* (5th ed.). Upper Saddle River, NJ: Pearson Education, Inc. pp. 407–409.

6 **Answer: 4** **Rationale:** The description of the lesions matches psoriasis, a common disease of T-cell–mediated autoimmune response that occurs worldwide. The best nurse's response is one that reassures, gives correct information, and allows the client to express feelings or concerns. It also begins assessing the client's existing knowledge of the disease to begin planning for teaching and management. **Cognitive Level:** Analyzing **Client Need:** Physiological Adaptation **Integrated Process:** Communication and Documentation **Content Area:** Adult Health **Strategy:** Look for the option that assures the client and encourages expression of fears and concerns. **Reference:** LeMone, P., Burke, K., & Bauldoff, G. (2011). *Medical-surgical nursing: Critical thinking in patient care* (5th ed.). Upper Saddle River, NJ: Pearson Education, Inc., pp. 407–409.

7 **Answer: 1** **Rationale:** Melanomas tend to have asymmetry (A), border irregularity (B), color variegation (C), diameter (D) greater than 6 mm (or ¼ inch), and are elevated or evolving (E). The ABCDE rule can be applied to any skin condition, but malignant melanoma is the most severe and has changes in all of the rules. Although sun-exposed areas are the site in 90% of Caucasians, non–sun-exposed areas are often the site in clients with darker skin. **Cognitive Level:** Applying **Client Need:** Physiological Adaptation **Integrated Process:** Nursing Process: Assessment **Content Area:** Adult Health **Strategy:** Acronyms can help in remembering concepts. Recall the critical words in the ABCDE rule of asymmetry, border, color, diameter, and elevation or evolving. This will help to evaluate the options. **Reference:** LeMone, P., Burke, K., & Bauldoff, G. (2011). Medical-surgical nursing: Critical thinking in patient care (5th ed.). Upper Saddle River, NJ: Pearson Education, Inc., p. 430.

8 **Answer: 2** **Rationale:** Restrictive jewelry and clothing are removed immediately from the burn victim to prevent circumferential constriction of the torso and extremities when edema formation begins. Assessment of the fingers and interference with first aid treatment may or may not require removal of jewelry, but the primary reason is to prevent a tourniquet effect. Prevention of infection is a priority in the acute phase of burn injury, which is after the emergent stage. **Cognitive Level:** Applying **Client Need:** Physiological Adaptation **Integrated Process:** Nursing Process: Implementation **Content Area:** Adult Health **Strategy:** Note the critical word in the question is *priority*. Meaning that the correct action is more important than the others, even if all would be technically correct. To help make a selection, recall what nursing actions are needed to prevent complications from an expected physiological response to burns. **Reference:** LeMone, P., Burke, K., & Bauldoff, G. (2011). *Medical-surgical nursing: Critical thinking in patient care* (5th ed.). Upper Saddle River, NJ: Pearson Education, Inc., p. 465.

9 **Answer: 4** **Rationale:** A superficial-thickness burn such as a sunburn involves only the epidermal layer of the skin. The color ranges from pink to bright red and usually no blisters form. This is the greatest risk besides dehydration unless the children are wearing sunscreen. The next action that the nurse should take is to determine whether the children are wearing sunscreen. Skin cancer can develop later in life because of sunburns. Nevi are one type of skin lesion but are not triggered by sun exposure or heat. Sunlight would not cause full-thickness burns. **Cognitive Level:** Applying **Client Need:** Health Promotion and Maintenance **Integrated Process:** Nursing Process: Assessment **Content Area:** Child Health **Strategy:** Visualize the scenario presented in the question and use the process of elimination to choose the most likely answer that represents an ordinary sunburn. **Reference:** LeMone, P., Burke, K., & Bauldoff, G. (2011). *Medical-surgical nursing: Critical thinking in patient care* (5th ed.). Upper Saddle River, NJ: Pearson Education, Inc., p 452.

10 **Answer: 3** **Rationale:** Tanning and sun exposure can increase susceptibility to skin cancer, and not all individuals use a sunscreen or consider tanning as having serious consequences. Assessment of foods, cosmetics, and environmental factors are all aimed at assessing for allergies, which have a greater tendency to be characterized by a rash than a new and pigmented lesion. **Cognitive Level:** Analyzing **Client Need:** Health Promotion and Maintenance **Integrated Process:** Nursing Process: Assessment **Content Area:** Adult Health **Strategy:** Consider what problem the nurse is assessing for. Choose the answer that gathers data related to risk factors, and eliminate each of the incorrect choices because they all focus on allergies. **Reference:** LeMone, P., Burke, K., & Bauldoff, G. (2011). *Medical-surgical nursing: Critical thinking in patient care* (5th ed.). Upper Saddle River, NJ: Pearson Education, Inc., p. 430.

References

D'Amico, D., & Barbarito, C. (2012). *Health & physical assessment in nursing* (2nd ed.). Upper Saddle River, NJ: Pearson Education, Inc.

Ignatavicius, D. D., & Workman, M. L. (2013). *Medical-surgical nursing: Critical thinking for collaborative care* (7th ed.). Philadelphia: W. B. Saunders Company.

Kee, J. L. (2010). *Laboratory and diagnostic tests* (8th ed.). Upper Saddle River, NJ: Pearson Education.

Lehne, R. (2010). *Pharmacology for nursing care* (7th ed.). St. Louis, MO: Saunders.

LeMone, P., Burke, K., & Bauldoff, G. (2011). *Medical-surgical nursing: Critical thinking in patient care* (5th ed.). Upper Saddle River, NJ: Pearson Education.

Lewis, S., Dirksen, S., Heitkemper, M., & Bucher, L., & Camera, I. (2011). *Medical surgical nursing: Assessment and management of clinical problems* (8th ed.). St. Louis, MO: Elsevier.

Longo, D., Fauci, A., Kasper, D., & Hauser, S. (2011). *Harrison's principles of internal medicine* (18th ed.). New York: McGraw-Hill.

McCance, K. L., & Huether, S. E. (2010). *Pathophysiology: The biologic basis for disease in adults and children* (6th ed.). St. Louis, MO: Mosby, Inc.

Osborn, K. S., Wraa, C. E., & Watson, A. (2010). *Medical surgical nursing: Preparation for practice*. Upper Saddle River, NJ: Pearson Education.

Porth, C., & Matfin, G. (2010). *Pathophysiology: Concepts of altered health states* (8th ed.). Philadelphia, PA: Lippincott Williams & Wilkins.

Smith, S. F., Duell, D. J., & Martin, B. C. (2012). *Clinical nursing skills: Basic to advanced skills* (8th ed.). Upper Saddle River, NJ: Pearson Education.

ANSWERS & RATIONALES

Hematological and Oncological Health Problems

15

NCLEX-RN® Test Prep

Use the accompanying online resource, NursingReviewsandRationales, to test yourself with hundreds of NCLEX®-style practice questions.

Objectives

➤ Define key terms associated with hematological and oncological health problems.
➤ Identify risk factors associated with the development of hematological and oncological health problems.
➤ Explain the common etiologies of hematological and oncological health problems.
➤ Describe pathophysiological processes associated with specific hematological and oncological health problems.
➤ Distinguish between normal and abnormal hematological and oncological health findings obtained from nursing assessment.
➤ Prioritize nursing interventions associated with specific hematological and oncological health problems.

Review at a Glance

achlorhydria absence of free hydrochloric acid in a pH maintained at 3.5
cheilosis presence of cracks in corners of mouth
factor VIII an alpha globulin that stabilizes fibrin clots
factor IX a vitamin-dependent beta globulin essential in stage 1 of intrinsic coagulation system as an influence on amount of thromboplastin available
ferritin an iron-phosphorus-protein complex that contains about 23% iron
hemoglobin electrophoresis a blood test that causes hemoglobin molecules to migrate in solution in response to electric currents to determine presence and percentage of hemoglobin

intrinsic factor a substance secreted by parietal cells of gastric mucosa that promotes absorption of vitamin B_{12}
mean corpuscular hemoglobin (MCH) a measurement of average weight (concentration) of hemoglobin in red blood cells
mean corpuscular hemoglobin concentration (MCHC) the ratio of weight of hemoglobin to volume of red blood cells
mean corpuscular volume (MCV) a measurement of size (volume) of red blood cells
nadir lowest point of bone marrow suppression following chemotherapy
neutropenia a decrease in neutrophils

paresthesias altered sensations such as numbness or tingling in extremities
pernicious anemia body's inability to absorb vitamin B_{12} because of a lack of intrinsic factor, a substance secreted by parietal cells of gastric mucosa
petechiae small, flat, purple or red spots on skin or mucous membranes caused by minute hemorrhage in dermis or submucous layer
Philadelphia chromosome characteristic chromosomal abnormality present in chronic myelogenous leukemia (CML)
pica craving to eat unusual substances such as clay or starch

plethora engorged or distended blood vessels causing a ruddy color of face, hands, feet, ears, and mucous membranes

proprioception ability to identify one's position in space; problems may include difficulty with balance and spinal cord damage

purpura hemorrhage into tissues as evidenced by bruising

Schilling test a vitamin B_{12} absorption test that indicates lack of intrinsic factor by measuring excretion of orally administered radionuclide labeled B_{12}

PRETEST

1 A client with anemia has a hemoglobin level of 6.5 grams/dL. The client is experiencing symptoms of cerebral tissue hypoxia. Which nursing intervention would be the most important in providing care?

1. Provide rest periods throughout the day.
2. Institute energy conservation techniques.
3. Assist in ambulation to the bathroom.
4. Check temperature of water prior to bathing.

2 The nurse is caring for a client experiencing renal failure as a complication from multiple myeloma. A family member asks what is causing the problem. The nurse's best response should include which information?

1. Proteins secreted by the abnormal plasma cells have caused the blood to thicken, resulting in renal failure.
2. Increased white blood cells and platelets have caused blood clots to form in the heart and blood vessels.
3. Healthy infection-fighting immunoglobulins are being produced in response to the myeloma progression.
4. The complications mean HIV is an additional worry but the medications should prevent the cell counts from dropping.

3 A client has a platelet count of 60,000/mm³. What precautions does the nurse need to include in the plan of care?

1. Not allowing visitors or staff with infections to have direct contact
2. Removing clutter and objects that could contribute to a fall
3. Checking for a positive Homan sign or calf tenderness
4. Encouraging foods like green, leafy vegetables

4 A 40-year-old client is referred to a hematologist with a tentative diagnosis of acute myelogenous leukemia (AML). The client's only symptom is fatigue. Which laboratory or diagnostic test would the nurse expect to be ordered first?

1. Liver function studies
2. Uric acid
3. Lumbar puncture
4. Bone marrow biopsy and aspiration

5 The nurse should recommend that a client with anemia increase intake of which foods that contain nutrients needed for erythropoiesis?

1. Milk, eggs, liver, and green, leafy vegetables
2. Apples, peanuts, oats, and cottage cheese
3. Cantaloupe, lima beans, and sweet potatoes
4. Dry yeast, grapefruit, and tuna fish

6 A client with iron deficiency anemia will receive an iron preparation by injection because the intravenous (IV) route is not possible for this client. The nurse expects the medication prescription to be written for which parenteral route?

1. Subcutaneous (SubQ) alternating with intramuscular (IM)
2. Deep gluteal intramuscular (IM) injection, using the Z-track method
3. Intramuscular in the deltoid to promote medication dissipation through muscle contraction
4. Subcutaneous injection with weekly site rotation

7 The nurse is applying pressure to a small bleeding laceration. Because the client has normal blood clotting, the nurse plans to safely release the pressure at which time?

1. During the platelet phase, which occurs seconds after the injury
2. During the clot retraction phase in 3–4 minutes
3. When fibrin reinforces the platelet plug in the coagulation cascade within 1–2 minutes
4. When the plasmin system produces fibrinolysis in clot dissolution in 5–7 minutes

8 A client has megaloblastic anemia along with some neurological symptoms. The nurse prepares to collect what specimen to verify the diagnosis of pernicious anemia?

1. Blood for storage of vitamin B_{12}
2. Gastric contents to test for pH
3. Urine for a 24-hour collection
4. Blood for detection of parietal cell and intrinsic factor antibodies

9 A client with a history of sickle cell anemia has recovered from an episode of sickling. At this time, the nurse plans to teach the client to avoid which conditions that may trigger another episode? Select all that apply.

1. Hypothermia
2. Dehydration
3. Bedrest
4. Excessive exercise
5. Infections

10 The nurse diligently assesses a neutropenic client diagnosed with leukemia for signs of infection. When questioned by a family member, the nurse uses which information as the best explanation as to why signs of infection may be absent or muted in this client?

1. Most infections are caused by organisms that are foreign pathogens.
2. The number of white blood cells (WBCs) drops rapidly and recovery time is slow.
3. Neutrophils necessary to produce an inflammatory response are inadequate in number or immature.
4. The immunoglobulins are reduced.

➤ *See pages 394–395 for Answers and Rationales.*

I. RISK FACTORS FOR HEMATOLOGICAL AND ONCOLOGICAL HEALTH PROBLEMS

A. **Lifestyle-related factors** such as smoking, alcohol consumption, and dietary or nutritional factors such as decreased intake of B vitamins and iron
B. **Risk factors for leukemia:** occupational and physical environment risk factors such as exposure to chemicals (such as benzene and arsenic) or large amounts of radiation; others are genetic factors, Down syndrome, viral etiology, and chemotherapeutic agents
C. **Risk factors for lymphoma:** viral exposure, genetics, ethnicity, and/or immune system compromise
D. **Risk factors for hematological cancers:** iatrogenic agents such as immunosuppressants and chemotherapy drugs
E. **Risk factors for anemia:** socioeconomic factors, such as poverty and inadequate nutrition

II. LEUKEMIA

A. **Overview**

1. Defined as a malignant neoplasm of blood-forming tissues including bone marrow, spleen, and lymph system
2. Characterized by an abnormal proliferation of immature white blood cells (WBCs or leukocytes) and their precursors that infiltrate bone marrow and peripheral blood as well as body organs and tissues

3. Types: categorized by type of WBC affected (granulocytic, lymphocytic, monocytic) and course and duration of disease (acute or chronic)
   a. Acute lymphocytic/lymphoblastic leukemia (ALL)
      1) Immature lymphocytes proliferate in bone marrow
      2) Abnormal leukemic cells resemble immature lymphocytes or lymphoblasts
      3) Most common in children ages 2–10 years
      4) A second rise in incidence occurs in middle age and in older adults
   b. Acute myelogenous or myelocytic leukemia (AML) or acute granulocytic leukemia (AGL)
      1) Immature granulocytes proliferate and accumulate in bone marrow
      2) Rate of incidence increases with age (especially over 50 years)
      3) Auer rods may be present in cytoplasm of myeloblasts; a standard diagnostic criterion for AML is that more than 30% of hematopoietic cells are myeloblasts
      4) Myelodysplastic syndrome, a hematological disorder of bone marrow, is referred to as pre-leukemia and may progress to AML; this syndrome has abnormal hematologic cell production and low peripheral blood counts
   c. Chronic lymphocytic leukemia (CLL)
      1) Abnormal incompetent lymphocytes proliferate, accumulate, and spread to other lymphatic tissue; is more gradual in onset
      2) Is more common in men and occurs most frequently between ages 50–70 years
   d. Chronic myelogenous leukemia (CML)
      1) Abnormal stem cells lead to an uncontrolled proliferation of granulocyte cells resulting in a marked increased in circulating blast cells, which can lead to leukostasis and intracerebral hemorrhage
      2) In most cases, a characteristic abnormality of chromosome 22 (referred to as **Philadelphia chromosome**) is present
      3) Occurs primarily between ages 30–50 years; incidence is slightly higher in men; and is more in gradual onset
4. Cause is usually unknown, but may be related to risk factors identified in previous section

B. **Pathophysiology**
   1. Abnormal or immature WBCs form but do not function properly; because of massive proliferation of abnormal immature cells, fewer normal WBCs are produced; abnormal cells continue to multiply and infiltrate, causing damage to bone marrow, spleen, lymph nodes, liver, kidneys, lungs, gonads, skin, and central nervous system (CNS)
   2. Normal bone marrow becomes diffusely replaced with abnormal or immature WBCs, interfering with ability of bone marrow to produce other types of cells such as erythrocytes and thrombocytes; bone marrow becomes functionally incompetent with resulting bone marrow suppression
   3. Acute leukemia has a rapid onset, progresses rapidly, with a short clinical course; left untreated, death will result in days or months; symptoms relate to bone marrow depression, infiltration of leukemic cells into other organ systems, and hypermetabolism of leukemia cells
   4. Chronic leukemia has a more insidious onset with a more prolonged clinical course; asymptomatic early in disease; life expectancy may be more than 5 years; symptoms relate to hypermetabolism of leukemia cells infiltrating other organ systems; cells are more mature and function more effectively
   5. Signs and symptoms include anemia, infection from inadequate functional WBCs, hemorrhage from thrombocytopenia, shortness of breath, fatigue, malaise, weakness, weight loss, decreased activity tolerance, bone or joint pain, headaches, visual disturbances, anorexia, fever, petechiae or other ecchymosis, gingival bleeding, epistaxis, pallor, generalized lymphadenopathy, hyperuricemia, splenomegaly, increased WBC count, and hepatomegaly

C. Nursing assessment

1. Assessment includes breath sounds, activity tolerance, pain, nutrition, vital signs, oral mucosa, signs of bleeding or infection, and enlargement of spleen, liver, or lymph nodes

2. Infection is a common presenting factor in acute leukemia, but signs and symptoms may be absent because of **neutropenia** (a decrease in neutrophils); CNS manifestations are most common in lymphocytic leukemia

3. Hemoglobin, hematocrit, platelet count, and granulocyte count will drop consistently during chemotherapy, reaching its lowest point 5–7 days after initiation of therapy; counts will remain low for 7–10 days and will slowly begin rebounding, platelets first, then WBCs, then red blood cells (RBCs)

4. Diagnostic tests: complete blood count (CBC), electrolytes, and cultures (if infection present); bone marrow biopsy and aspirate is the only definitive diagnostic test

D. Nursing management

1. Medications include analgesics to control pain, antiemetics for nausea, and chemotherapeutic regimens including radioactive drugs such as sodium radioiodine (Iodotope)

2. Large doses of chemotherapy are often given at one time (called induction therapy) for certain types of leukemia such as AML

3. Other types of treatment: bone marrow transplant, biological therapies such as interferons and interleukins, and alternative treatments

4. Bone marrow biopsy
   a. Assess coagulation factors before procedure
   b. Posterior iliac crest, anterior iliac crest, and sternum are preferred locations
   c. After procedure, apply firm pressure for 5 minutes and observe puncture site for hemorrhage hourly for at least 4 hours

5. Protect from infection (see Box 15-1 for neutropenic precautions), especially in **nadir** period (lowest level of bone marrow function from suppression following chemotherapy); identify risk of infection by calculating the client's absolute neutrophil count (ANC): WBC × (% bands + % segs) = ANC (needs to be 1,000 or greater)

6. Prevent bleeding (soft toothbrush, fall prevention, safety with razors)

7. Prevent fatigue secondary to anemia, plan adequate rest periods, limit visitors if necessary

8. Maintain hydration and nutrition, evaluate weight loss

9. Stomatitis (inflammation of mouth) is common, therefore daily oral assessments and good oral hygiene should be performed

10. Encourage and assist client and family to discuss concerns and fears

11. If chemotherapy regimen is likely to cause alopecia, discuss options for regarding hair before drug therapy begins optimally

---

Practice to Pass

A client is being discharged following induction therapy for acute myelogenous leukemia (AML). He is in his nadir period. What type of education will be needed? What type of clinical follow-up should be expected over the next 7–10 days?

Box 15-1	
Neutropenic Precautions	• Use meticulous hand hygiene. • Provide oral hygiene after meals and at bedtime. • Screen all visitors and staff for colds or infections. • Monitor vital signs every 4 hours. • Prohibit fresh fruit or flowers, plants, and standing water. • Change intravenous (IV) tubing every 24 hours. • Avoid certain medications that may mask fever, such as acetaminophen (Tylenol) and ibuprofen (Advil). • Administer antibacterial/antifungal/antiviral therapy as prescribed.

III. LYMPHOMA

A. Overview

1. Defined as a group of malignant neoplasms that affect lymphatic system
2. Hodgkin's disease is a malignant disorder of lymph nodes that is characterized by presence of Reed-Sternberg cell
3. Non-Hodgkin's lymphomas are a broad group of neoplastic disorders that affect lymphatic system and include all lymphomas except Hodgkin's disease
4. Cause is unknown or associated with predisposing factors

B. Pathophysiology

1. *Hodgkin's disease (HD)*
   a. Reed-Sternberg cells (malignant cells) replace normal cells; these are giant cell mutations of T-lymphocytes that are present in lymph node when diagnosed with HD
   b. Originates in one lymph node and then spreads to adjacent structures through lymph system
   c. Eventually infiltrates other tissues including liver, spleen, lungs, bone marrow, and ureters
   d. Peaks in 2 age groups: 15–35 years of age, and then again from 55–75 years of age; occurs twice as often in men than women
2. *Non-Hodgkin's lymphoma*
   a. Cells that make up lymphoid tissue become abnormal and eventually crowd out normal cells within specific regions of lymph nodes; there are no Reed-Sternberg cells
   b. Lymphoma usually originates outside lymph nodes and becomes disseminated rapidly
   c. Incidence increases between the ages of 50–70; men are more frequently affected than women
3. Has an insidious onset; diagnosis usually occurs from pressure exerted by large nodes on surrounding tissues and/or obstruction or infiltration of lymphoma into vital organs such as kidney, lung, or spleen
4. Staging is based on Cottswold Staging Classification System
   a. Stage I: limited to 1 lymph node region, lymphoid structure, or extra-lymphatic site
   b. Stage II: involvement of 2 or more lymph node regions on same side of diaphragm or localized extra-lymphatic involvement
   c. Stage III: involvement of lymph node regions or structures on both sides of diaphragm; may involve spleen or localized extranodal disease
   d. Stage IV: diffuse or disseminated extra-lymphatic disease
5. Signs and symptoms include painless unilateral or bilateral lymph node enlargement; cervical generally involved first, then axillary and inguinal (most easily assessed since they are more superficial); clients with more advanced disease often present with weight loss, night sweats, malaise, chills, pruritus, anorexia, nonproductive cough, dyspnea, and renal failure

C. Nursing assessment

1. Assessment includes lymph nodes, presence or absence of pain, nutritional status, weight, activity level and tolerance, respiratory status, and kidney function
2. Diagnostic tests: CBC, blood urea nitrogen (BUN) and creatinine; lymph node biopsy is the only definitive diagnosis of either Hodgkin's or non-Hodgkin's lymphoma (via surgical incision or needle aspirate); lymphangiogram (radiologic exam after infusion of a blue oil–based dye into lymphatic system to determine extent of involvement)

Practice to Pass

Discuss the similarities and the differences between Hodgkin's (HD) and non-Hodgkin's lymphoma. How is the care of the client with HD the same or different from the care of the client with non-Hodgkin's lymphoma?

D. Nursing management

1. Medications include combination chemotherapy for both Hodgkin's and non-Hodgkin's disease, depending on stage
2. Radiation therapy
3. Postprocedure care following lymphangiogram
    a. Instruct client that urine, veins of lower extremities, and dorsal skin of feet may have a blue-green discoloration from dye excretion for 2–5 days
    b. Monitor for signs of dye-based complications: cough, dyspnea, pleuritic pain, hemoptysis
4. Protect from infection and monitor and maintain normal body temperature
5. Prevent or decrease pain
6. Maintain adequate nutrition and hydration

IV. MULTIPLE MYELOMA

A. Overview

1. Defined as plasma cell neoplasms or related disorders with proliferation and collection of immunoglobulin or plasma cells
2. Affects mostly men 50–69 years of age; more prominent in African Americans
3. Cause is unknown; however, some studies suggest that multiple myeloma reflects an inappropriate response to an antigen or a virus-like particle; genetics may be involved

B. Pathophysiology

1. Malignant plasma cells arise from 1 clone of B cells, proliferate within hematopoietic tissue, and then infiltrate rest of bone to produce osteolytic lesions; substances secreted by malignant plasma cells produce systemic effects and involve bone marrow, causing major complications

2. Subsequent bone destruction leads to hypercalcemia and pathologic fractures
3. Proliferation of plasma cells crowds marrow space, usually inhibiting production of RBCs
4. Plasma cells also synthesize and secrete an abnormally small number of immunoglobulins, increasing risk of infection
5. In some cases, a marked increase in IgG or occasionally IgA increases blood viscosity, leading to occlusion of small blood vessels

6. A hallmark of multiple myeloma is production of an abnormal immunoglobulin (M component) indicated by elevated blood levels and presence of Bence Jones protein in urine
7. Signs and symptoms
    a. Gradual, insidious onset with recurrent infections, especially pneumonia
    b. Pain is a major problem as bony destruction begins and lytic bone lesions occur
    c. Cord compression may occur from vertebral collapse
    d. Diffuse osteoporosis with a negative calcium balance may also be seen
    e. Renal stones occur with demineralization

    f. Hypercalcemia can also cause neurological disturbances (confusion, depression), gastrointestinal (GI) distress, altered musculoskeletal status, fluid and electrolyte imbalance, and altered cardiopulmonary function

    g. Renal disease may develop as a result of renal calculi and toxic effect of Bence Jones protein on renal epithelial cells

C. Nursing assessment

1. Assessment includes symptom analysis of pain, history of fractures, recurring pneumonia, kidney problems, musculoskeletal problems, or cardiovascular complications

Practice to Pass

A hospitalized client with multiple myeloma who has bone metastasis was just started on long-acting morphine sulfate (MS Contin) tablets. In preparation for discharge, what important information should the nurse review with the client and significant other?

2. Diagnostic tests: electrolytes, chest x-ray (CXR), CBC, BUN, creatinine, computerized tomography (CT) scan, IgE, urinalysis

D. Nursing management

1. Medications
   a. Analgesics to manage pain
   b. Antimicrobial therapy in the presence of positive blood cultures
   c. Melphalan (Alkeran) and cyclophosphamide (Cytoxan) are common chemotherapeutic agents used to manage the condition; thalidomide (generic) and lenalidomide (Revlimid) may also be used
   d. Hypercalcemia is managed with use of steroids, IV hydration, diuretics, calcitonin (Calcimar), etidronate disodium (Didronel), gallium nitrate (Ganite), and pamidronate disodium (Aredia)
2. There is no cure for multiple myeloma, so treatment is often palliative; autologous and allogenic bone marrow transplants are also an option
3. Maintaining adequate hydration is of primary concern; fluids are administered to attain a urinary output of 1.5–2 L/day
4. Weight bearing, range of motion (ROM), and ambulation helps bone to reabsorb calcium; ambulation is most significant in lowering calcium level
5. Radiation therapy is usually limited to clients with disabling pain or those with spinal cord compression
6. Blood transfusions are often indicated to manage resulting anemia
7. Gallium nitrate (Ganite) is contraindicated with renal insufficiency (creatinine greater than 2.5 mg/dL)
8. Manage pain if metastasis occurs, instructing client on how to take medication prior to severe pain and possible side effects

V. THROMBOCYTOPENIA

A. Overview

1. Defined as a platelet count less than 100,000/mm^3; is most frequent cause of abnormal bleeding
2. Hemorrhage from minor trauma and spontaneous bleeding can occur when platelet count falls below 20,000/mm^3
3. Fatal GI, cerebral, and pulmonary hemorrhage can occur if count drops below 10,000/mm^3
4. Causes include unknown reasons, diseases (anemias, systemic lupus erythematosus, acquired immunodeficiency syndrome [AIDS]), sequelae to viral infections, chemotherapy or radiation, hypersplenism or splenomegaly, coronary bypass or autotransfusion, and heparin therapy

B. Pathophysiology

1. Relates to 3 basic mechanisms: accelerated platelet destruction or consumption, defective platelet production, or disordered platelet distribution
2. *Immune (or idiopathic) thrombocytopenia purpura* (ITP) occurs when destruction of platelets is greatly accelerated

   a. Destruction is believed to be caused by body's immune system and is therefore categorized as an autoimmune disorder
   b. Acute ITP is more common in children, while chronic ITP is more common in adults
   c. Platelets become coated with antibodies from an autoimmune response mediated by B lymphocytes; although platelets function normally, they are recognized by spleen as foreign and destroyed
   d. Platelet circulation time is decreased to 1–3 days

3. *Secondary thrombocytopenia* is a condition in which there is a defect in platelet production; this defect may occur as a result of:
    a. Medications such as thiazide diuretics, acetylsalicylic acid (ASA), ibuprofen (Advil), indomethacin (Indocin), naproxen sodium (Anaprox), sulfonamides, quinidine sulfate (Quinidex), cimetidine (Tagamet), digoxin (Lanoxin), furosemide (Lasix), heparin sodium, morphine sulfate, and vitamins C and E
    b. Spices: ginger, cumin, turmeric, cloves, garlic
    c. Viral or bacterial infections
    d. Bone marrow disorders
    e. Chemotherapy and radiation therapy
4. *Disordered platelet distribution* occurs when large numbers of platelets are sequestered in spleen; occurs as a result of lymphoma, portal hypertension, and hypothermia during heart surgery
5. Signs and symptoms include decreased platelet count; prolonged bleeding time; **purpura** (hemorrhage into tissues as evidenced by bruising); ecchymosis (flat or raised areas of discoloration of skin or mucous membranes caused by subcutaneous bleeding); **petechiae** (small, flat, purple or red spots on skin or mucous membranes caused by minute hemorrhage in dermis or submucous layer); weakness and fatigue

C. **Nursing assessment**
1. Assessment
    a. Evaluation of skin for signs of hemorrhage and symptom analysis of any bleeding episodes; look for petechiae and purpura on commonly affected areas (anterior thorax, arms, and neck); other common types of bleeding are epistaxis, menorrhagia, hematuria, and GI bleeding
    b. Activity tolerance (may be reduced from a secondary anemia)
    c. Home medications used, including herbal products
    d. Recent infections
2. Diagnostic tests: CBC, platelet count, coagulation studies including prothrombin time (PT) and partial thromboplastin time (PTT), bone marrow exam

D. **Nursing management**
1. Medications include steroids to suppress immune response in ITP; immunoglobulin has been shown to have a temporary therapeutic effect in immune response disorders
2. Initiate thrombocytopenic precautions (see Box 15-2)
3. Focus client education primarily on risk for bleeding
4. Platelet transfusions may be given when platelet counts fall below 20,000/mm^3, but are of little benefit in ITP
5. Educate clients about Cushingoid side effects of steroid therapy, such as adiposity, edema, capillary fragility, and excessive hair growth
6. Treatment may consist of a splenectomy, especially in ITP

Box 15-2	
Thrombocytopenic Precautions	• Avoid intramuscular (IM) or subcutaneous injections. • Avoid use of acetylsalicylic acid (aspirin) or aspirin-containing products. • Avoid use of toothbrushes and razors. • Avoid invasive or traumatic procedures. • Avoid rectal temperatures and suppositories. • Assess for signs of bleeding (skin, mouth, nose, feces, and urine). • Guaiac all stool, urine, and emesis. • Pad side rails if necessary. • Avoid venipuncture (clients usually have a triple-lumen central line in place for blood sampling, medication administration, and blood product transfusion). • Administer stool softeners as necessary.

VI. HEMOPHILIA

A. Overview

1. Defined as a group of hereditary clotting factor disorders characterized by prolonged coagulation time that results in prolonged and sometimes excessive bleeding
2. Hemophilia A and B are X-linked recessive disorders transmitted by female carriers, displayed almost exclusively in males (see Figure 15-1)

B. Pathophysiology

1. *Hemophilia A* (classic hemophilia) is a deficiency in **factor VIII** (an alpha globulin that stabilizes fibrin clots); deficiency is determined by first measuring PTT; a factor VIII deficient plasma substrate is then mixed with client's plasma and degree of correction in PTT is determined and compared to degree of correction obtained by normal plasma
2. *Hemophilia B* (Christmas disease) is a deficiency in **factor IX** (a vitamin-dependent beta globulin essential in stage 1 of intrinsic coagulation system as an influence on amount of thromboplastin available); deficiency is determined by first measuring PTT; a factor IX deficient plasma substrate is then mixed with client's plasma and degree of correction in PTT is determined and compared to degree of correction obtained by normal plasma
   a. Despite the difference in factor deficiency, hemophilia A and B are clinically identical
   b. Clients with hemophilia A and B form platelet plugs at site of bleeding, but clotting factor deficiency impairs coagulation response and capacity to form a stable clot
   c. With a factor level less than or equal to 5% of normal (moderate hemophilia), bleeding result from trauma or surgery
   d. Spontaneous bleeding can occur with factor level activity below 1% (severe hemophilia) resulting in hemarthrosis with joint deformity and potential disability
3. *Von Willebrand disease* is a deficiency of von Willebrand factor (vWF) and platelet dysfunction seen in both genders
   a. Factor VIII has 3 properties, pre-coagulant activity, antigenic activity, and von Willebrand factor activity
   b. It is classified as an autosomal dominant trait factor VIII defect; in hemophilia A, vWF is normal, but in von Willebrand disease, vWF is characteristically low (less than 40% of control sample activity)
4. Signs and symptoms
   a. Prolonged clotting times
   b. Subcutaneous ecchymosis, bleeding from gums, hematomas, and hemarthrosis (joint bleeding, swelling, and damage)
   c. Slow oozing of blood from minor cuts, with onset of bleeding being delayed for several hours, or even days after injury
   d. GI bleeding, evidenced by hematemesis (vomiting blood), occult blood in the stools, gastric pain, or abdominal pain

Practice to Pass

Both the client with hemophilia and the client with thrombocytopenia have a nursing diagnosis of Risk for Injury: Hemorrhage. How do these 2 medical diagnoses differ in their nursing interventions? How are they similar?

Figure 15-1

Genogram illustrating inheritance pattern for hemophilia A and B, which are X-linked recessive characteristics. Females carry the gene, but males express the gene and develop the disorder

◯ = Normal female   ◖ = Hemolytic carrier female

☐ = Normal male   ◼ = Hemophiliac male

       e. Urinary tract bleeding evidenced by hematuria

       f. Pain or paralysis resulting from pressure of hematomas on nerves

C. Nursing assessment

    1. Includes assessment of bleeding, pain, skin, and oral mucosa; perform a symptom analysis of any bleeding episodes, infections, or difficulty in controlling bleeding; question use of over–the–counter drugs and herbal products

     2. Diagnostic tests: PTT is prolonged (intrinsic clotting pathway); PT or international normalized ratio (INR), fibrinogen level and platelet count are normal; bleeding time is prolonged in von Willebrand's disease; CBC, guaiac stool, and urinalysis (UA) may be ordered

D. Nursing management

    1. Medications include replacement of deficient factor

       a. Hemophilia A: cryoprecipitate containing 8–100 units of factor VIII per bag at 12-hour intervals until bleeding ceases

       b. Hemophilia B: plasma or factor IX concentrate given every 24 hours or until bleeding ceases

       c. Von Willebrand's disease: cryoprecipitate containing 8–100 units of factor VIII per bag at 12-hour intervals until bleeding ceases

    2. Referral for genetic counseling is essential

    3. Never give acetylsalicylic acid (aspirin) to a client with hemophilia

    4. Stop topical bleeding as quickly as possible by applying direct pressure or ice, packing area with gel foam or fibrin foam, and applying topical hemostatic agents such as fibrin

    5. When joint bleeding occurs, totally rest the joint, apply ice, and administer hemophilia factors

    6. Treatment may consist of plasmapheresis and/or prothrombin complexes for development of antibody inhibitors against specific coagulation factor

VII. ANEMIA

A. Overview

    1. Defined as a condition where hemoglobin content of blood is insufficient to satisfy bodily needs

    2. Caused by decrease in circulating RBCs, but may also be caused by accelerated hemolysis, decreased production, or high numbers of reticulocytes; other causes include side effects of medications, menstruation, GI bleeding

B. Pathophysiology

    1. Anemia reduces oxygen-carrying capacity of blood, producing tissue hypoxia

    2. Basic classifications of anemia are nutritional, hemolytic, and bone marrow depression; see Box 15-3 for types of anemias within each classification

---

Box 15-3	**Nutritional Anemias**
	• Iron-deficiency anemia
Classification of	• Vitamin B_{12} anemia
Selected Anemias	• Folic acid anemia
	Hemolytic Anemias
	• Sickle cell anemia
	• Thalassemia
	• Acquired hemolytic anemia
	• Glucose-6-phosphate dehydrogenase anemia
	Bone Marrow Depression Anemia
	• Aplastic anemia

3. Another classification is anemia of chronic disease (ACD), which results from chronic infection, chronic immune activation, or malignancy and is thought to protect body by limiting amount of available iron to potentially harmful pathogens
   a. Ferritin level may be normal or high but total iron-binding capacity (TIBC) is reduced because body has stored iron as ferritin
   b. Treatment for ACD is to treat underlying condition; administration of iron is *not* recommended, as it makes more iron available to potential pathogens
4. Nutritional anemia results from nutrient deficiencies that disrupt erythropoiesis or hemoglobin synthesis
   a. *Iron-deficiency anemia*
      1) Supply of iron is inadequate for optimal formation of RBCs because of excessive iron loss from bleeding, decreased dietary intake, or malabsorption
      2) Adequate iron in RBCs is essential since oxygen molecule attaches to it
      3) Erythrocytes are small (microcytic with RBC diameter less than 6) and pale (hypochromic); **mean corpuscular volume (MCV)**; measures size) is decreased and **mean corpuscular hemoglobin (MCH)** or **mean corpuscular hemoglobin concentration (MCHC)** (calculated value of hemoglobin present in RBC compared to its size), is decreased; MCV, MCH, and MCHC should be analyzed only when hemoglobin is low
      4) An average diet supplies body with 12–15 mg/day of iron, of which only 5–10% is absorbed
      5) Iron is stored in body as **ferritin**, an iron-phosphorus-protein complex that contains about 23% iron; it is formed in intestinal mucosa, when ferritin iron joins with protein apoferritin; ferritin is stored primarily in reticuloendothelial cells of liver, spleen, and bone marrow
      6) Normal iron excretion is less than 1 mg/day through urine, sweat, bile, feces, and from desquamated skin cells; an average woman loses 0.5 mg of iron daily or 15 mg monthly during menstruation (most common cause of iron deficiency in women, while GI bleeding is most common cause in men)
      7) Develops slowly through 3 phases: body's stores of iron for erythropoiesis are depleted; insufficient iron is transported to bone marrow; and iron deficient erythropoiesis begins, allowing small hemoglobin-deficient cells to enter peripheral circulation in large numbers; iron is needed on hemoglobin so oxygen molecule will attach
      8) Signs and symptoms develop gradually with client not seeking attention until hemoglobin drops to 7–8 grams/dL; manifestations include fatigue, weakness, shortness of breath, pallor (ear lobes, palms, and conjunctiva), brittle spoonlike nails; **cheilosis** (cracks in corners of mouth); smooth sore tongue; dizziness, hypoxia, and **pica** (craving to eat unusual substances such as clay or starch)
   b. *Vitamin B$_{12}$ deficiency anemia*
      1) Impairs cellular division and maturation especially in rapidly proliferating RBCs
      2) Macrocytic (megaloblastic) anemia (RBC diameter greater than 8)
      3) **Pernicious anemia** is body's inability to absorb vitamin B$_{12}$ because of a lack of **intrinsic factor**, a substance secreted by parietal cells of gastric mucosa
      4) Laboratory exam shows an increase in MCV and MCHC
      5) Gastric secretion analysis reveals **achlorhydria** (absence of free hydrochloric acid in a pH maintained at 3.5)
      6) Inevitably develops after total gastrectomy, with 15% of clients developing pernicious anemia after partial gastrectomy or gastrojejunostomy, and increased incidence following gastric bypass surgery
      7) Lack of vitamin B$_{12}$ alters structure and disrupts function of peripheral nerves, spinal cord, and brain

8) Clients with this anemia tend to have fair hair coloring or become prematurely gray

9) Signs and symptoms include pallor or slight jaundice, weakness, smooth sore beefy red tongue, diarrhea, **paresthesias** such as numbness or tingling in the extremities, impaired **proprioception** (ability to identify one's position in space) which may progress to difficulty with balance and to spinal cord damage)

c. *Folic acid deficiency anemia*

1) Required for DNA synthesis and normal maturation of RBCs

2) Macrocytic (megaloblastic) anemia (RBC diameter greater than 8); MCV high with low hemoglobin

3) Causative etiology: poor nutrition, malabsorption syndrome, medications that impede absorption (oral contraceptives, antiepileptics, methotrexate [MTX]), alcohol abuse, and anorexia

4) Signs and symptoms include pallor, progressive weakness, fatigue, shortness of breath, and palpitations; GI symptoms are similar to B_{12} deficiency, but usually more severe (anemia, glossitis, cheilosis, and diarrhea); neurological symptoms seen in B_{12} deficiency are not seen in folic acid deficiency and therefore assist in differentiation

C. **Nursing assessment**

1. Assessment includes symptom analysis of activity tolerance, skin color, nails, oral assessment, GI and nutritional assessment; neurological assessment is indicated in vitamin B_{12} anemia

2. Diagnostic tests: CBC, MCV, MCH, MCHC; parietal cell and intrinsic factor antibodies

3. 24-hour urine for **Schilling test**; indicates if a client lacks intrinsic factor by measuring excretion of orally administered radionuclide labeled B_{12}

D. **Nursing management**

1. Iron-deficiency anemia

a. Medications include oral iron preparations before meals if tolerated and nausea does not occur; vitamin C enhances absorption, while antacids inhibit absorption; intramuscular (IM) iron dextran (Infed) should be administered using Z-track technique to prevent tattooing of skin

1) Parenteral iron is given to those who have an intolerance to iron preparations, habitually forget medications, or have continued blood loss

2) Because of high risk of allergic reaction, first dose should be infused slowly with concurrent and careful client assessment

b. Increase amount and number of iron-rich foods, such as beef, chicken, egg yolk, pork loin, turkey, and whole-grain breads and cereals

c. Monitor for safety and injury if severe anemia occurs because of tissue and cerebral hypoxia

2. Vitamin B_{12} deficiency anemia

a. Medications include parenteral replacement of vitamin B_{12} IM; required for life for clients lacking intrinsic factor

b. Teach clients with insufficient dietary intake to increase intake of foods such as eggs, meats, and dairy products

3. Folic acid deficiency anemia

a. Medications include oral folic acid supplements indefinitely with malabsorption or impaired folic acid metabolism

b. In malnourishment, foods containing folic acid should be added, such as green, leafy vegetables, broccoli, organ meats, eggs, and milk

Practice to Pass

What is the primary difference between pernicious anemia and anemia caused by a folic acid deficiency? How are the 2 similar?

VIII. SICKLE CELL ANEMIA

A. Overview

1. Defined as a hereditary, chronic form of hemolytic anemia
2. Affects African Americans; 8% are heterozygous (carriers) for sickle cell anemia thereby inheriting one affected gene (sickle cell trait); 1% are homozygous, inheriting a defective gene from each parent—these clients have sickle cell anemia and are likely to experience sickle cell crisis
3. Caused by an autosomal genetic defect (one gene affected) that results in synthesis of hemoglobin S (see Figure 15-2)

B. Pathophysiology

1. Produced by a mutation in beta chain of hemoglobin molecule through a substitution of amino acid valine for glutamine in both beta chains
2. When there is decreased plasma oxygen tension, hemoglobin S causes RBCs to elongate, become rigid, and assume a crescent sickled shape, causing cells to clump together and obstruct capillary blood flow, causing ischemia and possible tissue infarction
   a. Conditions likely to trigger a sickle cell crisis include hypoxia, low environmental and/or body temperature, excessive exercise, high altitudes, or inadequate oxygen during anesthesia
   b. Other causes include elevated blood viscosity or decreased plasma volume, infection, dehydration, and/or increased hydrogen ion concentration (acidosis)
3. With normal oxygenation, sickled RBCs resume their normal shape
4. Repeated episodes of sickling and unsickling weaken cell membranes, causing them to hemolyze and be removed
5. A vasoocclusive crisis begins with sickling in microcirculation and leads to a cascade of events:
   a. Vasospasm creates a logjam effect, which brings blood flow through vessels to a stop
   b. Thrombosis and infarction of local tissue occur
   c. Crisis results, which is extremely painful and can last from 4–6 days
6. Sickle cell trait is a generally mild condition that produces few, if any, manifestations
7. Signs and symptoms include anemia with sickled cells noted on a peripheral smear; general manifestations similar to those of hemolytic anemia (pallor, jaundice,

Practice to Pass

The nurse sees a child with sickle cell anemia in the outpatient clinic who is planning to fly to Florida during spring vacation. What should the nurse teach the client and his parents to prevent the client from experiencing a crisis while away?

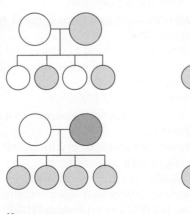

Figure 15-2

Inheritance pattern for sickle cell anemia

Key:

◯ Normal

◯ Sickle cell trait: heterozygous defective genes

● Sickle cell anemia: homozygous defective genes

fatigue, and irritability); large joints and surrounding tissue may become swollen during crisis; priapism (abnormal, painful continuous erection of penis) may occur if penile veins are obstructed

C. **Nursing assessment**

1. Assessment includes symptom analysis of activity tolerance, skin color, swelling of joints, and degree of pain if any

 2. Diagnostic tests: **hemoglobin electrophoresis**, a blood test that causes hemoglobin molecule to migrate in solution in response to electric currents, determines presence and percentage of hemoglobin S and is used for a definitive diagnosis; CBC

D. **Nursing management**

1. Medications include folic acid supplements (to meet increased metabolic demands of bone marrow) and analgesics

2. During a crisis, hydration therapy is essential to improve blood flow, reduce pain, and prevent renal damage

3. Hydration therapy as well as scheduled transfusions will decrease number of painful crisis episodes

4. For clients experiencing a pain crisis, treatment includes rest, oxygen, use of IV opioids, and hydration

IX. POLYCYTHEMIA (POLYCYTHEMIA VERA)

A. **Overview**

1. Defined as an increase in number of circulating RBCs and concentration of hemoglobin in blood; also known as polycythemia vera, PV, or myeloproliferative red cell disorder

2. Bone marrow stimulates an overproduction of RBCs, WBCs, and platelets thereby increasing blood viscosity, blood volume, and congestion of tissues and organs with blood

3. Can be a primary or secondary disorder

4. Causes include primary—unknown; secondary—erythropoietin-secreting tumors, Cushing's disease, end-stage renal disease, hypoxemia, and long-term dialysis

B. **Pathophysiology**

1. *Primary polycythemia*

a. Most common in Caucasian men of European Jewish ancestry

b. Is a neoplastic stem cell disorder characterized by overproduction of RBCs, certain WBCs, and platelets

c. Erythrocytosis causes increased blood volume and viscosity with liver and spleen congestion

d. Thick, slow-moving blood becomes an ideal environment for acidosis and clotting, with resultant tissue and organ infarction secondary to thrombi

2. *Secondary polycythemia*

a. Most common form of PV

b. Excess of erythropoiesis that arises as a response to an abnormal increase in erythropoietin

c. Abnormally high levels of erythropoietin may also be produced because of hypoxemia, in turn caused by:

1) Prolonged exposure to high altitudes

2) Systemic disorders that affect oxygenation (chronic obstructive pulmonary disease [COPD], heart failure [HF])

3) Hypoventilation secondary to morbid obesity

4) Long-term smokers: "smokers' erythrocytosis"

3. Signs and symptoms

a. **Plethora** (engorged or distended blood vessels causing a ruddy color of face, hands, feet, ears, and mucous membranes)

   b. Engorgement of retinal veins (bloodshot eyes) and sublingual veins
   c. Splenomegaly (primary PV only)
   d. Hepatomegaly, headache, a feeling of fullness in head, dizziness, weakness, fatigue on exertion, visual disturbances, hypertension, hypermetabolism, epigastric distress, and backache
   e. Pruritis that does not respond to antihistamines
   f. Manifestations of vascular disease (angina, intermittent claudication, cerebral insufficiency)

C. **Nursing assessment**
   1. Includes symptom analysis of pain, itching, skin color, and palpation of spleen or liver
   2. Diagnostic tests: high erythrocyte count (8–12 million/mm^3); decreased MCHC; increased leukocytes, thrombocytes, and total blood volume

D. **Nursing management**
   1. Medications include antineoplastic agents (but side effects are often worse than the disease); radioactive phosphorus (may cause generalized suppression of hematopoiesis with resultant anemia, leukopenia, or thrombocytopenia)
   2. Encourage smoking cessation in clients who smoke
   3. Manage underlying chronic condition (COPD, HF) with supportive measures and appropriate drug therapy

X. BETA THALASSEMIA

A. **Overview**
   1. Inherited defect in alpha and beta chain synthesis, which is involved in adult hemoglobin
   2. Defined as a microcytic-hypochromic hemolytic anemia
   3. Depression of beta-chain synthesis results in RBCs having a decreased amount of hemoglobin; most erythroblasts are destroyed by mononuclear phagocytes
   4. Two types, major and minor, which depend on heterozygosity
   5. Most common in certain ethnicities: African American, Greek, Italian, and some Arab and Sephardic Jew cultural groups

B. **Pathophysiology**
   1. *Beta thalassemia (minor and major)*: moderate (minor) or severe (major) depression of beta-chain synthesis, resulting in RBCs with a reduced amount of hemoglobin
   2. Signs and symptoms (minor)
      a. Mild to moderate microcytic-hypochromic anemia
      b. Mild splenomegaly
      c. Bronze coloring of skin
      d. Hyperplasia of the bone marrow
   3. Signs and symptoms (major)
      a. Severe anemia with significant cardiovascular burden
      b. High-output heart failure
      c. Hepatomegaly from hemosiderosis
      d. Splenomegaly due to extramedullary hematopoiesis and increased destruction of RBCs
      e. Spinal impairment
      f. Bone marrow hyperplasia that causes a characteristic facial deformity—widening of nasal bridge, mandible, and maxilla

C. **Nursing assessment**
   1. Assess familial history
   2. Clinical manifestations: anemia, bronze skin, mild splenomegaly (minor) or severe anemia, heart failure and hepatomegaly/splenomegaly (major)
   3. Diagnostic tests: newborn screening, blood smears, hemoglobin electrophoresis

D. Nursing management
1. Manage blood transfusions
2. Assist with iron chelation therapy in combination with hypertransfusion
3. Manage pre- and postoperative care of patients undergoing splenectomy

Case Study

The client is a 62-year-old female who has been a diabetic since age 25 and takes insulin twice daily. Over the last 2 months, she has had difficulty recovering from a cold, experiences periods of extreme fatigue, lost 10 pounds, and has a low-grade temperature of 100°F. Blood studies and a bone marrow biopsy and aspirate led to a diagnosis of acute lymphocytic leukemia (ALL). Currently the client is hospitalized with a triple-lumen Hickman catheter in place and is undergoing chemotherapy with vincristine (Oncovin), daunorubicin (Cerubidine), and prednisone.

Assessment data reveals the client is oriented to person, place, and time; has headache and dizziness upon standing; slight numbness and tingling of lower extremities; petechiae cover arms, chest, and upper thighs; skin color pale; recoil is less than 6 seconds, with dry mucous membranes. A small ulcerated area is present on outer aspect of right ankle; Hickman site is clean and dry but slightly red; no obvious dyspnea but reports shortness of breath upon exertion; lung sounds clear; sputum slightly yellow in color; vital signs: pulse 90; blood pressure 140/84 lying and 128/72 standing; respirations 20 and regular; lab work: white blood count (WBC) 9,000/mm³; red blood count (RBC) 2.23/mm³; hemoglobin 8.8 grams/dL; hematocrit 26%; platelets 12,000/mm³; WBC differential: segs 10%; bands 1%; lymphocytes 60%; glucose: 250 mg/dL; albumin 2.4 grams/dL; calcium 8.0 mEq/L.

1. What are the most important nursing diagnoses, and how should they be prioritized?

2. What is the relationship between the client's absolute neutrophil count (ANC) and the risk for infection?

3. How will the nurse know the client is developing infection?

4. What effect will the client's diabetes have on her treatment course?

5. How should the nurse prepare the client for discharge from the hospital?

For suggested responses, see page 467.

POSTTEST

1 A client with anemia due to chemotherapy has a hemoglobin level of 7.0 grams/dL. Which client manifestations would indicate to the nurse that the client has tissue hypoxia related to anemia? Select all that apply.

1. Dizziness
2. Thirst and polyuria
3. Nail beds that are pale
4. Fatigue and weakness
5. Dyspnea

2 A medical record indicates that a client has a positive Philadelphia chromosome. The nurse plans care considering the needs of the client with which disorder?

1. Acute myeloid leukemia (AML)
2. Hairy cell leukemia
3. Chronic myeloid leukemia (CML)
4. Chronic lymphocytic leukemia (CLL)

3 A nurse caring for a client who has just experienced a bone marrow biopsy and aspiration should assess for which of the following as the most serious complication postprocedure?

1. Bleeding
2. Infection
3. Shock
4. Splintering of bone marrow fragments

4 For the client diagnosed with iron deficiency anemia, the nurse should recommend an increased intake of which of the following foods?

1. Fresh citrus fruits
2. Milk and cheese
3. Organ meats
4. Whole grain breads

5 The nurse would interpret that a client is most severely at risk for bleeding when which laboratory test result is noted?

1. Neutrophils are 50%.
2. Lymphocytes are 30%.
3. Platelets are less than 20,000/mm^3.
4. Basophils are 0.

6 The nurse conducting an in-service on the hematology unit is comparing the pathophysiology of acute and chronic leukemias. The nurse reminds coworkers that which feature is common to both types?

1. Compensatory polycythemia stimulated by thrombocytopenia
2. Unregulated accumulation of white blood cells in the bone marrow
3. Increased blood viscosity resulting from an overproduction of white cells
4. Reduced plasma volume in response to a reduced production of cellular components

7 The nurse should include which information in client education for a client with sickle cell trait?

1. Avoid fluid loss or overhydration.
2. Triggering conditions are highly likely to initiate a sickle cell crisis.
3. The client can expect to experience chronic anemia.
4. Genetic counseling may be helpful before starting a family.

8 A client with pancytopenia seeks care at a clinic because of large areas of ecchymosis on the skin. The nurse should caution the client to avoid using which medications that can alter platelet function?

1. Acetylsalicylic acid (aspirin), dipyridamole (Persantine), and naproxen (Aleve)
2. Milk of magnesia (MOM), heparin (Liquaemin), and quinidine sulfate (Quinidex)
3. Senna (Senokot), furosemide (Lasix), and phenytoin (Dilantin)
4. Acetaminophen (Tylenol), sulfonamides, and penicillins

9 A male client newly diagnosed with hemophilia asks the nurse what problems he can expect to develop because of the disease. What is the nurse's best response?

1. "Try not to worry excessively. The disease usually affects females, and males only get mild cases."
2. "You may have joint bleeding, swelling, and damage because the bleeding causes inflammation in the joints and tissues."
3. "Since you have excess Von Willebrand factor, you may bleed more than normal for dental extractions or surgery."
4. "Don't worry about future complications yet. If you take extra vitamin K and vitamin B$_{12}$, your problems will be postponed."

10 A client enters the clinic reporting a sore mouth. Physical assessment reveals a beefy red tongue. The nurse would next assess for what other manifestations, suspecting the client may have pernicious anemia? Select all that apply.

1. Pallor or slight jaundice
2. Weakness and trouble with proprioception
3. Diminished short-term memory
4. Paresthesias such as numbness or tingling
5. Diet deficient in green, leafy vegetables

➤ See pages 395–397 for Answers and Rationales.

ANSWERS & RATIONALES

Pretest

1 **Answer: 3** **Rationale:** Cerebral tissue hypoxia is commonly associated with dizziness. The greatest potential risk to the client with dizziness is injury, especially with changes in position, so assistance with ambulation is important. Planning for periods of rest and consuming energy are important for someone with anemia because of his or her fatigue level, but most important is safety. Water temperature is not relevant to the issue of cerebral perfusion in this client. **Cognitive Level:** Analyzing **Client Need:** Physiological Adaptation **Integrated Process:** Nursing Process: Implementation **Content Area:** Adult Health **Strategy:** Review the problems associated with cerebral hypoxia. Prioritize the nursing actions needed for a safe and effective care environment. **Reference:** LeMone, P., Burke, K., & Bauldoff, G. (2011). *Medical-surgical nursing: Critical thinking in patient care* (5th ed.). Upper Saddle River, NJ: Pearson Education, pp. 1078–1079.

2 **Answer: 1** **Rationale:** Major complications of multiple myeloma include bone pain, hypercalcemia, renal failure, anemia, and impaired immune responses that are a result of bone marrow involvement. The systemic effects of paraproteins secreted by the malignant plasma cells may cause a hyperviscosity of body fluids, causing renal failure. **Cognitive Level:** Applying **Client Need:** Physiological Adaptation **Integrated Process:** Nursing Process: Implementation **Content Area:** Adult Health **Strategy:** If the answer is not clear, begin by eliminating the options that are not correct for multiple myeloma. **Reference:** LeMone, P., Burke, K., & Bauldoff, G. (2011). *Medical-surgical nursing: Critical thinking in patient care* (5th ed.). Upper Saddle River, NJ: Pearson Education, pp. 1102–1103.

3 **Answer: 2** **Rationale:** Thrombocytopenia is a platelet count less than 100,000/mL. This client is at risk of spontaneous bleeding and easy bruising, although the client is not at the severe level of below 20,000/mL. The client needs to be protected from trauma such as falls. **Cognitive Level:** Analyzing **Client Need:** Reduction of Risk Potential **Integrated Process:** Nursing Process: Planning **Content Area:** Adult Health **Strategy:** First determine what the platelet count indicates. Then decide what nursing order is appropriate. **Reference:** LeMone, P., Burke, K., & Bauldoff, G. (2011). *Medical-surgical nursing: Critical thinking in patient care* (5th ed.). Upper Saddle River, NJ: Pearson Education, p. 1107.

4 **Answer: 4** **Rationale:** Bone marrow biopsy and aspirate is the only definitive diagnosis of acute myelogenous leukemia (AML). The presence of Auer rods is diagnostic for AML. The presence of leukemic cells in the spinal fluid is more common in acute lymphocytic leukemia (ALL). Uric acid and lactic dehydrogenase levels may be elevated in AML, but this is not diagnostic for the disease. **Cognitive Level:** Applying **Client Need:** Reduction of Risk Potential **Integrated Process:** Nursing Process: Assessment **Content Area:** Adult Health **Strategy:** Consider what body system is affected by acute myelogenous leukemia (AML). What diagnostic test is most applicable? **Reference:** LeMone, P., Burke, K., & Bauldoff, G. (2011). *Medical-surgical nursing: Critical thinking in patient care* (5th ed.). Upper Saddle River, NJ: Pearson Education, p. 1087.

5 **Answer: 1** **Rationale:** Milk, eggs, liver and green, leafy vegetables are all foods that contain high levels of protein, folic acid, iron, and vitamin B_{12} and that are needed for erythropoiesis. The foods listed in the other options are grouped in such a way as to provide lesser amounts of these nutrients. **Cognitive Level:** Applying **Client Need:** Health Promotion and Maintenance **Integrated Process:** Nursing Process: Implementation **Content Area:** Adult Health **Strategy:** Which food list contains the best sources of needed nutrients? Although good sources are included in all the options, recognize that one option contains more protein, minerals, and needed vitamins than the others. **Reference:** LeMone, P., Burke, K., & Bauldoff, G. (2011). *Medical-surgical nursing: Critical thinking in patient care* (5th ed.). Upper Saddle River, NJ: Pearson Education, pp. 1077–1078.

6 **Answer: 2** **Rationale:** Iron dextran can be given intravenously or via deep intramuscular (IM) injection. A test dose for allergic response should be given before starting the therapy. The gluteal muscle is the best route for IM administration since the muscle is large and highly vascular. The Z-track method is preferable to prevent tattooing of the skin and tissue necrosis caused by infiltration into the subcutaneous tissue.

Cognitive Level: Applying **Client Need:** Pharmacological and Parenteral Therapies **Integrated Process:** Nursing Process: Implementation **Content Area:** Adult Health **Strategy:** The core issue of the question is knowledge of the properties of injectable iron and how this impacts on administration. Review this medication if the question was difficult. **Reference:** LeMone, P., Burke, K., & Bauldoff, G. (2011). *Medical-surgical nursing: Critical thinking in patient care* (5th ed.). Upper Saddle River, NJ: Pearson Education, pp. 1077–1078.

7 **Answer: 3** **Rationale:** In hemostasis, after vascular spasm, platelet aggregation immediately forms a platelet plug at the site of bleeding, but fibrin reinforces the platelet plug in the next step. Pressure can be safely released once the fibrin clot is formed—usually in 1–2 minutes. Clot retraction and clot dissolution occur in later phases of the process. **Cognitive Level:** Applying **Client Need:** Physiological Adaptation **Integrated Process:** Nursing Process: Implementation **Content Area:** Adult Health **Strategy:** Apply knowledge of the blood-clotting process to clinical actions. **Reference:** LeMone, P., Burke, K., & Bauldoff, G. (2011). *Medical-surgical nursing: Critical thinking in patient care* (5th ed.). Upper Saddle River, NJ: Pearson Education, pp. 883–884.

8 **Answer: 4** **Rationale:** Pernicious anemia is caused by the body's inability to absorb vitamin B_{12}. This is caused by a lack of intrinsic factor in the gastric juices or surgical removal of the terminal ileum where the vitamin is absorbed. The Shilling test, a 24-hour urine test for excretion of vitamin B_{12}, is seldom used today because detection of parietal cell and intrinsic factor antibodies (a blood test) is now possible for a definitive diagnosis of pernicious anemia. Blood testing for vitamin B_{12} and gastric pH are not done to diagnose pernicious anemia. **Cognitive Level:** Applying **Client Need:** Reduction of Risk Potential **Integrated Process:** Nursing Process: Planning **Content Area:** Adult Health **Strategy:** Use nursing knowledge and the process of elimination to answer the question. Note the similarity between the words *parietal cell* and *intrinsic factor* in the correct option with the words pernicious anemia in the stem of the question. **Reference:** LeMone, P., Burke, K., & Bauldoff, G. (2011). *Medical-surgical nursing: Critical thinking in patient care* (5th ed.). Upper Saddle River, NJ: Pearson Education, p. 1072.

9 **Answer: 1, 2, 4, 5** **Rationale:** In sickle cell anemia, if hypoxemia develops, the hemoglobin is deoxygenated and crystallizes into rod and chain shapes, deforming the erythrocyte into a crescent shape. Cells clump together, obstructing capillary blood flow. Conditions likely to trigger sickling include low body temperature, hypoxia, excessive exercise, dehydration, infections, or acidosis. Bedrest, which conserves energy, would not be a trigger. **Cognitive Level:** Applying **Client Need:** Physiological Adaptation **Integrated Process:** Teaching and Learning **Content Area:** Adult Health **Strategy:** Consider what conditions can predispose the client to problems. Notice that several options are similar and since the instructions are to select all that apply, choose the similar options if guessing. **Reference:** LeMone, P., Burke, K., & Bauldoff, G. (2011). *Medical-surgical nursing: Critical thinking in patient care* (5th ed.). Upper Saddle River, NJ: Pearson Education, p. 1073.

10 **Answer: 3** **Rationale:** Leukemic cells do not function as mature WBCs and are ineffective in the inflammatory and immune processes. This provides the best explanation. In the absence of an effective immune system, many infections are caused by normal flora. The function of WBCs is impaired in the client with leukemia, not just the number of WBCs. The client is at not high risk of infection because of reduction in immunoglobulins. **Cognitive Level:** Analyzing **Client Need:** Physiological Adaptation **Integrated Process:** Nursing Process: Diagnosis **Content Area:** Adult Health **Strategy:** Relate the function of neutrophils to the inflammatory process. What is expected if the counts are low? **Reference:** LeMone, P., Burke, K., & Bauldoff, G. (2011). *Medical-surgical nursing: Critical thinking in patient care* (5th ed.). Upper Saddle River, NJ: Pearson Education, p. 1084.

Posttest

1 **Answer: 1, 3, 4, 5** **Rationale:** Cerebral tissue hypoxia is commonly associated with dizziness, faintness, and headache. Recognition of cerebral hypoxia is critical since the body will attempt to shunt oxygenated blood to vital organs and away from the skin. Dyspnea, weakness, fatigue, and pallor may be observed. **Cognitive Level:** Applying **Client Need:** Physiological Adaptation **Integrated Process:** Nursing Process: Assessment **Content Area:** Adult Health **Strategy:** Recall first how hemoglobin causes reduced oxygen to the tissues and symptoms of hypoxia. Look for options that describe findings caused by hypoxia. **Reference:** LeMone, P., Burke, K., & Bauldoff, G. (2011). *Medical-surgical nursing: Critical thinking in patient care* (5th ed.). Upper Saddle River, NJ: Pearson Education, p. 1069.

2 **Answer: 3** **Rationale:** Approximately 95% of clients with chronic myeloid leukemia (CML) are Philadelphia chromosome-positive. This represents a translocation of the long arms of chromosomes 9 and 22. The other types of leukemia are not characterized by the Philadelphia chromosome. **Cognitive Level:** Applying **Client Need:** Physiological Adaptation **Integrated Process:** Nursing Process: Diagnosis **Content Area:** Adult Health **Strategy:** Specific knowledge is needed to answer this question. If you need to make an educated guess, consider that chromosome changes are most likely present in a chronic condition. **Reference:** LeMone, P., Burke, K., & Bauldoff, G. (2011). *Medical-surgical nursing: Critical thinking in patient care* (5th ed.). Upper Saddle River, NJ: Pearson Education, p. 1087.

3 **Answer: 1** **Rationale:** The risk for bleeding is of greatest risk since a large-bore needle is used to perform the biopsy and aspiration. Many of these clients often have an altered clotting capability. While the risk of infection is also a consideration, the procedure is performed under sterile conditions and is less of a concern than hemorrhage. Shock and bone marrow fragments are not of concern postprocedure. **Cognitive Level:** Applying **Client Need:** Physiological Adaptation **Integrated Process:** Nursing Process: Assessment **Content Area:** Adult Health **Strategy:** Any biopsy carries similar risks. Consider the additional problems a client who needs a bone marrow study may experience. **Reference:** LeMone, P., Burke, K., & Bauldoff, G. (2011). *Medical-surgical nursing: Critical thinking in patient care* (5th ed.). Upper Saddle River, NJ: Pearson Education, p. 890.

4 **Answer: 3** **Rationale:** Organ meats, green, leafy vegetables, and egg yolks are a good source of iron. Whole grain breads also contain iron, but not in as high a quantity as organ meats. Vitamin C, found in citrus fruits, facilitates absorption of iron but does not contain iron. Milk and cheese are high in calcium, but not iron. **Cognitive Level:** Applying **Client Need:** Health Promotion and Maintenance **Integrated Process:** Nursing Process: Implementation **Content Area:** Adult Health **Strategy:** The critical word in the question is *iron*. Use knowledge of diet therapy to determine which foods have highest iron value. **Reference:** LeMone, P., Burke, K., & Bauldoff, G. (2011). *Medical-surgical nursing: Critical thinking in patient care* (5th ed.). Upper Saddle River, NJ: Pearson Education, p. 1077.

5 **Answer: 3** **Rationale:** Neutrophils, lymphocytes, and basophils relate to the white blood cells, which are involved in protecting the client against infection. A platelet count lower than 20,000/mm³ increases the client's risk for severe bleeding because of reduced platelets to assist in the clotting cascade to form a clot. **Cognitive Level:** Analyzing **Client Need:** Reduction of Risk Potential **Integrated Process:** Nursing Process: Diagnosis **Content Area:** Adult Health **Strategy:** Recall the normal values of common laboratory tests. For this question, look for a result that relates to *bleeding*—a clue word in the question. **Reference:** LeMone, P., Burke, K., & Bauldoff, G. (2011). *Medical-surgical nursing: Critical thinking in patient care* (5th ed.). Upper Saddle River, NJ: Pearson Education, p. 1105.

6 **Answer: 2** **Rationale:** Leukemia is a result of erratic production of white blood cells (WBCs) by the bone marrow, which replace normal marrow components, and it can arise from both lymphocytic and myeloid etiologies. WBCs are often immature and incapable of performing their expected function(s). Although the malignancies present with proliferation of different cells, they all arise from unregulated WBCs in the bone marrow. **Cognitive Level:** Analyzing **Client Need:** Physiological Adaptation **Integrated Process:** Nursing Process: Diagnosis **Content Area:** Adult Health **Strategy:** Select the option that relates to both acute and chronic leukemia. **Reference:** LeMone, P., Burke, K., & Bauldoff,

G. (2011). *Medical-surgical nursing: Critical thinking in patient care* (5th ed.). Upper Saddle River, NJ: Pearson Education, pp. 1086–1087.

7 **Answer: 4** **Rationale:** Sickle hemoglobin is transmitted by recessive inheritance. Sickle cell trait is generally a mild condition that produces few if any manifestations. A client with sickle cell trait is a carrier of the disease and should have genetic counseling to determine presence of the hemoglobin S. The client with sickle cell trait would not go into a sickle cell crisis under conditions of dehydration. The client is at minimal risk, and would only go into crisis under conditions of extreme stress. The sickle cell trait does not commonly cause anemia. **Cognitive Level:** Applying **Client Need:** Health Promotion and Maintenance **Integrated Process:** Nursing Process: Planning **Content Area:** Adult Health **Strategy:** Consider the differences between sickle cell trait and sickle cell anemia. **Reference:** LeMone, P., Burke, K., & Bauldoff, G. (2011). *Medical-surgical nursing: Critical thinking in patient care* (5th ed.). Upper Saddle River, NJ: Pearson Education, pp. 1073–1074.

8 **Answer: 1** **Rationale:** Acetylsalicylic acid (aspirin), dipyridamole (Persantine), and naproxen (Aleve) can affect platelet aggregation and should be avoided in a client with bleeding tendencies. Generally, the nonsteroidal anti-inflammatory drugs (NSAIDs) and aspirin-containing products interfere with platelet function while acetaminophen is safe. The other medications listed would not increase the risk for bleeding by altering platelet function. **Cognitive Level:** Applying **Client Need:** Physiological Adaptation **Integrated Process:** Nursing Process: Implementation **Content Area:** Adult Health **Strategy:** Recall that to be the correct answer, all parts of the option must be correct. Eliminate any option that contains one or more drugs that do not affect platelets. **Reference:** LeMone, P., Burke, K., & Bauldoff, G. (2011). *Medical-surgical nursing: Critical thinking in patient care* (5th ed.). Upper Saddle River, NJ: Pearson Education, p. 927.

9 **Answer: 2** **Rationale:** Hemophilia is a group of hereditary clotting factor disorders characterized by prolonged coagulation time that results in prolonged and sometime excessive bleeding, often into joint spaces and tissues. It is an X-linked recessive characteristic transmitted by female carriers, and displayed almost exclusively in males. Although the client will have bleeding risks with dental work and surgery, there is not excess Von Willebrand factor. Vitamins will not help address the condition. **Cognitive Level:** Applying **Client Need:** Physiological Adaptation **Integrated Process:** Communication and Documentation **Content Area:** Adult Health **Strategy:** Consider that an honest, accurate answer that prepares the client to manage the disease is the best response. **Reference:** LeMone, P., Burke, K., & Bauldoff, G. (2011). *Medical-surgical nursing: Critical thinking in patient care* (5th ed.). Upper Saddle River, NJ: Pearson Education, pp. 1108–1111.

10 **Answer: 1, 2, 4** **Rationale:** The sore, beefy red tongue is very suspicious of pernicious anemia. The nurse should assess for other findings including altered sensations such as numbness or tingling in the extremities, and difficulty identifying one's position in space (proprioception), which may progress to difficulty with balance and spinal cord damage. Pallor and jaundice may be observed, but memory is not affected. The etiology is malabsorption of vitamin B_{12} rather than dietary deficiencies. **Cognitive Level:** Applying

Client Need: Physiological Adaptation **Integrated Process:** Nursing Process: Assessment **Content Area:** Adult Health **Strategy:** Identify that the sore, beefy red tongue may indicate pernicious anemia. Next consider what other findings are expected, recalling also general symptoms common to all forms of anemia. **Reference:** LeMone, P., Burke, K., & Bauldoff, G. (2011). *Medical-surgical nursing: Critical thinking in patient care* (5th ed.). Upper Saddle River, NJ: Pearson Education, p. 1072.

References

Adams, M., Holland, L., & Bostwick, P. (2011). *Pharmacology for nurses: A pathophysiologic approach* (3rd ed.). Upper Saddle River, NJ: Pearson Education.

Ignatavicius, D., & Workman, M. (2013). *Medical-surgical nursing: Critical thinking for collaborative care* (7th ed.) Philadelphia: W. B. Saunders Company.

Itano, J. K., & Taoka, K. N. (2005). *Core curriculum for oncology nursing* (4th ed.). Philadelphia, PA: W. B. Saunders.

Kee, J. L. (2010). *Laboratory and diagnostic tests* (8th ed.). Upper Saddle River, NJ: Pearson Education.

LeMone, P., Burke, K., & Bauldoff, G. (2011). *Medical-surgical nursing: Critical thinking in patient care* (5th ed.). Upper Saddle River, NJ: Pearson Education.

McCance, K., & Huether, K. (2010). *Understanding pathophysiology: The biologic basis for disease in adults and children* (6th ed.) St. Louis, MO: Elsevier.

Osborn, K. S., Wraa, C. E., & Watson, A. (2010). *Medical surgical nursing: Preparation for practice.* Upper Saddle River, NJ: Pearson Education.

Porth, C. (Ed.). (2011). *Essentials of pathophysiology* (3rd ed.). Philadelphia, PA: Lippincott Williams & Wilkins.

Porth, C., & Matfin, G. (2010). *Pathophysiology: Concepts of altered health states* (8th ed.). Philadelphia, PA: Lippincott Williams & Wilkins.

Wagner, K. D. (2009). Alterations in red blood cell function and hemostasis. In K. D. Wagner, K. Johnson, & M. Hardin-Pierce (Eds.), *High acuity nursing* (5th ed.). Upper Saddle River, NJ: Pearson Education.

Wilkes, G. M., & Burke, M. B. (2012). *Oncology nursing drug handbook.* Boston, MA: Jones and Bartlett.

Wilson, B. A., Shannon, M. T., & Shields, K.M. (2012). *Pearson nurse's drug guide 2012.* Upper Saddle River, NJ: Pearson Education.

16

Genetic and Developmental Health Problems

Chapter Outline

Risk Factors for Genetic and Developmental Health Problems

Trisomy 21 (Down Syndrome)

Turner Syndrome

Klinefelter Syndrome

Phenylketonuria (PKU)

Huntington's Disease

Marfan Syndrome

Albinism

Cystic Fibrosis (CF)

Cleft Lip or Palate

NCLEX-RN® Test Prep

Use the accompanying online resource, NursingReviewsandRationales, to test yourself with hundreds of NCLEX®-style practice questions.

Objectives

➤ Define key terms associated with genetic and developmental health problems.

➤ Identify risk factors associated with development of genetic and developmental health problems.

➤ Identify common etiologies of genetic and developmental health problems.

➤ Describe the pathophysiological processes associated with genetic and developmental health problems.

➤ Distinguish between normal and abnormal genetic and developmental health findings obtained from nursing assessment.

➤ Prioritize nursing interventions associated with specific genetic and developmental health problems.

Review at a Glance

autosomal all chromosomes other than sex (XX or XY) chromosomes; in normal human cells, there are 22 pairs of autosomal chromosomes and 2 pairs of sex chromosomes

carrier a person who has 1 affected and 1 unaffected autosome; they have no clinical disease but can pass on gene to offspring

choreiform a rapid and jerky body motion that is involuntary

chromosome protein structures consisting of DNA that map out cell functions of within body; 23 pairs

congenital a condition present since birth; causes are genetic, environmental, or multifactorial

gamete one of two cells created by meiosis; male (spermatozoon) and female (ovum)

gene genetic material (DNA) responsible for programming body function and characteristics; basic unit of inheritance

genotype entire genetic makeup of a person, such as a pattern of genes on chromosomes

heterozygous distribution of zygote for autosomal dominant presentation; only 1 abnormal autosomal has to be present (e.g., Marfan syndrome)

homozygous malformation created with autosomal recessive presentation; both abnormal chromosomes must be present (e.g., cystic fibrosis)

karyotype pictorial analysis of chromosomes of a person

malformation abnormal development process in utero leading to defect in organ or region of body

meiosis two stages of separating to create 2 gametes that can then combine to have both parent traits within a new zygote

mitosis stages of separation to create a new daughter cell in order to replace older cells for normal growth and replacement

mosaicism a person with presence of cells from 2 different genetic materials

multifactorial combination of causes for congenital defect (i.e., environmental plus gene abnormality)

nondisjunction an abnormal separation during meiosis; instead of a pair of gametes there is a trisomy (3) or monosomy (1) combination
steatorrhea foul-smelling stool containing undigested fat
syndrome a congenital defect associated with a characteristic set of anomalies (e.g., Down syndrome)

translocation after a chromosome breaks, a transfer of all or a part of chromosome to another chromosome leading to a severe or fatal defect
trisomy a condition in a chromosome where there are 3 chromosomes instead of a chromosome pair in cell (e.g., trisomy 21)

X-linked an inherited gene disorder located on X-chromosome (e.g., Duchenne muscular dystrophy)
zygote end product of parent cells (male/female) joining during reproduction

PRETEST

1 Which response by the nurse is best when the daughter of a woman with Huntington's disease asks why the client should be given thickened liquids?

1. "Your mother is at risk for dehydration."
2. "Your mother is at risk for aspiration of regular consistency liquids into the airway."
3. "Your mother may have difficulty chewing because of fatigue."
4. "Your mother may have pain on swallowing and this will minimize this risk."

2 The pediatric nurse assigned to a hospitalized infant with Down syndrome plans care to aid the infant in meeting which of Erikson's developmental stages?

1. Initiative vs. self doubt
2. Industry vs. inferiority
3. Autonomy vs. shame and doubt
4. Trust vs. mistrust

3 The nurse should monitor the adolescent who has Marfan syndrome for which potentially lethal complication?

1. Aortic rupture
2. Retinal detachment
3. Hyperextended joints
4. Seizure

4 The parent of a child born with albinism type I asks the nurse how this happened. What feature of the genetics of this disorder would the nurse include in a response?

1. Autosomal dominant
2. Autosomal recessive
3. X-linked
4. Multifactorial

5 A priority nursing intervention for the infant with cleft lip is which of the following?

1. Monitoring for adequate nutritional intake
2. Teaching high-risk newborn care
3. Assessing for shallow respirations
4. Preventing injury

6 The nurse explains to a parent of a child with cystic fibrosis that the parent should administer the pancrelipase (Pancrease) how often?

1. Three times daily
2. After each loose stool
3. Upon arising in the morning
4. With each meal and snack

7 A child is noted to have a very short stature, webbed neck, and low posterior hairline. The nurse will expect which of the following health problems?

1. Turner syndrome
2. Down syndrome
3. Marfan syndrome
4. Klinefelter syndrome

8 A child with cleft palate begins pulling on his left ear, is irritable, and begins to run a temperature of 102°F. Based on these findings, the nurse would next assess the child for signs of which of the following?

1. Pneumonia
2. Urinary tract infection (UTI)
3. Otitis media
4. Cellulitis

9 The nurse concludes that a male child with a karyotype showing XXY is a candidate for which of the following?

1. Turner syndrome
2. Klinefelter syndrome
3. Down syndrome
4. Marfan syndrome

10 The nurse explains to the mother of an infant born with phenylketonuria (PKU) that the infant requires a low phenylalanine diet to prevent which of the following complications?

1. Irreversible brain damage
2. Kidney failure
3. Blindness
4. Neutropenia

➤ *See pages 416–417 for Answers and Rationales.*

I. RISK FACTORS FOR GENETIC AND DEVELOPMENTAL HEALTH PROBLEMS

A. **Miscarriage**: genetic defects cause 60% of spontaneous abortions (miscarriages)

B. **Maternal and paternal influences**
  1. Familial: tends to run in certain families or ethnic groups
  2. With each subsequent offspring, incidence may increase, although each pregnancy should be viewed as an independent event
     a. Endocrine: higher incidence of type 2 diabetes mellitus in Native American families
     b. Cardiac: ventral septal defect has increased reoccurrence among siblings
     c. Hematology: Mediterranean descent increases risk for glucose-6-phosphatase deficiency (G6PD), thalassemia

C. **Age**
  1. Increased age of sperm, ova, or **gametes** (1 or 2 cells created by meiosis)
     a. Parents over 35 years of age; both mother and father increase incidence of abnormal **zygote** (end product of parent cells joined during reproduction) such as **trisomy** (a condition in which there are 3 chromosomes instead of a pair in a cell)
     b. **Autosomal** (all chromosomes other than sex [XX or XY]): dominant disorders such as Marfan syndrome
  2. Adolescent: younger age of mother leads to increased risk
     a. Factors related to hormonal changes
     b. Dietary insufficiency of protein, iron
     c. Risk-taking behaviors: smoking, drugs

D. **Nutrition**
  1. Malnutrition leads to poor cell formation
  2. Folic acid deficiency is a known factor in spina bifida
  3. Low protein increases risk of congenital heart disease
  4. Iron-deficiency anemia and small for gestational age (SGA)

E. **Environment**
1. Teratogens: interfere with fetal development
   a. Drugs
      1) Tobacco increases incidence of congenital defects
      2) Alcohol exposure leads to fetal alcohol syndrome (FAS)
      3) Drugs, such as phenytoin (Dilantin), lead to a higher incidence of congenital malformation
   b. Radiation leads to increase risk of **nondisjunction** (an abnormal separation) during **meiosis** (2 stages of separating to create 2 gametes)
   c. Infection
      1) Can interfere with fetal development
      2) Rubella leads to increased risk of microcephaly
      3) Cytomegalovirus (CMV) leads to increased risk of optic atrophy
2. Oxygen deprivation
   a. Smoking leads to increased possibility of prematurity
   b. Maternal hypertension can lead to birth complications and cerebral palsy
F. **Multifactorial (combination of causes for a congenital defect)**
1. Combination of all of the above: disruption in utero plus hereditary predisposition, such as cleft lip or palate

Practice to Pass

What is the rationale for developing a family tree (pedigree) as a part of family planning?

2. Genetic predisposition that leads to **malformation** (abnormal development process in utero leading to defect in organ or region of body)
   a. Approximately 5–10% of cancers have a **gene** (genetic material [DNA]) marker
   b. Positive human leukocyte antigen-B (HLA-B) allele in children with type 1 diabetes mellitus

II. TRISOMY 21 (DOWN SYNDROME)

A. **Overview**
1. Defined as a chromosome disorder involving the 21st chromosome (3 copies instead of 2)
2. **Syndrome** (a congenital defect associated with a characteristic set of anomalies) is a predisposition for:
   a. Congenital heart disease: atrial ventricular canal; 40–50% have improper development of separate atria and ventricles on left and right, which can cause heart failure (HF)
   b. Leukemia, 30 times higher incidence
   c. Hypothyroidism, 20 times higher incidence
   d. Hirschsprung disease, higher incidence
B. **Pathophysiology**
1. Malformation involves 21st **chromosome** (23 pairs of protein structures consisting of DNA that map out functions of cells within body)
   a. **Trisomy**

   1) Nondisjunction: causes 92–95% of Down syndrome; zygote contains 3 chromosomes instead of normal pair at chromosome 21; increased incidence with paternal or maternal age
   2) **Mosaicism** (presence of cells from 2 different genetic materials in same person)—causes 1–3% of Down syndrome; trisomy occurs during **mitosis** (stages of separation to create a new daughter cell); leads to some normal and abnormal cell lines; milder form of the syndrome
   b. **Translocation** (after a chromosome breaks, a transfer of all or part of a chromosome to another chromosome leading to a severe or fatal defect)
   1) Causes 3–5% of Down syndrome
   2) Zygote has exchanged materials from break in chromosome 21
   3) No increased risk with age, but does have a 5–15% risk of reoccurrence

2. Signs and symptoms
  a. Physical characteristics
    1) Hypotonia: lack of general muscle tone
    2) Hyperflexibility: able to flex joints beyond 180 degrees
    3) Wide space between first and second toe
    4) Transverse palmar crease: (horizontal crease across palm) or plantar crease in foot is present in clients with Down syndrome (see Figure 16-1)
    5) Low-set ears: normal is along an imaginary line from eye to top of ear
    6) Epicanthal folds: folds of skin along external to internal edge of eye
    7) Depressed nasal bridge
    8) High, arched, narrow palate and protruding tongue
  b. Intellectual characteristics: moderate to severe mental retardation; emphasis is on concrete and individualized operations
  c. Sensory deficits include myopia, hyperopia, and strabismus
C. Nursing assessment
  1. Assessment
    a. Early detection (look for physical attributes in newborn nursery)
    b. Family assessment
      1) Use tool to measure family strengths Apgar, family profile
      2) Assess grieving process: denial, nonacceptance of diagnosis; depression; unable to care for self or others; withdrawal, not speaking with family; anger; being unreasonable with nursing staff
    c. Physical characteristics: muscle strength and flexibility, appearance and distinguishing features, growth and development, sensory status, respiratory and cardiac status for possible complications
  2. Diagnostic tests include genetic screen to detect cause of abnormal chromosome 21
    a. Prenatal: amniocentesis to identify chromosome 21; chorionic villi sampling
    b. Postnatal: chromosome 21, detection of trisomy
D. Nursing management
  1. Development
    a. Goal: promote optimal development; infant may develop at a slower rate with smaller steps; involve family in setting goals for child
    b. Interventions should be planned according to developmental level

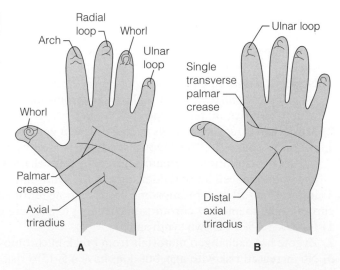

Figure 16-1

Characteristic palm markings. A. Normal individual, B. Individual with Down syndrome

1) Infant
   a) Cognition: Piaget's sensorimotor: Denver Developmental Screening Test (DDST) or comparable developmental screening tool to determine baseline level; monitor progression; enroll in infant stimulation program
   b) Social: Erickson's trust vs. mistrust: assessment of family, cultural, and feeding interaction to reinforce a positive family bond; refer to social services if suspect abuse/neglect
2) Toddler
   a) Cognition: Piaget's sensorimotor, continue to promote sensory stimulation; reinforce realistic expectations/goals
   b) Social: Erickson's autonomy vs. shame and doubt, unsuccessful toilet training can lead to child abuse; anticipatory guidance in relation to temper tantrums
3) Preschool
   a) Cognition: Piaget's preoperational support; involvement in child's early education program
   b) Social: Erickson's initiative vs. self-doubt, allow for successes within an integrated school program

Practice to Pass

Why is it important to understand child development in the client with Down syndrome?

4) School-age
   a) Cognition: will usually remain in Piaget's concrete formations; give simple, visual cues for any teaching during hospitalizations
   b) Social: Erickson's industry vs. inferiority; inclusion programs are beneficial for schools and the child; after school activities
5) Adolescence: social, Erickson's identity vs. role confusion; must involve in teen activities; information on reproduction and puberty at their level
6) Adult: job placement; level of living independence; parent or guardianship and living will issues need to be resolved

2. Monitor for respiratory infections (especially in infant); because of large protruding tongue and hypotonia, child has an increased incidence of respiratory complications or compromise
   a. May be detected by vital signs (increased respiratory rate, fever), congestion, and inability to tolerate feedings
   b. Prevent infection by liquefying secretions with humidifier; use saline and bulb syringe to suction secretions

Practice to Pass

Why is it important to determine the cause of trisomy 21?

3. Cardiac defects: monitor for heart failure by assessing urine output (minimum 1–2 mL/kg/hr), edema formation, activity and feeding tolerance; note change in color, cyanosis
4. Provide postoperative care for child with correction of heart defect
5. Priority nursing diagnoses: Delayed Development, Impaired Parenting, Risk for Ineffective Airway Clearance, Ineffective Tissue Perfusion, Decreased Cardiac Output

III. TURNER SYNDROME

A. Overview
1. Defined as a deletion or abnormal X on chromosome 45; there are a total of 45 chromosomes with 22 somatic pairs and only 1 sex chromosome (45, XO)
2. Turner syndrome predisposes client to hypothyroidism, aortic coarctation, renal structure anomalies, and behavior and learning disturbances

B. Pathophysiology
1. Female phenotype with incidence 1:2,500 female births
2. Not clear but thought to be nondisjunction or fragmented X
3. The only monosomy that is viable, yet 99% are spontaneously aborted
4. Signs and symptoms
   a. Newborn: low posterior hairline, lymphedema of feet and legs, and webbed neck

  b. Child: short stature; growth slows after age 3; below 3% on growth chart
   1) No development of secondary sex characteristics during puberty
   2) Lack of or nonfunctioning ovaries
   3) Wide-spaced nipples
   4) Short 4th metacarpals
   5) "Shield-like" chest with underdeveloped breasts
   6) Normal intellectual development
   7) Frequent urinary tract infections (UTIs)

C. Nursing assessment
 1. Assessment includes any signs or symptoms of renal, cardiac, or thyroid dysfunction
  a. Renal: note any UTIs
  b. Cardiac: aortic coarctation, decrease in lower extremity blood pressure
  c. Hypothyroidism: intolerance to cold, weight gain, lethargy, hair loss, enlarged thyroid gland
 2. Early recognition: note physical characteristics in newborn nursery
 3. Assessment of family and cultural characteristics, noting strengths of family
 4. Additional assessment: growth charts (height and weight), observance of sex characteristics, physical characteristics
 5. Diagnostic tests
  a. Labs: blood urea nitrogen (BUN), creatinine (CR) for kidney function
  b. Radiology: voiding cystourethrography, cystoscopy
  c. Prenatal genetic testing before birth
  d. Genetic **karyotype** (pictorial analysis of a person's chromosomes after birth)

D. Nursing management
 1. Medications include (as appropriate) estrogen prior to age 12 years and progesterone for secondary sexual characteristics
 2. Monitor nonverbal and verbal suggestion of hopelessness; encourage verbalization
 3. Encourage teen support group
 4. Early detection: note characteristics at birth in order to initiate genetic counseling for family
 5. Genetic counseling: educate on defect, sex-linked chromosome disorder; determine type of malformation for family planning, if possible
 6. Nursing priority diagnoses: Disturbed Body Image, Ineffective Sexuality Patterns, Impaired Family Processes

Practice to Pass

How is it possible for the client with Turner syndrome to not be diagnosed until adolescence?

IV. KLINEFELTER SYNDROME

A. Overview
 1. Defined as a polysomic **X-linked** (an inherited gene disorder located on X-chromosome) chromosome defect with 1 or more extra X-chromosomes in **genotype** (entire genetic make-up) of individual male
 2. Associated with increased parental age (maternal or paternal)
 3. Incidence: 1:850 male births

B. Pathophysiology
 1. During meiosis, nondisjunction of X- and Y-chromosome causes disorder
 2. With an increase in Xs, there is an increase in mental retardation
 3. Usually occurs as presence of extra chromosome 47; for example, additional X and possibly Y chromosomes 47-XXY 48-XXYY
 4. Signs and symptoms
  a. Tall, lean body with disproportionately long legs to trunk
  b. Small or undescended testicles and sterility
  c. Gynecomastia
  d. Sparse facial hair and voice does not change at puberty
  e. Normal intellectual development, may have delay in language

      f. Abnormalities include scoliosis, dental abnormalities, cardiac abnormalities and pulmonary disease

C. Nursing assessment

    1. Assessment includes sexual characteristics, growth chart (height and weight), and reproductive history

    2. Early recognition of physical characteristics that may be delayed until puberty

    3. Family and cultural assessment

D. Nursing management

    1. Medication, including testosterone

    2. Support child and family through diagnosis: verbalize positive attributes; demonstrate parenting; provide anticipatory developmental and safety guidance; support constructive discipline

    3. Early child development program: use face position and eye contact; stimulate cognitive development; monitor for achievement of physical, cognitive, and psychosocial milestones

    4. Genetic counseling: family planning and family support and/or referral

    5. Encourage support of teens: identify effective ways to express anger or frustration; identify community resources; educate about sterility; encourage peer support

    6. High priority nursing diagnoses: Disturbed Body Image, Impaired Family Processes, Risk for Impaired Development

Practice to Pass

Explain nondisjunction as the cause of Klinefelter syndrome.

V. PHENYLKETONURIA (PKU)

A. Overview

    1. Defined as a metabolic disorder with a defect in enzyme phenylalanine hydroxylase that metabolizes phenylalanine, leading to accumulation of phenylalanine and other metabolites

    2. Autosomal recessive disorder with **homozygous** presentation (malformation created with autosomal recessive presentation; both chromosomes must be present) (see Figure 16-2)

    3. If untreated, will lead to severe mental retardation, seizures, and death

    4. Incidence is 1:15,000 and carrier state can be detected; is more common in Caucasians

Figure 16-2

Phenylketonuria: Autosomal Recessive Gene Pattern (Both Chromosomes Present)

A.

		Carrier father	
		D	d
Carrier	D	DD	Dd
mother	d	dD	dd

B.

		Carrier father	
		D	d
Disease	D	DD	Dd
mother	D	DD	Dd

C.

		Normal father	
		d	d
Disease	D	Dd	Dd
mother	D	Dd	Dd

D.

		Normal father	
		d	d
Carrier	D	Dd	Dd
mother	d	dd	dd

DD = Disease   D = disease gene
dD, Dd = Carrier   d = normal gene
dd = No risk

B. Pathophysiology

1. Enzyme phenylalanine hydroxylase is absent, which converts phenylalanine to tyrosine
2. Tyrosine is needed by body for melanin pigment and for hormones epinephrine and thyroxin
3. Phenylalanine is responsible for growth; accumulation of serum phenylalanine leads to irreversible central nervous system damage and mental retardation
4. Increased metabolites in blood (phenylpyruvic acid and phenylacetic acid) are excreted in urine, causing a musky odor and phenylketonuria (PKU)
5. Signs and symptoms
   a. Musky odor to urine
   b. Neuromuscular development delay
   c. Failure to thrive
   d. Mental retardation by age 6 months
   e. Acute episodes may include possible seizures, vomiting, and development of eczematous rashes

C. Nursing assessment

1. Assessment includes growth and development, urine, nutritional status, skin, and signs of dehydration
2. Diagnostic tests (done after 24 hours of protein-containing fluids)
   a. Newborn screen: blood specimen taken after 48 hours but within 7 days of birth (if taken earlier, should be repeated at 1–2 weeks of age); phenylalanine levels over 10–15 mg/dL leads to brain damage
   b. Electroencephalography (EEG)

D. Nursing management

1. Newest recommendation is to maintain low phenylalanine diet for life
   a. Breastfeeding possible if phenylalanine levels are monitored
   b. Phenylalanine level must be maintained between 2–6 mg/dL
   c. Dietary products: Pro-Phree and Phenex-1 are examples of low-phenylalanine products
   d. Avoid high-protein foods (especially meat and dairy products), which are highest in phenylalanine; as well as aspartame
   e. Older child can exchange some vegetables, but should maintain minimal meat consumption
   f. Adolescent females and child-bearing women should adhere to diet to prevent congenital anomalies (low birth weight, mental retardation, and microcephaly)
2. Monitor growth and development
   a. Must maintain adequate nutrition with an extremely limited diet
   b. Educate family on importance of maintaining routine primary health care visits for screening and growth assessment
3. Monitor phenylalanine levels
   a. Phenylalanine at dangerous levels if greater than 15 mg/dL
   b. Increased stress, illness, growth spurts will trigger increased phenylalanine levels
   c. Most common manifestation is vomiting leading to dehydration
   d. Maintain seizure precautions
4. Plan for genetic counseling with the family through genetic screening to assess offspring **carrier** (one affected and one unaffected autosome) and by future pregnancy planning (see Table 16-1 again)
5. Female with PKU at puberty
   a. Counseling on secondary sexual development
   b. Counseling on family planning if mother has disorder
      1) If partner is carrier, 2:4 chance of reoccurrence; if partner is not a carrier, all offspring will be carriers (see Table 16-1 again)
      2) Instruct on strict control of diet if planning pregnancy

Practice to Pass

A client and her husband are carriers of the phenylketonuria (PKU) allele. She asks the nurse what the risk is that their children will present with the disease. How should the nurse respond?

6. Priority nursing diagnoses: Risk for Injury related to seizure activity and increased phenylalanine levels; Deficient Knowledge related to diet therapy; Risk for Impaired Development related to CNS damage

VI. HUNTINGTON DISEASE

A. Overview

1. Defined as a rare, inherited disease caused by degeneration in cerebral cortex and basal ganglia; defect on chromosome 4; also called Huntington's chorea
2. An autosomal dominant disease inheritance pattern with **heterozygous** (only 1 abnormal autosomal has to be present) presentation (see Figure 16-3)
3. Usually evident between 25–55 years of age; has a 5 in 100,000 occurrence; occurs in all ethnic groups, with life expectancy about 10 years

B. Pathophysiology

1. Degeneration in cerebral cortex and basal ganglia causes a deficient inhibitory neurotransmitter system and neurotransmitters are lost; especially gamma-aminobutyric acid (GABA)
2. GABA is an inhibitory transmitter of central nervous system (CNS) that inhibits specific target pathways to slow increased activity in these pathways
   a. A deficiency of GABA causes increased neural excitation and is associated with epilepsy, anxiety disorders, depression
   b. Receptors are concentrated in 2 areas, including limbic system (controlling emotional behaviors) and locus ceruleus (controlling arousal)
3. An imbalance in basal ganglia occurs between dopamine and acetylcholine, and GABA; acetylcholine is decreased but dopamine not affected (unlike Parkinson's disease)
   c. **Choreiform** (rapid and jerky body motion that is involuntary) movements result from deficient neurotransmitter inhibition
4. Degeneration in cerebral cortex leads to progressive increase in labile emotions caused by decrease in GABA and may include violent behavior changes and dementia
5. Alleles inherited from father results in onset later in life than if inherited from mother
6. Other physiologic changes
   a. Lesions may occur in putamen, corpus striatum, and thalamus
   b. Frontal lobes of brain atrophy, enlarge, and change lateral ventricle structure
   c. Neurons in certain areas of brain are reduced
7. Symptoms begin between age of 25–55 years
8. Signs and symptoms
   a. Movement: choreiform movements and athetosis (slower movements than choreiform)
   b. Intellect: progressive degeneration, impaired memory and judgment

Figure 16-3

Huntington's Disease: Autosomal Dominant Gene Pattern (Only One Chromosome Present)

A.   Normal father
              d   d
Disease D | Dd | Dd |
mother   d | dd | dd |

B.   Disease father
              D   d
Disease D | DD | Dd |
mother   d | dD | dd |

DD, Dd, dD = Disease   D = disease gene
dd = No risk   d = normal gene

    c. Severe dementia with impulsiveness, paranoia, delusions, and hallucinations, neurosis, verbal and emotional outbursts, irritability, suicidal tendency, and personality changes

C. Nursing assessment

  1. Assessment includes memory, ability to follow commands, ability to perform activities of daily living (ADLs) and degree of movement problems, mental status, history of recent changes in personality and level of consciousness, ability to stay on task

  2. Diagnostic tests

    a. Diagnosis made by clinical manifestations and family history

    b. No prognostic lab studies to treat or predict disease

    c. Positive gene marker on DNA testing for conclusive diagnosis

    d. Magnetic resonance imagery (MRI) to assess brain involvement

D. Nursing management

  1. Medications include antipsychotics (such as phenothiazines and Butyrophenones) and antidepressants

  2. Genetic counseling

    a. Autosomal dominance requires only 1 affected autosome (see Figure 16–3); there is a 2:4 reoccurrence if 1 parent has Huntington's disease and a 3:4 reoccurrence if both parents have disease

    b. Ethical considerations in testing gene presence: variance in age of presentation; disorder is currently not curable; family planning issues

  3. Nutrition

    a. Establish baseline and monitor for weight loss; increase calories and protein to support increased activity level

    b. Maintain good oral hygiene

    c. Impaired swallowing could lead to aspiration: maintain in upright position during eating; give small amounts at one time; give thickened liquids

Practice to Pass

What are the ethical implications of early diagnosis by identifying gene marker 4 in offspring of the client with Huntington's chorea?

  4. Long-term care

    a. Monitor family for issues related to behavior control

    b. Suicide precautions may be necessary

    c. Drug and alcohol abuse are common and should be monitored

    d. Institutionalization when home care no longer possible

  5. Controversial therapies: fetal brain tissue transplants have been moderately successful, but ethical issues exist related to source of transplant

  6. Future therapies: possible gene replacement therapy to replace abnormal gene on chromosome 4

  7. Priority nursing diagnoses: Deficient Knowledge, Imbalanced Nutrition: Less than Body Requirements, Risk for Aspiration, Ineffective Family Coping

VII. MARFAN SYNDROME

A. Overview

  1. Defined as a connective tissue disorder caused by atrophy of neurons in specific areas of brain; involves chromosome 15

  2. An autosomal dominant inheritance pattern disorder with heterozygous presentation; no carrier status; incidence is 1:10,000

  3. A **congenital** (present since birth) disorder with 25% spontaneous mutations

B. Pathophysiology

  1. A mutation occurs of frillin-1, a connective tissue protein found in body tissue

  2. Defect is in elastic fibers of connective tissues causing long, thin extremities, hyperextendable joints, and spinal deformities

   3. Associated defects
      a. Aortic aneurysm: most common cause of early death; weakness within aorta leads to dilation and rupture
      b. Optic lens disorders: dislocated optic lens, retinal detachment, cataracts, glaucoma, and myopia

   4. Signs and symptoms
      a. Tall, lean body with thin fingers (arachnodactyly) and winged scapula
      b. Vision disturbances
      c. Musculoskeletal deformities: pectus excavatum, curvature of thoracic spine, hyperextensibility of joints, scoliosis
   5. Often associated with sports-related cardiac arrest
C. **Nursing assessment**
   1. Assessment includes growth and development, proportioned body, visual examination, range of motion, scoliosis screening, auscultation of abdomen for pulse, blood pressure, cardiac status
   2. Diagnostic tests: genetic screening, MRI if aneurysm suspected
D. **Nursing management**
   1. Medications include beta blockers for cardiac problems
   2. Community and school education: support automated external defibrillator (AED) implementation, health physical prior to participation in athletic events, and scoliosis screening
   3. Sensory: note any change in vision and encourage yearly eye exams
   4. Cardiac
      a. Monitor cardiac status: auscultation of abdomen, pulse, vital signs
      b. Aortic valve replacement may be indicated
      c. Maintain blood pressure within normal limits
   5. Genetic counseling: include discussion about family planning and risk of recurrence, and parent and child education on risks for associated anomalies
   6. Priority nursing diagnoses: Risk for Decreased Cardiac Output, Disturbed Sensory Perception: Visual, Disturbed Body Image, Deficient Knowledge

VIII. ALBINISM
A. **Overview**
   1. Defined as a lack of skin pigmentation caused by absence of tyrosinase (needed for melanin synthesis)
   2. An autosomal recessive chromosomal disorder with homozygous presentation; incidence is 1:17,000 individuals
   3. Two types include type I (oculocutaneous) and type II (less pigmented)
B. **Pathophysiology**
   1. Autosomal recessive disorder; both parents are carriers; there is 25% chance of mutation, 25% chance not carrying gene, and 50% chance of having carrier status; risk is unchanged with each subsequent pregnancy
   2. Individuals are deficient in tyrosinase, an enzyme needed to synthesize melanin, but have a normal number of melanocytes
   3. Type I: *oculocutaneous*
      a. Defect in tyrosinase; client is unable to convert tyrosine to dopa; results in lack of melanin synthesis
      b. Associated visual problems
         1) Foveal hypoplasia can occur; abnormal retinal development because of lack of pigment
         2) Transillumination: iris lacks sufficient pigment to screen light coming into eye

3) Associated vision disturbances: nystagmus, strabismus, myopia, hyperopia, photophobia

4. Type II: *less pigmented*; client may have slight pigmentation but there are no ocular or integument variations

5. Syndromes associated with albinism; Hermansky-Pudlak syndrome (HPS)

   a. Syndrome of albinism including bleeding tendencies

   b. Can include lung (pulmonary fibrosis) and bowel (inflammatory bowel disease)

   c. Bleeding problems result from malfunction of platelets and include nosebleeds, bruising, or severe bleed during surgery or childbirth

   d. Client will have normal results in prothrombin time (PT), partial thromboplastin time (PTT); may lack von Willebrand factor (less than 70% occurrence, higher risk of bleed)

6. Signs and symptoms

   a. Lack of pigment in skin, hair, eyes: pale or pink skin, white or yellow hair, and light-colored or pink eyes

   b. Vision assessment: may reveal low vision (20/50); legal blindness at 20/200; visually evoked potential (VEP) may be done for young infant

C. Nursing assessment

1. Nursing assessment: visual exam, presence of any extraocular movements, and ability to read because of nystagmus; inspection of color in skin, hair, and eyes

2. Diagnostic tests: none

D. Nursing management

1. Symptomatic care: screen vision; avoid sun exposure and use maximum sunscreen; wear sunglasses; have frequent checks for potential melanoma; corrective visual wear or aids with dark lenses

2. Genetic counseling: teach parent and child about potential for future children with albinism; genetic screening of family

3. Cultural competency: dispel myths related to mixed ethnicity or inbreeding as cause; educate about genetics as cause

4. Priority nursing diagnoses: Deficient Knowledge, Risk for Impaired Skin Integrity, Risk for Impaired Sensory Perception

IX. CYSTIC FIBROSIS (CF)

A. Overview

1. Defined as an autosomal recessive chromosome disorder with exocrine gland dysfunction, which manifests in multiple body systems; incidence is 1:2,000; affects mostly Caucasians

2. Multisystem involvement: respiratory, pancreatic, liver, and gastrointestinal (GI); severity of symptoms varies on an individual basis; goal is to increase longevity

B. Pathophysiology

1. Homozygous presentation: chromosome 7 defect affecting single gene on long arm of chromosome that encodes for cystic fibrosis transmembrane regulator (CFTR)

2. Primary feature is lack of function of chloride channels: failure to open or absence of channels

3. Defective protein inhibits transport of sodium chloride, leading to an increased viscosity of secretions and an increase of sodium chloride (NaCl) in sweat

4. System pathophysiology

   a. Respiratory tract

      1) Decreased ciliary function and increased thickness of mucous secretions occurs

      2) Decreased function of alveoli and alveolar plugs leads to repeat infections and chronic obstructive pulmonary disease (COPD)

          a) COPD leads to cor pulmonale (right-sided heart failure caused by respiratory problems) and chronic hypoxemia

          b) *Pseudomonas aeruginosa* and *Staphylococcus aureus* are common organisms that resist antibiotics, leading to drug-resistant pneumonia

       3) Sinus tract disease with polyps and chronic thick mucus

    b. Gastrointestinal

       1) Thick secretions block ducts leading from pancreas to duodenum

       2) Malabsorption occurs because digestive enzymes don't reach food; predominantly affects fats and fat-soluble vitamins A, D, E, K; leads to malnutrition if untreated

    c. Pancreas: damage to Islets of Langerhans causes an increased incidence of type 1 diabetes mellitus

    d. Liver: biliary obstruction leads to cirrhosis and gallbladder disease

  5. Signs and symptoms

    a. Respiratory

       1) Frequent pneumonias (methicillin-resistant *staphylococcus aureus* [MRSA] leads to high mortality rate)

       2) Productive cough with thick, foul-smelling secretions

       3) Clubbing of nails from chronic hypoxemia

       4) Persistent sinusitis for adolescent

       5) COPD leads to chronic high CO_2 level

    b. Nutrition

       1) Large protruding abdomen

       2) Infant: failure to thrive

       3) Older child: osteomalacia (rickets), abnormal clotting times, and malnourishment

    c. Newborn: ileus related to thick mucus from meconium

    d. Infant: rectal prolapse because of thick stools and **steatorrhea** (foul-smelling stool containing undigested fat)

    e. Older child: diabetes-related disorders if diabetic ketoacidosis unchecked; delayed secondary sexual characteristics

    f. Young adult

       1) Females: thick cervical secretions lead to decreased fertility

       2) Males: sterile or minimal sperm production related to blocked seminal ducts

C. Nursing assessment

  1. Nursing assessment includes: respiratory status, vital signs, lung sounds, sputum analysis, abdominal size, stool characteristics, sexual characteristics, reproductive history, daily weight, and growth chart

  2. Diagnostic tests

    a. Classic NaCl sweat test (2–5 times greater than normal)

    b. Newborn screen: decreased trypsin (pancreatic enzyme) level in stool indicates CF; normal is positive in small amounts (screen is required in most states)

    c. Prenatal and carrier status screening is available

    d. Arterial blood gases (ABGs) or pulse oximetry

    e. Chest x-ray (CXR) and pulmonary function studies (PFS)

D. Nursing management

  1. Medications include bronchodilators, antibiotics as needed, corticosteroids, dornase alfa (Pulmozyme) to reduce mucus viscosity (aerosol), annual immunizations, and pancrelipase (Pancrease) by mouth

  2. Nursing interventions

    a. Respiratory

       1) Administer oxygen (O_2) as needed: use caution with O_2 administration; chronically high CO_2 can alter respiratory drive

       2) Assess respiratory status

3) Teach proper administration of inhalers and O$_2$: separate administration of corticosteroids from other inhalers; administer corticosteroids last
4) Monitor for side effects of medications, particularly tachycardia

5) Increase fluids to liquefy secretions
6) Chest physiotherapy: postural drainage and percussion with vibration to loosen and clear secretions; flutter device and huffing procedure as an aid to expectoration; perform after bronchodilation
7) Treat pulmonary infections; there is increased risk for antibiotic-resistant microorganisms; it is important to monitor therapeutic response
b. Pancreas

1) Pancreatic enzyme replacements such as pancrelipase (Pancrease) must be given before each meal or snack
2) Note stool characteristics (steatorrhea) to determine absorption
3) Assess growth while hospitalized; monitor daily weights at same time and using same scale
3. Chronic degenerative disease
a. Lung/heart transplant is current trend to treat irreversible lung/heart disease
b. Developmental issues
1) Support adolescents who struggle with sexuality and chronic illness
2) Monitor parental characteristics of overprotection
3) Discuss end-of-life issues as they arise
4. Genetic counseling
a. Provide anticipatory guidance to parents of a child with CF regarding future pregnancies
b. Encourage genetic counseling for the client with CF
c. Update client on therapies for gene replacement as they become available
5. Priority nursing diagnoses: Failure to Thrive, Impaired Growth and Development, Impaired Gas Exchange, Risk for Infection, Impaired Family Processes, Deficient Knowledge

X. CLEFT LIP OR PALATE

A. Overview
1. Cleft lip is defined as a vertical opening (cleft) in upper lip
2. Cleft palate is defined as a fissure in roof of mouth creating a passageway between mouth and nose
3. Most common craniofacial malformation
4. Cleft lip and palate can be together or separate, unilateral or bilateral, and complete or incomplete
5. Cause is **multifactorial** and is associated with various syndromes (e.g., Pierre Robin's)
B. Pathophysiology
1. Interruption in development, leading to lack of fusion or rupture of palate or lip; occurs at 6–8 weeks' gestation for cleft lip (CL) and 8–12 weeks gestation for cleft palate (CP)
2. Cleft lip may involve external nares, nasal cartilage, nasal septum, and alveolar process
3. Cleft palate may involve uvula and soft palate

4. Signs and symptoms include visual defect, crusting on cleft, swallowing air, vomiting, difficulty sucking, expulsion of formula through nose (cleft palate), aspiration, difficulty with speech, otitis media

C. Nursing assessment
1. Cleft lip apparent at birth: unilateral, bilateral, or complete
2. Cleft palate needs more thorough assessment in newborn
   a. Biuvula or split uvula is indicative of a cleft
   b. Note any feeding difficulties; is at high risk for aspiration
3. Overall assessment: nutritional status, abdominal distention, lung sounds (aspiration), signs of infection at site, weight, speech and dental (when older), hearing

D. Nursing management
1. Cleft lip: surgical repair recommended and can occur as a young infant (approximately 2 months)
2. Cleft palate
   a. Team approach with stages of repair occurring as young infant through adolescence
   b. Coordination of team
      1) Orthodontist: oral–pharyngeal development and dentition
      2) Speech and language therapist: develop sucking and treat altered speech
      3) Otolaryngologist: assesses and treats chronic otitis related to abnormal connection between Eustachian tube and posterior oropharynx
      4) Audiologist: chronic otitis leads to hearing loss
      5) Plastic surgeon: repairs craniofacial anomalies
      6) Social worker: monitors financial and emotional needs
3. Preoperative nursing interventions
   a. Nutrition: assess adequate intake; encourage parent to provide modified nipple or supplemental tube feeding, assess if child can adequately suck; monitor to prevent aspiration of formula or breast milk; feed in sitting position
   b. Oropharyngeal (CP): understand and educate family on orthodontic hardware for infant or child; monitor effectiveness of speech therapy for coordinating speech and adequate sucking
   c. Hearing: frequently monitor for hearing loss; listen to family for reports of delayed or altered speech
4. Postoperative nursing interventions
   a. Prevent damage to surgical site
      1) Child with repair of cleft lip is not to be placed prone
      2) Keep objects away from mouth
      3) Elbow restraints: monitor for skin breakdown to area restrained
      4) Educate family to keep child's hands away from face if restraints off
      5) Cleanse area with prescribed solution, usually peroxide (H_2O_2) and sterile water (H_2O); follow current agency protocol
      6) Lubricate lip with antibiotic ointment
      7) Devices such as Logan bar or bow to relieve tension on incision site
   b. Monitor for adequate fluid and nutrition intake; weigh daily
   c. Monitor for incisional pain
5. Growth and development
   a. Monitor family for positive bonding with infant: it is important to bring newborn with cleft to parent soon after delivery; connect families early with support group and repair team
   b. Monitor child for positive self-image
   c. Genetic counseling for familial tendencies
6. Priority nursing diagnoses: Imbalanced Nutrition: Less than Body Requirements, Risk for Impaired Parenting, Acute Pain (postoperative), Risk for Aspiration

Practice to Pass

Why is it important to assess for a biuvula in the newborn?

Case Study

A 6-month-old male infant is admitted to the nursing unit with the diagnosis of recurrent pneumonia. On admission, the client has a respiratory rate of 50, heart rate of 170, and a temperature of 102°F. The client is retracting substernally with bilateral wheezes and rhonchi. The mother states that this is her son's third admission since birth for pneumonia. She also mentions that he hasn't been gaining weight like her older child had at 6 months of age.

1. How is this consistent with cystic fibrosis?

2. What tests could be ordered to confirm the diagnosis?

3. What nursing interventions could alleviate the respiratory distress?

4. What is the rationale behind the poor weight gain?

5. What teaching needs to be done with the family about the respiratory component of cystic fibrosis before the child goes home? What genetic counseling should occur for the family?

For suggested responses, see pages 467–468.

POSTTEST

1 A 16-year-old client comes to the health care provider's office for a physical examination, which is required to join the high school basketball team. He is a tall, lean male with long, slender fingers. His mother is concerned about his health because she has heard about high school athletes dying on the basketball court during games. The nurse interprets that the parent could be referring to which congenital anomaly and associated life-threatening defect?

1. Down syndrome and atrial-ventricular (AV) canal
2. Marfan syndrome and aortic dilation
3. Phenylketonuria (PKU) and seizures
4. Turner syndrome and hypothyroidism

2 The nurse should plan to teach the parent of a client with albinism about which preventive health care measure?

1. Ulcerative colitis diet
2. Use of a high sun protection factor (SPF) sunblock
3. Hair loss monitoring
4. Monitor for growth retardation

3 A woman who has just been diagnosed with Huntington's disease asks the nurse if her children are likely to develop this disorder also. What should the nurse include in a response?

1. If the mother alone has the disease, the children have a 50% chance of inheriting the same disorder.
2. Both parents must have the disease for the offspring to inherit the same disorder.
3. The disorder is a spontaneous disruption of the neurotransmitters with no inheritance principles.
4. If the mother has the disease, the children have a 1:4 chance of inheriting the same disorder.

4 The symptoms in a client with cystic fibrosis (CF) have progressed rapidly over the past 2 years. Presently, the client is in the emergency department with significant respiratory distress. What physical characteristics should the nurse expect to see in the client? Select all that apply.

1. Low-set ears and long slender fingers
2. Increased anteroposterior chest diameter (barrel chest)
3. Clubbed fingernails
4. Bibasilar crackles on auscultation
5. Chronic cough

5 The nurse explains to parents of an infant with cystic fibrosis (CF) that the foul-smelling, frothy characteristic of stools results from the presence of large amounts of which of the following?

1. Sodium and chloride
2. Undigested fat
3. Semidigested carbohydrates
4. Lipase, trypsin, and amylase

6 A client with cystic fibrosis (CF) is in obvious respiratory distress with circumoral cyanosis. What factor should the nurse consider when administering oxygen with a prn order for this client?

1. Children with cystic fibrosis (CF) respond poorly to oxygen administration.
2. Administration of oxygen could decrease respiratory drive.
3. The higher the flow rate of oxygen, the better the child will breathe.
4. Oxygen should only be administered via face mask.

7 The parents of a baby with Down syndrome are seeking genetic counseling. The baby has been identified as having trisomy of chromosome 21. The nurse would include which information when counseling the clients about the risk of conceiving another child with trisomy 21? Select all that apply.

1. The risk increases with maternal age.
2. There is no risk of a second child with Down syndrome.
3. The risk is 1 in 4 since there is already a child with Down syndrome.
4. The age of the father is a bigger risk factor than the mother's age.
5. If the mother is 45 years old, the risk is 3–5%.

8 Nursing care of an adolescent client with Klinefelter syndrome focuses mainly on which problem?

1. Changes in fluid and electrolyte balance
2. Body image issues
3. High risk for complications
4. Difficulty with movement

9 A 16-year-old girl comes to the clinic because she has not begun to menstruate like all of her friends. She is short and shows no signs of secondary sex characteristics. She reports swollen hands and feet, has skin folds in the neck, and has a low hairline. How would the nurse best address the client's concerns?

1. "Don't worry. Many girls are late developing. Just wait a little longer."
2. "There must be something really wrong considering what you have told me. Let's see what the doctor says."
3. "We recommend that girls with problems like yours have chromosomal studies to find the reason and begin treatment."
4. "You have a severe chromosomal problem. There is no treatment but you could consider yourself lucky not to get periods."

10 The nurse would use which explanation in telling the mother of a child who is postoperative for cleft lip repair about the importance of keeping the elbow restraints in place?

1. "Your child could pull out his or her nasogastric tube."
2. "Your child might dislodge his or her intravenous catheter."
3. "Your child may aspirate formula."
4. "Your child may disrupt the lip suture line."

➤ *See pages 417–419 for Answers and Rationales.*

POSTTEST

ANSWERS & RATIONALES

Pretest

1 **Answer: 2** **Rationale:** An individual with Huntington's disease develops chorea (rapid, jerky movements) and might have difficulty swallowing liquids, which could lead to the potential of aspiration of thin liquids. Death usually results from aspiration pneumonia or another infection. Thickened liquids will not help dehydration and are not needed because of fatigue or pain. **Cognitive Level:** Applying **Client Need:** Physiological Adaptation **Integrated Process:** Teaching and Learning **Content Area:** Adult Health **Strategy:** Eliminate the incorrect options after identifying the risks reduced by providing thickened liquids. **Reference:** LeMone, P., Burke, K., & Bauldoff, G. (2011). *Medical-surgical nursing: Critical thinking in patient care* (5th ed.). Upper Saddle River, NJ: Pearson Education, pp. 1534–1535.

2 **Answer: 4** **Rationale:** The child with Down syndrome will go through the same first developmental stage of trust vs. mistrust, only at a slower rate. Therefore, the nurse should concentrate on developing a bond between the primary caregiver and the child. The other stages listed occur after infancy. **Cognitive Level:** Applying **Client Need:** Health Promotion and Maintenance **Integrated Process:** Nursing Process: Planning **Content Area:** Foundational Sciences **Strategy:** Specific knowledge of developmental stages is needed to answer the question. Note that the client is an infant to pick the first developmental stage, which sets the stage for how the infant will relate to the world after birth. **Reference:** Ball, J., Bindler, R., & Cowen, K. (2010). *Child health nursing: Partnering with children and families* (2nd ed.). Upper Saddle River, NJ: Pearson Education, p. 132.

3 **Answer: 1** **Rationale:** The connective tissue disorder of Marfan syndrome can include weakened arterial walls that can lead to aortic rupture or dissection, which is the primary cause of death for the disorder. Retinal detachment and hyperextensible joints are not life threatening. Seizure activity represents a neurological problem. **Cognitive Level:** Applying **Client Need:** Physiological Adaptation **Integrated Process:** Nursing Process: Assessment **Content Area:** Child Health **Strategy:** The critical words in the question are *potentially lethal*. Evaluate 2 options easily because they are not life threatening and then recall that Marfan disease is a connective tissue disorder rather than a neurological disorder to make a final selection. **Reference:** LeMone, P., Burke, K., & Bauldoff, G. (2011). *Medical-surgical nursing: Critical thinking in patient care* (5th ed.). Upper Saddle River, NJ: Pearson Education, p. 1004.

4 **Answer: 2** **Rationale:** Albinism type I is an autosomal recessive disorder. Both parents must be carriers for the child to inherit the congenital disorder. One parent would have the disease in an autosomal dominant trait. X-linked traits tend to manifest in male children. A multifactorial disorder is affected by both genetics and environment. **Cognitive Level:** Applying **Client Need:** Physiological Adaptation **Integrated Process:** Teaching and Learning **Content Area:** Foundational Sciences **Strategy:** Use general nursing knowledge to answer the question. Recall that when options are opposites, one of them must be incorrect. **Reference:** LeMone, P., Burke, K., & Bauldoff, G. (2011). *Medical-surgical nursing: Critical thinking in patient care* (5th ed.). Upper Saddle River, NJ: Pearson Education, p. 394.

5 **Answer: 1** **Rationale:** The infant with cleft lip is unable to create an adequate seal for sucking. The child is at risk for inadequate nutritional intake as well as aspiration. Although newborn care and injury prevention are general nursing interventions for all clients, the priority need is one that meets basic physiological needs and considers pathophysiology. **Cognitive Level:** Applying **Client Need:** Physiological Adaptation **Integrated Process:** Nursing Process: Implementation **Content Area:** Foundational Sciences **Strategy:** Consider Maslow's hierarchy when prioritizing. Recall that physiological needs are a priority before safety needs. **Reference:** Ball, J., Bindler, R., & Cowen, K. (2010). *Child health nursing: Partnering with children and families* (2nd ed.). Upper Saddle River, NJ: Pearson Education, pp. 1129–1130.

6 **Answer: 4** **Rationale:** Pancrelipase (Pancrease) should be given with each meal and snack so it is available before food enters the duodenum. Pancrelipase, a drug that is a pancreatic enzyme, allows a diet with normal amounts of fat and protein. The dose and product type are individualized for each client. The drug is not given to treat loose stools. Administering it more than once per day is partially correct in that meals are eaten 3 times per day, but this option is nonspecific as to timing with food and does not account for intake of snacks. **Cognitive Level:** Applying **Client Need:** Pharmacological and Parenteral Therapies **Integrated Process:** Teaching and Learning **Content Area:** Child Health **Strategy:** Recall the role of the enzyme in aiding digestion in order to help focus on the option that is most accurate. **Reference:** LeMone, P., Burke, K., & Bauldoff, G. (2011). *Medical-surgical nursing: Critical thinking in patient care* (5th ed.). Upper Saddle River, NJ: Pearson Education, p. 1133.

7 **Answer: 1** **Rationale:** Short stature, nonpitting lymphedema of the hands and feet, webbed neck, and low posterior hairline are the key assessment features in Turner syndrome. If the child is diagnosed early in age, proper treatment with growth hormone can be offered to the family. Down syndrome is characterized by low-set ears and epicanthal folds. Physical manifestations in Marfan syndrome include a tall, thin build, "pigeon chest," and arachnodactaly. The male with Klinefelter syndrome tends to have wider hips and some breast development. **Cognitive Level:** Applying **Client Need:** Physiological Adaptation **Integrated Process:** Nursing Process: Assessment **Content Area:** Child Health **Strategy:** The question describes one of these genetic disorders. If guessing, eliminate the ones known to be incorrect. Otherwise, specific nursing knowledge is needed to answer the question. **Reference:** LeMone, P., Burke, K., & Bauldoff, G. (2011). *Medical-surgical nursing: Critical thinking in patient care* (5th ed.). Upper Saddle River, NJ: Pearson Education, p. 1637.

8 **Answer: 3** **Rationale:** The child with cleft palate has communication between the oropharnyx and the Eustachian tube. The child is at high risk for recurrent ear infections. The symptoms described are common with otitis media regardless of the congenital abnormality. Pneumonia is a respiratory infection, but no specific respiratory symptoms are listed. The child with urinary tract infection (UTI) would report painful urination, which is not one of the symptoms described. The child with cellulitis would not be pulling on his ear. **Cognitive Level:** Analyzing **Client Need:** Physiological Adaptation **Integrated Process:** Nursing Process: Assessment **Content Area:** Child Health **Strategy:** Read the symptoms carefully. The phrase *pulling on his left ear* is a clue to the location of the infection. Recall also the pathophysiology of cleft palate in making a selection. **Reference:** LeMone, P., Burke, K., & Bauldoff, G. (2011). *Medical-surgical nursing: Critical thinking in patient care* (5th ed.). Upper Saddle River, NJ: Pearson Education, p. 1606.

9 **Answer: 2** **Rationale:** The child with Klinefelter has an extra X chromosome. The karyotype shows the pictorial analysis of the total chromosomes of a cell (or an individual), which in this case is XXY. X is the karyotype for Turner syndrome. A trisomy 21 is the karyotype for Down syndrome. Marfan is an autosomal dominant disorder with a mutation rather than aneuploidy. **Cognitive Level:** Applying **Client Need:** Physiological Adaptation **Integrated Process:** Nursing Process: Diagnosis **Content Area:** Child Health **Strategy:** Recall that *karyo-* refers to the nucleus of a cell. In this question, if the word *karyotype* is unfamiliar, relate your answer to the extra X chromosome. **Reference:** LeMone, P., Burke, K., & Bauldoff, G. (2011). *Medical-surgical nursing: Critical thinking in patient care* (5th ed.). Upper Saddle River, NJ: Pearson Education, p. 152.

10 **Answer: 1** **Rationale:** The child with phenylketonuria (PKU) must maintain a strict low-phenylalanine diet to prevent central nervous system damage, seizures, and eventual death. The child lacks phenylalanine hydroxylase, an enzyme needed to metabolize phenylalanine. Kidney failure, blindness, and neutropenia are not

involved in PKU. **Cognitive Level:** Applying **Client Need:** Physiological Adaptation **Integrated Process:** Teaching and Learning **Content Area:** Child Health **Strategy:** Recall that phenylketonuria (PKU) tests are routinely done on all newborns. Specific nursing knowledge is needed to answer this question. **Reference:** Ball, J., Bindler, R., & Cowen, K. (2010). *Child health nursing: Partnering with children and families* (2nd ed.). Upper Saddle River, NJ: Pearson Education, pp. 1307–1308.

Posttest

1 **Answer: 2** **Rationale:** The physical characteristics of the client are consistent with Marfan syndrome. This connective tissue disorder can involve the heart—specifically the aorta—and can lead to a fatal aortic aneurysm. Clients with Down syndrome are typically not tall and lean; they tend to be shorter in height and of average build. Clients with phenylketonuria (PKU) have an inborn error of metabolism and require a low phenylalanine diet. Turner syndrome is a chromosomal anomaly with the absence of one X chromosome, and hypothyroidism is a disorder in which the thyroid gland produces less than required triiodothyronine (T3) and thyroxine (T4) for bodily metabolism. **Cognitive Level:** Analyzing **Client Need:** Physiological Adaptation **Integrated Process:** Nursing Process: Assessment **Content Area:** Child Health **Strategy:** Consider the physical characteristics given in the question. After you have identified the disorder, what is the life-threatening aspect? **Reference:** LeMone, P., Burke, K., & Bauldoff, G. (2011). *Medical-surgical nursing: Critical thinking in patient care* (5th ed.). Upper Saddle River, NJ: Pearson Education, pp. 1293, 1004.

2 **Answer: 2** **Rationale:** Without melanin production, the child with albinism is at risk for severe sunburns. Maximum sun protection should be taken, including use of hats, long sleeves, minimal time in the sun, and high sun protection factor (SPF) sunblock, to prevent any problems. It is unnecessary to alter the diet because there is not an associated risk of ulcerative colitis; hair loss and growth retardation are not of concern. **Cognitive Level:** Applying **Client Need:** Health Promotion and Maintenance **Integrated Process:** Nursing Process: Planning **Content Area:** Child Health **Strategy:** This question asks about preventive health maintenance. Eliminate the options that do not apply to albinism. **Reference:** LeMone, P., Burke, K., & Bauldoff, G. (2011). *Medical-surgical nursing: Critical thinking in patient care* (5th ed.). Upper Saddle River, NJ: Pearson Education, pp. 393–394.

3 **Answer: 1** **Rationale:** Huntington's disease is an autosomal dominant disorder needing only 1 chromosome to be present. The risk of transmission of the chromosome 4 defect is 2:4 incidences if 1 parent has the disease, meaning 2 children will have the disorder and 2 will not. If both parents have it, 3 of the 4 children will have the disease and 1 will not. **Cognitive Level:** Analyzing **Client Need:** Health Promotion and Maintenance **Integrated Process:** Nursing Process: Assessment **Content Area:** Child Health **Strategy:** The core issue of the question is the risk of developing a disease with an autosomal dominant disorder. Use principles of genetics and recall that this is an autosomal dominant disorder to make a selection. **Reference:** LeMone, P., Burke, K., & Bauldoff, G. (2011). *Medical-surgical nursing: Critical thinking in patient care* (5th ed.). Upper Saddle River, NJ: Pearson Education, pp. 1534–1535.

4 Answer: 2, 3, 4, 5 Rationale: The child with cystic fibrosis (CF) is chronically hypoxic because of progression of chronic obstructive pulmonary disease (COPD). Clubbing of nail beds occurs after 6 months of inadequate oxygenation, which is characteristic of children with CF. The client will have a chronic cough, bibasilar crackles, barrel chest, and possibly signs of right-sided heart failure. Low-set ears are seen with Down syndrome, and long slender fingers are seen with Marfan syndrome. **Cognitive Level:** Applying **Client Need:** Physiological Adaptation **Integrated Process:** Nursing Process: Assessment **Content Area:** Child Health **Strategy:** Look for respiratory system findings. Do not choose abnormalities for other syndromes. **Reference:** LeMone, P., Burke, K., & Bauldoff, G. (2011). *Medical-surgical nursing: Critical thinking in patient care* (5th ed.). Upper Saddle River, NJ: Pearson Education, pp. 1250–1251.

5 Answer: 2 Rationale: The client with cystic fibrosis (CF) poorly absorbs fats because of the thick secretions blocking the pancreatic duct. The lack of natural pancreatic enzyme leads to poor absorption of predominantly fats in the duodenum. Foul-smelling, frothy stool is termed *steatorrhea*. **Cognitive Level:** Applying **Client Need:** Physiological Adaptation **Integrated Process:** Teaching and Learning **Content Area:** Child Health **Strategy:** Recall that in cystic fibrosis (CF), the pancreatic insufficiency results in digestive problems, causing the stool described in the question. Consider the role of the exocrine pancreas in digestion. Do not be fooled by an option with pancreatic-sounding names. **Reference:** LeMone, P., Burke, K., & Bauldoff, G. (2011). *Medical-surgical nursing: Critical thinking in patient care* (5th ed.). Upper Saddle River, NJ: Pearson Education, p. 1249.

6 Answer: 2 Rationale: Clients with cystic fibrosis (CF) develop chronic obstructive pulmonary disease (COPD) and chronic carbon dioxide retention (hypercapnia), becoming dependent on hypoxia to drive the respiratory system. Too much oxygen will decrease the body's stimulus to breathe; therefore, the nurse should monitor the respiratory status of a client with cystic fibrosis for potential apnea. **Cognitive Level:** Applying **Client Need:** Basic Care and Comfort **Integrated Process:** Nursing Process: Implementation **Content Area:** Child Health **Strategy:** Consider the chronic obstruction with cystic fibrosis (CF) and apply knowledge of safe oxygen administration. **Reference:** LeMone, P., Burke, K., &

Bauldoff, G. (2011). *Medical-surgical nursing: Critical thinking in patient care* (5th ed.). Upper Saddle River, NJ: Pearson Education, pp. 1249–1250.

7 Answer: 1, 5 Rationale: The risk of Down syndrome increases with the age of the mother since the oocytes have been formed since birth. The risk is 1 in 1,300 at 25 years and increases to 1 in 30 at 45 years. Since males produce sperm throughout their life, the paternal age is not thought to be a factor. If the child had translocation of the 21st chromosome, there would be no relation to maternal age but a high recurrence risk if the mother was a carrier. This information is important to disclose to the family in genetic counseling. **Cognitive Level:** Applying **Client Need:** Health Promotion and Maintenance **Integrated Process:** Teaching and Learning **Content Area:** Child Health **Strategy:** Specific nursing knowledge is needed to answer this question. Apply knowledge of birth defects and risks. **Reference:** LeMone, P., Burke, K., & Bauldoff, G. (2011). *Medical-surgical nursing: Critical thinking in patient care* (5th ed.). Upper Saddle River, NJ: Pearson Education, pp. 133–134.

8 Answer: 2 Rationale: The adolescent client with Klinefelter syndrome is a tall, lean male with no secondary sex characteristics. Body image is the appropriate problem for the adolescent client after taking into account growth and developmental considerations. Fluid and electrolyte imbalance and mobility issues are not of concern, and high risk for complications is too vague to be of use for this client. **Cognitive Level:** Applying **Client Need:** Psychosocial Integrity **Integrated Process:** Nursing Process: Planning **Content Area:** Child Health **Strategy:** The core issue of this question is an understanding of the key growth and developmental concerns of an adolescent client with an inherited disorder that affects physical appearance. Use these concepts and the process of elimination to make a selection. **Reference:** LeMone, P., Burke, K., & Bauldoff, G. (2011). *Medical-surgical nursing: Critical thinking in patient care* (5th ed.). Upper Saddle River, NJ: Pearson Education, p. 1637.

9 Answer: 3 Rationale: It is recommended that girls who have lymphedema, delayed puberty, and are below the 5th percentile in height have chromosomal studies. This client has the appearance of Turner syndrome. It needs to be confirmed and treated. Statements that ignore the client's concerns or increase the client's fear (even if technically correct) are not helpful. **Cognitive Level:** Applying **Client Need:** Physiological Adaptation **Integrated Process:** Communication and Documentation **Content Area:** Child Health **Strategy:** The problems of this client are greater than delayed puberty. Choose an option that gives true information. **Reference:** LeMone, P., Burke, K., & Bauldoff, G. (2011). *Medical-surgical nursing: Critical thinking in patient care* (5th ed.). Upper Saddle River, NJ: Pearson Education, p. 1637.

10 Answer: 4 Rationale: For optimal appearance and healing of the suture line for cleft lip repair, the child should not be allowed to touch the mouth. **Cognitive Level:** Applying **Client Need:** Management of Care **Integrated Process:** Communication and Documentation **Content Area:** Child Health **Strategy:** Consider the need for postoperative healing, remembering that the principle of restraints

is to use the least restraint for the shortest time. **Reference:** LeMone, P., Burke, K., & Bauldoff, G. (2011). *Medical-surgical nursing: Critical thinking in patient care* (5th ed.). Upper Saddle River, NJ: Pearson Education, pp. 78–79.

References

Ball, J., Bindler, R., & Cowen, K. (2012). *Pediatric nursing: Caring for children* (5th ed.). Upper Saddle River, NJ: Pearson Education.

LeMone, P., Burke, K. M., & Bauldoff, G. (2011). *Medical-surgical nursing: Critical thinking in patient care* (5th ed.). Upper Saddle River, NJ: Pearson Education.

McCance, K., & Huether, K. (2010). *Understanding pathophysiology: The biologic basis for disease in adults and children* (6th ed.). St. Louis, MO: Elsevier.

Porth, C., & Matfin, G. (2010). *Pathophysiology: Concepts of altered health states* (8th ed.). Philadelphia, PA: Lippincott Williams & Wilkins.

Wilson, B., Shannon, M., & Shields, K. (2012). *Pearson nurse's drug guide 2012.* Upper Saddle River, NJ: Pearson Education.

17 Multisystem Health Problems

Chapter Outline

Risk Factors for Multisystem
   Health Problems
Shock

Trauma
Disseminated Intravascular
   Coagulopathy (DIC)

Acute Respiratory Distress
   Syndrome (ARDS)

NCLEX-RN® Test Prep

Use the accompanying online resource,
NursingReviewsandRationales, to test
yourself with hundreds of NCLEX®-style
practice questions.

Objectives

➤ Define key terms associated with multisystem health problems.
➤ Identify risk factors associated with development of multisystem
   health problems.
➤ Explain etiologies of multisystem health problems.
➤ Describe pathophysiological processes associated with specific
   multisystem health problems.
➤ Distinguish between normal and abnormal multisystem findings
   obtained from nursing assessment.
➤ Prioritize nursing interventions associated with multisystem health
   problems.

Review at a Glance

acute respiratory distress syndrome (ARDS) a form of acute respiratory failure with respiratory insufficiency and inefficient gas exchange

anaphylactic shock shock resulting from an immune response to presence of antigens; a form of distributive shock

antigen a foreign substance introduced into body that triggers antibody production and can cause allergic reactions

bacteremia presence of bacteria within bloodstream

cardiac tamponade compression of heart muscle by excess fluid or blood within pericardial sac

cardiogenic shock type of shock caused by abnormal cardiac functioning or "pump failure"

contusion a bruising of tissue

disseminated intravascular coagulopathy (DIC) a disorder of coagulation in which body alternately clots and hemorrhages in response to injury; body's clotting substance reserves are overwhelmed resulting in massive hemorrhaging

fibrinolysis process in which thrombi (clots) are broken down

hypovolemic shock type of shock caused by a decrease in circulating volume as a result of actual fluid or blood loss

laceration any tearing or slicing of flesh and possibly underlying fleshy structures

metabolic acidosis a condition caused by abnormal decrease in bicarbonate concentrations within body; body's pH becomes acidic

neurogenic shock type of shock that results from a decrease in sympathetic control of vasomotor responses, usually as a result of spinal injury; a form of distributive shock

obstructive shock type of shock in which ventricles are not able to fill or empty appropriately because of a block in flow of blood from heart

pulse pressure difference between systolic and diastolic pressure readings; normally about 30–40 mmHg

pulsus paradoxus a notable decrease in pulse upon inspiration

shock state of inadequate perfusion and oxygenation to vital organs and tissues throughout body

septic shock type of shock that occurs in response to release of endotoxins from bacteria, generally Gram-negative; a form of distributive shock

toxic shock syndrome a form of septic shock that occurs most commonly in women who utilize tampons while menstruating; *Staphylococcus aureus* is generally thought to be bacteria involved

trauma a physical injury caused by outside forces

PRETEST

1 A client involved in a motor vehicle crash presents with a BP 100/50, pulse 100, respirations 28–32/minute and labored, and temperature 98.4°F orally. The anterior chest has obvious rib fractures, and breath sounds are absent in this area. The client's trachea is deviated to the left side of the neck. The nurse concludes that the client is probably experiencing which type of pneumothorax?

1. Spontaneous
2. Tension
3. Iatrogenic
4. Open

2 A client is brought to the emergency department after a near-drowning incident with submersion for an undetermined amount of time. The client has since regained consciousness and is alert and oriented, but anxious. Vital signs are BP 120/72, pulse 92, respirations 26, temperature 98.0°F orally. Pulse oximetry indicates SaO_2 of 93% on 4 L/min of oxygen via nasal cannula. The nurse concludes that the client is at greatest risk to develop which of the following?

1. Cardiogenic shock
2. Spontaneous pneumothorax
3. Renal failure
4. Acute respiratory distress syndrome (ARDS)

3 A client was brought to the emergency department after a motorcycle crash. The client is awake with intermittent confusion and reports moderate to severe thirst and left thigh pain. Vital signs are BP 100/60, pulse 112, respirations 28, and temperature 98.4°F orally. Capillary refill is 3 seconds and urine output is 30 mL/hour. The client has an obvious pelvic deformity and the left thigh is distended. A diagnosis of hypovolemic shock is established. The nurse interprets by these findings that the client is in which phase of shock?

1. Initial phase
2. Compensatory phase
3. Progressive phase
4. Irreversible phase

4 A client reports difficulty breathing and generalized weakness after experiencing chest pain for almost 1 hour the previous night. On exam, the client's skin is pale and diaphoretic, breath sounds are equal with crackles noted throughout all lung fields, capillary beds are dusky, and jugular venous distention is present. Vital signs are BP 98/50, pulse 118 and thready to palpation, respirations 26 and labored, temperature 98.6°F orally. The nurse prepares to take action for which suspected condition?

1. Obstructive shock
2. Neurogenic shock
3. Hypovolemic shock
4. Cardiogenic shock

5 A client who took the third dose of a prescribed antibiotic arrives at the urgent care clinic. The client is weak, diaphoretic, reports difficulty breathing and itching, and appears flushed. The nurse obtains a dose of epinephrine for the provider considering that the client is likely experiencing which form of shock?

1. Septic
2. Anaphylactic
3. Hypovolemic
4. Neurogenic

6 A client arrives in the emergency department after a fall of approximately 10 feet. The initial body point of contact was the upper back, and the client reports sharp pain in this area with movement. The nurse suspects which primary type of injury?

1. Head injury
2. Spleen injury
3. Cervical spine injury
4. Liver injury

7 A client reports chest pain, rapid heart beat, and difficulty breathing. On exam, heart sounds are muffled. Which assessment findings by the nurse would support a diagnosis of cardiac tamponade? Select all that apply.

1. Deviated trachea
2. Weak peripheral pulses
3. Absent breath sounds to the lower lobes
4. Diminished or absent carotid or femoral pulses during inspiration
5. Blood pressure 94/72 during inspiration, 10 mmHg lower systolic than the blood pressure on expiration

8 A client who sustained a penetrating bowel injury has several possible problems that need to be addressed in planning future care. Which potential problem would receive priority by the nurse in developing the client's plan of care?

1. Constipation
2. Peritonitis
3. Paralytic ileus
4. Intestinal adhesions

9 A client seeks treatment for a laceration to the forehead sustained in a fight. The client reports no loss of consciousness but is confused and has a strong alcohol odor on the breath. The emergency department nurse prepares the client for which priority diagnostic assessments?

1. Skull x-ray and urine alcohol
2. MRI of the brain and blood alcohol
3. Blood alcohol and glucose
4. Electroencephalography (EEG) and blood alcohol

10 A client has a suspected femoral fracture from an injury sustained 3 hours ago. There is gross swelling to the left thigh, and the skin is tight and bruised. The client reports numbness and tingling in the toes. What other assessments would the nurse expect to make if compartment syndrome exists? Select all that apply.

1. Toes cool and dusky
2. Bounding pulses distal to the fracture
3. Pain in the leg unrelieved by opioid analgesics
4. Inability to move the ankle and toes in the affected leg
5. Changes in level of consciousness (LOC)

➤ *See pages 448–450 for Answers and Rationales.*

I. RISK FACTORS FOR MULTISYSTEM HEALTH PROBLEMS

A. Shock

1. Hypovolemic shock
   a. Hemorrhagic: trauma (internal and external), aneurysm dissection, disseminated intravascular coagulopathy (DIC)
   b. Nonhemorrhagic: burns, vomiting, diarrhea, inadequate intake, excessive sweating, severe third-spacing of body fluids (such as edema, ascites)
2. Cardiogenic shock: myocardial infarction (MI; most common), cardiac dysrhythmias (heart block, supraventricular tachycardia [SVT], atrial fibrillation), electrolyte imbalances, cardiac tamponade, cardiomyopathy, cardiac valve disease, cardiac surgery, pericarditis, genetic anomalies

3. Obstructive shock: cardiac tamponade, pulmonary embolism, obstructive valve disease, tension pneumothorax, pulmonary hypertension
4. Distributive (*normovolemic*)
   a. Anaphylactic shock: antibiotic therapy, immunizations, food, animal or chemical exposure (sensitization must occur prior to event), allergies, new drug therapy, insect bites, venomous bites
   b. Septic shock: trauma, surgical procedures of gastrointestinal (GI) and urinary tracts, therapy involving invasive devices and procedures (IVs, urinary catheter, tracheal intubation), burns, immunosuppressed states (cancer, HIV, AIDS, steroid therapy), diabetes, tampon usage, older adulthood

B. Trauma
1. Factors predisposing a person to traumatic injury are limitless
2. Certain lifestyle patterns, hobbies, and professions greatly increase risk such as fire and police personnel, motorcycling, farm workers, construction workers, electricians; high impact sports such as football, skiing, racing; and ingesting alcohol or controlled substances while operating equipment
3. Exposure to forces of acceleration, deceleration, or various forces of thrust and energy upon an inadequately protected person because of failure to use safety devices such as seat belts or harnesses or nonadherence to standard safety procedures

C. Disseminated intravascular coagulopathy (DIC): shock, complications of pregnancy, hemolytic reactions, trauma, metabolic acidosis

D. Acute respiratory distress syndrome (ARDS): shock, trauma, major insult to any organ system, characterized by reduced perfusion to major organs, massive infection

II. SHOCK

A. Overview
1. **Shock**: state of inadequate perfusion and oxygenation to vital organs and tissues throughout body; it cannot be defined as a single specific disease
2. Manifests itself as a syndrome within many diseases or traumatic injuries that may be life threatening
3. The body normally maintains perfusion to cells by cooperation of:
   a. The pumping mechanism of the heart
   b. An intact vascular "highway" that facilitates blood flow
   c. An adequate amount of oxygenated blood that is exchanged at the capillary level with metabolic wastes
   d. An intact clotting cascade (intrinsic and extrinsic)
4. A disruption of any component within this system results in an algorithmic attempt to compensate, which manifests itself in classic signs and symptoms of shock
5. Types of shock are labeled as hypovolemic (may be either hemorrhagic or nonhemorrhagic), cardiogenic, obstructive, or distributive (anaphylactic and septic)
6. Cause is usually related to a major insult to body
7. Hemodynamic concepts that are basic components of vascular homeostasis are important in identifying and treating shock states (see Figure 17-1)
   a. Stroke volume (SV): amount of blood that is ejected from left ventricle into aorta with each ventricular contraction
   b. Cardiac output (CO): amount of blood pumped from left ventricle every minute; calculated by equation *Stroke volume × Heart rate = CO*
   c. Systemic vascular resistance (SVR): amount of resistance provided by vascular bed against flow of blood ejected from left ventricle; when sympathetic nervous system (SNS) is stimulated in response to a threat, vasoconstriction occurs, increasing SVR

Figure 17-1

Algorithmic flow of the
basic hemodynamic
responses to forms of shock

Decreased perfusion

$\downarrow$CO = $\downarrow$MAP
Compensatory mechanisms
$\uparrow$SV × $\uparrow$HR = $\uparrow$SVR

↓

Continued decreased perfusion

Compensatory mechanisms
$\uparrow$SV × $\uparrow$HR = $\uparrow$CO + $\uparrow$SVR = $\uparrow$MAP

↓

Continued decreased perfusion

Overwhelmed *compensatory mechanisms*
$\downarrow$CO = $\downarrow$MAP

    d. Mean arterial pressure (MAP): average pressure maintained within arterial system of body; calculated by $CO \times SVR$
        1) When any component increases, MAP increases; conversely, with any decrease, there is a drop in MAP
        2) An increase or decrease in intravascular volume affects MAP in a parallel manner
  8. Regardless of cause of shock, reactions and symptoms will generally follow same course with a few notable signs defining the particular type of shock or underlying cause
  9. It is important to *first* identify that shock is occurring rather than to identify particular type

B. Pathophysiology
  1. Shock is a syndrome that manifests itself as a result of body's attempts to achieve homeostasis in direct response to a perfusion and oxygenation insult
  2. Origin of the insult may differ, but compensatory mechanisms for all types are similar (see Box 17-1)
    a. *Initial phase of shock* (mild)
        1) A decline in circulating blood volume (500 mL or less) activates baroreceptors in vascular system to note decline in MAP; SNS activity is activated; beta receptors are stimulated to increase oxygen (O_2) consumption of cardiac muscle
        2) Catecholamines (epinephrine and norepinephrine notably) are released, creating vasoconstriction in areas that can more easily undergo periods of ischemia, such as fat, bone, and skin; SVR is increased as a result
        3) Bronchodilation and increased CO occurs as a result of beta-receptor stimulation
        4) Few objective physical assessment findings are noted because vasoconstriction is minimal and little anaerobic activity occurs

Neurologic

- Hypoxia with decreasing volume and systemic pressure
- Cerebral edema with severe, continuing hypoxia
- Circulatory collapse as sympathetic nervous system (SNS) stimulation is lost

Respiratory

- Bronchodilation and increase in respiratory rate in response to hypoxic status at cellular level
- Diminished respirations as a result of continued hypoxia to pulmonary tissue

Cardiac

- Increase in rate and contractility as a result of SNS stimulation in response to decreasing volume
- Decreasing blood pressure as shock progresses
- Diminished perfusion to heart itself as a result of continued hypoxia

Gastrointestinal

- Ischemia as a result of shunting of blood to heart, lungs, and brain
- Ulcer and paralytic ileus may occur as a result of prolonged ischemia

Renal

- Ischemia as a result of compensatory shunting to heart, lungs, and brain
- Release of renin in response to decreased renal perfusion and decreased glomerular filtration, which results in decreased urine production in an effort to raise BP
- Tubular necrosis with prolonged renal hypoxia and renal failure

Integumentary

- Vasoconstriction with SNS stimulation
- Edema occurs in late shock as a result of fluid shifting to the interstitial spaces

b. *Compensatory phase of shock* (moderate shock)
   1) With volume loss of 25–30%, more intense compensatory measures are initiated; MAP continues to decline
   2) Cardiac contractility, rate, and peripheral vasoconstriction increase
   3) In an attempt to shunt blood flow to vital organs (heart, lungs, brain), blood flow to kidneys, liver, GI tract, and extremities declines
   4) Capillary pressure decreases allowing fluid shifts from interstitial spaces into blood vessels to expand circulating volume
   5) Decreased renal perfusion initiates renin-angiotensin-aldosterone (RAA) system, causing thirst and an increased reabsorption of water and sodium
   6) Objective findings become apparent

c. *Progressive phase of shock* (severe or decompensated)
   1) As shock continues to progress, compensatory mechanisms from previous phase continue unchecked, worsening the status
   2) Volume loss of 35–50% occurs because of hemorrhage or fluid leakage
   3) Continued vasoconstriction worsens an already hypoxic state of cells and tissues
   4) As cells die because of hypoxia, they release destructive enzymes and proteins into surrounding tissues, increasing oncotic pressure in interstitial space, and decreasing circulating volume even further
   5) Body shifts from aerobic to anaerobic respiration at cellular level and lactic acid is produced as a byproduct; **metabolic acidosis** (acid–base imbalance

caused by an abnormal decrease in serum bicarbonate concentrations, shifting pH of body to acidotic state)

    6) Dramatic physical changes in assessment parameters occur

  d. *Irreversible phase of shock*

    1) Despite restoration of circulating volume or stabilization of vital signs (VS), death will occur

    2) Microcirculation has been compromised beyond repair, resulting in widespread cellular death that eventually encompasses tissues of vital organs

    3) Symptoms displayed during shock are part of "survival" physiology initiated in response to disease or injury

    4) Systemic changes are closely correlated with advancing SNS stimulation and byproducts of that stimulation

3. Overall course of shock states is very similar; however, underlying cause may vary the pathological processes

  a. Four types of shock: hypovolemic, cardiogenic, obstructive, and distributive (including anaphylactic, septic, and neurogenic)

  b. Anaphylactic, septic, and neurogenic shock are known as *distributive* forms of shock because although intravascular volume is adequate, it is distributed within body in a manner that does not sustain perfusion and oxygenation

  c. Hypovolemic shock

    1) Is caused by a reduction of more than 15% in circulating volume

    2) Loss of volume is from obvious hemorrhaging, extracellular fluid and/or plasma loss from burns, peritonitis, or ruptured aneurysms

    3) Fluids can also be lost from GI tract because of severe vomiting, diarrhea, or gastric suctioning

    4) Inadequate intake, excessive sweating, diuretic usage, and interstitial shifting (third-spacing) associated with processes such as liver disease and severe protein wasting may cause this form of shock

    5) Loss of circulating volume causes an inadequate MAP, activating SNS and initiating compensatory mechanisms

    6) Signs and symptoms (see Table 17-1)

  d. Cardiogenic shock

    1) Is caused by abnormal cardiac functioning or "pump failure"

    2) There is adequate intravascular volume; however, cellular perfusion and oxygenation is inadequate because of inability of heart to move blood throughout body with acceptable force

Table 17-1   **Clinical Manifestations of Hypovolemic Shock**

	Initial	Compensatory	Progressive	Irreversible
Subjective	Reports pain and thirst; sensorium intact	Anxious; restless; reports greater thirst; episodes of confusion	Confused; restless; agitated	
Objective	Tachycardia; respirations baseline; normotensive; fleshtone or pallor of extremities; skin dry or slightly moist; capillary refill < 3 sec; normal or slightly decreased urine output; ABGs normal	Hypotension; tachycardia; tachypnea; skin cool, pale, and dry or diaphoretic; capillary refill < 4–6 sec, urine output less than 30 mL/hr; ABGs indicate trend toward metabolic acidosis	Profound hypotension; tachycardia with weak or nonpalpable peripheral pulses; cardiac dysrhythmias; tachypnea; skin pale, dusky, and/or mottled capillary beds without refill, blanching; ABGs: metabolic acidosis; diminished or absent urine output; no purposeful movement	Severe hypotension; tachypnea with shallow depth; diminishing air exchange with crackles; cardiac dysrhythmias; skin ABGs—profound metabolic acidosis; anuria; comatose

Table 17-2	Clinical Manifestations of Cardiogenic Shock
	Signs and Symptoms
Subjective	Restless Agitated
Objective	Hypotension Tachycardia with weak, thready pulse Cardiac dysrhythmias Decreased or narrowed pulse pressure Tachypnea with labored depth and crackles Jugular venous distention (JVD) Skin cool and moist Circumoral cyanosis Nail beds dusky

3) Most common and dangerous cause of cardiac failure is MI; cardiomyopathy, cardiac tamponade, valve disease, and dysrhythmias are contributing factors
4) A decrease in MAP stimulates SNS, which stimulates beta receptors of heart and increases cardiac O_2 consumption, thus placing greater stress on cardiac tissue
5) Distal vascular beds become congested with deoxygenated blood creating the hallmark nail bed cyanosis with this form of shock
6) Increased SVR occurs from the pooling that occurs in the periphery
7) Pressure is then exerted on left ventricle, causing pulmonary congestion as fluid cannot exit lungs to left ventricle
8) Signs and symptoms (see Table 17-2)

e. **Obstructive shock**
1) Results from an inability of cardiac ventricles to fill or empty appropriately because of an obstruction in blood flow from heart; cardiac preload is decreased and severely compromised; may be difficult to diagnose
2) There is an increased pressure on right side of heart and an inadequate blood return
3) This form of shock is differentiated from cardiogenic shock because heart can pump adequately and is not necessarily diseased; it is some "obstruction" outside of heart that compromises perfusion; trauma may create obstructions
4) Pulmonary embolism (PE) is most common cause of obstructive shock; damage to alveoli from embolus in lung creates an increasing pressure on right side of heart because blood cannot enter lung easily from right ventricle; with suspected PE, signs and symptoms of shock should be correlated to obstruction
5) Signs and symptoms often correlate with right-sided heart failure: jugular venous distention (JVD), hepatomegaly, and edema (see Box 17-2)

f. **Distributive shock**
1) **Anaphylactic shock**
   a) Results from an overwhelming immune response to an allergen or **antigen** (a foreign substance introduced into body that causes body to produce antibodies)
   b) This form of shock is particularly catastrophic and requires aggressive and immediate intervention as circulatory collapse is rapid
   c) Associated with administration of antibiotics or exposure to a foreign protein; parenteral medication administration routes are more prone to cause true anaphylaxis than oral routes

Box 17-2	**Signs and Symptoms**
Clinical Manifestations of Obstructive Shock	Anxiety
	Somnolence
	Hypotension
	Tachycardia
	Tachypnea with dyspnea
	Jugular venous distention (JVD)
	Pallor
	Pericardial friction rub
	Muffled heart sounds or gallop (S_3)
	Chest pain
	Decreased to absent urinary output
	Possible signs and symptoms of a pneumothorax
	Possible open chest wound or fractured ribs
	Possible diminished or absent breath sounds
	Possible whistling or rushing sounds with inspiration
	Possible tracheal deviation

     d) On exposure to an antigen, body's immune system produces an antibody specific to allergen

     e) With subsequent exposure, a reaction occurs wherein large amounts of histamines are released into blood stream in response to foreign body

     f) Histamines cause marked dilation in arterioles as well as increasing capillary permeability

     g) There is a profound fluid shift into interstitial spaces from intravascular compartment, creating edema (third-spacing)

     h) Overwhelming vasodilation and pooling of circulating blood in periphery causes a precipitous drop in MAP; vasodilation produces characteristic skin flushing and warmth

     i) Laryngeal edema may occur, and bronchospasms further compromise pulmonary function and airway clearance

     j) Signs and symptoms (see Box 17-3)

  2) Septic shock

     a) Is most often associated with release of endotoxins from Gram-negative bacteria into bloodstream, although it may also be caused by some Gram-positive bacteria; massive vasodilation occurs in response to pathogen's release of toxins into bloodstream

     b) An initial infection occurs and progresses to **bacteremia**, (presence of bacteria in blood); sepsis follows in most instances

     c) Some shock states may be present without obvious bacteremia if a localized infection is large enough to generate a sufficient toxic release

     d) **Toxic shock syndrome** is a form of septic shock that occurs most often in menstruating women who use tampons and is often caused by *Staphylococcus aureus*; blood cultures may not always be positive with this form of septic shock

     e) As pathogens release their poison into blood stream, inflammatory process and immune system respond to destruction of blood cells and presence of bacteria

Box 17-3	**Signs and Symptoms**
Clinical Manifestations of Anaphylactic Shock	Marked restlessness
	Anxiety
	Severe itching and difficulty swallowing
	Hypotension
	Tachycardia
	Tachypnea with wheezing and possible stridor
	Diminished breath sounds
	Hypersalivation and/or drooling
	Generalized urticaria
	Edema (focusing on orbital and facial components)
	Cardiac dysrhythmias
	Skin cool and moist
	Flushing
	Abdominal cramping
	Emesis

Practice to Pass

A 23-year-old woman who has suffered no apparent injury or recent illness is diagnosed as being in shock. What predisposing risk factor would be investigated and why?

f) Initial presentation is generally with a fever and flushing that is not seen in other forms of shock

g) Disseminated intravascular coagulopathy (DIC) is associated with this form of shock and is reviewed later in this chapter

h) Signs and symptoms (see Table 17-3)

3) **Neurogenic shock**

a) Occurs as a result of decreased SNS control of vasomotor responses; parasympathetic stimulation is unchecked, allowing peripheral vasodilation to occur, thereby decreasing MAP

b) This form of shock is somewhat rare and generally associated with significant spinal trauma

c) Because neurogenic shock is often associated with trauma, it is important to remember to rule out hypovolemic shock initially, even in the absence of obvious volume loss or bleeding

d) Signs and symptoms (see Box 17-4)

Table 17-3 Clinical Manifestations of Septic Shock

Early Shock	Late Shock
Sensorium intact with restlessness and agitation	Somnolence to coma
Nausea; possible abdominal tenderness	Cardiac dysrhythmias
Normotensive	Hypotension
Tachycardia	Tachycardia
Tachypnea	Tachypnea with laboring and shallow depth
Skin flushed, warm and moist	Skin cool and pale
Moderate to severe hyperthermia	Normothermic to hypothermic (indicates decreasing basal metabolic rate)
Shivering	Decreased to absent urinary output
Emesis	
Exudate from wound sources	

Box 17-4	**Signs and Symptoms**
Clinical Manifestations of Neurogenic Shock	Level of consciousness varies according to underlying cause
	Hypotension
	Bradycardia followed by tachycardia (especially in brain and spinal trauma)
	Skin flushed followed by pallor and coolness
	Possible hypothermia
	Decreased to absent urinary output
	Respiratory rate depends on cause of shock

Note: Traumatic injuries and central nervous system depressants vary the objective findings accordingly.

    4. General signs and symptoms are common to all forms of shock (see Figure 17-2)

C. Nursing assessment

    1. Assessment criteria for each category

        a. *Hypovolemic shock*

            1) Assessment includes symptom analysis of pain and thirst, level of consciousness (LOC), VS, skin color and temperature, capillary refill, urine output (UO), evidence of coping (or lack of), cardiac rhythm, heart and lung sounds, movement, peripheral pulses, and presence of risk factors

            2) Diagnostic tests

                a) Hemoglobin and hematocrit (H&H): includes baseline and serial monitoring to reflect changes; H&H levels with whole blood loss will reflect a decrease; an increase in H&H will occur when majority of fluid lost is within vascular system (such as with dehydration and third-spacing)

                b) Urinalysis may indicate presence of blood secondary to direct injury or indirect "shaking" of kidney during traumatic incident

                c) Arterial blood gases (ABGs): normal to metabolic acidosis

                d) Type and cross match (TXM): in preparation for blood administration

                e) Coagulation studies such as partial thromboplastin time (PTT), prothrombin time (PT)

        b. *Cardiogenic shock*

            1) Assessment includes preexisting cardiac dysfunction such as MI or trauma and other risk factors; VS; heart rhythm; pulses; lung sounds; heart sounds; presence of edema; skin color and temperature; capillary refill and color of nail beds; mentation; UO; differentiate damage from MI versus cardiac tamponade by noting signs of tamponade such as JVD without pulmonary congestion and by presence of a pericardial friction rub; this is an important distinction because treatment for tamponade must be instituted immediately

            2) Diagnostic tests

                a) H&H levels may be decreased with a long medical history of heart disease from chronic renal hypoperfusion

                b) Cardiac enzymes, isoenzymes, and troponin may be elevated as a result of cardiac tissue damage

                c) Chest x-rays (CXR) may indicate cardiomegaly and pulmonary edema

                d) Electrocardiogram (EKG) 12-lead

                e) ABGs: metabolic acidosis

        c. *Obstructive shock*

            1) Assessment includes risk factors and predisposing diagnoses such as thrombophlebitis, deep vein thrombosis (DVT), and risk factors for DVT such as smoking

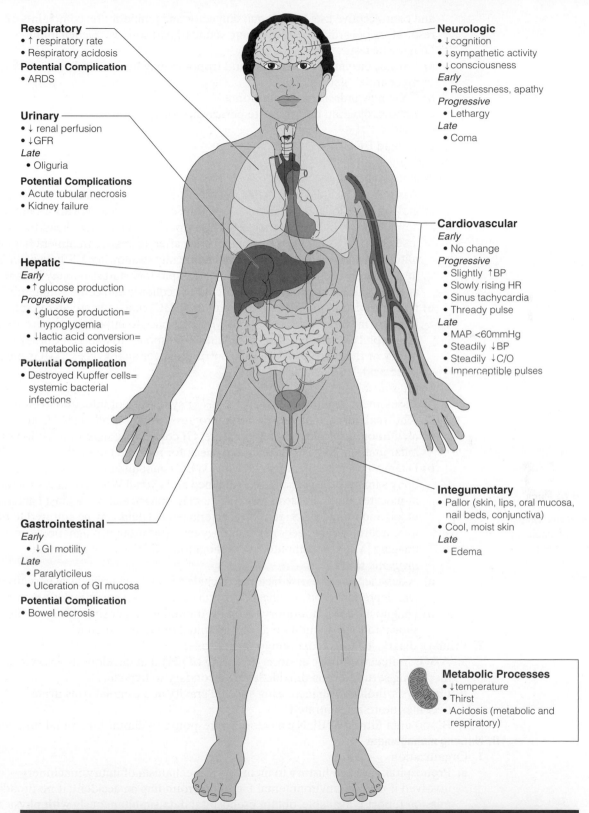

Respiratory
- ↑ respiratory rate
- Respiratory acidosis

Potential Complication
- ARDS

Urinary
- ↓ renal perfusion
- ↓GFR

Late
- Oliguria

Potential Complications
- Acute tubular necrosis
- Kidney failure

Hepatic
Early
- ↑ glucose production

Progressive
- ↓glucose production= hypoglycemia
- ↓lactic acid conversion= metabolic acidosis

Potential Complication
- Destroyed Kupffer cells= systemic bacterial infections

Gastrointestinal
Early
- ↓ GI motility

Late
- Paralyticileus
- Ulceration of GI mucosa

Potential Complication
- Bowel necrosis

Neurologic
- ↓cognition
- ↓sympathetic activity
- ↓consciousness

Early
- Restlessness, apathy

Progressive
- Lethargy

Late
- Coma

Cardiovascular
Early
- No change

Progressive
- Slightly ↑BP
- Slowly rising HR
- Sinus tachycardia
- Thready pulse

Late
- MAP <60mmHg
- Steadily ↓BP
- Steadily ↓C/O
- Imperceptible pulses

Integumentary
- Pallor (skin, lips, oral mucosa, nail beds, conjunctiva)
- Cool, moist skin

Late
- Edema

Metabolic Processes
- ↓temperature
- Thirst
- Acidosis (metabolic and respiratory)

Figure 17-2

Multisystem effects of shock

and contraceptive use; VS; edema; skin color and temperature; complaints of respiratory or cardiac problems; lung sounds; heart sounds; trachea midline

    2) Diagnostic tests

       a) Cardiac enzymes, isoenzymes, and troponin may be elevated secondary to myocardial tissue damage

       b) CXR may indicate pneumothorax

       c) Echocardiogram may indicate pericarditis or valve disease

       d) ABGs

       e) 12-lead EKG

  d. *Distributive shock*

    1) Anaphylactic shock

       a) Assessment includes preexisting exposure to medication, foods with high allergic potential (iodine-containing foods, coarse wheat products, various nuts), animals, insect bites and other risk factors; perform a thorough head-to-toe assessment to locate source of bite or sting after aggressive treatment has been initiated; assess mentation, itching and difficulty swallowing, VS, lung sounds, heart sounds, edema, GI complaints, and respiratory status; in many instances anaphylactic shock progresses to circulatory collapse and coma within minutes

       b) Diagnostic tests: complete blood counts (CBC) may indicate an overall increase in white blood cells (WBC) in response to inflammatory process; eosinophil counts may also be elevated in response to allergens; other laboratory or radiology tests are noncontributory for anaphylaxis; ABGs determine acid–base balance

    2) *Septic shock*

       a) Assessment includes preexisting signs or symptoms of infection even if current treatment for an infection is in progress; assess for other risk factors; VS; mentation; skin color and temperature; GI complaints; signs of infection or inflammation; UO; vaginal exam to check for retained tampon

       b) Diagnostic tests: CBC shows elevated WBC count initially; as shock progresses, body's immune response is overwhelmed and overall WBC count decreases; monocytes may increase in response to macrophage activity against bacteria; blood and wound C&S identifies bacteria (spinal fluid may be cultured to diagnose neurological infections); radiology tests (ultrasound, magnetic resonance imaging [MRI], or computerized tomography [CT]); coagulation studies

    3) *Neurogenic shock*

       a) Assessment includes risk factors to include traumatic injury, central nervous system depressants, and anesthesia; VS; skin color and temperature; UO; mentation

       b) Diagnostic tests: laboratory testing is limited in diagnosing this form of shock; radiology studies may reveal spinal or cranial trauma

2. Primary diagnostic tests (common to most forms)

  a. ABGs: reflect metabolic acidosis (lowering of pH) that develops as a result of increasing serum carbon dioxide levels secondary to hypoxia

  b. Urinalysis: indicates an increasing specific gravity and osmolality as urine becomes more concentrated

  c. Blood urea nitrogen (BUN): increases in response to diminishing renal function

D. Nursing management

1. Organization

  a. Prehospital: baseline history to include VS, mechanism of injury, machinery involved if trauma, environmental factors surrounding an accident; if no preadmission report is available, obtain prehospital data simultaneously with physical assessments and interventions

  b. Specialty personnel within hospital should be organized before arrival of a trauma victim in shock if possible, and include respiratory therapists, radiology

> **Practice to Pass**
>
> A client presents with a diagnosis of cardiogenic shock. What diagnostic value is the most accurate for gauging the severity of shock and why?

personnel (to include CT), additional nursing support, surgeons, anesthesiologists, orthopedists, and radiologists

    c. Ancillary units such as intensive care unit (ICU) and operating room (OR) need to be notified of a potential admission

    d. In many facilities a trauma protocol (team approach) is initiated within emergency department so that care is delivered in an organized manner; nurses may be assigned to an anatomical area or to a procedure, becoming "IV nurse" or "thoracic nurse"

2. General treatment measures

    a. Maintain life support by instituting basic life support guidelines

    b. Supine position with spinal alignment maintained (all head injuries are considered spinal injuries also until ruled out as negative)

    c. Airway should be secured, protected, and supplemental oxygen should be initiated using as appropriate delivery device according to client's overall assessment

    d. Immediately initiate an appropriate IV access, usually an 18-gauge catheter for peripheral IV

    e. Initiate continuous cardiac and SaO_2 (pulse oximetry) monitoring and prepare for frequent VS assessments

    f. Maintain stabilization to all deformities and prevent hypothermia by covering client

    g. All clients suspected of shock should have insertion of an indwelling urinary catheter to accurately measure UO; do not attempt to place in presence of obvious pelvic deformity or active bleeding from urethra

    h. Sympathomimetic medications may be prescribed for inotropic and vasoconstricting effects, such as epinephrine (Adrenalin), dopamine (Intropin), isoproterenol (Isuprel), and amiodarone (Cordarone), as well as glucose to rule out hypoglycemia

        1) A positive inotropic effect provides for increased cardiac contractility

        2) Sympathomimetics stimulate $beta_1$ receptors, creating an increase in O_2 consumption by heart

        3) Sympathomimetics may not be given to those in cardiogenic shock or with serious heart disease secondary to cardiac stress they create

3. *Hypovolemic shock*

    a. Medications include sympathomimetics, vasopressors, and drugs to treat acid–base and electrolyte imbalances

    b. Place client in a supine position with legs elevated (modified Trendelenburg or shock position) to increase cerebral blood flow; keep neck and obvious deformities stabilized; avoid this position, however, if a head injury is suspected

    c. Prepare for potential application of antishock trousers (inflatable pantlike devices that compress lower half of body to enhance circulation to heart, lungs, and brain)

    d. Gain IV access by inserting at least 2 large-bore IV cannulas (18-gauge or larger)

        1) Insert lines on admission to enable rapid fluid resuscitation; avoid jugular and subclavian veins if possible

        2) Intraosseous infusions may need to be initiated in cases of severe burns or in pediatric clients

    e. Initiate IV fluids

        1) Crystalloids (isotonic or balanced solutions such as normal saline [NS] and lactated Ringer's [LR]) may be initiated to treat mild shock

        2) Moderate to severe shock may require administration of colloidal solutions to expand plasma volume; however, beware that coagulation disorders may develop as well as hypersensitivity reactions

        3) Colloidal solutions also increase oncotic pressure in intravascular space, which may predispose client to circulatory overload, pulmonary edema, and allergic reactions

     f. Blood, a type of colloid, is also given with caution

       1) Infection as well as hemolytic reactions are a concern

       2) Obtain a type and crossmatch lab specimen to identify blood type; however, universal O-negative blood should be requisitioned if time does not allow for specific matching and hospital protocol allows

       3) Monitor VS every 15 minutes; a febrile reaction (fever) usually indicates a reaction

     g. In severe, unremitting shock, autotransfusions may be administered, in which client's own blood is collected using special equipment and is reinfused

4. *Cardiogenic shock*

     a. Medications include agents to correct acid–base and electrolyte imbalances, cardiac agents such as amiodarone (Cordarone) or positive inotropic agents may be used

     b. Typically, sympathomimetic agents that stimulate alpha and beta receptors indiscriminately are avoided due to increased O_2 demand they place on cardiac tissue

     c. Place client in a supine position or with slight leg elevation if systolic blood pressure (BP) is low; this position is contraindicated in clients experiencing respiratory distress associated with pleural effusion

     d. Obtain IV access, however, clients experiencing cardiogenic shock may have fluids restricted

5. *Obstructive shock*

     a. Medications include vasopressors such as norepinephrine (Levophed)

     b. Prepare for insertion of a thoracostomy tube to relieve a tension pneumothorax

     c. Prepare for pericardiocentesis to relieve cardiac tamponade

     d. Provide supportive treatment with fluids

6. *Distributive shock*

     a. *Septic shock*

       1) Medications include positive inotropes and broad spectrum antibiotics; empirical antibiotic therapy is often initiated before C&S results are available, but all cultures should be collected before starting antibiotic therapy

       2) Prepare to administer crystalloid fluids

     b. *Anaphylactic shock*

       1) Medications include crystalloids, sympathomimetics (specifically epinephrine) as well as antihistamines, vasopressors, and glucocorticoids; use sympathomimetics cautiously in clients with heart disease

       2) Aerosol treatments for bronchodilation may be given for bronchospasm

       3) Maintain client in a supine position and do not overheat with excessive sheets and blankets

     c. *Neurogenic shock*

       1) Medications include IV fluids (crystalloids) and vasopressors; this type of shock may or may not respond well to fluid therapy

       2) Place client in a supine position, maintaining skeletal alignment in presence of suspected spinal trauma

7. Reassessment

     a. Nursing management of all forms of shock includes continuous, accurate monitoring of client's status to identify improvement or deterioration, including VS, UO, and laboratory results

     b. Clients experiencing shock are also at great risk for GI ulcers secondary to GI ischemia, and ARDS

     c. Various monitoring devices may include central venous pressure, pulmonary artery or capillary wedge pressure, or intracranial pressure

     d. Signs of resolution of a shock state include stable VS with signs of adequate perfusion, improved and/or adequate UO, alert and oriented LOC, H&H within normal parameters or improving, and pH within normal limits

Practice to Pass

A client presents with a diagnosis of septic shock. When would antibiotics be initiated and what classification of therapy would be given?

III. TRAUMA

A. Overview
1. **Trauma** is defined as physical injury to body from external forces; there are many predisposing factors and all parts of body are vulnerable
2. Trauma may range from simple to complex, depending on organs and systems involved
3. Injury is generally a result of accelerating forces (for example, gunshot wound) or decelerating forces (such as impact from motor vehicle crash
4. Injuries may be blunt, penetrating, or shearing in nature
5. Body organs and tissues may also experience traumatic injury from medical procedures and treatment
6. Effects that an injury may have on a person cannot be predicted with certainty, so care must be approached in an algorithmic, organized, and rapid manner

B. Pathophysiology
1. *Skull/brain trauma*
   a. Trauma to skull may take form of soft tissue or bone injury and is often associated with acceleration and deceleration of great velocity
   b. Scalp and face have an extensive vascular system so that wounds may bleed in copious amounts; if this is combined with other areas of hemorrhage, a hypovolemic state may occur
   c. Intracranial hemorrhages may be classified by location in relation to protective meningeal coverings of brain; dura (outer), arachnoid (middle), and pia mater (internal); hemorrhaging may also occur within any other area within brain itself forming an intracerebral hematoma
   d. Subdural (below brain's lining) or epidural (above brain's lining) hematomas may develop; these may be acute in nature or develop over course of hours
      1) Subdural hematomas are common and usually from venous tissue bleeding
      2) Epidural hematomas usually result from arterial bleeding (usually middle meningeal artery)
   e. Symptoms of brain injury closely relate to amount and location of damage and may be diffuse or specific in nature
   f. *Closed* trauma to head may occur with or without skull fracture; there is no passage formed by injury between brain and atmosphere
      1) Hemorrhage within brain creates pressure; as pressure elevates, increased force created by bleeding leads to more injury; hypoxemia increases cerebral blood flow in response to rising CO_2 levels, creating more swelling
      2) Brain injury itself may suppress vital functions such as ventilation, worsening the hypoxic state
      3) Depending on location of injury, sensory and motor function may be impaired, reflected in paresthesias, paralysis, and an altered sensorium (leaving client open to further injury)
      4) Injuries that hemorrhage rapidly and profusely may cause a "shift" of brain as pressure is exerted
   g. *Open* head injuries are those in which integrity of cranial cavity is compromised, leaving a passage for material (such as bacteria) to move from atmosphere to brain; however, swelling that occurs may be lessened with an open-head injury
      1) This type of trauma may also result in brain tissue swelling and hemorrhage; many of symptoms will be same as those seen with closed head injury (depending on location) and extent
      2) Open head injuries tend to be more focal in nature rather than diffuse
   h. Injuries to protective tissues of brain pose a unique problem of infection (bacteria may be introduced, resulting in meningitis)

    i. Trauma to ear, sinus, and eye may also provide potential routes for infection to brain and must be investigated

    j. Facial bone injury may be isolated or complicate a skull injury

        1) Mandibular and maxillary fractures are generally a result of blunt or crushing forces to facial area and pose a unique problem to airway management

        2) Trauma to facial nerves may also be present

    k. Orbital fractures, often seen with fractures of zygomatic bones, may also involve damage to eye sphere itself

    l. All fractures of face, with or without hemorrhaging, should be viewed with suspicion, and cranial integrity should be verified

2. *Cervical/neck trauma*

    a. Cervical and neck trauma should automatically be suspected with head injuries, falls, or injuries to chest and upper back

    b. May involve soft tissue and/or cervical portion of spinal column

    c. Great vessel injury to carotid arteries or jugular veins is life threatening in nature, and a hypovolemic state may be immediate and profound

    d. Damage to trachea may occur simultaneously with great vessel injury and may result in either mechanical blocking of air, or diminished air exchange secondary to active hemorrhaging

    e. Cervical spinal injuries involve vertebrae from C1 to C8; suspect these injuries when there is head injury or injury that involves hyperflexion (bending forward) of neck, such as motor vehicle crashes where head moves forward first and then "whips" back

    f. Traumatic injuries that strike top of head and push head down into body (axial loading) should also be suspected of creating spinal injuries (see Figure 17-3)

    g. Depending on specific location and whether cord itself is transected (complete severance), a variety of symptoms may occur as innervation of various organs and structures is disrupted

    h. Higher cord damage may result in cessation of vital life functions such as respiration

    i. Lower cervical cord injury may also mimic higher lesions because of paralysis of other functions; therefore, it is of higher priority to carry out emergency interventions than to try to diagnose *specific* location of injury

3. *Chest trauma*

    a. Injuries to chest most often result from blunt or penetrating trauma

    b. Bone injury may occur to surrounding protective cage of chest, with or without trauma to underlying tissues and organs; however, cardiac and pulmonary injury should always be ruled out when there is enough force to injure bony structures encasing these organs

    c. With significant chest injuries, air exchange and tissue perfusion may be profoundly impaired; a hypovolemic state may be created as a result

    d. Great vessel injury is another potential complication of chest trauma and may result in severance or tearing of these structures

    e. Significant heart problems

        1) Cardiac tamponade results when heart is compressed by excess fluid or blood in pericardial sac

            a) An ensuing decrease in CO leads to cardiogenic or obstructive shock, which progresses rapidly and is a medical emergency

            b) A hallmark sign of cardiac tamponade is **pulsus paradoxus** or paradoxical pulses, a notable decrease in pulse upon inspiration

            c) Pulse pressure (difference between systolic and diastolic BP, about 30–40 mmHg) also begins to diminish in tamponade

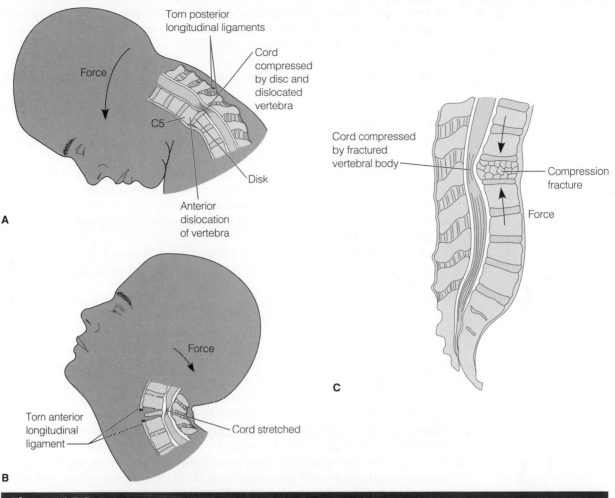

Figure 17-3

Spinal injury mechanisms. A. Compression of cord, B. Stretching of cord, C. Compression fracture.

2) To differentiate MI from cardiac tamponade in initial assessment, be aware that JVD will occur in tamponade without concurrent pulmonary congestion that occurs with heart failure from MI; a friction rub may also be auscultated in tamponade

3) A **contusion**, or bruising, occurs when cardiac tissue itself is injured as opposed to pericardial area; contusions should always be suspected when there is cardiac tamponade

4) A preexisting cardiac condition may further complicate the scenario because of diseased heart's inability to tolerate additional stress

f. Significant lung problems

1) Pneumothorax: an emergent condition in which air leaks into pleural space, either through lung itself (closed) or from outside atmosphere (open)

a) Negative pressure within pleural space becomes equal to atmosphere, resulting in collapse of area of lung involved

b) A pneumothorax may be spontaneous in nature and not evolve from an injury; however, most occur because of blunt or penetrating trauma to pleural space

2) Tension pneumothorax: if pleural cavity becomes open to outside atmosphere through penetrating trauma to chest, a tension pneumothorax might result
   a) Wound itself becomes a valve, allowing air to enter chest cavity and none to escape
   b) Increasing pressure may cause a shift of mediastinum away from side of injured lung
   c) Trachea also deviates to side of unaffected lung, a hallmark sign of tension pneumothorax
   d) Increasing pressure on unaffected lung compromises an already impaired gas exchange
3) Hemothorax: a collection of blood in pleural space from blunt or penetrating trauma; hemorrhage into pleural cavity impairs gas exchange and potentially causes a significant source of hypovolemia
4) Flail chest: occurs when 2 or more ribs are fractured in 2 areas, resulting in chest wall instability
   a) With inspiration and expiration, this segment moves paradoxically to rest of chest; on inspiration segment moves inward, while on expiration, it may appear to bulge
   b) Paradoxical movement mechanically impairs normal expansion of lungs and is often associated with underlying pulmonary injuries such as a contusion or pneumothorax

4. *Abdominal trauma*
   a. Injury to abdomen may cause many complications because of numerous organs and major blood vessels located within abdominal cavity
   b. If a specific determination of organ involved cannot be made initially, basic life support and shock management should take precedence
   c. After a specific diagnosis is made of injured organ(s), the functional limitation of organ(s) should be considered and included in continuing plan of care
   d. Any rupture of an abdominal organ should include focus on spillage of organ contents into abdominal cavity that may result in infectious or chemical peritonitis
      1) Liver: injuries may result from blunt or penetrating trauma
         a) Liver has a large reservoir of blood, so significant injury may cause a hypovolemic crisis
         b) Contusions and hemorrhaging may be insidious in nature and signs and symptoms may not initially appear
         c) Liver injury should be suspected with lower rib fractures, pulmonary trauma, and thoracic and abdominal injuries
      2) Pancreas: injury to pancreas from trauma carries a high risk of other associated injuries because of its location; hypovolemia may result and injury to surrounding organs from released pancreatic fluids containing digestive enzymes
      3) Spleen: injury to spleen may result from blunt or penetrating forces and is a significant source of hemorrhaging
         a) As a part of lymph system, spleen is not essential to maintenance of vital life functions and may be removed
         b) Acute injury may result in hypovolemia
         c) Injury in clients who have previously enlarged spleen, such as pregnant women and those with mononucleosis, occurs more easily
      4) Bowel: bowel injury may be specific to small or large intestines
         a) Both areas may be injured by blunt or penetrating sources, however, large bowel, or colon, is more often associated with abdominal trauma
         b) Trauma to colon is frequently associated with peritonitis from intracolonic bacteria being released into abdominal cavity

    5) Stomach: injury to stomach is a rare finding in trauma, probably because of its location within protective shell of rib cage

      a) Penetrating injuries, such as gunshots, comprise majority of gastric injuries associated with trauma

      b) Because of its anatomical location, injury to spleen is very often associated with stomach trauma and can rapidly lead to death due to hemorrhage; assess for an enlarging abdomen

      c) Damage may cause spillage of gastric juices and air into surrounding cavities

5. *Genitourinary trauma* (closely associated with abdominal trauma)

  a. Renal trauma: kidneys are well protected by spinal column and ribs, however, traumatic injury may result from blunt or penetrating forces

    1) Because kidneys are somewhat "free-floating" they can be jostled, resulting in hematuria with minimal trauma

    2) Renal system is also prone to significant damage because of diminished blood flow secondary to shock

    3) Suspect injury to the renal system, even when no hematuria is present, when there is identified abdominal, thoracic, or pulmonary trauma

    4) Most renal injuries are minor in nature, but profound blood loss may occur with vessel tearing or rupture

    5) Injuries to ureter are very rare and are usually penetrating in nature

  b) Bladder trauma: is most often associated with blunt trauma; however, penetrating injury may result from external forces and fractures of pelvis

    1) Bladder rupture occurs most often when bladder is distended or full at time of injury

    2) While bladder is not viewed as a significant source of bleeding, bladder injury should be assessed when there are pelvic injuries that may cause gross hemorrhaging; its location near great pelvic vessels warrants high levels of attention in assessment

  c) Urethral trauma is somewhat uncommon and is usually associated with blunt injury in males

    1) "Saddle"-type injuries may occur in both females and males if symphysis pubis impacts an object while decelerating, such as a steering column or cross beam

    2) Pelvic fractures are often associated with urethral injury

6. *Fractures*

  a. A break in continuity of any bone is considered a fracture

  b. Fractures result when bone cannot withstand mechanical forces being exerted upon it; force may be direct or indirect in nature, such as spontaneous fractures (these occur when body weight upon standing is sufficient to injure weakened bone)

  c. When integrity of bone is broken, there is hemorrhaging within site that begins the inflammatory process

  d. Swelling causes pain and reduces movement of surrounding muscles and tissues

  e. Severe fractures may impinge on nerves and/or may compromise blood flow to extremity involved

    1) Compartment syndrome can occur: any excess swelling or pressure that constricts blood flow to muscles and nerves

    2) Hypoxemia and cellular death may result at site and distal to injury, creating a potential loss of limb

  f. Fractures near great vessels that tear or rupture as a result of injury may also cause secondary hemorrhaging, creating a hypovolemic state

  g. Large bone fractures such as pelvis or femur may create a hypovolemic state due to blood loss from bone itself

   h. *Spinal fractures*
  1) Fractures to spinal column at cervical level generally result from deceleration and acceleration, which flex, hyperextend, or rotate neck
  2) Penetrating or crushing injuries are more common below cervical spine
  3) Vertebral fractures may completely sever spinal cord, resulting in paralysis below fracture site
  4) Disruption of blood supply to cord may also cause permanent damage
  5) Extent and location of fracture determines degree of system impairment, which results from damage to neural pathways from spinal cord to organs and tissues they control
  6) Injury to spine may also be seen in posttraumatic states when ligaments and bones are unstable and subsequently move

   i. *Pelvic fractures*
  1) Occur most often in older adults from low-velocity falls; these are generally closed and nondisplaced
  2) In younger, healthier people, high-velocity deceleration injuries to pelvis are seen as a result of motor vehicle accidents and falls
  3) These fractures may be a significant source of hemorrhage and may signal additional trauma to abdominal and urinary organs
  4) Pelvic fractures and other long bone fractures are prone to release of fat, potentially forming a life-threatening fat embolus

   j. *Acetabulum, hip, and proximal femur fractures*
  1) Proximal portion of femur meets pelvis at acetabulum and forms the hip; this area of the body is prone to fracture in older adults from falls or pathologic fractures, which occur as a result of porous bone density
  2) Femur is largest bone in body and contains a significant amount of blood stored in shaft; a large amount of force is needed to break this bone, and as such, assessment for other pelvic and knee injuries should be done
  3) Because of their close location to femoral vessels, injuries to these bones may also result in injury to arteries, veins, and nerves; hypovolemia may be of significant concern
  4) Peripheral blood flow and neurological function of lower extremities may be severely compromised

   k. *Soft tissue injuries*
  1) Are those injuries resulting in damage to tissues and their underlying vasculature
  2) These may be crushing in nature or as a result of a puncture or **laceration** (injuries to soft tissue from a tearing or slicing of skin and possibly underlying fleshy structures)
  3) May also be seen in industrial settings where liquid or air is used under high pressure; substance is introduced to tissues at great volumes and under tremendous pressure and tissues are crushed, altering circulation in area
  4) Bone or ligament and tendon involvement is usually not seen when tissue injury is a primary diagnosis
  5) Hemorrhage into surrounding tissue at site of injury results in diminished perfusion to area that may cause tissue necrosis or delayed healing

C. Nursing assessment
1. Multisystem injury that threatens life or limb requires rapid and sequential assessment and intervention for a successful outcome
2. Each primary assessment phase will correspond with an immediate intervention if an injury is discovered
   a. Remember also that there are generally multiple members of a trauma team who assess and intervene almost simultaneously

Practice to Pass

A client presents with a small caliber gunshot wound to the lower left lateral chest with signs and symptoms suggesting a pneumothorax and shock. No other injury is noted. What type of shock and pneumothorax is suspected and why?

> **b.** A secondary assessment occurs after life-threatening injuries are addressed and airway, breathing, and circulation (ABCs) are restored

> **3.** Treatment for a "higher" level system, such as airway, should never be postponed in order to complete entire assessment sequence

4. Many hospitals use rapid assessment forms that allow for a determination of intensity or severity of a trauma client's condition; these tools provide great assistance in organizing common needs of clients at differing levels of acuity

5. Assessment

    a. Prearrival: VS; focused injury findings; neurological status (to include if victim has lost consciousness); machinery involved (includes type and caliber of weapon); current medications, medical history, and allergies; safety belt use; mechanism of injury and time of injury, environmental factors such as chemical spills

>   **b.** If no report is available prior to client's arrival, gather pertinent information simultaneously while assessing client's condition; obtain tetanus immunization status if wounds are present; *treatment should never be delayed because of missing or incomplete history*

    c. Obtaining data about circumstances of injury is important to rule out secondary and delayed manifestations of an injury; however, life support is carried out in a consistent manner for all trauma victims

    d. Upon arrival

>   **1)** Assess airway and adequate ventilation by inspection and auscultation; note abnormalities such as absence of breathing or inadequate ventilations and irregular depth or rate

>   **2)** Maintain cervical spine stabilization

        3) Assess for vomitus or debris in mouth

        4) Assess for flail segments of ribs, diminished or absent breath sounds, presence of a deviated trachea (trachea is "pushed" to one side rather than midline in anterior neck), and sounds of any air movement through a wound

        5) Assess cardiac activity through gentle palpation of carotid pulse and/or auscultation

        6) Assess cardiac rhythms via a cardiac monitor, noting any dysrhythmias

        7) Assess for distant heart sounds, pericardial friction rub and distended jugular veins

        8) Assess for obvious sources of hemorrhage, including urethral meatus and rectum

>   **9)** Assess for signs and symptoms of shock, specifically hypovolemic or cardiogenic shock (give close attention to diminishing UO, as pulse and BP may not alter dramatically until late in shock state)

>   **10)** Assess neurological status including LOC, pupil size in millimeters and response to light, peripheral posturing, sensation, mobility, symmetry of movement, and paralysis

>   **11)** Be sure to assess client's back while maintaining cervical and spinal alignment; use "log-roll" technique

        12) Rectal exam performed by provider; loss of rectal tone may be assessed in presence of spinal cord injury

        13) Assess for fractures with special attention provided to thoracic, pelvic, and femoral areas; assess for pain, shortening, and external rotation of affected leg commonly found in hip fractures; assess for fracture variations and locations, numbering sites if there are multiple injuries; crushing injuries may mask displaced bones, but may be threatening in and of themselves; areas of gross distention may produce a *compartment* or tourniquet effect at site and distal to injury, blocking blood flow and producing a limb-threatening emergency

6. Diagnostic tests
   a. H&H: hypovolemic shock is always a significant risk with trauma; decreasing levels and rate of deterioration may indicate severe hemorrhaging
   b. WBC: may elevate with inflammatory response to trauma or in response to blood in abdominal cavity, indicating a source of hemorrhage
   c. Cardiac enzymes: elevation indicates cardiac tissue damage has occurred
   d. Blood alcohol and/or toxicology screen: traumatic injuries are often associated with alcohol ingestion or substance use
      1) Severe intoxication compromises airway clearance and respiratory effort
      2) Client is at more risk for injury; assess carefully to differentiate diminished mentation caused by injury from that brought on by intoxication or an abnormal glucose
   e. Glucose testing: hyperglycemia may be mistaken for alcohol intoxication because of the pungent, fruity smell of the breath and the confusion clients typically exhibit
   f. ABGS: indicates respiratory failure and acid-base imbalances; used to direct supplemental oxygen therapy
      1) Respiratory failure is indicated by a PaO_2 less than 60 mmHg or a $PaCO_2$ greater than 50 mmHg
      2) If failure is acute in nature, pH (normal 7.35–7.45) will fall as CO_2 is retained
   g. EKG: may reveal dysrhythmias requiring treatment or procedural interventions
   h. Urinalysis: microscopic hematuria may indicate minor to significant genitourinary trauma

D. **Nursing management**
   1. Prearrival
      a. Organize ancillary staff (additional nursing support, respiratory and radiology personnel and any other medical consultants) based on client's status
      b. Equipment: organize equipment to include resuscitative equipment (crash cart with airway management equipment and medications), IV access equipment and fluid, urinary catheterization equipment, bandaging supplies, sterile water and basins, lab specimen collectors and other supplies as needed for procedures such as cricothyrotomy, thoracostomy, thoracotomy, peritoneal lavage, and pericardiocentesis
   2. Standard interventions
      a. Maintain airway, circulation, and neurological assessment (see Table 17-4)

Practice to Pass

A client presents with a cast on the lower left arm because of a fracture from falling. The upper-left arm is severely bruised and distended, and the client is complaining of severe "pressure" to this area. What emergent condition could be related to the client's injuries?

Table 17-4 **Nursing Management of Trauma**

Airway	Circulation	Neurological
• Establish and maintain adequate airway • Use supplemental oxygen • Remove debris with tongue depressor and suction • Utilize airway supplements such as oropharyngeal or endotracheal tubes • Utilize nasal intubation if cervical injury suspected • Prepare for thoracostomy (chest tube) if needed	• Monitor for cardiac dysrhythmias • Prepare to administer medications and perform procedures specific to dysrhythmia, such as defibrillation • Prepare for a thoracotomy if necessary • Pericardiocentesis may be needed if cardiac tamponade is evident • Monitor vital signs every 5–15 minutes	• Assess neurological status every 15 minutes as needed • Medications include osmotic diuretics and steroids for cerebral edema; antibiotics for open head injury • Maintain immobile and aligned cervical spine while neurological assessment is unstable • Restrict fluids if level of consciousness is changing and shock is not evident • Use hyperventilation to lower cerebral edema • Control seizures

b. Assistance with ventilation using supplemental O_2

c. Maintain cervical spine alignment at all times in supine position until an appropriate diagnosis is made

d. Cardiac monitoring and continuous or intermittent VS monitoring to include pulse oximetry

e. Establish intravenous (IV) access; 2 large-bore IV catheters (18 gauge or larger) are usually inserted

f. Manage shock state

g. Splint and support obvious deformities; slightly elevate legs in absence of head injury, cardiac decompensation or pulmonary edema or congestion

h. Monitor intake and output accurately
1) Insert indwelling urinary catheter when accurate measurements are required
2) Do not insert a catheter when there is bleeding from urethral meatus or obvious hip and pelvic deformity until bladder injury is ruled out

i. Document all assessments, interventions, and responses

3. Fractures

a. Medications include analgesics and antibiotics, which may be given prophylactically for open wounds

b. Support and split obvious fractures without manipulating or "reducing" (bending a fracture into alignment) bone, utilizing pillows, folded linens, and tape

c. Release constricting garments or splints without manipulating fractured area; frequently perform neurovascular checks distal to site of injury

d. Ice may be applied to cool area, avoiding direct contact with skin or injured area

e. With an open or suspected open fracture, apply sterile, saline-soaked gauze until area is thoroughly cleansed

4. Hemorrhage

a. Treat obvious sources of external hemorrhage by direct pressure applied through moist, sterile bandages

b. A hemothorax may contain over 1 liter of blood and may be a significant source of volume loss; a thoracostomy tube may be inserted and an autotransfusion may be performed

c. Bleeding from within abdomen and retroperitoneum may occur with or without abdominal distention and rigidity until late in shock state; peritoneal lavage may be performed to determine presence of blood

d. Fractures of the pelvis and femur are also capable of producing profound hypovolemic states; intravascular volume is restored by infusing crystalloids or colloids (including blood) and by administering sympathomimetics

IV. DISSEMINATED INTRAVASCULAR COAGULOPATHY (DIC)

A. Overview

1. **Disseminated intravascular coagulopathy (DIC)** is a complex and abnormal response of body's normal clotting mechanisms to an injury

2. Clotting processes are accelerated and normal clothing substances become depleted, leaving client vulnerable to massive hemorrhaging

3. DIC may become a complicating side effect in some forms of shock, most commonly with septic shock; it also occurs secondary to other disorders but does not occur alone

4. It is associated with a high mortality rate

5. Causes of DIC include sepsis, shock, malignant neoplasms, liver disease, metabolic disorders, circulatory disorders, gynecological conditions, spinal or brain injuries, transfusion reactions, and immune disorders including venomous bites

B. Pathophysiology

1. In healthy people, homeostasis is maintained between vessel injury and bleeding when an appropriate size clot forms; clotting only becomes a problem when no injury has been sustained or when hemorrhaging depletes client's reservoir of clotting factors

2. Intrinsic and/or extrinsic clotting pathways are activated in response to a traumatic injury

3. Thromboplastin is released from damaged cells and platelets begin to adhere to damaged vessel or blood cell forming a "barrier" to prevent further hemorrhaging and injury

4. A plug of fibrinogen and fibrin is stabilized at site of injury through normal clot formation process; clot or plug then undergoes **fibrinolysis** (process by which a clot is broken down)

5. Fibrinolysis may occur immediately or days after an injury and causes release of fibrin degradation products (FDPs) and fibrin degradation fragments (FDFs); in healthy clients or those with only minor injuries, this process is restricted to area of injury

6. Clients with massive tissue and cellular damage, such as traumatic or shock states, deplete clotting factors because they are used up in an attempt to prevent further hemorrhage

7. This cycle becomes self-defeating in that circulating fibrin clots become widespread throughout body's intravascular volume, often causing widespread thrombosis (blood clots in bloodstream)

8. Thrombi indicate to body that further damage is occurring and body responds by releasing more clotting factors that are also consumed until, finally, massive hemorrhaging occurs; circulating FDPs also have an anticoagulant effect, worsening the scenario

9. Client hemorrhages at a life-threatening level, while extensive clotting occurs at same time in an unrelenting cycle

10. Signs and symptoms
    a. Decreased BP and peripheral pulses
    b. Purpura, ecchymosis, petechiae

    c. Cyanosis and bleeding that may range from mild oozing around catheter and IV sites and oral mucosa to profound volume loss noted by hematuria or occult blood in stool or vomitus
    d. Intraabdominal bleeding may manifest itself with pain, distention, and rigidity
    e. Hypoxemia, dyspnea, and air hunger
    f. Neurologic symptoms: confusion, decreased LOC, seizures
    g. Renal symptoms: oliguria
    h. GI symptoms: nausea, vomiting
    i. Epistaxis
    j. Seizures
    k. Pain in chest, muscles, back, and abdomen

C. Nursing Assessment

1. Assessment
    a. Risk: any client who presents with frank hemorrhaging without obvious injury, predisposing conditions such as shock or septicemia, or those requiring transfusion of blood products
    b. Assessment includes VS, pulses, respiratory and cardiac status, assessment of all orifices and venipuncture sites, symptom analysis of pain, skin color, capillary refill, mentation, UO, and GI complaints

2. Diagnostic tests
   a. PT, international normalized ratio (INR) PTT, FDPs or FDFs: elevated
   b. D-dimer test will be elevated
      1) Serial testing is very important and assists in determining diagnosis of DIC as opposed to other bleeding disorders
      2) A steady increase in these values indicates ongoing, massive clot breakdown rather than a lack of clotting factors
   c. Routine labs such as CBC, electrolyte panel, BUN, and creatinine
D. Nursing management
1. Medications include heparin (in some clients) to neutralize effects of circulating thrombin
   a. Administer heparin with great care and only when extreme circumstances warrant its use
   b. Generally is administered when DIC is not rapidly reversed by treating underlying cause or in clients who are threatened by bleeding or massive thrombus formation
2. It is important to treat underlying cause of DIC as quickly as possible and treat for any shock state that precipitated crisis
3. Fresh frozen plasma and cryoprecipitate are administered to replace clotting factors
4. Monitor coagulation tests not only for diagnosis, but for treatment

V. ACUTE RESPIRATORY DISTRESS SYNDROME

A. Overview
1. **Acute respiratory distress syndrome (ARDS)** is acute respiratory failure caused by many factors such as shock, trauma, burns, bacterial or viral pathogens, aspiration of fluids, and toxic injury
B. Pathophysiology
1. Alveolar walls are severely impaired; pulmonary capillaries are injured or there is damage to alveolar lining
2. Result is increased permeability of alveolar blood vessels, which allows fluid to accumulate in alveolar spaces and alveoli become airless; a tremendous strain is placed on heart and cardiac complications are likely
3. Fluid in alveoli causes a decrease in surfactant and increased surface tension, leading to a loss of lung compliance, decreased ventilation, and hypoxia; lungs become stiff and noncompliant because of alveolar collapse
4. As alveoli are damaged, hypoxia and eventually cell injury and death occur
   a. Inflammatory reactions can occur as alveoli and capillaries are damaged
   b. Inflammation causes release of cytokines that leads to damage of nearby capillaries and alveoli
   c. Hyaline membranes form inside alveoli and further hinder exchange of O_2 and CO_2
5. A spontaneous pneumothorax can occur
6. Supplemental oxygen does not improve condition (a hallmark of ARDS)
C. Nursing assessment
1. Assessment includes respiratory distress (tachypnea, use of accessory muscles, marked dyspnea), lung sounds (crackles or rhonchi), abnormal ABGs (hypoxia and/or hypercapnia), cyanosis, retractions, agitation, and confusion (late stage)
2. Diagnostic tests: CXR (large, diffuse infiltrates or "white outs" with normal heart size), ABGs (PaO_2 less than 50 mmHg and respiratory alkalosis), PFS (decreased lung compliance; reduced vital capacity, minute volume, and functional vital capacity), and pulmonary artery pressure monitoring for diagnostic purposes (normal pressures will be evident in ARDS versus elevated pressures in pulmonary edema)

D. Nursing management

1. Medications
   a. Nitrous oxide for its analgesic effect or to dilate blood vessels and improve oxygenation
   b. Nonsteroidal anti-inflammatory drugs (NSAIDs), interleukin-1 receptor antagonists, neutrophil inhibitors, or corticosteroids to reduce inflammation
   c. Lung surfactants: beractant (Survanta), calfactant (Infasurf), and colfosceril (Exosurf Neonatal) to lower surface tension of alveoli and prevent alveolar collapse; this action restores pulmonary compliance and oxygenation
   d. Antibiotics if an infection is suspected as cause
   e. Heparin to prevent complications of ARDS such as thrombophlebitis, pulmonary embolus, or disseminated intravascular coagulopathy (DIC)
   f. Sedatives or skeletal muscle relaxants such as pancuronium bromide (Tubocurarine) to control agitation associated with mechanical ventilation
2. Foremost therapy is to treat cause
3. Main form of therapy is endotracheal intubation and mechanical ventilation
   a. Continuous positive airway pressure (CPAP) or positive-end expiratory pressure (PEEP) is often used to keep alveoli open and improve gas exchange
   b. PEEP has been associated with decreased CO, lung injury caused by high mechanical pressure known as barotrauma; and decreased VS, especially a drop in BP; monitor lung sounds
4. Maintaining a prone position may improve oxygen perfusion
5. Monitor pulmonary arterial pressures through use of a pulmonary artery (Swan-Ganz) catheter
6. Maintain adequate fluid and nutritional status
7. Monitor oxygen saturation and signs of a pneumothorax, which is a complication of ARDS

Case Study

A trauma victim presents to the emergency department after a motor vehicle crash in which the prehospital report indicates that the car steering wheel was broken and no seat belt was worn. Vital signs are BP 100/58, pulse 116, respirations 26 and labored, temperature 97.2°F oral. The client is intermittently confused and is lethargic. There is a 6-inch laceration to the frontal scalp. Pupils are equal and reactive. Upon exam, there is a large ecchymotic area to the right anterior chest and paradoxical movement is noted. Breath sounds are absent to the right base, anteriorly and posteriorly. The right leg is externally rotated and shortened.

1. What fundamental interventions would be initiated immediately upon arrival based on this information?

2. What procedures would potentially be performed?

3. What phase and type of shock is suspected on presentation? What diagnostic values would contribute to determining the phase and type?

4. What are the potential injuries that are most highly suspected of contributing to the shock state?

5. What physical finding would cause concern when determining whether to place a urinary catheter for accurate output monitoring?

For suggested responses, see page 468.

POSTTEST

1 A client is transported by ambulance to the emergency department (ED) with suspected chest and spinal injuries after a motor vehicle crash. Upon admission of the client to the ED, the nurse determines that which of the following is a priority intervention?

1. Preparing spinal traction to align head and spinal cord
2. Checking interior of the mouth for broken teeth or other injuries
3. Applying pressure to areas of gross bleeding
4. Auscultating and inspecting chest for the presence of pneumothorax or tamponade

2 A client who sustained trauma has been admitted to the emergency department. The nurse analyzes the hemoglobin and hematocrit (H&H) levels to monitor for which type of shock state?

1. Hypovolemic
2. Cardiogenic
3. Anaphylactic
4. Distributive

3 A 57-year-old man who sustained a large myocardial infarction develops acute respiratory distress syndrome (ARDS) as a complication. The client is intubated and mechanically ventilated with positive end expiratory pressure (PEEP). The nurse becomes most concerned about which finding while the client is on PEEP?

1. Sinus tachycardia of 125 beats per minute
2. Anxiety
3. Blood pressure of 88/52
4. Temperature of 100.5°F

4 A client has developed hypovolemic shock. The nurse would use which physiological indicator when prioritizing the ongoing plan of care?

1. Urine output
2. Skin turgor
3. Range of mobility
4. Temperature

5 A client who was an unrestrained passenger in a motor vehicle crash is brought by ambulance to the trauma unit. She was thrown sideways against the right side of an older car that has standard hand cranks for the window. Her abdomen is distended and painful to touch, hematocrit and hemoglobin (H&H) are low, and BP is 80/50. What should be the nurse's major concern?

1. Head injury
2. Spontaneous pneumothorax
3. Ruptured liver or spleen
4. Ruptured kidney

6 A client who sustained a head injury from a blow to the head 10 hours ago is brought to the emergency department in a lethargic state with 1 pupil larger and sluggish in responding to light. The computed tomography (CT) scan shows a venous bleed and subdural hematoma. The nurse would look to what changes or assessments as indicators of worsening neurological status? Select all that apply.

1. Further loss of consciousness (LOC)
2. Lowering of systolic blood pressure
3. Bradycardia
4. Projectile vomiting occurring without warning
5. Papilledema on fundoscopic examination

7 A client presents to the emergency department with a gunshot wound to the upper anterior left chest. Which assessment would the nurse perform next after the primary survey has been completed with stabilization of life-threatening injuries?

1. Patency of the airway
2. Secondary injuries such as extremity fractures
3. Chest excursion and gas exchange
4. Constipation and smoking history

8 When evaluating the status of a client who is recovering from hypovolemic shock after administration of blood products and other colloids, which indicators would the nurse use to determine whether the client has had the best outcome?

1. Vital signs, hematocrit and hemoglobin (H&H), and coagulation tests within normal limits
2. Vital signs and a hematocrit and hemoglobin (H&H) level within normal limits and a urinalysis without hematuria
3. Vital signs and a hematocrit and hemoglobin (H&H) level within normal limits and a negative C-spine x-ray
4. Vital signs and neurological exam within normal limits

9 The nurse assesses a client who sustained a fracture of the femur 16 hours ago for which complication for which the client is at greatest risk?

1. Disuse syndrome
2. Fat embolism syndrome
3. Reflex sympathetic dystrophy
4. Infection

10 The nurse determines that a successful outcome measurement for a client who experienced open trauma to the head includes which of the following?

1. Recall of the actual event of injury
2. Loss of consciousness of no greater than 24 hours
3. Absence of signs of meningitis
4. Absence of pain

➤ *See pages 450–451 for Answers and Rationales.*

POSTTEST

ANSWERS & RATIONALES

Pretest

ANSWERS & RATIONALES

1 **Answer: 2** **Rationale:** All forms of pneumothorax may progress to the extent that tension develops within the affected lung space and exerts pressure on the unaffected lung. A deviated trachea is a classic sign of tension pneumothorax. **Cognitive Level:** Analyzing **Client Need:** Physiological Adaptation **Integrated Process:** Nursing Process: Assessment **Content Area:** Adult Health **Strategy:** Look for the abnormal manifestations and reflect on the mechanism of injury to determine the problem. **Reference:** LeMone, P., Burke, K., & Bauldoff, G. (2011). *Medical-surgical nursing: Critical thinking in patient care* (5th ed.). Upper Saddle River, NJ: Pearson Education, pp. 1207–1208.

2 **Answer: 4** **Rationale:** Aspiration of any liquid into the lungs places the client at risk for development of acute respiratory distress syndrome (ARDS). Assessments to evaluate the onset of this syndrome should focus on the respiratory system and diminishing oxygen saturation despite increasing supplemental oxygen. Cardiogenic shock, spontaneous pneumothorax, and renal failure are not immediate concerns. **Cognitive Level:** Analyzing **Client Need:** Physiological Adaptation **Integrated Process:** Nursing Process: Assessment **Content Area:** Adult Health **Strategy:** The clues are the near-drowning situation and the poor respiratory status. Recall that with drowning, there is aspiration of water into the lungs. **Reference:** LeMone, P., Burke, K., & Bauldoff, G. (2011). *Medical-surgical nursing: Critical thinking in patient care* (5th ed.). Upper Saddle River, NJ: Pearson Education, pp. 1215–1216.

3 **Answer: 2** **Rationale:** During the compensatory phase of shock, the body attempts to correct the progression of a decrease in intravascular volume through an increase in pulse and respiration and the subjective sensation of thirst. Shunting of blood begins to occur from organs not vital for immediate survival. Renal blood flow is diminished, and urinary output falls. Blood pressure is decreasing but adequate for current homeostasis. Thirst is a response to decreased blood volume. **Cognitive Level:** Analyzing **Client Need:** Physiological Adaptation **Integrated Process:** Nursing Process: Diagnosis **Content Area:** Adult Health **Strategy:** Consider that tissue perfusion is still being maintained as evidenced by mentation and urine output of 30 mL/hr, although the heart rate and blood pressure indicate moderate severity of shock. **Reference:** LeMone, P., Burke, K., & Bauldoff, G. (2011). *Medical-surgical nursing: Critical thinking in patient care* (5th ed.). Upper Saddle River, NJ: Pearson Education, pp. 253–255.

4 **Answer: 4** **Rationale:** Myocardial infarction is the most common cause of cardiac damage resulting in cardiac insufficiency or "pump failure" leading to cardiogenic shock. Jugular venous distention and pulmonary congestion are consistent with heart failure. The client has no underlying condition that obstructs blood flow from exiting the heart; spinal cord injury is the cause of neurogenic shock; and there are no indications of fluid or blood loss to signal hypovolemic shock. **Cognitive Level:** Analyzing **Client Need:** Physiological Adaptation **Integrated Process:** Nursing Process: Diagnosis **Content Area:** Adult Health **Strategy:** All the options are for a type of shock. Determine the origin from the situation. **Reference:** LeMone, P., Burke, K., & Bauldoff, G. (2011). *Medical-surgical nursing: Critical thinking in patient care* (5th ed.). Upper Saddle River, NJ: Pearson Education, pp. 258–259.

5 **Answer: 2** **Rationale:** The client is exhibiting symptoms of a generalized, IgE-mediated reaction to the administration of an antibiotic, and sensitizing dosages have already occurred as reported by the client. The history of repeated exposure to an allergen, combined with the difficulty breathing, itching, and flushing, should direct the nurse to a diagnosis of anaphylaxis. The first line intervention is epinephrine. More information would be needed to determine whether this client is developing septicemia or septic shock. There is no supporting evidence in the client's situation for hypovolemic or neurogenic shock. **Cognitive Level:** Applying **Client Need:** Physiological Adaptation **Integrated Process:** Nursing Process: Planning **Content Area:** Adult Health **Strategy:** Read the client situation of receiving a few doses of an antibiotic and then developing symptoms of a problem. **Reference:** LeMone, P., Burke, K., & Bauldoff, G. (2011). *Medical-surgical nursing: Critical thinking in patient care* (5th ed.). Upper Saddle River, NJ: Pearson Education, pp. 260–261.

6 **Answer: 3** **Rationale:** Cervical spine injuries can result from an acceleration–deceleration mechanism involving the upper spine. The client did not report hitting his head, but head injuries may be suspected as secondary occurrences when there are spinal injuries. Liver and spleen injuries are not likely to be the primary problem with this mechanism of injury. **Cognitive Level:** Analyzing **Client Need:** Physiological Adaptation **Integrated Process:** Nursing Process: Diagnosis **Content Area:** Adult Health **Strategy:** Consider the history of fall and the impact to the upper back. Use knowledge of anatomy and pathophysiology when eliminating the incorrect options. **Reference:** LeMone, P., Burke, K., & Bauldoff, G. (2011). *Medical-surgical nursing: Critical thinking in patient care*

(5th ed.). Upper Saddle River, NJ: Pearson Education, pp. 1480–1481.

7 **Answer: 2, 4, 5** **Rationale:** Paradoxical pulses (pulsus paradoxus) is a hallmark sign of cardiac tamponade. As pressure is exerted on the left ventricle from fluid, the natural increase in pressure from the right ventricle during inspiration diminishes cardiac output. Narrowed pulse pressure, hypotension, and weak pulses are also manifestations of cardiac tamponade. A deviated trachea is a sign of a tension pneumothorax, and atelectasis is not associated with tamponade. **Cognitive Level:** Analyzing **Client Need:** Physiological Adaptation **Integrated Process:** Nursing Process: Assessment **Content Area:** Adult Health **Strategy:** Recall that in cardiac tamponade, there is rising intracardiac pressure resulting in decreased diastolic filling and decreased cardiac output. Consider what manifestations will be observed because of these events. **Reference:** LeMone, P., Burke, K., & Bauldoff, G. (2011). *Medical-surgical nursing: Critical thinking in patient care* (5th ed.). Upper Saddle River, NJ: Pearson Education, pp. 998–999.

8 **Answer: 2** **Rationale:** Penetrating injury to the bowel releases intracolonic material into the peritoneal cavity, predisposing the individual to a serious infection that may progress to septicemia. While a paralytic ileus is of concern any time the abdominal cavity has been accessed via surgery, injury, or administration of certain medications. It is not of the life-threatening nature that occurs with peritonitis. Peritonitis may cause the occurrence of a paralytic ileus. Constipation and intestinal adhesions are not immediate concerns. **Cognitive Level:** Applying **Client Need:** Physiological Adaptation **Integrated Process:** Nursing Process: Planning **Content Area:** Adult Health **Strategy:** Consider which option poses a potential for life-threatening complications. When narrowing the options to 2, determine which one needs the most immediate intervention. **Reference:** LeMone, P., Burke, K., & Bauldoff, G. (2011). *Medical-surgical nursing: Critical thinking in patient care* (5th ed.). Upper Saddle River, NJ: Pearson Education, p. 259.

9 **Answer: 3** **Rationale:** Many traumatic injuries occur as a result of the slowed responses and judgment associated with alcohol intoxication. Hyper- or hypoglycemia may exhibit similar signs and symptoms of intoxication so it is necessary to assess both values. Skull x-rays are noncontributory for brain injuries unless there is an obvious or highly suspected fracture. The client reports no loss of consciousness but a CT scan may be done if head injury in addition to the laceration is suspected. An MRI is not appropriate at this time. An electroencephalography (EEG) measures the electrical brain waves to determine brain death or some type of seizure and abnormal cerebral activity. **Cognitive Level:** Analyzing **Client Need:** Reduction of Risk Potential **Integrated Process:** Nursing Process: Assessment **Content Area:** Adult Health **Strategy:** Note that blood alcohol levels appear in many options. Both tests in the option must be appropriate for the option to be correct. Consider what etiology besides alcohol intoxication may cause this client's symptoms. **Reference:** LeMone, P., Burke, K., & Bauldoff, G. (2011). *Medical-surgical nursing: Critical thinking in patient care* (5th ed.). Upper Saddle River, NJ: Pearson Education, pp. 243–245.

10 **Answer: 1, 3, 4** **Rationale:** Compartment syndrome results from swelling or pressure that constricts blood flow to muscles and nerves. Hemorrhage and shifting of intra-vascular fluid to the interstitial spaces creates a tourni-quet effect, compromising circulation at the site of injury and distally. Unrelieved pain, signs of compro-mised arterial circulation, sensory loss, and motor weak-ness are important symptoms. Nerve symptoms develop within 30 minutes of ischemia, and muscle weakness develops in 2–4 hours. Level of consciousness (LOC) is not affected with compartment syndrome. **Cognitive Level:** Applying **Client Need:** Physiological Adaptation **Integrated Process:** Nursing Process: Assessment **Content Area:** Adult Health **Strategy:** Consider that when circulatory changes occur with musculoskeletal trauma, there is an increased likelihood of compartment syndrome. Read each option carefully and use the process of elimination to make a selection. **Reference:** LeMone, P., Burke, K., & Bauldoff, G. (2011). *Medical-surgical nursing: Critical thinking in patient care* (5th ed.). Upper Saddle River, NJ: Pearson Education, pp. 1310–1311.

Posttest

1 **Answer: 2** **Rationale:** The client's airway is priority in all phases of life support. Remember ABCs (airway, breathing, circulation) for priority setting. A trauma team usually consists of many people, and others can be assessing less critical areas. Spinal traction is not the same as immobilizing the cervical spine, which is another priority of care. **Cognitive Level:** Analyzing **Client Need:** Management of Care **Integrated Process:** Nursing Process: Implementation **Content Area:** Adult Health **Strategy:** Remember ABCs (airway, breathing, and circu-lation) to prioritize your answer. **Reference:** LeMone, P., Burke, K., & Bauldoff, G. (2011). *Medical-surgical nursing: Critical thinking in patient care* (5th ed.). Upper Saddle River, NJ: Pearson Education, p. 243.

2 **Answer: 1** **Rationale:** Hematocrit and hemoglobin (H&H) levels will continue to decrease with ongoing hemorrhaging, indicating the aggressiveness of interven-tions to replace intravascular volume in hypovolemic shock. Cardiogenic shock would not be characterized by a drop in H&H, nor would anaphylactic or distributive shock. **Cognitive Level:** Applying **Client Need:** Physiological Adaptation **Integrated Process:** Nursing Process: Evalua-tion **Content Area:** Adult Health **Strategy:** Identify what mechanism causes the hemoglobin and hematocrit (H&H) to steadily fall. Recall what happens to the blood volume and blood pressure if this occurs to make a selection. **Reference:** LeMone, P., Burke, K., & Bauldoff, G.

(2011). *Medical-surgical nursing: Critical thinking in patient care* (5th ed.). Upper Saddle River, NJ: Pearson Education, pp. 260–261.

3 **Answer: 3** **Rationale:** Barotrauma (decreased cardiac output and damage to lung tissue) is a complication of positive end expiratory pressure (PEEP). A drop in blood pressure is associated with a decrease in cardiac output. The sinus tachycardia may be a compensatory mechanism to raise the BP or a response to the acute respiratory dis-tress syndrome (ARDS). Anxiety is expected with intu-bation, and the small temperature elevation may or may not indicate a serious problem. **Cognitive Level:** Analyzing **Client Need:** Physiological Adaptation **Integrated Process:** Nursing Process: Diagnosis **Content Area:** Adult Health **Strategy:** The clue is to select an option that is of concern with the positive end expiratory pressure (PEEP). The other options are related to the client's status but not necessarily to the PEEP. **Reference:** LeMone, P., Burke, K., & Bauldoff, G. (2011). *Medical-surgical nursing: Critical thinking in patient care* (5th ed.). Upper Saddle River, NJ: Pearson Education, pp. 264–266.

4 **Answer: 1** **Rationale:** All forms of shock diminish perfu-sion to the renal system. A decreasing output is indica-tive that the kidneys may be losing function as a result of significant tubular necrosis. Skin turgor will generally reflect circulating volume but is not a precise indicator. Range of mobility is irrelevant to circulating volume. Temperature could elevate with fluid volume loss but is again an imprecise indicator. **Cognitive Level:** Applying **Client Need:** Physiological Adaptation **Integrated Process:** Nursing Process: Planning **Content Area:** Adult Health **Strategy:** Consider which assessment will give the best information related to blood volume and circulation. **Reference:** LeMone, P., Burke, K., & Bauldoff, G. (2011). *Medical-surgical nursing: Critical thinking in patient care* (5th ed.). Upper Saddle River, NJ: Pearson Education, pp. 264–266.

5 **Answer: 3** **Rationale:** A distended, painful abdomen with signs of hypovolemic shock and a low hematocrit and hemoglobin (H&H) should trigger the nurse to con-sider a ruptured liver. Although a ruptured kidney could also occur, the major concern would be the liver because of its vascular nature. A head injury or pneu-mothorax should be assessed, but they are not expected injuries given the mechanism of injury. **Cognitive Level:** Analyzing **Client Need:** Physiological Adaptation **Integrated Process:** Nursing Process: Assessment **Content Area:** Adult Health **Strategy:** The manifestations and history suggest trauma and hemorrhage. What body area is most likely injured? **Reference:** LeMone, P., Burke, K., & Bauldoff, G. (2011). *Medical-surgical nursing: Critical thinking in patient care* (5th ed.). Upper Saddle River, NJ: Pearson Education, p. 243.

6 **Answer: 1, 3, 4, 5** **Rationale:** Subdural hematomas are formed most often from venous tissue bleeding and are more common than other forms of brain injury. They have a high mortality because of secondary brain injury due to edema and increased intracranial pressure (ICP). Signs of increased ICP include projectile vomiting, deteriorating level of consciousness (LOC), papilledema (swelling of the optic disk) or, in late stages, the Cushing's triad (increased systolic blood pressure, widening pulse pressure, and bradycardia). A drop in systolic blood pressure would suggest blood loss from hemorrhage, not worsening neurological state. **Cognitive Level:** Applying **Client Need:** Physiological Adaptation **Integrated Process:** Nursing Process: Assessment **Content Area:** Adult Health **Strategy:** Recall the signs of increased intracranial pressure (ICP) after considering that the ICP would rise because of accumulating blood in the subdural space. **Reference:** LeMone, P., Burke, K., & Bauldoff, G. (2011). *Medical-surgical nursing: Critical thinking in patient care* (5th ed.). Upper Saddle River, NJ: Pearson Education, p. 1439.

7 Answer: 2 Rationale: A secondary assessment or survey occurs once the airway, breathing, and circulation (primary survey) are assessed and interventions are begun. Life-threatening injuries located during the primary assessment must be stabilized prior to reviewing for additional injuries or wounds. Airway and breathing assessments have already been done. Assessing for constipation and smoking is not a priority at this time. **Cognitive Level:** Applying **Client Need:** Physiological Adaptation **Integrated Process:** Nursing Process: Assessment **Content Area:** Adult Health **Strategy:** Remember airway, breathing, circulation (ABCs). Utilize principles of conducting a secondary survey to recall what step comes after the client is stabilized from the life-threatening injury. **Reference:** LeMone, P., Burke, K., & Bauldoff, G. (2011). *Medical-surgical nursing: Critical thinking in patient care* (5th ed.). Upper Saddle River, NJ: Pearson Education, pp. 243–244.

8 Answer: 1 Rationale: Administering colloidal solutions may diminish the blood's ability to coagulate by reducing platelet adhesion while expanding the intravascular volume needed in severe shock states. Normal test results for coagulation are reassuring findings. Vital signs within established parameters indicate support of vital functions. Acceptable hematocrit and hemoglobin (H&H) levels substantiate and support perfusion at a cellular level as well as resolution of volume loss. The presence or lack of hematuria is not a viable indicator of the level of shock states or their resolution. **Cognitive Level:** Analyzing **Client Need:** Physiological Adaptation **Integrated Process:** Nursing Process: Evaluation **Content Area:** Adult Health **Strategy:** Differentiate between the physiological effects of intravenous crystalloids and colloids. What is the desired client response? **Reference:** LeMone, P., Burke, K., & Bauldoff, G. (2011). *Medical-surgical nursing: Critical thinking in patient care* (5th ed.). Upper Saddle River, NJ: Pearson Education, pp. 261–262.

9 Answer: 2 Rationale: Fat is more easily expressed from the larger bones such as the hip and femur when they are fractured. A time frame of 16 hours does not suggest disuse syndrome. Reflex sympathetic dystrophy is not a sequelae of a long bone fracture. Infection can be associated with any trauma, but not specifically with a femur fracture. **Cognitive Level:** Applying **Client Need:** Physiological Adaptation **Integrated Process:** Nursing Process: Assessment **Content Area:** Adult Health **Strategy:** The critical word in the question is *femur*. Consider what serious complication may follow a fracture of a long bone such as the femur. **Reference:** LeMone, P., Burke, K., & Bauldoff, G. (2011). *Medical-surgical nursing: Critical thinking in patient care* (5th ed.). Upper Saddle River, NJ: Pearson Education, pp. 1311–1314.

10 Answer: 3 Rationale: An injury to the protective tissues of the brain poses a risk for infection in that bacteria can be introduced, especially with an open injury. Successful treatment would avoid the development of meningitis. A concussion to the head could produce permanent retrograde amnesia. Loss of consciousness for no more than 24 hours is not a successful outcome by itself; the ultimate outcome for this client should be eventual function and absence of infection. The brain itself has no pain receptors. **Cognitive Level:** Analyzing **Client Need:** Physiological Adaptation **Integrated Process:** Nursing Process: Evaluation **Content Area:** Adult Health **Strategy:** The critical words *open trauma* relate to the body's protective barriers being breeched in the trauma. Consider what can enter the body to select an answer. **Reference:** LeMone, P., Burke, K., & Bauldoff, G. (2011). *Medical-surgical nursing: Critical thinking in patient care* (5th ed.). Upper Saddle River, NJ: Pearson Education, pp. 1465–1468.

References

Copstead-Kirkhorn, L., & Banasik, J. (2010). *Pathophysiology* (4th ed.). Philadelphia, PA: Saunders.

Kee, J. (2009). *Laboratory and diagnostic tests and nursing implications* (8th ed.). Upper Saddle River, NJ: Pearson Education.

LeMone, P., Burke, K., & Bauldoff, G. (2011). *Medical-surgical nursing: Critical thinking in patient care* (5th ed.). Upper Saddle River, NJ: Pearson Education.

McCance, K., & Huether, K. (2010). *Understanding pathophysiology: The biologic basis for disease in adults and children* (6th ed.) St. Louis, MO: Elsevier.

Porth, C., & Matfin, G. (2010). *Pathophysiology: Concepts of altered health states* (8th ed.). Philadelphia, PA: Lippincott Williams & Wilkins.

Wagner, K., Johnson, K., & Hardin-Pierce, M. (2010). *High acuity nursing* (5th ed.). Upper Saddle River, NJ: Pearson Education.

Wilson, B., Shannon, M., & Shields, K. (2012). *Pearson nurse's drug guide 2012.* Upper Saddle River, NJ: Pearson Education.

ANSWERS & RATIONALES

Appendix

➤ Practice to Pass Suggested Answers

Chapter 1

Page 7: *Suggested Answer*—Beclomethasone (Vanceril) is a steroid; a common yet concerning side effect in children is growth retardation. A child's asthma may require a medication on a daily basis as strong as corticosteroids. A decline in growth in height and weight has been documented while children are on continuous steroid therapy, and these parameters should be monitored monthly.

Page 9: *Suggested Answer*—Corticosteroids such as prednisone are often used for exacerbations of COPD with effective results. A side effect, however, is fluid retention, which could easily occur in a cardiac client with a history of CHF. Careful monitoring of intake and output, weight, presence of edema, and lung sounds should be done to identify early signs of CHF should they occur.

Page 14: *Suggested Answer*—Either the antibiotic is not the correct treatment for the type of organism causing the pneumonia or the pneumonia is viral in nature. A culture and sensitivity should be obtained to identify the causative organism and to ensure sensitivity of the antibiotic to the organism. If the problem is viral pneumonia, antibiotics will not usually help anyway. Any time fever persists after 72 hours of antibiotic therapy, additional considerations should be made.

Page 15: *Suggested Answer*—Remember that 2 groups at risk for tuberculosis are the disadvantaged and HIV-positive individuals. This client carries those risk factors and could be HIV-positive without knowing at this time. Also, females with sexually transmitted infections (STIs) often test positive for resistant strains of TB.

Chapter 2

Page 37: *Suggested Answer*—The fact that she has coronary heart disease (CHD) does not mean she has had damage (injury) to the heart muscle itself. CHD indicates blockage in the arteries that bring blood to the heart and supply the needed oxygen. She can live with CHD without having a heart attack if she modifies her lifestyle behaviors that lead to CHD. The symptoms of a heart attack need to be explained

(nausea, vomiting, crushing chest pain, shortness of breath, diaphoresis) as well as the difference between angina and a myocardial infarction.

Page 38: *Suggested Answer*—The nurse should explain to the client that having stable angina does not mean that the client will have a heart attack. As long as the causes of the pain are known and it stops with rest or responds to nitroglycerin, it should not cause permanent injury to the heart. However, if the pain changes in duration or intensity, or if the number of attacks increases, a health care provider should be seen as soon as possible. During an angina attack, if the pain stays longer, is more intense, or does not respond to rest or nitroglycerin, call for emergency help.

Page 41: *Suggested Answer*—An example of an acceptable response might be: "I understand that you feel that way, but now that you are here we can help you. Try to take deep, even breaths. We will give you some medication to help with the pain." Explain the prescribed procedures and what appears to be happening. Also explain that the feeling is normal when someone is having chest discomfort and shortness of breath. Do not offer false reassurance that everything will be all right when it may not.

Page 48: *Suggested Answer*—The nurse should explain that the client has been very ill and it will take some time for his body to return to normal. The provider should talk to him about follow-up care. It is important that he follow the directions and rehabilitation schedule and not try to return to work too soon or further problems or complications may develop. An appropriate explanation and comparison for clients with heart problems is to compare it to a broken leg. The broken bone cannot always be seen, but it's still there and takes time to heal. The crutches are often the only reminder of the problem. The heart needs time to heal also and the signs and symptoms experienced are the only reminders of the problem. The client should check with the provider as to when the proper time is to return to work.

Page 57: *Suggested Answer*—The nurse should go immediately to the room and assess the client. If he is unresponsive and pulseless, call a code and call for the crash cart and defibrillator. If the client is awake, alert, and talking, check the monitor leads for proper connection. Chaotic activity could be caused by ventricular fibrillation, interference, a disconnected lead wire, a loose monitor pad, or activity such as bathing or respiratory percussion. Regardless, the client should always be assessed first.

Page 61: *Suggested Answer*—Inform the client that close follow-up care is needed. The disease progression must be monitored with various tests, as well as how well the client tolerates the progression. If signs of heart failure begin, the client will be treated with medication to help the heart beat more effectively. If angina occurs, clients often respond to beta blockers and nitroglycerin. Sometimes it is necessary to have a valve replaced. That is a decision that the client and the doctor must make together. The client must know that prior to any invasive procedure (including dental procedures), prophylactic antibiotics may be prescribed to prevent infection from getting to the valve and causing further problems or complications.

Chapter 3

Page 75: *Suggested Answer*—Discuss what the client means by forgetting medicines and making up the dose at the next medication time. It would be very helpful to determine which medications the client is taking in this manner—prescription drugs, an over-the-counter medicine, or an herbal product. The nurse should review the medication schedule and purpose of each medication with the client and appropriate family members. The primary outcome is to have the client's blood pressure reading be less than 140/90. Ask the client and family members if the medication schedule is convenient. The nurse should ask if the client is experiencing any side effects, and if so, which medications are involved, how long they have been present, and whether the client has notified the prescriber. Writing medication schedules on a card or adding medications to a weekly medication box may reduce confusion about drug schedules. Determine if the client can adequately read and see the medication labels in order to read the dosage and times. If the client cannot read, pictures or a video describing what is to be done and how should be provided. If the client cannot see to read the drug names, the nurse can develop specific directions and use big numbers to indicate the time of day the medicine is to be taken. In addition, a referral to a home health agency for supervisory visits focused on medication adherence might be helpful. Time for client questions should be provided.

Page 77: *Suggested Answer*—The focus of the plan of care is to assist the client in preventing and reducing risk factors. Suggest the following:

- Avoid sitting or standing in one place for prolonged periods of time. Frequently, support hose will help manage venous congestion.
- Avoid the use of round garters and the wearing of tight abdominal garments, which constrict blood flow.
- Elevate the legs while sitting if venous congestion is a problem.
- Begin a walking program per provider's instructions and gradually increase distance up to 1 mile.
- Lose weight, if overweight or obese. A referral to a weight reduction program within the community may help.

- Add bulk to the diet to eliminate constipation to prevent straining and follow a healthy-heart diet low in sodium, cholesterol, and fat.
- Stop smoking and limit caffeine if these are present factors. Cardiac disease such as heart failure, myocardial infarction, and cardiomyopathy are risk factors for PVD and that PVD can lead to a thrombus or emboli.
- Maintain a normal blood pressure and having it monitored frequently if hypertension exists.

Page 79: *Suggested Answer*—The family should be commended on their concern and the nurse should identify that their concern is very important. Explain that surgery to repair an aneurysm is major surgery and should not be considered lightly. The major complications are hemorrhage, stroke, and possibly death. Explain that an aneurysm that is not growing larger or leaking is often better left alone. The client should be compliant in having MRIs every 6 months and keeping weight and blood pressure under control. Surgery is usually recommended when the aneurysm is at 5 cm (or greater) or shows signs of rapid growth or hemorrhage. Stress the point that the surgery will be a major operation for a 70-year-old person; therefore, careful consideration should be made when the time is appropriate. The family should be instructed to seek medical advice if the back pain worsens or continues.

Page 83: *Suggested Answer*—Smoking is a primary cause of Buerger's disease, whereas genetics or unknown etiology is associated with Raynaud's disease. Raynaud's disease affects women more than men, while Buerger's affects mostly men. Raynaud's is usually triggered by stress or cold temperatures, while smoking triggers Buerger's disease. Raynaud's disease involves the digits mostly and more commonly the hands, while Buerger's disease usually affects the lower extremities. The blue-white-red color changes in the hands are classic for Raynaud's disease, while intermittent claudication is associated with Buerger's disease. Clients with either disease should stop smoking to limit the events and protect the extremities from cold injury during an event.

Chapter 4

Page 102: *Suggested Answer*—Encourage discussion of concerns and major goals of rehabilitation based on the client goals. These may include improved mobility, maintenance of range of motion, self-care, bladder and bowel control, improved communication, optimal family functioning, and prevention of complications and repeated stroke. Stress that the goal of rehabilitation is to allow the client to learn his or her strengths and improve on limitations. The family should be encouraged to support rehabilitative efforts and refrain from offering to "do things" for their loved one. Explain that an acute care setting usually offers a lot of assistance during the acute phase versus a rehabilitation facility that encourages clients to perform their own ADLs under supervision.

Page 110: *Suggested Answer*—Consult and follow the facility's Infection Control Policies and Procedures. Isolation is no longer recommended in most cases. Careful "standard precautions" are always important to protect the client and nurse with the exception of meningococcal meningitis. Proper hand hygiene, use of gloves, and proper disposal of waste products should be initiated. Small infants and pregnant women should always avoid any potential risk.

Page 113: *Suggested Answer*—Review the procedure with the client to assess understanding and emphasize that there is no pain involved; provide open-ended questions to encourage discussion; recommend washing hair to decrease oil and avoid gels or hairspray; no sedatives or hypnotics should be administered beforehand, except as part of the EEG study; do not allow client to fast before study or to use stimulants like caffeinated drinks or coffee; clarify with provider if any routine medications are to be held; explain what the placement of the electrodes means.

Page 115: *Suggested Answer*—

- Ineffective Airway Clearance, Ineffective Breathing Pattern, Impaired Gas Exchange
- Impaired Physical Mobility
- Self-Care Deficit
- Imbalanced Nutrition: Less than Body Requirements
- Constipation, Diarrhea, Urinary Retention
- Risk for Infection
- Risk for Impaired Skin Integrity
- Impaired Verbal Communication (if tracheostomy)
- Pain
- Anxiety
- Powerlessness

Page 119: *Suggested Answer*—Assess the nature of the swallowing difficulty. Is the client having difficulty swallowing liquids and/or solids or chewing his food?

- Sit the client upright to eat and at least 30–45 minutes after eating.
- Observe the client swallow a sip of water; note coughing during and after eating.
- Observe as the client projects the tongue and moves it back and forth; refer to speech therapist for thorough evaluation; assist client to erect sitting position.
- Stay with the client while eating; cut food in small bites.
- Teach the client to think through the act of swallowing: close lips with teeth together, move the tongue up to the roof of the mouth with food on it; swallow with head bent forward.
- Try soft foods and thickened liquids.
- Massage client's face and neck muscles before eating.

Chapter 5

Page 139: *Suggested Answer*—The most effective way to increase joint mobility and maintain joint function is to participate in a regular exercise program and implement measures that decrease joint stress. The regular exercise program should be developed in collaboration with a physical therapist and include isometric exercises, PROM, and AROM. Some examples of measures that will decrease joint stress include pacing activities, performing activities when sitting if possible, using a splint for hands and wrists, and relaxation techniques. Water aerobics are significantly helpful, especially to elderly clients.

Page 140: *Suggested Answer*—To determine appropriate drug therapy in a client diagnosed with gouty arthritis it is important to know if elevated uric acid levels are related to increased production of uric acid or decreased excretion. A 24-hour urine specimen is collected to determine if the client is excreting normal levels of uric acid, 200–750 mL/24 hrs. A level that exceeds 750 mL/24 hrs indicates that production of uric acid is increased; levels below 200 mL/24 hrs indicate that excretion of uric acid is impaired.

Page 142: *Suggested Answer*—Bone deformities occur in Paget's disease as a result of excessive bone remodeling. Normal bone marrow is replaced with vascular, fibrous connective tissue and bones eventually enlarge. Often one of the first symptoms of Paget's disease is increased head size.

Page 145: *Suggested Answer*—The following factors differentiate these bone tumors; growth rate, age of onset, tissue origin, and location. All 3 bone tumors are classified as primary bone tumors: chondrosarcomas are characterized by slow growth; Ewing's sarcomas and osteosarcomas are characterized by rapid growth; Ewing's sarcomas metastasize to the lung tissue. Chondrosarcomas occur more frequently in adult males, the other 2 primary bone tumors occur more often in young males during periods of optimal growth, 10–25 years of age. The tissue of origin for osteosarcomas is the metaphysis of long bones and they are usually found in the distal femur, proximal tibia, and proximal humerus following an injury. The tissue of origin for chondrosarcomas is cartilage located in the pelvis, femur, and humerus. Ewing's sarcomas originate in the nerve tissue within the bone marrow, located in the pelvis, humerus, ribs, and femur.

Page 149: *Suggested Answer*—

Nursing diagnosis: Deficient Knowledge related to cast care

Goal: Client and significant other will care for cast correctly and report problems to health care provider for early intervention.

Interventions: Instruct client and caregiver on the following:

- Report increase in pain, decrease in movement, changes in color, coolness of fingers, loss of sensation, and/or increased swelling.
- Apply ice directly over fracture for first 24 hours.
- Elevate the cast on pillows and expose to air while drying.
- Check areas of skin at cast edges for skin breakdown, provide padding as needed.
- Do not place any objects in the cast; use a blow dryer on cool setting for itching.

- Report drainage or odor from cast.
- Wear a sling to support the arm.
- Keep cast dry; cover with a plastic bag during bathing.

Chapter 6

Page 162: *Suggested Answer*—Explain to the client that open-angle glaucoma is a treatable condition and that blindness is not an inevitable result. Careful physician monitoring of intraocular pressure along with strict adherence to the medical regimen (e.g., use of prescribed beta adrenergic eye drops, miotics, and/or carbonic anhydrase inhibitors) will preserve sight.

Page 163: *Suggested Answer*—Postoperative instructions should include the importance of strict compliance with the administration of prescribed eye drops, keeping the eye covered between administration of eye drops, the need to avoid bending over, and the importance of sleeping on the non-operative side.

Page 166: *Suggested Answer*—The macula is an area in the center of the retina that receives light from the center of the visual field. It is the center of greatest visual acuity. Degeneration of the macula occurs when the outer layer of the retina deteriorates or "fails" and waste products build up. These waste products cause death of retinal cells and loss of vision.

Page 167: *Suggested Answer*—Retinal detachment occurs when the retina (the inner layer of the eye) pulls away from the choroid (middle layer). The retina is the sensory part of the eye that is essential for sight. When it separates, damage and/or death occurs to the nerve cells and loss of vision occurs. Retinal detachment is a medical emergency and requires surgical correction. However, surgical procedures like scleral buckling along with photocoagulation can reattach the retina and preserve sight.

Page 171: *Suggested Answer*—The nurse should urge the mother to avoid allowing the child to lie down while drinking from a bottle since this position increases the risk of acute otitis media. In addition, the mother should be advised that exposure to tobacco smoke in the home poses risks for otitis media.

Page 178: *Suggested Answer*—The nurse should discuss with the client the availability of various types of speech generators as well as the possibility of learning esophageal speech. Surgical procedures to restore speech such as tracheoesophageal puncture (TEP) in conjunction with a prosthesis are also available.

Chapter 7

Page 187: *Suggested Answer*—Although the indigestion of GERD and that associated with a heart attack can feel very similar, angina usually feels like a tightness or heaviness, associated with shortness of breath, sweating, lightheadedness, and sometimes nausea. The discomfort of GERD will be centered more around mealtime with stress and other factors increasing the acidity in the stomach. Instruct the client not to let indigestion unrelieved by medicine continue without seeking medical attention.

Page 188: *Suggested Answer*—Prevention of a peptic ulcer includes caution in the use of nonsteroidal anti-inflammatory drugs (NSAIDs), including acetylsalicylic acid (aspirin); avoiding excessive physiologic and psychologic stress; and avoiding cigarettes and too much caffeine. Additional risk factors are a positive family history for ulcers as well as type O blood. Clients should always be aware of side effects of any over-the-counter (OTC) and prescription medications, which could cause ulcers also. High stress levels add to the risk as well as spicy, hot foods unless the client is already accustomed to them.

Page 192: *Suggested Answer*—Assessment criteria used for any client with possible dehydration are appropriate, including assessing for skin turgor and sunken eyeballs, dry skin, dry mucous membranes, dark amber urine with decreased output, and reports of thirst. Lab data would include a high hematocrit level, increased blood urea nitrogen (BUN), increased specific gravity of urine, hypernatremia, and hypokalemia.

Page 195: *Suggested Answer*—An unrelieved obstruction that is accompanied by such significant symptoms needs immediate attention. The condition could worsen with increased distention, change in level of consciousness, electrolyte imbalances, and increased pain, especially if the bowel ruptures or peritonitis occurs.

Page 196: *Suggested Answer*—The lack of fever and normal WBC would help in determining a diagnosis of appendicitis. Rebound tenderness should be checked and an IV started. Without any further symptoms and no rebound tenderness, the condition may be only a stomach virus and the IV fluids will cause improvement in the pain within 24 hours. Remember, however, if appendicitis is an appropriate diagnosis, sudden cessation of the pain could mean the appendix ruptured.

Chapter 8

Page 210: *Suggested Answer*—Determination of ascites can be made through objective observation of the size and contour of the abdomen, weight gain, firmness to the abdomen, taunt skin over the abdomen, distant, low-pitched bowel sounds, intake greater than output, and daily increase in abdominal girth. Subjectively, the client may report fullness or back pain. Lab data should include serum albumin, protein, electrolytes, and tests specific to the cause such as liver function tests for cirrhosis or hepatitis.

Page 211: *Suggested Answer*—In alcoholic (Laënnec's) cirrhosis, scarring of the liver occurs such as in biliary cirrhosis but there is also fat accumulation. Both of these (scarring and fat accumulation) cause a decrease in the function of the liver. The alcohol is transformed to acetaldehyde, which begins the process of altering hepatic function. The acetaldehyde inhibits the removal of proteins from the liver and alters metabolism of vitamins and minerals. Ammonia is unable to be metabolized, therefore a serum level is high (hence the odor). Failure of the liver to work properly can lead to a GI bleed. A client who has alcoholism often forfeits good meals for drinking either because of lack of appetite, lack of money (money spent on alcohol instead of food), or remaining in a stuporous state and failing to eat. Blood pressure (BP) elevates in the client because of portal hypertension and can often reach stroke range.

Page 213: *Suggested Answer*—Hepatitis A and E can be prevented by avoiding contaminated food and water, by avoiding situations in which one might come in contact with food handlers who do not use the necessary precautions. The client also should avoid contact with possibly contaminated shellfish. Hepatitis B, C, and D may be avoided by preventing contact with contaminated blood and body fluids. This includes needles, syringes, pooled blood, and unprotected sexual activity. A vaccine for hepatitis A and B is available for prophylaxis. Immunoglobulin may be given after exposure to hepatitis A, B, and D.

Page 215: *Suggested Answer*—Nursing diagnoses would include Pain, Imbalanced Nutrition: Less than Body Requirements, and Risk for Deficient Fluid Volume. If cholecystitis occurs and surgery is necessary, additional diagnoses would be Risk for Infection; Impaired Skin Integrity; and Risk for Impaired Gas Exchange. Nursing interventions would include keeping the client NPO, administering pain medication as needed, administering oral bile acids or dissolvers, monitoring lab work, assessing for pain, stool characteristics, GI complaints, and nutritional status. Teaching should be instituted when appropriate about eating less fat-containing foods and losing weight.

Page 218: *Suggested Answer*—Because these 3 diagnoses have similar elevated lab work, the nurse should be able to differentiate specific symptoms and lab work related to each.

Cholecystitis: A classic symptom is pain radiating to the back or right shoulder, intolerance to fat-containing foods, and fever. Remember, - *itis* signifies inflammation, and fever is usually present. Lab work specific for cholecystitis is elevated direct bilirubin and alkaline phosphatase with a normal serum amylase.

Pancreatitis: A classic symptom is fever and pain radiating to the back and is relieved by sitting up, leaning forward, flexing the left leg, or by walking. Classic lab findings are elevated amylase and lipase levels.

Cirrhosis: Pain is usually not present, but ascites are characteristic as are spider angiomas, palmar erythema, and hepatomegaly. Specific lab work indicating cirrhosis is elevated liver function tests (alanine aminotransferase [ALT], aspartate aminotransferase [AST], alkaline phosphatase, gamma-glutamyl transpeptidase [GGT]).

The symptoms of jaundice and clay-colored stools can be present in all 3 as well as an elevated bilirubin level.

Chapter 9

Page 234: *Suggested Answer*—Essential information to provide the client newly diagnosed with hypothyroidism includes the following:

- Take thyroid medications as prescribed; do not abruptly discontinue.
- Take medications 1 hour before or 2 hours after meals for optimal absorption.
- Monitor weight and report changes as instructed.
- Do not use iodized salt or drugs containing iodine.
- Avoid excessive intake of foods such as cabbage, turnips, spinach, and carrots because these foods inhibit the thyroid hormone (TH) utilization.
- Consume adequate fluids, at least 2,000 mL, or as prescribed.
- Consume a high-fiber diet to avoid constipation.
- Obtain adequate rest.
- Maintain skin integrity by proper care of dry skin.

Page 236: *Suggested Answer*—Because there is a high risk of damage to the parathyroid glands during a thyroidectomy, the client should be monitored for hypoparathyroidism. Manifestations are attributed to hypocalcemia and include tetany, muscle spasms, positive Chvostek's sign, positive Trousseau's sign, a decreased serum calcium level, and increased serum phosphorus level.

Page 239: *Suggested Answer*—Fluid volume excess is a complication of Cushing's disease as a result of excess cortisol which leads to sodium and water reabsorption. Interventions would include the following:

- Weigh client daily at the same time, using the same scale.
- Measure and record intake and output every 8 hours; compare with previous 72 hour totals to identify trends.
- Monitor heart rate, blood pressure, respirations, lung sounds.
- Assess for jugular vein distention and peripheral edema.
- Educate client about fluid restriction as prescribed.

Page 240: *Suggested Answer*—In Addison's disease, an insufficient amount of glucocorticoids and mineralocorticoids leads to fluid volume deficit, hyperkalemia, and hyponatremia. Instructions on nutritional management of Addison's disease would include the following:

- Consume a diet high in sodium and low in potassium; high-potassium foods to avoid include fruits, vegetables, chicken, liver, tuna, and turkey.
- Consume at least 3,000 mL of fluid daily, or as prescribed.
- Do not skip meals.
- Weigh self daily and report changes as instructed.

Page 243: *Suggested Answer*—Chronic diabetes insipidus will require lifelong replacement of antidiuretic hormone (ADH). Failure to replace the water loss can result in severe hypovolemia and hypernatremia. Instructions would include the following information:

- Treatment is lifelong.
- Take antidiuretic hormone as prescribed.
- Consume fluids as prescribed.
- Wear MedicAlert bracelet.
- Signs and symptoms of diabetes insipidus.

Chapter 10

Page 258: *Suggested Answer*—Obtain history of present illness: duration of symptoms, history of kidney stones, previous UTI, kidney or bladder disease; past history of diabetes, hypertension, allergies, pregnancy; last menstrual period, use of birth control methods, date of last sexual contact, history of new sex partner; assess recent medication use including antibiotics; family history of kidney disorders; inquire about diet: caffeine or carbonated drinks and water intake. Instructions should include the following: take medication as prescribed; explain indications of medications and side effects; increase water intake to at least 8 glasses of water per day; avoid food or beverages that contribute to urine acidity, which may promote bacterial growth; explain the importance of follow up urinalysis to assure resolution of infection; and teach women hygiene measures to prevent contamination or irritation.

Page 260: *Suggested Answer*—Teach the client factors that increase the risk of stone formation (male, Caucasian race, prior or family history, medications such as vitamins A, C, and D, antacids with calcium, gout) and what they can do to minimize this risk; emphasize increasing fluid intake and dietary restrictions (such as limiting foods high in vitamin D, purines, oxalate, acidic, and alkaline foods) to prevent further stone formation; teach the client about signs and symptoms of urinary tract infection; demonstrate how to strain all urine and save any stones for further analysis.

Page 261: *Suggested Answer*—Polycystic kidney disease is a hereditary disease and causes cysts to form in the kidney thereby causing the kidney to enlarge; these cysts may obstruct and ultimately destroy kidney tissue; common symptoms include flank pain, blood in the urine, infection, and stones.

Page 263: *Suggested Answer*—Glomerular filtration rate is the amount of fluid filtered from the blood into the capsule per minute; this rate is influenced by 3 factors: total surface area available for filtration, permeability of the filtration membrane, and the net filtration pressure; the normal GFR in both kidneys is 120–125 mL/min in adults; one advantage of a high GFR is that it allows the kidneys to rapidly filter waste products from the body and it allows the body fluid to be filtered and processed by the kidney many times a day;

glomerulonephritis causes a decreased GFR which leads to azotemia and activation of the RAA system; this in turn causes sodium and water retention and edema.

Page 268: *Suggested Answer*—Fluids are usually limited in CRF, especially if dialysis is being done; the more fluid consumed, the sooner dialysis will be needed and edema will be evident; the client should learn the amount of fluid allowed in a 24-hour period and how this should be distributed, accounting for medicine administration; provide an explanation that fluids are usually offered based on total allowance rather than randomly with each meal; explain that research has indicated that lowering protein in CRF slows disease progression and decreases common signs of uremia such as anorexia, nausea, and vomiting.

Chapter 11

Page 280: *Suggested Answer*—There is a familial tendency to develop hypospadias, but no gene has yet been identified. Therefore, the client's sons may, but the risk is less than 50%. Assurance should be given to the parents that if the son does have the condition, surgery can be performed to correct the situation.

Page 281: *Suggested Answer*—Nonsteroidal anti-inflammatory drugs (NSAIDs) should have been discontinued 10 days preoperatively. Additionally, clients with BPH should avoid taking OTC allergy medications, as they can induce urinary retention from spasm of the bladder sphincter.

Page 284: *Suggested Answer*—Testicles are comprised of tiny tubelike structures (seminal vesicles and vas deferens). If a lumpectomy were performed, any cancer present would escape into the tube systems and begin growing there, thus spreading the cancer. The inguinal route of surgery allows the testicle to be removed intact and prevent cancer seeding into the tissues surrounding the tumor.

Page 290: *Suggested Answer*—The first mammogram should be performed between the ages of 35 and 40, with yearly mammograms beginning at 40 according to the American Cancer Society's recommendations. She should have a mammogram now and yearly from this point on.

Page 292: *Suggested Answer*—Doxycycline is a tetracycline and therefore contraindicated during pregnancy (Pregnancy Category D drug). Tetracycline is known to cause discoloration of tooth enamel. A pregnancy test must be performed. If the client is pregnant, withhold the doxycycline and notify the provider of the client's pregnancy. Expect the provider to order a different medication such as azithromycin (Zithromax).

Chapter 12

Page 309: *Suggested Answer*—The nurse should know that allergies to dust, mold, grasses, pollens, and spores trigger a type I hypersensitivity response that is localized rather than systemic. Systemic type I hypersensitivity would lead to anaphylaxis. In a localized type I hypersensitivity, cell-bound IgE in the bronchial tree, nasal mucosa, and conjunctival tissues come in contact with the allergen and releases histamine and chemical mediators that produce the symptoms of asthma, rhinitis, and conjunctivitis. A good explanation for the mother is to inform her that small doses of the agent to which the child is allergic will be given in order to help the body develop antibodies. These antibodies will then build the immune system so that her child will react less or perhaps not at all when the allergen is introduced. Calm her fears about a severe reaction by explaining that the dose is usually diluted and will be slowly increased in strength to prevent major complications. Also inform her that the child will be monitored during the time immediately after receiving the injection for any complications.

Page 310: *Suggested Answer*—An autoimmune disease is when the body no longer recognizes self as self, but instead identifies and targets self as nonself. The basis of the immune system is that it has the ability to recognize self vs. nonself in order to target any foreign cell or particle. In essence, the body turns on itself in an autoimmune disease. In rejection of an organ tissue, the body recognizes the tissue as foreign and the immune system responds as it should to any foreign particle, rejecting its presence in the body. Although the desired outcome is for the body not to reject the tissue, the immune system is working correctly in this situation. Immunosuppressant drugs are given to stop the body from rejecting the donor organ tissue.

Page 310: *Suggested Answer*—The presence of antihistamines would prevent the test from producing true positive or negative results. When an allergen comes in contact with the individual, the response is for the immune system to release histamine and other chemicals (inflammatory symptoms). If an antihistamine is on board, the release of histamine will be blocked and a reaction may not occur.

Page 311: *Suggested Answer*—The mildest and most common symptoms would be dry, itchy, red rash on the back of the hands and fingers. Blistering and weeping may occur along with swelling. These symptoms constitute an irritant contact dermatitis. A true type I immediate hypersensitivity reaction would occur within 5 to 30 minutes and stop when the gloves were removed. Immediate itching and swelling of the fingers or hand occurs. The gloves should not be snapped because the latex can adhere to the particles of starch powder inside the gloves and inhalation of the powder aerosol may provoke symptoms also.

Page 312: *Suggested Answer*—Individuals exhibiting a true anaphylaxis are usually highly sensitive individuals and the reactions, which may be mild or severe, develop in minutes (almost instantaneous). Second, anaphylactic shock is always a potential concern for anyone exhibiting anaphylactic symptoms. The effects may involve the respiratory or cardiac system along with vasodilation and fluid loss from the vascular system.

Page 316: *Suggested Answer*—In a client who has been exposed to HIV, antibodies may not be produced for 6 weeks to 6 months after the initial infection (known as seroconversion). The ELISA test identifies HIV antibodies. Therefore, depending on the timing of infection and antibody production, an ELISA may return negative initially but return positive later on. Hence, a second ELISA is often conducted to confirm a suspicion of positive HIV results. To actually confirm the diagnosis of positive HIV, a Western blot antibody test, which is more reliable than ELISA, is conducted once a positive ELISA has been obtained.

Chapter 13

Page 326: *Suggested Answer*—Clients with immune deficiency disorders, clients receiving chemotherapy, or clients receiving long-term corticosteroid therapy are often those who contract opportunistic infections. In all of these states, the immune system, which normally defends against pathogens, is suppressed and unable to perform normally.

Page 331: *Suggested Answer*—Some viruses enter the host cell and insert their genome into the chromosome of the host, remaining in a latent, nonreplicative state for long periods of time. A virus can remain communicable during recurrence. Stress increases the recurrence of latent or recurrent viruses. The lack of symptoms may be problematic in that the client is contagious and does not know it. Also, a virus can recur and be more virulent than the first time, without a cure.

Page 332: *Suggested Answer*—Bacteria may be described as cocci (spherical), bacilli (rod-shaped), clavate (club-shaped), or spirochetal (corkscrew-shaped). Staining characteristics include Gram-positive or Gram-negative characteristics. Typically, Gram-negative organisms are more virulent. Bacteria may also be classified as aerobic (requiring oxygen) or anaerobic (not needing oxygen).

Page 336: *Suggested Answer*—Corticosteroids are immunosuppressants and therefore enhance growth of fungal skin infections. A fungal infection as well as tuberculosis will be exacerbated if a corticosteroid is used.

Page 341: *Suggested Answer*—Intestinal obstruction can occur with helminth infestation and can be a life-threatening event. The organisms may also affect other organs: cestodes (brain), nematodes (alveoli), and trematodes (blood vessels, intestines, liver, or lungs).

Chapter 14

Page 353: *Suggested Answer*—Sunburn is a minor burn injury of the superficial layer of the skin. Sporadic, intense sunburns are more damaging to the skin than everyday exposure with use of a sunscreen. Use of sunscreens and limiting sun exposure to the less hazardous hours of the day (before 10:00 a.m. and after 3:00 p.m.) can prevent sunburn. Recurrent sunburn can lead to other skin disorders such as early skin aging, seborrheic keratosis, basal and squamous cell carcinoma, and malignant melanoma.

Page 356: *Suggested Answer*—Instruct the client to wash the skin with a mild soap and water at least twice a day to remove accumulated oils. Eat a regular, well-balanced diet. Exposing the skin to sun may help but sunburns should be avoided; get regular exercise and sleep. Do not squeeze the pimple; this causes the material to go deeper into the skin and usually the pimple gets larger and infected. The client should be instructed to be patient because treatment for acne can take months for a noticeable difference.

Page 357: *Suggested Answer*—Stress the importance of good nutrition and cleanliness through good handwashing and proper disposal of dressings. Teach the client never to squeeze or try to open the infected area. Teach the client signs and symptoms that should be reported to a health care provider such as fever, swelling, redness, pain, and drainage. Teach the importance of taking the full course of medication that has been prescribed.

Page 360: *Suggested Answer*—HSV 2 is a herpes simplex virus that usually involves the genitalia and skin below the waist in sexually active individuals. Explain the natural history of the disease with emphasis on recurrent episodes, asymptomatic viral shedding, and sexual transmission. Antiviral therapy can be used on an episodic basis or as suppressive therapy. Stress the importance of use of condoms during sexual intercourse, but the need to abstain from all sexual activity when lesions or prodromal symptoms are present.

Page 361: *Suggested Answer*—Do not share linens; use a clean towel and washcloth daily. Carefully dry between the toes. Do not wear the same pair of shoes every day, and avoid wearing rubber or plastic-soled shoes. Wear cotton socks that are changed frequently. Educate on the use of talcum powder and that over-the-counter fungal powder/spray should be used twice daily or prescribed medication for at least 2 weeks even though the symptoms have disappeared. Inquire if others in the family have the same symptoms. Educate on cleaning bathing surfaces after each bath/shower.

Chapter 15

Page 380: *Suggested Answer*—Since the client is in his nadir period, he is experiencing pancytopenia with all of his blood counts being affected. He is at high risk for infection and will require education on a neutropenic diet, limiting exposure to others, taking his temperature orally every 4 hours, and the importance of hand hygiene, especially washing hands after toileting. The client is also at risk for hemorrhage, secondary to a low platelet count. The client should be educated to avoid aspirin and aspirin-containing products, avoid straining to have a bowel movement, and use electric razors while shaving. He can expect frequent lab work, transfusions with red cells and platelets, as well as possible antibiotic and antifungal administration.

Page 382: *Suggested Answer*—Both Hodgkin's and non-Hodgkin's arise from the lymph nodes and then disseminate throughout the body. Hodgkin's disease usually affects younger people, while non-Hodgkin's lymphoma occurs in the middle to later years. The causative etiology for both is unknown; however, chemical exposure may be a causative agent. Hodgkin's disease is classified by the presence of Reed-Sternberg cells, which don't occur in non-Hodgkin's lymphoma. Both clients are diagnosed by lymph node biopsy. Depending on bone marrow invasion, both clients are at risk for infection and bleeding. Depending on the stage of the disease, the client may need surgery only, surgery and radiation, therapy, or surgery, radiation, and chemotherapy. The chemotherapeutic protocols are unique for each of the diagnoses.

Page 383: *Suggested Answer*—With bone involvement the client is at risk for developing hypercalcemia. The family should learn the importance of maintaining mobility and to ensure the client ambulates with assistance due to her increased risk for falling. The role of hydration also needs to be emphasized, and the family needs to know the importance of an intake and output record. The family should understand the signs and symptoms of hypercalcemia, and the importance of reporting these to the client's provider. Finally, the family should be educated on the administration of long-acting morphine and the importance of administering it on a specific schedule to avoid breakthrough pain.

Page 385: *Suggested Answer*—Both platelets and factor VIII play an important role in clot formation; therefore, the client with a decreased platelet count is just as susceptible to hemorrhage as the client with a factor VIII deficiency. The client with thrombocytopenia is at greater risk for spontaneous hemorrhage, and the problem is usually treated with platelet transfusions, except in idiopathic thrombocytopenia purpura (ITP), when the treatment of choice is steroid therapy. The client with factor VIII deficiency usually receives scheduled factor VIII infusions and is at greater risk of bleeding into the joints. Both clients need to be educated on bleeding and safety precautions.

Page 388: *Suggested Answer*—Both pernicious anemia and folic acid deficiency are macrocytic (megaloblastic) anemia. Pernicious anemia is caused by a deficiency in vitamin B_{12}, usually caused by a lack of intrinsic factor, while folic acid deficiency is caused by a deficiency of folic acid. Both present with a smooth, sore, beefy, red tongue, while pernicious anemia presents with paresthesias, which distinguishes it from folic acid deficiency.

Page 389: *Suggested Answer*—The nurse should educate the client and his parents about the importance of adequate hydration during their vacation since dehydration will increase intravenous viscosity, triggering a crisis. The client should also be encouraged to take rest breaks while at any water or amusement parks, since extreme body heat and excessive exercise can trigger an event. Since high altitude can trigger a sickling episode, the nurse should discuss the feasibility of using ground transportation to get to the vacation destination.

Chapter 16

Page 401: *Suggested Answer*—The pedigree can demonstrate the risk for congenital defects in future offspring. The pedigree can also establish patterns of inheritance and what diseases the family is prone to develop.

Page 403: *Suggested Answer*—The child with Down syndrome is following the same pattern of development as peers of a similar age, but at a slower pace. The family needs anticipatory guidance as the child nears each phase of development. Erickson's stages of development can still be identified and need the same attention. Helping the client deal with social concerns as well as sexual questions should consist of fair treatment.

Page 403: *Suggested Answer*—There are 3 known types of chromosome 21 abnormalities; nondisjunction, translocation, and mosaicism. Translocation has a 5–15% chance of reoccurrence and should be considered in future family planning. Prevention of another child with trisomy 21 may be an option.

Page 404: *Suggested Answer*—The adolescent with Turner syndrome has no development of secondary sex characteristics and growth is below standard level. Because these clinical manifestations don't occur until adolescence, the diagnosis and treatment may be delayed.

Page 405: *Suggested Answer*—Nondisjunction is an abnormal separation during meiosis. This can lead to interference with fetal development. In nondisjunction, one zygote receives too many alleles and the other too few. Examples are trisomy 21, monosomy in Turner syndrome, and Klinefelter syndrome (which can be trisomy or multiple additions of X and possibly Y). In particular, Klinefelter syndrome is an X-linked defect with one or more extra X chromosomes in a genotype; e.g., XXY, XXXY.

Page 406: *Suggested Answer*—Refer to Figure 16-2 (p. 000) for autosomal recessive patterns. The risk of having children with PKU is 1:4, 2:4 risk of being carriers, and 1:4 risk being normal.

Page 408: *Suggested Answer*—At present there is no cure for Huntington disease and no predictor of when symptoms will begin. If a client knows he or she has a disease, but no control over when and how it will develop, it can be an overwhelming piece of information. Yet a client has the right in family planning to know what might potentially be passed along to his or her children.

Page 413: *Suggested Answer*—The newborn with biuvula has a cleft palate that could possibly go undetected. The child with a cleft needs to be referred for treatment and prevent complications such as otitis media, aspiration, and speech impairment. Sometimes the biuvula is the only obvious physical characteristic.

Chapter 17

Page 429: *Suggested Answer*—In the absence of illness or injury, a woman in the childbearing years would have the predisposing risk factor of utilizing tampons for menstruation. A thorough assessment of recent menstruation and sanitary product utilization would be indicated. The concern for toxic shock syndrome is high in light of her age.

Page 432: *Suggested Answer*—Arterial blood gases (ABGs) are the most accurate measure of progressing shock. All forms of shock are a syndrome that result in inadequate perfusion and oxygenation of tissues. As shock progresses, anaerobic respiration replaces aerobic. Lactic acid production builds, causing metabolic acidosis. ABGs measure the pH of the blood. Other tests that may be ordered are creatinine phospholinase (CPK) and isoenzymes and troponin level, but these determine heart damage, not shock.

Page 434: *Suggested Answer*—A broad-spectrum antibiotic is usually begun initially as soon as the diagnosis is made. A narrow-spectrum antibiotic cannot be initiated until the culture and sensitivity returns, which then confirms the actual diagnosis. It is imperative to collect all cultures prior to the start of any antibiotic. Failure to collect all specimens can and most likely will result in improper treatment or incorrect diagnosis.

Page 440: *Suggested Answer*—An open hemothorax is suspected. A bullet wound provides an opening to the outside atmosphere so the development of a tension pneumothorax is possible. A tension pneumothorax is a life-threatening medical emergency. Bleeding within the pleural space could provide a significant source of hemorrhage so the shock state is hypovolemic in nature.

Page 442: *Suggested Answer*—Swelling from edema and bleeding may create a tourniquet-like effect, creating compartment syndrome. The nurse should assess circulation to the lower arm: pulses, capillary refill, color of extremities, and have client rank his or her pain. The physician should be notified immediately so that the casts can be removed or the client may need surgery.

Page 443: *Suggested Answer*—Necessary staff should be summoned including additional nursing support, as well as respiratory and radiology personnel. In a smaller institution or one that has on-call personnel, a representative from neurology and perhaps radiology should be made available. Resuscitative equipment should be ready including airway management equipment; an intravenous line should be primed and ready to infuse; cardiac monitor readied; suction available; a catheterization tray on hand; and typical wound care supplies available. Although most trauma rooms will be stocked with these supplies, a quick survey decreases time once the client arrives.

Page 444: *Suggested Answer*—A D-dimer test is indicated for a differential diagnosis. This test measures fibrin fragments, which elevate during clot breakdown. A steady increase in these values indicates ongoing clot breakdown rather than a lack of clotting factors.

Page 444: *Suggested Answer*—ARDS often occurs suddenly and is extremely fatiguing for the client. A client already stressed because of an acute MI doesn't need the additional respiratory stress, nor can the body tolerate extreme respiratory difficulty for long periods. Insufficient oxygenation coupled with a heart that has impaired circulation could be fatal. Treatment should be quick in order to prevent further complications.

➤ *Case Study Suggested Answers*

Chapter 1

1. Give the mother an explanation about the action of each drug and any specific side effects. Montelukast (Singulair) carries few side effects, headaches being the most common. Stress that this medication should be taken every day, regardless of the event of an asthma attack. Explain the difference between the maintenance inhaler nedocromil (Tilade) and the rescue inhaler albuterol (Ventolin). Be sure the mother understands that the maintenance drug is given every day and the albuterol is a rescue inhaler that is given only if an attack occurs and should be used immediately. If the attack does not stop within 30–60 minutes, the albuterol drops plus saline can be used via nebulization. Specific instructions on using a nebulizer and mixing the saline with albuterol should be given to the mother before discharge. The rescue inhaler as well as the nebulizer can cause extreme nervousness in clients. Provide explanations about how to use the inhaler (complete exhalation; administering the correct number of puffs while inhaling to the count of 10), correctly cleaning the mouthpiece, and checking for fullness of the canister.

2. Explain that asthma is an inflammation of the airways that leads to constriction (or closing) of the bronchi, but this constriction is reversible with medications. The closing of the bronchi causes clients to feel like they cannot get enough air, which can be very frightening. The wheezing that can be heard when these clients breathe is also due to the closing of the bronchi; the air is trying to pass through a smaller opening than usual.

3. Usually the provider will give specific instructions on when to seek medical attention. However, standard protocol is to seek treatment when first the rescue inhaler and then the nebulizer have been used without any results. If the provider allows more than one nebulizer treatment, encourage the mother to give the allowed number of treatments before seeking immediate attention; explain that some attacks may take longer to stop than others. However, any time the child is having more frequent or more severe attacks, a provider should examine the child. Also, if attacks are occurring right after another or an attack is prolonged (status asthmaticus), immediate attention is necessary.

4. The child should be given a brief explanation of what asthma is in terms he or she can understand. If the child is extremely anxious during an attack, assurance should be given that he or she will always be able to breathe, but may not be able to get a good, deep breath. Address the child's fears and allow the child to voice his or her concerns. Explain that the higher the anxiety level, the more difficult it is to breathe.

5. Triggers are stimuli that produce the initial inflammatory response that proceeds to the asthma attack, causing mucosal edema, mucous secretion, and inflammation of the airways. Triggers cause the bronchospasm and can be specific allergies (mold, dust, pollen, etc.) or such things as cold air, strong odors, high altitude, intense exercise, and emotional stress. An individual may also find other unusual triggers that are not common to all people with asthma.

Chapter 2

1. Begin by assessing the ABCs—airway, breathing, and circulation. He has an open airway and is breathing adequately. Assess circulation by checking pulse (apical and radial) and blood pressure and placing client on the monitor to assess heart rhythm. Assess the level of pain on a pain scale of 1 to 10, with 10 being the worst pain. Assess the duration and location of the pain (does it radiate?) and have the client describe the pain in his own words. Listen to his heart sounds; note any abnormal sounds such as murmur, friction rub, or S_3 or S_4 gallops. Assess his skin color and temperature; note capillary refill (should be less than 3 seconds). Listen to his lung fields anteriorly and posteriorly for crackles, rhonchi, or wheezes. Note any labored respirations or use of accessory muscles and ask whether he feels short of breath. Assess his abdomen and extremities for signs of swelling. Assess distal pulses.

2. The nurse would ask if he has had prior history of cardiac disease or episodes of angina, any previous heart attack, or history of coronary heart disease. Does he have a history of hypertension, hypercholesterolemia, or hyperlipidemia? The nurse needs to assess if he has a strong family history of cardiac problems. Is he diabetic? Has he ever had previous ECGs done and where? Who is his family doctor and does he have a cardiologist?

3. Laboratory data would include troponin, CK-MB, CBC with differential, complete chemistries (electrolytes, glucose, BUN/Cr, liver functions), PT and PTT, as well as a chest x-ray and 12-lead ECG at bedside. If necessary, ABGs or continuous pulse oximetry may be ordered.

4. Possible medications ordered include nitroglycerin (Nitrostat, NTG) sublingual 0.4 mg or nitroglycerin IV drip, titrated to pain and/or systolic blood pressure of 100 mmHg; nitroglycerin paste (Nitro-Dur) 1 or 2 inches to chest wall; acetylsalicylic acid (aspirin) as an antiplatelet drug to prevent clots; and morphine sulfate

2 to 5 mg IV push if nitroglycerin is not effective in relieving chest pain or if BP is too low. After the initial chest pains are relieved, a beta blocker, nitrate, and/or calcium channel blocker would probably be ordered.

5. The nurse should look for inverted T waves and depressed S–T segments as a sign of ischemia; elevated S–T segments as a sign of injury; Q waves in 2 contiguous leads as a sign of infarct of undetermined age; tachycardia that may be present because of the effects of pain and anxiety; any abnormal rhythm or ectopic beats such as PVCs as a sign of irritability.

Chapter 3

1. Since the client has had several colds, the provider should assess what medications, both prescription and over the counter (OTC), the client took during these periods of illness and whether they are still being used. Many OTC products can cause an increase in blood pressure (BP). Second, data should be collected on whether the client has ever had a sudden increase in BP before; if so, what was the reason (if known), and what was done about it? It is always suggested to verify that the client is indeed compliant with medicine administration and diet. It would be helpful to know if a family member has been visiting the health care provider with the client in order to relay accurate information. Last, verify that the instructions about correct dose and time of administration are being followed by the client.

2. The family and client should be counseled on what is meant by a high BP value and the possible complications (stroke, death, etc.). If medications are not being taken correctly, educate on each medication—what it is for, how much should be taken, and setting up a dosing schedule that meets the needs of the client. Explain what side effects can occur and the consequences of skipping a dose. If diet is a concern, educate the client on low-sodium foods and the relationship of sodium to BP. Using the readings from the Council on Aging, establish a normal BP range that is safe for the client. Be sure the family knows how to monitor the BP as well as when to report to a provider.

3. Essential information includes drug name, dosage, and time for administration, need to assess pulse and/or blood pressure prior to taking the medication, reason for taking the medication, and side effects that need to be reported to the provider. Report any chest pain or problems with respirations. Some medications require the client to move slowly when changing positions to avoid lightheadedness. Emphasis should be placed on not "making up" a missed medication; rather wait until the next time the medicine is due to take the dose prescribed unless instructed otherwise. Parameters for low pulse and BP reading should be provided as well.

4. Priority of care is decreasing the BP to a range acceptable for the client. Once this is established, priorities include:

- Teaching the client and family about the medication regime
- Awareness of the possibility of compliance issues
- Assisting the client in maintaining compliance through clear instructions; make accommodations for clients with poor eyesight and those who are unable to read or speak English
- Implementing the plan to form a partnership with the client, the significant others, and the health team for support, information, and care

5. Essential hypertension is usually from an unknown cause and is also termed primary hypertension. It occurs in a majority of hypertensive clients (about 95%). Secondary hypertension is usually related to a disease process and is often easier to control because control of the disease will often regulate the BP. It is important to understand that in essential hypertension the left ventricle (the power chamber of the heart) must work harder to overcome the resistance it encounters when blood is pumped out. When the ventricle must continuously work hard, the muscle will hypertrophy (or stiffen); this can cause heart problems later on. When the heart is unable to adjust to the hypertension, the kidneys become involved in an effort to regulate the pressure. One of the serious concerns is that there are rarely obvious symptoms, and often there are no symptoms at all. A headache or nosebleed may occur when the pressure rises extremely high.

Chapter 4

1. Anticipated signs and symptoms of Parkinson's disease include resting tremors, stooped posture, masklike face, soft monotone voice, drooling, poor balance, shuffling propulsive gait, rigidity, insomnia, weight loss, constipation, depression, and dementia. In addition, the client might be withdrawn, uncooperative, and noncompliant because of his reluctance to be at the facility.

2. A priority nursing diagnosis for the client is Impaired Physical Mobility, as well as Risk for Injury. The client with Parkinson's disease has difficulty initiating ambulation, is unsteady, and often has difficulty stopping and righting himself if he begins to fall. Safety should be a primary goal in the care of this client. Other diagnoses would include Self-Care Deficit, Imbalanced Nutrition: Less than Body Requirements, Risk for Constipation, Noncompliance, Interrupted Thought Processes, Hopelessness, and Powerlessness.

3. It would be best to schedule physical therapy to coincide with peak drug action. Planned rest periods should be a part of the client's daily routine to allow him to prevent fatigue and frustration during physical therapy. An explanation should be given about the importance of physical therapy.

4. A good approach to handling the client with Parkinson's disease who has become upset would be to:

- Acknowledge to him that you recognize he is frustrated and upset.
- State that you are sorry if it seemed you were trying to rush him.
- Encourage and praise him for his efforts to maintain independence. Stress that you recognize it is important for him.
- Allow him as much time as he needs to dress.

5. Some specific instructions to assist with mobility problems are:
   - Daily exercise to maintain function: walking, swimming, and stretching
   - Stretching and posture exercises as suggested by physical therapy
   - Take big steps and lift legs
   - Think about stepping over an object for episodes of "freezing"

Chapter 5

1. Emergency nursing care for the client with a fracture includes:
   - Immobilizing the fracture: Anything sturdy can be used to immobilize the fractured area; belts can be used to secure the fracture to the hard surface. The extremity or limb should be placed in the same position on the area where it is to be immobilized.
   - Controlling any bleeding: Pressure should be held to control bleeding. If clean linens are available, these can be applied to the area. Firm pressure should be held constantly if an artery has been severed.
   - Cleaning the wound if there is an open fracture: Open fractures should be cleaned if possible and a moist, clean towel applied to keep the bone from drying.

2. The nurse should assess the 6 Ps: pain, paresthesia, pulses, pallor, polar, and paralysis; elevate the extremity and apply ice during the first 24 hours; keep the cast open to air and supported on pillow to allow for drying; assess for signs and symptoms of compartment syndrome during the first 48 hours.

3. Provide instructions to client and caregivers regarding cast care and complications to report.
   - Report increase in pain, decrease in movement, changes in color, coolness of fingers, loss of sensation, and/or increased swelling.
   - Apply ice directly over fracture for first 24 hours.
   - Elevate the cast on pillows and expose to air while drying.
   - Check areas of skin at cast edges for skin breakdown, provide padding as needed.
   - Do not place any objects in the cast; use a blow dryer on cool setting for itching.
   - Report drainage or odor from cast.
   - Wear a sling to support the arm.
   - Keep cast dry; cover with a plastic bag during bathing.

- Instruct the client to expect pain, especially during the first 24–48 hours. The client should also be instructed to use pain medicine at the first sign of pain and avoid waiting since this makes pain control more difficult.

4. Compartment syndrome is usually the reason for excruciating pain after 48 hours. Even with a crushing fracture, pain will begin to decrease within 48 hours if a cast has been applied and the area is immobilized. Swelling and pressure account for the excruciating pain and should be relieved immediately.

5. Notify the physician immediately. The cast will need to be removed to assess the limb. Then elevate the extremity and apply ice to relieve the edema. Next, assist with bivalving the cast or prepare client for fasciotomy as indicated. Usually, the relief of the edema and pressure relieves the pain. If not, analgesics should be administered. Remember to obtain a surgical permit before medication is administered in the event of surgery. An explanation of the problem should be given to the client and family, especially if pain medicine is being held.

Chapter 6

1. Assessment findings in acute Ménière's disease include the symptoms outlined in the case study as well as hypotension, diaphoresis, and nystagmus. The vertigo may be so severe that the client becomes immobilized and may even fall to the floor.

2. Medical interventions for acute attacks may include the use of anticholinergics (e.g., scopolamine [Isopto Hyoscine], atropine [Isopto Atropine]), antiemetics (e.g., prochlorperazine [Compazine], meclizine [Antivert]), and central nervous system (CNS) depressants (e.g., diazepam [Valium]) to control the nausea, vomiting, and symptoms of motion sickness. Bed rest should be initiated as well as fluid and electrolyte replacement if necessary.

3. Diagnostic tests include audiometry, x-rays, and computed tomography (CT) scans of the vestibule, and an electronystagmography (ENG) test battery including caloric ice water testing. In addition, an auditory dehydration test that uses glycerine or fast-acting diuretics to dehydrate the inner ear is often used. Acute, temporary improvement in symptoms following this test is considered diagnostic of Ménière's disease.

4. Ménière's disease is a chronic disorder of the inner ear that presents with 3 major symptoms: dizziness (vertigo), ringing in the ears (tinnitus), and hearing loss. The cause of the disorder is unknown and usually affects only one ear. The symptoms appear to be caused by the accumulation of fluid in a part of the inner ear known as the membranous labyrinth. Factors that cause acute symptoms include increased sodium intake, stress, allergies, and premenstrual fluid retention.

5. Discharge instructions for clients with Ménière's disease should include:
   - The signs of impending attacks (e.g., feeling of fullness in the ear, increasing tinnitus, dizziness, nausea, and/or vomiting)
   - Avoidance of attack triggers (e.g., stress, fatigue, blinking lights, loud noises, and/or quick or jerky body movements)
   - The need for adequate rest and sleep as well as relaxation techniques
   - Safety measures to utilize if attacks occur while driving
   - Sodium-restricted diets
   - The avoidance of substances causing vasoconstriction (e.g.., tobacco, alcohol, and caffeine)

Chapter 7

1. Questions would include the following:
   - What caused you to come to the health facility?
   - Have you been vomiting? What other symptoms have you had? When did these start?
   - How many bowel movements do you usually have a day?
   - Have you had this problem before?
   - What are your usual dietary habits?
   - How much weight have you lost? Over what period of time?
   - Are you able to care for yourself?
   - Have you noticed blood or mucus in your bowel movements?
2. Objective data should include observation of color, consistency, and character of stools; level of pain; relationship between diarrhea and mealtime; abdominal palpation to determine areas of tenderness; check for rebound tenderness as an indication of peritonitis or appendicitis; monitor hemoglobin, hematocrit, WBC, serum Na, K, and Cl.
3. Social history information that would assist in her plan of care would be identification of job or family stress; use of cigarettes or alcohol; and presence of family or support systems. Stress factors have been known to aggravate the exacerbation of symptoms. Cigarettes and alcohol also are aggravating symptoms. The client will need to depend on family and/or social support systems as a part of her adjustment to home care.
4. Nursing measures would include administering antidiarrheal medications as ordered, teaching good skin care, monitoring and encouraging fluid intake, being sure the client has easy access to the bedpan or bathroom, supplying room deodorizers as necessary, and weighing the client daily.
5. Other nursing measures include administering corticosteroids or immunosuppressants as prescribed, implementing a low-fiber diet, promoting rest, using antianxiety measures (planned rest periods, decreasing excess stimuli if pain medicine is administered, allowing

privacy if diarrhea occurs), and preparing for surgery if indicated. In addition, explain the disorder, complications that can occur and prevention techniques, type of medications used and possible side effects, and how to lower stress.

Chapter 8

1. The risk factors present for pancreatic cancer in this client are age and cigarette smoking. Other risk factors include industrial chemicals, environmental toxin exposure, high-fat diet, pancreatitis, and diabetes mellitus.
2. The likely location of the pancreatic tumor based upon the symptoms of pain when supine, jaundice, and weight loss, is the body of the pancreas. The jaundice could be significant of cancer of the head of the pancreas, but the pain when supine does not correlate. There are usually no symptoms if the cancer is in the tail of the pancreas.
3. The primary preoperative nursing interventions are:
   - Evaluate physical and psychological status. Create a collaborative care plan, which includes physical, psychological, and spiritual interventions.
   - Determine client's acuity level.
   - Provide a teaching plan for client and family for postoperative care.
   - Explain that client may be cared for in the intensive care unit for a period of time.
   - Provide comfort measures through proper positioning and administration of pain medication as needed.
   - Monitor and maintain nausea and vomiting.
   - Assess lab work as ordered.
4. The primary postoperative nursing interventions are:
   - Monitor respiratory status.
   - Monitor renal output.
   - Monitor cardiac status.
   - Prevent wound infections.
   - Maintain patency of the gastric suction.
   - Administer pain medications at regular intervals.
   - Monitor blood chemistries.
   - Watch for complications of hemorrhage, hypovolemic shock, and hepatorenal failure.
5. The prognosis for this client is poor—nearly all pancreatic cancer is fatal within the first year; 85% of cases are not diagnosed until too late because symptoms are nonspecific and onset is slow. Although this type of cancer is rare (3–4% of the cancers in United States), it is more likely to occur in adults 50–70 years of age.

Chapter 9

1. Diabetes mellitus at a young age occurs when pancreatic beta cells are destroyed and cannot secrete insulin properly to control glucose (sugar). The glucose builds up in the bloodstream; this is called hyperglycemia. Normally, a certain amount of glucose is produced by the beta cells, then the body uses what glucose it needs

and stores what it does not. With diabetes, the increased level of glucose spills into the urine. Glucose acts to draw fluid with it, resulting in increased urination and thirst. A third problem is hunger. The body needs insulin to use carbohydrates (CHOs) for energy. When the body cannot use CHOs, it uses protein and fat, which causes the hungry feeling and results in weight loss.

2. The most important symptoms are the 3 Ps (polyphagia, polyuria, polydipsia), the signs of hypoglycemia (nervousness, weakness, faint feeling, and possible coma), and the signs and symptoms of diabetic ketoacidosis (fruity breath, a change in respirations, extreme fatigue, nausea, and vomiting).

3. Although type 1 DM is often familial, it is considered an autoimmune disease and may occur without any family history. Explain what an autoimmune disease is and that diabetes at age 16 may be from genetics, environmental, or immunological factors. Calm the mother by including her in the teaching sessions and allowing her to ask questions and share concerns.

4. Explain what peak time means and what the time is for each type of insulin. Explain that the most likely time for a hypoglycemic reaction is 2–4 hours after taking regular insulin and 6–8 hours after taking NPH insulin. Be sure she understands that she has to consider both peak times if the medications are mixed in the morning.

5. The client will most likely experience symptoms of hyperglycemia. The goal of maintaining her glucose values within a normal range should be emphasized, especially since adolescents do not always eat healthy foods. Without frightening her, stress the long-term consequences of DM. At the same time, factors that affect her glucose level, such as exercise, over- or undereating, and stress, could cause her glucose to drop and therefore she should know the symptoms of hypoglycemia. Instructions should be given to her about taking candy, fruit, or a regular cola if her glucose level does drop, especially during school hours.

Chapter 10

1. L. J. is experiencing metabolic acidosis, which is common in ARF. Hydrogen ions, which are high in acidosis, are unable to be eliminated along with other metabolic wastes. Remember, if the pH is low, H^+ ions are high. The pH and bicarbonate are both low and the carbon dioxide is normal, which indicates metabolic acidosis.

2. The hyperkalemia could cause cardiac dysrhythmias. The normal potassium level is 3.5 to 5.0 mEq/L and the heart does not tolerate values too low or too high.

3. L. J. is in the maintenance phase of ARF. Most of the signs and symptoms presented by L. J. are typical of this phase. The initial phase has very few manifestations and hopefully the recovery phase shows renal improvement. This phase should last from 1 to 2 weeks.

4. L. J. could possibly experience CHF or pulmonary edema. The edema, crackles, and low urine output are

suggestive of these disorders. The strain placed on the heart by the ARF episode could also trigger a cardiovascular event.

5. The diet should not be high in sodium because of the retention of fluid being experienced by the client. The low sodium is of least concern in his present state. Sodium supplements may be used to exchange potassium, thereby increasing sodium and lowering potassium levels. The main dietary restriction is protein and high carbohydrates should be given to accommodate for the low proteins.

Chapter 11

1. General anesthesia is usually used. A low abdominal incision is made. The prostate is resected and lymph nodes are also obtained. If it appears that the prostate capsule has been invaded with cancer, additional tissue around the prostate may be removed. Postoperative pain medication is provided. An indwelling urinary catheter will be in place.

2. The pathology report of the tissue removed (the prostate gland, surrounding tissue if taken, and lymph nodes) reveals the extent of the disease. Additional scans may also be utilized to stage the disease.

3. Prostate cancer in older adults is a very slow-growing cancer, and conservative treatment is utilized because of the expectation that the client's eventual demise will result from a cause other than the prostate cancer. The younger the client is at diagnosis, the more likely it is that the cancer is an aggressive form that will require more aggressive treatment. Another factor in determining what type of anesthesia to use is based on the surgical procedure and the age of the client.

4. Radiation therapy and chemotherapy will most likely be required after the surgery.

5. Stage 3 prostate cancer indicates that the cancer is outside the capsule of the prostate and may also be in the seminal vesicles. It has not spread to the lymph nodes or other organs.

Chapter 12

1. Immediate assessment should focus on airway patency (respiratory rate, depth, lung sounds, any dyspnea or stridor). The client is exhibiting initial signs of possible anaphylaxis (type I hypersensitivity reaction). Although his blood pressure (BP) is within normal limits (WNL), it is on the lower side and with tachycardia, the nurse should be proactive at this time. The welts definitely indicate a localized reaction, and his anxiety may or may not be related to anaphylaxis. If the airway is not patent, oxygen should be administered and an oropharyngeal or nasopharyngeal airway instituted immediately.

2. The nurse should first determine what the client's normal BP range is and then identify how he reacted to

bee stings in the past for comparison. If the client runs a much higher BP than this, the nurse may be concerned that hypotension is developing. Individuals allergic to a specific insect often react similarly when bitten or stung by other insects. This reaction may be typical for this client when venom is injected. If this response is exaggerated, the nurse should again be proactive and monitor the client closely. The reaction may be caused by the multiple stings of the hornets.

3. Drug therapy would involve topical and oral antihistamines and possibly corticosteroids. Epinephrine should be on hand for administration if airway management or severe edema presents.

4. The wife should be informed that her husband apparently has a type I hypersensitivity reaction to insect bites and stings (if he has presented with similar symptoms to bees) and that he probably always will respond in this fashion. Explain that each subsequent episode may be more exaggerated because the body has become sensitized to the allergen. Emphasize that the massive amount of welts is probably caused by the number of hornet stings, as hornets swarm and attack in large numbers. Calm the wife by explaining that the antihistamines will help with his symptoms and that he may be sleepy because of the antihistamines.

5. This client needs to be instructed on the following:
   - Have a "bee sting kit" available at all times, which includes a prefilled syringe of epinephrine (Epi-pen). The wife should be taught how to administer the Epi-pen. If the kit contains an inhaler, teach her on the use of the inhaler also.
   - Have antihistamine lotion and tablets available.
   - Have corticosteroid lotion available.
   - Teach her the symptoms of a true anaphylactic reaction and when to bring the client in by ambulance versus trying to drive him.
   - Discuss strategies to avoid allergens as much as possible.
   - Purchase a MedicAlert bracelet that should be worn at all times.
   - Encourage the wife to have an alternate plan if a local ambulance service is not available where she lives.
   - Demonstrate and have her return demonstrate steps to take when an anaphylactic reaction occurs: open the airway, place the client in high-Fowler's position, count the respirations, calm the victim.

Chapter 13

1. This is classified as a hospital-acquired infection and is probably related to the surgical procedure. Proper hand hygiene and use of aseptic technique in changing the dressing are the best interventions.

2. A culture and sensitivity of the wound is the diagnostic test. If this is positive, an antibiotic showing sensitivity will be ordered. If this is negative, other tests will be ordered. Complete blood count (CBC), blood culture and sensitivity, and chest x-ray (CXR) to rule out sepsis or pneumonia are recommended.

3. A white blood count (WBC) and differential should be analyzed. If an infection as described here is present, bacteria are the most likely cause. The WBC will probably be elevated with elevated neutrophils (since the onset is new).

4. Vancomycin (Vancocin) is the recommended treatment because it has bactericidal and bacteriostatic action. It interferes with cell membrane synthesis in multiplying organisms. It is active against both Gram-positive and Gram-negative organisms.

5. Neurotoxicity, ototoxicity, nephrotoxicity, fever, and chills are adverse effects. "Red neck syndrome" can be reduced by slowing the infusion.

6. Quinupristin and dalfopristin (Synercid); linezolid (Zyvox), or the synergistic effect of vancomycin (Vancocin) and gentamycin (Garamycin) are effective against vancomycin-resistant *Staphylococcus aureus* (VRSA). Daptomycin (Cubicin) is also effective with MRSA.

Chapter 14

1. The nurse should inquire as to when the eruption began, the appearance, and where the rash is located. Questions should be asked about any pain, itching, or burning around the area before the blisters appeared. The nurse should inquire about a history of chickenpox and any other medical diagnoses that may have compromised her immune status. A thorough review of all medications she is currently taking would be indicated, as some drugs also depress the immune system.

2. The nurse should thoroughly examine the skin for characteristic lesions and distribution. A determination should be made as to whether the involvement is dermatomal or unilateral and whether there is ophthalmic involvement. If the eyes are involved, emergency treatment and referral is indicated. Assessment for pain management is also essential as this can be very painful, especially for an elderly client.

3. Herpes zoster is caused by a reactivation of the varicella virus (chickenpox) that remained dormant in the basal ganglia after an episode of chickenpox. It is a viral infection usually involving the skin of a single dermatome and usually resolves within about 2 weeks. An antiviral medication will be necessary to shorten the duration of the disease, help lessen the itching, and control the pain.

4. The goal of therapy is suppression of pain, inflammation, and infection. Use of over-the-counter nonsteroidal anti-inflammatory drugs (NSAIDs) is recommended for pain and fever. Oral antiviral medications are available: valacyclovir HCL (Valtrex), famciclovir (Famvir), and acyclovir (Zovirax). Antipruritic medications such as corticosteroids or antihistamines will decrease itching and scratching.

5. Wet compresses using Burow's solution or cool tap water can be used for a soothing effect. Avoid scratching the area to prevent secondary infection. Stress keeping follow-up appointments in 3 days and again a week later to monitor the disease. Fever, chills, increased pain, or drainage should be reported promptly. The client needs to isolate herself from neonates, pregnant women, and immunosuppressed persons. Explain that she is contagious to those persons who have never had chickenpox. The disease usually resolves, but there may be scarring at the site of the lesions.

Chapter 15

1. Nursing diagnoses should be prioritized as follows:
   - Risk for Infection related to decreased circulating granulocytes secondary to acute lymphocytic leukemia and decreased ability to heal properly secondary to diabetes mellitus.
   - Risk for Injury: bleeding related to decreased circulating platelets secondary to acute lymphocytic leukemia.
   - Ineffective Airway Clearance related to increased phlegm, decreased secondary defenses, prolonged bed rest, and age.
   - Imbalanced Nutrition: Less than Body Requirements related to increased metabolism secondary to acute lymphocytic leukemia.
   - Impaired Oral Mucous Membranes related to the effect of chemotherapeutic medications and neutropenia.
   - Ineffective Role Performance related to recent cancer diagnosis.
   - Anticipatory Grieving related to fear of impending death secondary to recent cancer diagnosis.

   Since infection is the number one cause of death in these clients and the client's circulating granulocytes are decreased (absolute granulocyte count [AGC] = 990), the risk for infection is more life threatening than the other diagnoses and therefore is listed first. Since she is already experiencing petechiae and her platelet count is decreased ($12,000/mm^3$), bleeding becomes the second most life-threatening complication and should be considered second. Her weight loss of 10 pounds makes Imbalanced Nutrition an important diagnosis.

2. The client's absolute granulocytes/neutrophil count (AGC or ANC) is extremely low. The AGC is calculated by taking the WBC (% bands + % segs) and normally should be greater than 1,000. In this case: 9,000 (0.01 + 0.10) = 990, makes the client extremely susceptible to opportunistic infection. When the client's granulocytes are decreased, the client will lose first line of defense against infection. Neutrophils are the first cells to arrive at a site of infection; they engulf the invading organism and trigger the inflammation response. These clients are highly susceptible to life-threatening infections and often do not produce the normal response to infection. Fever may be the only sign of infection in these clients.

3. Monitor for manifestations of infection, which include elevated temperature, chills, throat pain, chest pain, cough, burning on urination, rectal or vaginal itching or irritation. Monitor vital signs and oxygenation every four hours. Assess for temperature spikes with chills, tachypnea, tachycardia, restlessness, change in PaO_2, and hypotension. Although the body temperature is usually elevated in infection, clients with leukemia may have an altered response and sepsis may be present before abnormal vital signs occur. Hypotension is usually a late symptom of sepsis. The presence of yellow-colored sputum and redness to the Hickman catheter are concerning since these are significant signs of infection.

4. Part of the client's treatment protocol includes prednisone. Steroid therapy will cause an increase release of glycogen from the liver thereby increasing the glucose level in the blood. As a result, the client will require frequent glucose monitoring and sliding scale insulin to regulate her diabetes. This will create an increase in the number of invasive procedures, since both capillary blood glucose monitoring and insulin injects will require a needle stick. Because of the underlying leukemia diagnosis, the client is more susceptible to infection, and with her diabetes diagnosis, she is susceptible to delayed healing. The nurse should use meticulous skin preparation for this client, and keep capillary blood glucose testing to a minimum. The nurse may consider discussing accessing a blood sample from the Hickman, but due to the small sample required, the risk may outweigh the benefit.

5. Primary caregiver support and place of discharge needs to be determined early in the hospital stay. Many clients are discharged at the completion of their chemotherapy induction to nadir at home. The nurse also needs to begin teaching the primary caregiver about Hickman catheter maintenance as well as preparation of the home to decrease infection exposure. Subcutaneous injection technique also needs to be assessed since the client will be discharged on insulin as well as other medications such as filgrastim (Neupogen), epoetin alfa (Procrit), and daunorubicin (Cerubidine).

Chapter 16

1. Cystic fibrosis (CF) is a multisystem disease. Respiratory compromise, recurrent pneumonia, and failure to thrive (FTT) are all symptoms of CF. The client has thick, increased viscosity of secretions, decreased ciliary function, decreased alveolar function and alveolar plugs that lead to repeat infections and long-term chronic obstructive pulmonary disease (COPD). *Pseudomonas* and *Staphylococcus* are the most common organisms and are often resistant to antibiotics. The gastrointestinal tract is also involved and malabsorption occurs due to blockage of the ducts leading from the pancreas to the duodenum. Fats and fat-soluble vitamins are not

absorbed and malnutrition can occur. In an infant, this is manifested as failure to thrive.

2. The test most commonly performed to confirm CF is the sweat chloride test revealing an elevated sodium chloride level. The defective protein inhibits transport of sodium chloride and these electrolytes are excreted in the sweat. The nurse could also refer to pulmonary function tests to determine the level of respiratory compromise. Hypoxia is chronic because of the COPD and can lead to cor pulmonale (right-sided congestive heart failure from a respiratory cause). Arterial blood gases (ABGs) or pulse oximetry are usually also conducted. In the newborn screen, a decreased trypsin in the stool indicates pancreatic insufficiency or cystic fibrosis.

3. Medications the nurse may administer would be bronchodilators such as albuterol (Ventolin), corticosteroid such as beclomethasone (Vanceril), and dornase alfa (Dnase) to decrease the viscosity of respiratory mucus. Antibiotics may also be ordered. Other interventions include administering low dose oxygen, chest physiotherapy (CPT), and suctioning as needed.

4. The client with CF has plugging of the pancreatic duct, which leads to decrease in absorption of fats, carbohydrates, and protein. The malabsorption leads to failure to thrive.

5. The family needs to be able to perform CPT, respiratory aerosol treatments, and know the potential side effects of those treatments. The family also must be able to recognize the signs and symptoms of infection and respiratory distress. Teaching the client concerning signs of hypoxia and use of a pulse oximetry is useful to avoid frequent visits to a health care provider. The nurse should also stress the need to keep the child's immunization status current to avoid other infections that may be exaggerated in CF. The nurse can review with the family what an autosomal recessive pattern is and if both parents are carriers what is the chance of reoccurrence. The family can also have the disease diagnosed in the prenatal and perinatal period.

Chapter 17

1. Fundamental interventions would include maintaining spinal alignment, providing supplemental oxygen and maintaining the airway. Initiation of intravenous access (IV) with 2 large bore IV cannulas, control of scalp hemorrhage, and laboratory/radiology testing to include arterial blood gases, complete blood count, chemistry panel (glucose), urinalysis, blood alcohol, type and crossmatch for donor specific blood, and x-rays of cervical spine, chest, hip, and pelvis. Further assessment of the client would include heart sounds, respiratory status, cardiac monitoring, peripheral pulses, complaints voiced by the client, especially chest or leg pain. A thorough head-to-toe assessment would then need to be made.

2. A thoracostomy (chest tube) may be inserted for the diagnosis of pneumothorax. A CT scan or MRI may be performed for possible brain injuries. An indwelling urinary catheter would also be needed unless contraindicated.

3. The client is in the compensatory phase of hypovolemic shock. The rise in pulse and respiration, along with the change in level of consciousness are indications. ABGs indicate the level of cellular perfusion and acid–base balance that is affected by respiration at the cellular level. Hematocrit and hemoglobin levels are also useful in determining active blood loss for hypovolemic shock.

4. While the scalp is very vascular and will bleed profusely depending on the size of the laceration, the potential for pelvic and hip fractures constitute the greatest threat of hemorrhage from both the bone itself and the possible injury to great vessels in the femoral area. With a diagnosis of flail chest, the potential for a pneumothorax or hemothorax could contribute to the overall volume loss. The client could also suffer a cardiac contusion or a hematoma.

5. It is vitally important to maintain an accurate record of output; however, in the presence of pelvic or hip injury there may also be penetrating damage to the bladder. Bleeding from the meatus would indicate bladder trauma or actual urethral damage that would contraindicate the insertion of a urinary catheter.

Index

Page numbers followed by b indicate box; those followed by f indicate figure; those followed by t indicate table.

Chronic venous insufficiency, 68, 76
Circulation, assessment of, 150f
Cirrhosis, 205, 207, 208–211
Cleft lip/palate, 412–413
CLL (*See* Chronic lymphocytic leukemia [CLL])
Clonazepam (Klonopin), 13
Clonic seizures, 112
Closed fracture, 149t
Closed trauma, 435
Closed-angle glaucoma, 161, 162
Clostridium botulinum, 332t
Clostridium difficile, 332t
Clostridium tetani, 332t
Clotting mechanisms, 443–445
Clubbing, nail, 5
CML (*See* Chronic myelogenous leukemia [CML])
Cochlear implants, 169
Cogwheel rigidity, 91, 118
Cold caloric testing, 173
Coliform bacteria, 333t
Collateral circulation, 33, 39
Colon cancer, 197–198
Colonization, 323, 326
Colonoscopy, 198
Coma, myxedema, 226, 232, 234
Comminuted fracture, 149t
Compartment syndrome, 135, 151
Complement proteins, 332
Complete blood count (CBC), 328
Compound fracture, 149t
Compression atelectasis, 10
Compression fracture, 149t
Computed tomography (CT), 141, 173
Conductive hearing impairment, 160, 170, 170b
Congenital, 398, 408
Congenital defects (*See* Genetic and developmental health problems)
Congestive heart failure (CHF), 33, 42–48
    biventricular, 46
    compensatory mechanisms, 43, 43t, 44
    left-sided, 44–45, 44f
    nursing assessment, 46
    nursing management, 46–48
    overview, 42
    pathophysiology, 42–46, 42t
    right-sided, 45–46, 45f
    risk factors, 35
Conn syndrome, 225, 227, 237, 238, 239
Contact dermatitis, 307, 349, 364, 365b, 366–367
Continuous positive airway pressure (CPAP), 13
Contraction atelectasis, 11
Contusion, 420, 437
Convalescent stage of infection, 327
COPD (*See* Chronic obstructive pulmonary disease [COPD])

Cor pulmonale, 1, 5
Corneal abrasion, 164, 165
Coronary artery bypass grafting (CABG), 38
Coronary heart disease (CHD), 33, 35–37
Corticosteroids, 26, 115, 138, 146, 148
Cortisol, 237
Corynebacterium diphtheriae, 332t
Countershock, 57–58
Creatinine phosphokinase (CK or CPK), 40, 41t
CREST syndrome, 147
Creutzfeldt-Jacob disease, 343
CRF (*See* Chronic renal failure [CRF])
Crohn's disease, 184, 186, 191–192, 192f
Cryoextraction, 164
Cryptorchidism, 276
Cryptorchidism, 279
Curling's ulcer, 188
Cushing's disease, 225, 227, 237–238
Cushing's triad, 96
CVA (*See* Cerebrovascular accident [CVA])
Cyanosis, 5
Cyproheptadine, 239
Cystic fibrosis (CF), 1, 410–412
    medications, 9–10
    nursing assessment, 6
    nursing management, 9–10
    pathophysiology, 5
    risk factors, 3
Cystitis, 255, 258
Cytokines, 300, 308
Cytomegalovirus, 330t
Cytotoxic hypersensitivity reaction, 308
Cytotoxic T-cells, 212, 305f

D

Decerebrate, 91, 96, 96f
Decorticate, 91, 96, 96f
Defense mechanisms, 327
Defibrillation, 57
Degenerative arthritis, 135–136
Delayed hypersensitivity reaction, 308–309
Dementia, 125–126
Depolarization, 50
Dermatitis
    atopic, 349, 366, 367
    contact, 307, 349, 364, 365b, 366–367
    exfoliative, 349, 366
    seborrheic, 350, 366, 367
Dermatophyte, 349, 361
Developmental health problems (*See* Genetic and developmental health problems)
Diabetes insipidus (DI), 225, 228, 243–244

Graft-versus-host disease (GvHD), 300, 310
Gram-negative bacteria, 331
Gram-positive bacteria, 331
Grand mal seizures, 112
Granulation tissue, 148
Granulocytes, 303–304
Graves' disease, 225, 227, 229
Greenstick fracture, 149t
Growth hormone (GH), 241, 242
Guillain-Barré syndrome, 94, 114–115

H
H$_2$-antagonists, 148
H$_2$-blockers, 189
Haemophilus influenza, 333t
Halo brace, 108
Hashimoto's thyroiditis, 232
HCO$_3^-$, 5b
Head injuries, 435–436
Headache, 73, 97
Hearing aids, 169
Hearing impairment
    conductive, 160, 170, 170b
    sensorineural, 160, 168–169
Heart (*See also* Cardiac health problems)
    inflammatory diseases of, 35, 58–60
Heart blocks, 49t, 54t, 56–57, 56t
Heart disease (*See* Cardiac health problems)
Heart failure (*See* Congestive heart failure)
Heberden's node, 132, 136
Helicobacter pylori, 184, 186, 188, 189, 333t
Helminth infections, 340–341
Helper T cells, 305f, 315, 365f
Hematemesis, 184, 189
Hematological health problems, 376–397
    anemia, 386–388
    beta thalassemia, 391–392
    hemophilia, 385–386
    leukemia, 378–380
    multiple myeloma, 382–383
    polycythemia, 390–391
    risk factors, 378
    sickle cell anemia, 389–390
    thrombocytopenia, 383–384
Hematomas
    intracerebral, 98–99
    intracranial, 93, 97–100
Hematomyelia, 91, 104
Hematuria, 255, 258
Hemochromatosis, 205, 207
Hemodynamics, 68, 79
Hemoglobin electrophoresis, 376, 390

Hemophilia, 385–386, 385f
Hemophilia A, 385
Hemophilia B, 385
Hemorrhage, 443
Hemothorax, 1, 19–20, 438
Heparin, 22, 41
Hepatic encephalopathy, 205, 209
Hepatitis, 205, 207, 212–214
Hepatitis A, 207, 212, 212t, 329t
Hepatitis B, 207, 212, 212t, 329t
Hepatitis C, 207, 212, 212t, 329t
Hepatitis D, 207, 212, 212t, 329t
Hepatitis E, 207, 212, 212t, 329t
Hepatitis F, 212
Hepatitis G, 212
Hepatobiliary health problems, 205–224
    cholecystitis, 207, 216–217
    cholelithiasis, 207, 215–216
    cirrhosis, 207, 208–211
    hepatitis, 207, 212–214
    liver cancer, 207, 214–215
    nonalcoholic fatty liver disease, 208, 214
    pancreatic cancer, 208, 219–220
    pancreatitis, 208, 217–219
    risk factors, 207–208
Hepatoxicity, 16
Hernia, hiatal, 186, 190–191, 190f
Herniation syndromes, 95–96
Herpes, 293–294
Herpes simplex (HSV), 329t, 349, 357–358, 358, 359
Herpes zoster, 349, 358, 359
Heterozygous, 398, 407
Hiatal hernia, 186, 190–191, 190f
High-density lipoprotein (HDL), 36, 74
Hip fractures, 440
Histamine, 308, 428
Hives, 366
HMG-CoA reduction inhibitors (statins), 37
Hodgkin's disease, 381–382
Homozygous, 398, 405
Hormones (*See also* specific hormones)
    adrenal, 237
    fat-soluble, 278
    parathyroid, 234
    pituitary, 241
    thyroid, 228
Horner syndrome, 105
Host, 323, 326
Host-parasite interaction, 326
Human immunodeficiency virus (HIV), 312–318, 314f, 330t
Human papilloma virus (HPV), 293
Humoral immune response, 300, 306

Steroids, 7, 9
Stomach cancer, 197–198
Stomach injury, 439
Stool softeners, 38, 41, 148
Streptococcus, 334t
Streptokinase (Streptase), 41
Stress, hypertension and, 70
Stroke, 93, 100–102
Stroke volume, 33, 39, 423
Subarachnoid hemorrhage, 99
Subdural hematoma, 98
Sulfonylureas, 247
Superficial-thickness burns, 367
Suppressor T cells, 305f, 307
Supratentorial herniation syndromes, 96
Supraventricular rhythms, 52–53t
Surgery
    for aneurysm, 79f
    for angina pectoris, 38
    for benign prostatic hyperplasia, 282
    for breast cancer, 290
    for cataracts, 164, 164b
    for cleft lip/palate, 413
    for intractable pain, 123
    laryngectomy, 178
    for lung cancer, 24
    for Ménière's disease, 174
    for pancreatic cancer, 219
    for retinal detachment, 167
    for sinusitis, 176
    for sleep apnea, 13
Swan neck deformity, 133, 138
Swimmer's ear, 172
Synchronized cardioversion, 58
Syndrome, 399, 401
Syndrome of inappropriate antidiuretic hormone (SIADH), 226, 228, 243–244
Syphilis, 292–293, 292t, 337
Systemic lupus erythematosus (SLE), 135, 145–147
Systemic sclerosis, 135, 147–148
Systemic vascular resistance (SVR), 423
Systolic, 69, 71
Systolic dysfunction, 42

T
T lymphocytes (T cells), 304, 305f, 306–307, 328, 365f
T wave, 50t
Tamoxifen, 290
Tapeworms, 340
TB (*See* Tuberculosis [TB])
Telangiectasis, 133, 147
Tension pneumothorax, 19, 20

Teratogens, 401
Testicular cancer, 279, 283–284
Tetanus, 332t
Tetracycline, 286
Tetraplegia, 105t
Thalassemia, 386b
Theophylline, 9, 13
Thermal burns, 367
Thiazolidinediones, 247
Third spacing, 209
Third-degree heart block, 49t, 54t, 56t, 57
Throat (*See* Eye, ear, nose, and throat health problems)
Thromboangiitis obliterans: Buerger's disease, 83–84
Thrombocytes, 303
Thrombocytopenia, 209, 383–384, 384b
Thrombolytic therapy, 38
Thrombolytics, 41
Thrombophlebitis, 69, 71, 79–80
Thrombus, 69, 71
Thymus, 304, 305
Thyrocalcitonin, 228
Thyroid gland, 228
Thyroid hormone (TH), 228, 232
Thyroid hyperfunction disorders
    goiter, 227, 229
    Graves' disease, 227, 229
    hyperthyroidism, 228, 230f, 231t
    nursing assessment, 229
    nursing management, 229, 231–232
    overview, 228
    pathophysiology, 228–229
    risk factors, 227
    thyroid storm, 229
Thyroid hypofunction disorders
    Hashimoto's thyroiditis, 232
    hypothyroidism, 227, 231t, 233f, 234
    iodine deficiency, 232
    myxedema, 227, 232
    myxedema coma, 232, 234
    nursing assessment, 234
    nursing management, 234
    overview, 232
    pathophysiology, 232
    risk factors, 227
    signs and symptoms, 232
Thyroid storm, 226, 229
Thyroid-stimulating hormone (TSH), 228, 241
Thyroxine (T$_4$), 228
Tinea versicolor, 350, 361
Tinnitus, 73
Tiotropium bromide (Spiriva), 8, 8f, 9